Clinics in Developmental Medicine No. 193
THE DEVELOPING HUMAN BRAIN:
GROWTH AND ADVERSITIES

Clinics in Developmental Medicine No. 193

The Developing Human Brain: Growth and Adversities

FLOYD H. GILLES, MD
Children's Brain Center, Department of Pathology and Laboratory
Medicine, Neuropathology Section, Burton E. Green Professor of
Pediatric Neuropathology, Children's Hospital Los Angeles, and
Professor, Departments of Pathology (Neuropathology), Neurology,
and Neurosurgery, Keck School of Medicine, University of Southern
California, Los Angeles, CA, USA

MARVIN D. NELSON, JR., MD, MBA, FACR
Pediatric Neuroradiology, Chairman, Department of Radiology,
and John L. Gwinn Professor of Radiology, Children's Hospital
Los Angeles, and Professor of Radiology, Keck School of Medicine,
University of Southern California, Los Angeles, CA, USA

2012
Mac Keith Press

Editor: Hilary Hart
Managing Director: Ann-Marie Halligan
Production Manager: Udoka Ohuonu
Project Management: Prepress Projects Ltd

The views and opinions expressed herein are those of the authors and do not necessarily represent those of the publisher

First published in this edition 2012

British Library Cataloguing-in-Publication data
A catalogue record for this book is available from the British Library

The cover shows a magnetic resonance image of a living fetus in the uterus. The image illustrates the dependence of normal fetal brain development on a healthy placenta and umbilical cord.

ISBN: 978-1-908316-41-7

Typeset by Prepress Projects Ltd, Perth, UK
Printed by Latimer Trend and Company Ltd, Estover Road, Plymouth, Devon

Mac Keith Press is supported by Scope

CONTENTS

COLOR PLATE SECTION FOLLOWS p. 400

PREFACE

Acquired damage to the developing human brain occurs mainly during the second half of gestation—a critical developmental period. Most neuronal migration has already happened, but many other events will progressively unfold, resulting in complex interactions between naturally evolving and unexpected deleterious forces. This book comprehensively describes many normal developmental events in the human brain such as brain weight accretion, myelination, germinal subventricular tissue evolution and involution, angiogenesis, and gyrus formation, as well as some common adverse influences that may distort the course of these events.

Simultaneously in early development internal connections become functional without myelin and contribute to embryonic and fetal reflexes. Both normal and pathologic conditions, utilizing anatomic and radiologic comparisons, are illustrated. Because of widespread confusion about fetal and neonatal pathologic conditions, we have emphasized the specific history of each entity in order to more effectively delineate the evolution of current terms and concepts.

ACKNOWLEDGMENTS

FHG Over the years I have been fortunate to have had many esteemed mentors and colleagues. Among them I would like to acknowledge several whose teachings were of enduring personal significance. DN Buchanan and DB Clark introduced me to the world of pediatric neurology, and GF Vawter to that of pediatric pathology. R Lindenberg clarified the concept of the borderzone lesion and led me into neuropathology. R O'Rahily and PI Yakovlev illuminated the anatomic wonders of the developing human brain. Importantly, LW Swanson, more than any other neuroanatomist, unveiled for me a panoramic concept uniting the differing vertebrate neuroanatomies.

Finally, I would like to recognize my indebtedness to A Leviton for introducing me to the power of populations, to the role of biologic variability in human development, to statistical and epidemiologic tools, and to critical thinking applied to human disease.

MDN I would like to thank Floyd Gilles for inviting me to be a part of this project and for 24 years of learning and friendship. I have enjoyed every minute.

I would also like to thank my long-time associates and collaborators S Bluml and A Panigrahy for their contributions to Chapter 7 in this volume.

Lastly, thanks to PhDc Mary, the love of my life, and my fine sons Kevin and Andrew. I hope that they are as fortunate as I have been in finding professions and people that keep them interested, challenged, and learning for the rest of their lives.

Also to be recognized for their work in contributing to some chapters in this volume: BA Brody, JG Chi, EC Dooling, I Gonzalez-Gomez, HC Kinney, KCK Kuban, JE McLennan, SF Murphy, and CJ Tavaré.

We would also like to acknowledge our emendator and neuropathologist BW Zaias. Still, this volume would not have been possible without DA Prosak's oversight, assistance, and attention to detail.

1
INTRODUCTION

Book subject matter

The developing human brain has an innate beauty and inherent intricacy, and is extraordinary in its assemblage, sequence, and the complexity of its integrated parts and circuits. However, adverse fetal, maternal, or environmental events may hamper the remarkable process of development.

This book concentrates on human brain development in the last half of gestation and in neonates and infants—periods that are regarded as largely responsible for the acquisition of childhood functional neurologic deficits, generally known as 'cerebral palsy,' 'developmental delay,' and 'mental retardation.'[a] Section 1 covers selected topics in typical development, including growth in brain weight, ventricular surfaces, gyral development, myelinated tract development, magnetic resonance spectroscopy, and angiogenesis. Section 2 addresses the common aforementioned acquired brain abnormalities. Between the two sections, Chapter 9 details embryonic and fetal physiologic reactions to external stimuli. We have intentionally excluded discussion of infectious diseases, bilirubin encephalopathy, and malformations because they are well reviewed in recent texts of pediatric neuropathology.[1]

This book is based, in part, on the same database as the previous review, which discussed the epidemiology of fetal brain lesions [National Collaborative Perinatal Project (NCPP)].[2] We rely on some data from the NCPP but here have emphasized brain growth, pathology, and neuroimaging. The NCPP database remains the only large autopsy survey of late fetal brain lesions in infants for each of whom a large number of data (1200+ variables) such as maternal lifestyle, gestation, delivery, and neonatal potential antecedents had been collected in a priori fashion before death.

Brain growth and development

We emphasize the incredible manner and speed with which the embryonic and fetal brain generates, relocates, and unites substantial numbers of central nervous system neurons. If one assumes a large figure for this ultimate number (for instance, estimated at 10^{11}—L. Swanson, personal communication, 2009), then, during the first half of gestation, neuronal precursor cells develop in the ventricular zone, move to a new location, mature in very large numbers

---

[a]UK usage: learning disability.

(for example, many hundreds of thousands every second), and make innumerable correct connections. Neuronal production and movement is not random; on the contrary, it seems tightly genetically controlled. Even so, there is considerable variance in developmental rates, for both early and late events, such as increase in weight, gyrus formation, and myelination. Growth acceleration alters abruptly toward the end of the second trimester and the growth rate becomes maximal at the end of gestation.

Traditional accounts of embryonic, early, and late fetal development tend not to appreciate the significance of the end of the second trimester: by this time most (but not all) neuronal proliferation and migration has ceased, fundamental brain anatomy has been established, and multiple, relatively simple, physiologic responses are occurring.

At second-trimester completion, brain weight accretion is accelerating maximally. Primary gyri begin maturation and subdivision, forming distinctive individual patterns, which are not mirror images of those in the opposite hemisphere, whereas total surface area remains similar in both hemispheres throughout gestation. Gyral outward growth, in configurations unique to each hemisphere and probably to each individual, introduces considerable functional imaging difficulties. The variability in human gyral patterns has been known for more than a century. Concomitantly, myelination flow accelerates, maximizing almost a year later, in the second half of the first postnatal year. Early myelination occurs in groups and is related to vestibular connections to the upper cervical cord via the medial longitudinal fasciculus and cerebellum; auditory connections with the brainstem, inferior colliculus, and medial geniculate; and peripheral sensory systems ascending from body peripheral nerves and the spinal cord to the brainstem, cerebellum, diencephalon, and eventually to the isocortex. Surprisingly, the tractus and nucleus solitarius, vital brainstem sites of central pattern generators for respiratory, cardiac, and visceral function, myelinate very late. Also late to myelinate are the fornix, hippocampus, and cingulum, considering that they lie at the medial hemispheral edge, which is first to form during embryonic life. Again, there is great variability in timing for any individual tract.

Identifying significant associations between neonatal neurologic damage and its antecedents is problematic for several reasons: the complex interaction between two individuals (fetus and mother) and their environments may obscure antecedents, and the living neonate, with its immature nervous system, sometimes stubbornly refuses to yield adequately valuable diagnostic and prognostic information until long after the neonatal period.

Investigative studies

DECREASING AUTOPSY RATES
Widespread decreasing autopsy rates and an inability to retain autopsy tissue for future study, coupled with a serious decline in neuroanatomic training for physician trainees, have resulted in few population studies, leading to much uncertainty regarding the precise location of brain lesions as well as misunderstanding of pathologic processes. For instance, a commonly used term, 'periventricular,' denoting an anatomic location, is of little value and is nonspecific, as all brain and spinal cord is periventricular at some time during development, and also because

the term includes gray as well as white matter. Another frequently mentioned concept is the theorized vascular borderzone in deep fetal cerebral white matter to explain focal white matter lesions. Traditional borderzone lesions, lying between arterial beds, are well known to extend over some distance; they are not focal lesions in any sense and usually involve both gray and white matter. Moreover, not all necrosis is infarct, even though all infarction is necrosis. Further varied designations such as 'stroke,' 'brain attack,' 'frontoparietal,' or 'prefrontal' have no anatomic or pathologic specificity; they are of little worth in epidemiologic, statistical, or functional imaging studies. Neuroimaging terms are frequently conflated, which obscures meaning. For example, the term 'periventricular leukomalacia' (multiple focal white matter necroses, as originally defined)[3] is used to describe diffuse white matter astrocytosis, or diffuse neuroimaging changes, or focal white matter lesions. Finally, there is widespread lack of autopsy evaluation and correlation of neuroimaging descriptions and interpretations, a potential source of manifold ambiguities.

INTERPRETATION

Labels used as antecedents or 'causes' need to be precise. For instance, some 34 different pathologic abnormalities, ranging from hemorrhage to necrosis, have been attributed to anoxia, hypoxia, hypoxia–ischemia, and asphyxia. The absence of adequate definitions of these clinical states in most reports suggests the possibility of other potentially modifiable risk factors having been missed by an obstetrician or neonatologist.[4]

For these reasons, we emphasize selected historic features of each entity and consider the original author's interpretation. Many older studies were based on large autopsy populations, contributing much to our understanding; nevertheless, they recognized normal biologic variation often overlooked today. Even though anatomic, embryologic, and pathologic nomenclature may be cumbersome, the many noteworthy normal and abnormal events occurring during human nervous system development can be narrated in a perceptive style and enhance our understanding.

History of cerebral palsy

Over a century of intense neuroanatomic and neuropathologic work elapsed before Wallenberg introduced the term 'cerebral palsy' in 1886 to summarize the underlying clinical and anatomic aspects of brain damage in a child with a motor disability.[5] Within a few years, the term was in general use (Table 1.1),[6–8] and, more recently, ELGAN study investigators[9] developed an algorithm based on a reliable, standardized neurologic examination to subclassify these individuals.[10,11]

NEUROANATOMIC KNOWLEDGE UNDERLYING BRAIN FUNCTION

Neuroanatomic knowledge was slow in developing. Leeuwenhoek (1717) and Fontana (1779)[12] recognized the nerve fiber and axon; in 1761, Morgagni realized that a lesion in one hemisphere caused contralateral paralysis.[13] A century later, Rolando maintained that the cerebrum controls motor function, Gall identified the pyramid, and Ehrenberg, Valentin, and Koelliker described the nerve cell and its origin of nerve fibers.[12]

3

TABLE 1.1

Overview: history, anatomy, and multiple pathologies of 'cerebral palsy' (CP)

Year	Investigator	
Cerebral palsy		
1886	Wallenberg	Summarized the clinical and anatomic aspects of 'infantile cerebral palsy' and first used the term
1888	Lovett	Used the term 'cerebral palsy'
1888	Osler	Used the term 'cerebral palsy'
1893	Freud	'Infantile cerebral diplegia'
1897	Freud	History of CP; emphasized preterm birth in association with diplegia; spent much of his book discussing lesions acquired during development, failure of development, and developmental retardation, but apparently did not recognize malformations of brain as understood today. Explained CP spasticity from brainstem and cord pyramidal tract secondary atrophy
Anatomic knowledge		
Seventeenth century	Malpighi	Introduced the microscope to medicine
1717	Leeuwenhoek	Nerve fiber and axon
1761	Morgagni	Lesions of one hemisphere result in contralateral paralysis
1781	Fontana	Nerve fiber and axon
1799	Bichat	Brought histology to pathology
1809	Rolando	Cerebrum controls motor function
1810–19	Gall	Pyramid. Functional localization in brain
1820s	–	Achromatic compound microscope introduced
1833	Ehrenberg	Microscopic structure of nerve cell and fiber
1836	Valentin	Nerve cell, its nucleus, and nucleolus
1837	Purkynje	Cerebellar nerve cells
1839	Schwann	Cell theory and serious use of microscope in neurologic disease
1849	Koelliker	Nerve fibers originate from nerve cells
1849	Waller	Secondary degeneration
1851	Türck	Secondary anterograde atrophy in spinal cord after cerebral lesions
1856	Turner	Secondary anterograde atrophy in crus, pons, and pyramids. Crossed cerebellar atrophy. Understood trophic dependence of thalamus upon its ipsilateral cerebral cortex
1875	Erb	Described quadriceps reflex; arrest of pyramid development
1876	Raymond (Charcot trainee)	Special localization of motor function in internal capsule
1877	Flechsig	Delineated pyramidal tract in posterior limb of internal capsule
1883	Golgi	Neuronal syncitial net

Year	Investigator	
1887	His	Each neuron is a distinct unit
1888	Cajal	Each neuron is independent of other neurons
1891	Waldeyer	Neuron
1896	Babinski	Babinski's sign; prior descriptions in the 1850s by Vulpian and in 1893 by Remak. All three linked it to brain or pyramidal tract damage

Acquired defects: Central nervous system cerebral gray and white matter

1818	Abercrombie	Parturitional spinal cord injuries
1822	Pinel (the son)	Lobar sclerosis
1826	Denis	Mechanical birth injuries cause hemorrhages in newborn brain
1827	Cazauvielh	Multiple small cysts; two cases with larger cysts; small pallium
1829–37	Cruveilhier	Small brain. Hemiatrophy of brain
1830	Delpech	Small brain
1842	Henoch	Infantile cerebral atrophy
1853–70	Little	Abnormalities of birth and neonatal asphyxia. Recognized that the majority of stillborn infants, when resuscitated, recover unharmed
1855	Friedleben	65% of newborn autopsies revealed cerebral lesions; brain sclerosis and atrophy
1859–68	Heschl	Porencephaly; vascular affection in fetus
1862	Parrot	Intracerebral hemorrhages; cervical spinal cord injury
1868	Cotard	Partial atrophy of brain; diffuse lobar sclerosis; lesions in specific arterial beds
1870	Parrot	Upper spinal cord lesions
1882	Ross	Lobar sclerosis results from arterial emboli
1884	Strümpell	Acute infantile hemiplegia 'polioencephalitis'
1885	McNutt	Convolutional sclerosis; bilateral paracentral atrophy
1887	Abercrombie	Found embolus in artery leading to cerebral defect
1888	Lovett	60 cases of CP: Embolism and parenchymal hematomas important
1888	Osler	50 cases of CP: Partial or lobar sclerosis; paracentral in all; arterial occlusion
1888	Gowers	Birth palsies: Arterial thrombosis and embolism
1890	Sachs	Cerebral palsies of early life
1891	Freud	Choreatic form of CP
1893	Anton	Status marmoratus
1896	Schultze	Parturitional cysts and scars in medulla and spinal cord
1899	Bresler	Ulegyria
1958	Crome	Multicystic encephalopathy

TABLE 1.1 (continued)

Year	Investigator	
Acquired defects: Cerebral white matter only		
1850	Bednar	Focal cerebral necroses newborn brain are mostly deep white matter
1862	Parrot	Focal necroses in white matter–metabolic disorder
1865–7	Virchow	Focal necroses in white matter–infection
1904	Schmorl	Described 280 cases of focal necroses in white matter; summarized previous studies from 1862 (Parrot) to 1903 (Moebius, Vivius, Herschfeld, and Hlava)
1940–5	McClelland, Benda, Crome	White matter hypoplasia; (separately) delayed myelination

Compiled from data in Freud,[8] Yakovlev,[15] Gilles et al,[16] and Laird et al.[17]

Embryonic and fetal age

One traditional independent variable, estimated gestational age, has an error of several weeks. Furthermore, gestational age estimates, adjusted for 'correctness' of body length or weight, may be 'improved' but suffer seriously from the bias of selective loss of data (for instance, how do you deal with the excluded case?) and of dependent factors that may often contaminate the estimate. The major advantage of gestational age as an independent variable is that it is regularly sequenced throughout gestation and, once determined, is free of events occurring within the mother or infant. Various terms are commonly used: menstrual age (time from the last menstrual period) is approximately 2 weeks longer than the postovulatory age; gestational age (the mother's best estimate of when she was fertilized); and implantation age (the time of uterine wall blastocyst implantation)—about 7.5 days. The best assessment of embryonic or fetal age is the conceptional, postconceptional, or postovulatory age, which is approximately 2 weeks less than the menstrual age. Of course, the actual age in days cannot be known. For this book, we use postovulatory age when we know it or can estimate it. For the neuroimaging sections, specific gestational age was often ambiguous and the author's estimates were used, implying possible appreciable variation in gestational age of a particular function.

For embryonic material, we use postovulatory dates unless otherwise stated; for developmental stages, we use Carnegie staging.[14] In the remainder of the book, we use the original author's statements as to embryonic or fetal age unless there are obvious errors. Embryonic stages are based on the apparent developmental morphologic state and hence are not directly dependent on either chronologic age or size. Embryo length as a single criterion is not in itself sufficient to establish a stage, as length may vary concomitantly with development of the brain abnormality.

National Collaborative Perinatal Project

The National Institute of Neurological and Communicative Disorders and Stroke prospectively collected data throughout pregnancy and childhood for a large number of children in an attempt to ascertain modifiable maternal, fetal, or perinatal events that could account for aspects of childhood cerebral dysfunction. Thus, all clinical data were similarly prospectively collected in both groups of infants: those who subsequently died and those who survived.

The NCPP pathologic material includes several distinct populations. Cases with recorded gestational and survival ages and fresh brain weights numbered 1537: correlation of pathologic and epidemiologic data used 1100 brains, Yakovlev selected 425 individuals for whole-brain serial sectioning after celloidin embedding,[15] while the remainder were processed through paraffin. See our previous volume[2] for details of other subpopulations. Each serially sectioned brain was photographed in six planes, yielding some 2400 black-and-white prints. More than 100 000 slides were generated and are currently maintained at the US Armed Forces Institute of Pathology. Paraffin-processed brains were cut in a standardized fashion at approximately 3-mm intervals; each slab was photographed and multiple blocks were prepared. In excess of 30 000 color transparencies of whole brains and slabs, as well as multiple stains on sections from each block, were obtained.

OBSERVER VARIABILITY
To minimize observer variability in data ascertainment, two observers simultaneously reviewed each selected photograph and slide either grossly or with a double-headed microscope.[16] The data were recorded on standard check-off sheets abstracted from a matrix of approximately 700 possible combinations of brain site and disease process.

STUDY ASSUMPTIONS
Any study is based on assumptions and biases, some identified and many unrecognized. We acknowledged and tried to deal operationally with the following assumptions.

We assumed that all brains were abnormal, as most were derived from fetuses or infants in some way sufficiently abnormal to have aborted spontaneously or to have died shortly after birth. Thus, statements about acquisition of a brain structure compare 'early' and 'late' in a population of abnormal infants. On one hand, this assumption may exaggerate a risk factor contribution in some circumstances, but, on the other hand, it may diminish such a contribution to a morphologic condition if the existent risk factor is otherwise common to all dead children. While assuming that all brains were abnormal, still it cannot be denied that some brains approached what is considered to be 'normal.' Then again, in making judgments about the developing human brain, this is the best we can do.

The second assumption was that, in evaluating the development of an organ, growth could be measured in many ways. Growth is generally a continuous process; however, one cannot repeatedly sample a single growing fetus. This limits the best growth estimates to fetuses that died at different times in development. As each way of measuring growth has its own strengths in contributing to our understanding, each is valued. Although we use the traditional strategy of measuring growth against the independent variable of estimated gestational age, we also use, in some instances, other parameters as the independent variable.

Body weight and crown–rump length are two variables frequently used as abscissae and ordinates. Although they are easily ascertained at birth or autopsy, they have serious limitations. First, changes in body length and brain or body weight are unequal throughout gestation and tend to decrease near term, when greatest discrimination is desired (in comparison with degree of myelination, for instance). Thus, one would recognize only coarse discrepancies, probably even with the use of ratios such as body/brain weight. Second, factors potentially inhibiting or failing to support some brain growth component could also affect body weight or length; consequently, if weight or length is the independent variable, such factors could conceivably be overlooked. Third, the allometric relationship between brain and body part growth precludes meaningful analysis of growth itself.[17]

The following assumptions are associated. We assumed that recognizable structural abnormalities underlie some functional cerebral deficits, such as mental retardation or cerebral palsy, and that they appear during gestation, originating in events that altered the fetal and/or neonatal environment. These alterations constitute 'natural experiments,' usable when investigating disease etiology. This last point is important because appropriate experiments on an infant are inconceivable and direct extrapolation from experiments on subhuman primates is fraught with conceptual and ethical problems. It is hoped that maternal and perinatal factors, which contribute to perinatal cerebral morbidity, can be directly modifiable (even if exact etiologic mechanisms are not understood). A related assumption was that these structural abnormalities are separable from nervous system morphologic abnormalities allied with 'dying.' Extrapolation of conclusions from information about dead to living children must be done with care. We may strongly suspect comparable processes in live children, but, without additional evidence, one must restrain this conjecture.

Despite the societal definition, the process of death is rarely instantaneous. Even when cardiac action ceases, some cellular metabolic activities continue. Before final cardiostasis, there is considerable internal milieu discord from cardiovascular, respiratory, and metabolic instability. Thus, a wide variety of nervous system changes (for instance, neuropil vacuolization, cellular shrinkage, neuronal hyperchromia) potentially merely reflect those terminal events. Although acute terminal brain morphologic changes may be similar to those sustained during a survived insult, their equivalence has never been adequately demonstrated in the human. Further, one must assume that there are, most likely, quantitative and qualitative differences between insults damaging development in a surviving brain and those accompanying death. Termination of life may indeed be associated in some brains with abnormalities traditionally called 'ischemic' or 'hypoxic' neuronal change; this supports, but does not prove, a causal relationship. Consequently, the observation that both some hypoxia and brain damage occur with a difficult delivery does not identify an initiator and, even more importantly, prevents an adequate search for other potentially treatable antecedents coincident with difficult delivery. For our purposes, we found karyorrhexis, coagulative necrosis, macrophages, glial scars, intramural vascular deposits, and neuronal depletion to be of greater interest than acute neuronal changes.

Another assumption was that morphologic abnormalities commonly found in dead newborn brains are similar in nature, site, and rate to those found in brains of people afflicted with mental retardation and cerebral palsy. This supposition is difficult to resolve owing to a lack of adequate data. For the purposes of these studies, we postulated comparability, at least at some level, with two accompanying corollaries. There were almost no NCPP cases of storage disease, tumors, or progressive degenerative diseases, and it became clear that the majority of individuals with mental retardation or cerebral palsy do not have these conditions. Thus, the NCPP brain population was quite appropriate in this respect. The second obvious corollary is that brain abnormalities in institutionalized individuals likely differ qualitatively or quantitatively from the NCPP population.

RANGE OF ABNORMALITIES

The range of NCPP cerebral abnormalities reflected those encountered on any usual neonatal neuropathology service. There were few congenital malformations similar to those found in the brains of institutionalized individuals. Thus, this volume records observations in a general sense; it focuses mainly on topics such as myelination delay, intracranial hemorrhage, and telencephalic leukoencephalopathies rather than malformations or genetic or metabolic conditions.

The pathologist, when examining neonatal brains of differing gestational ages, should be aware that some adult criteria of abnormality are potentially misleading. For instance, macrophages in moderately cellular leptomeninges, perivascular cuffs of small mononuclear cells adjacent to ventricle, or large numbers of microglia-like cells in telencephalic structures are abnormal in the adult brain but are typical in the infant brain.

Lesions in neonatal brain range in complexity from simple loss of neural tissue (for instance, necrosis) to complex malformations arising from diverse mixtures of developmental arrests, migration abnormalities, and abortive repair attempts. Delay in acquiring an evolving brain component (such as myelin) characterizes another broad group of 'lesions.' This latter 'lesion,' and evaluation of its antecedents, likely has greater long-term social significance than the more dramatic lesions referred to above, as more children are at risk for more prevalent antecedents (such as malnutrition). Moreover, assessment of delayed nervous system development (in terms of weight, neuronal mass, complexity of dendritic tree and spine arborization, or myelination degree, for instance) presupposes that adequate standards, controlled for site and systemic disease, are available. Unfortunately, such standards that exist are largely unsatisfactory, most being based on small samples, anecdotal evidence, or populations limited by arbitrary case exclusion. A similar predicament applies to the phenomenon of fetal brain myelination: available tables are constructed from small case numbers or fail to estimate normal biologic variation within each tract as it myelinates (for example, time of onset or rate of myelination). Thus, one of our tasks is to identify histologic and pathologic clues in unmyelinated and/or myelinating brain tissue, the tactile and visual characteristics of which are distinct from tissue in adult brain and whose normal constituents and 'reacting' cells are still immature, not having reached their full capabilities.

At term, the brain is at its maximal growth rate; by the second year it will almost have tripled its birthweight. Deposition of a large amount of myelin in the last gestational weeks and during the first few neonatal months probably accounts for most of this weight gain. Importantly, then, this transient and unique tissue (myelinating white matter) is potentially vulnerable to multiple and heterogeneous insults, and thus estimation of its degree of maturation is crucial. Similarly, another transient tissue, germinal tissue lining the ventricular system, may be subject to distinctive damage.

REFERENCES

1. Golden JA, Harding BN, editors (2004) *Developmental Neuropathology*. Basel: International Society of Neuropathology.
2. Gilles FH, Leviton A, Dooling EC (1983) Developing Human Brain: Growth and Epidemiologic Neuropathology. Boston: John Wright-PSG Publishing Co.
3. Banker BQ, Larroche JC (1962) Periventricular leukomalacia of infancy. A form of neonatal anoxic encephalopathy. *Arch Neurol* 7: 386–410.
4. Gilles FH (1977) Lesions attributed to perinatal asphyxia in the human. In: Gluck L, editor. *Intrauterine Asphyxia and the Developing Fetal Brain*. Chicago: Year Book Medical Publishers, Inc, pp. 99–107.
5. Wallenberg A (1886) Ein Beitrag zur Lehre von den cerebralen Kinderlähmungen. *Jahrbuch für Kinderheilkunde* 24: 384–439.
6. Lovett R (1888) A clinical consideration of sixty cases of cerebral paralysis in children. *Boston Med Surg J* 26: 641–646.
7. Osler W (1888) The cerebral palsies of children. Med News (Phila) 2–5.
8. Freud S (1897) Die Infantile Cerebrallähmung, Vol. IX. In: Nothnagel, series editor. *Specielle Pathologie und Therapie*. Vienna: Holder.
9. O'Shea TM, Allred EN, Dammann O, et al; ELGAN study investigators (2009) The ELGAN study of the brain and related disorders in extremely low gestational age newborns. *Early Hum Dev* 85: 719–725.
10. Kuban KC, Allred EN, O'Shea M, Paneth N, Pagano M, Leviton A (2008) An algorithm for identifying and classifying cerebral palsy in young children. *J Pediatr* 153: 466–472.
11. Accardo PJ, Hoon AH Jr. (2008) The challenge of cerebral palsy classification: the ELGAN study. *J Pediatr* 153: 451–452.
12. Clarke E, O'Malley C (1996) *The Human Brain and Spinal Cord; A Historical Study Illustrated by Writings from Antiquity to the Twentieth Century*. San Francisco: Norman Publishing.
13. Morgagni G (1761) *The Seats and Causes of Diseases*. Translated by Alexander B. London: Johnson and Payne.
14. O'Rahilly R, Müller F (1994) *The Embryonic Human Brain: An Atlas of Developmental Stages*. New York: Wiley-Liss.
15. Yakovlev PI (1970) Whole brain histological sections. In: Tedeschi C, editor. *Neuropathology; Methods and Diagnosis*. Boston: Little, Brown, pp. 371–378.
16. Gilles FH, Winston K, Fulchiero A, Leviton A (1977) Histologic features and observational variation in cerebellar gliomas in children. *J Natl Cancer Inst* 58: 175–181.
17. Laird A, Barton A, Tyler S (1968) Growth and time: an interpretation of allometry. *Growth* 32: 347–354.

Section 1

2
BRAIN GROWTH

Introduction

There are two goals for this chapter. The first is to demonstrate the importance of recognizing brain development periods when the brain requires large amounts of metabolites necessary to support rapid growth of tissue. This makes it possible to estimate when the brain is most generally vulnerable to undernutrition, inborn errors of metabolism, radiation, endocrine imbalance, or amnion or maternal infection-induced inflammatory responses. In contrast, more particular vulnerabilities relate to distinct stages in brain development such as neurogenesis, neural migration, forebrain or hindbrain growth, gray matter or white matter maturation, dendritic sprouting, and synaptogenesis. The second goal is to provide the pediatric pathologist with 'normal' standards of brain development that are important in order to recognize deviations constituting abnormality.

The 'normal' newborn brain weight is 326 to 448g.[1] This chapter examines how the brain attains this weight while in utero and how brain weight changes during the first 2 years of life. Varying estimates as to when the brain attains full weight range from 2 years[2] to 25 years.[3] The weight of all brain components during the growing period must be considered, including the entire vascular bed and the intravascular blood necessary to support the brain's remarkable growth and activity.[4] Unfortunately, the argument of defining 'normal' brain weight as a ratio relative to some other body parameter (allometric relationship) or in association with specific gestational ages continues. If brain weight is defined as a ratio to body weight alone, adverse influences affecting both the brain and body are likely missed. On the other hand, defining brain weight as a function of gestational age may induce greater variation about the expected weight.

Mammalian embryonic and fetal growth proceeds at a much higher rate prenatally than postnatally. Growth consists of a proportional daily (or weekly) gain in mass (weight) and is a very complex process for each organ.[5] In the brain and its various subdivisions, new cells, axons, dendrites, neural supporting cells, and vasculature all individually contribute to weight gain with each component added during separate developmental times.

Brain growth is a dynamic process varying not only in time and space but also from one neural subdivision to another. During development, an individual's body size and shape change as a result of differential growth of body parts. Growth cannot be discussed without considering its relation to rate. As most human embryonic and fetal growth processes cannot be measured continuously, mathematical growth models are used. The advantage of such models is that growth curve characteristics such as maximum rate and points of inflection can be estimated. Growth rate is the percentage increase in weight and spatial dimensions per unit of time, and it varies over time, particularly for specific brain parts. Points of inflection reflect major changes in acceleration or deceleration of growth. The models also estimate unobserved values, smooth measurement values, and minimize stochastic errors.

The final utility of any growth model, aside from the quality of statistical curve fitting and the theoretical biologic significance of 'growth parameters,' lies in its ability to compress a large amount of data over a period of time (growth range) into a convenient formula. This in turn allows comparison of a new brain with the growth model or differing brain portions with each other.

As a fertilized ovum grows to a term fetus, many changes occur in form and shape secondary to local differentiation within the embryo or fetus. In the brain, these are due to growth changes in different parts. Whereas whole brain growth is merely the sum of growth of all its parts, individual parts increase or decrease in size relative to the whole brain or to each other. Overall, the final size a fetus achieves depends on embryonic cellular growth rate, available food materials, and duration of growth. Brain growth rate and final size are under genetic control,[6] given optimal nutritional environment and the absence of adverse events during the growth period (such as fetal or maternal infection). If any factors affecting growth are increased or decreased, the normal brain proportions will be correspondingly altered. During gestation and the first 2 years of life, the major proportion of mass of our most intricate functional system is attained, requiring only subtle and proportionate expansions to complete maturation. At term, the human fetal brain is making its greatest strides in acquiring weight.[7]

Intrauterine growth periods

BLASTOCYST IMPLANTATION PERIOD
The time from blastocyst implantation to just before establishment of intraembryonic circulation comprises the first 3 weeks of gestation (Carnegie stages 1–9),[8] when somites first appear. Fetal membranes are established and germ layers are laid down in the embryonic disc.[8] Stage 9 marks the primitive node and neural groove. Three major brain divisions are recognizable. The future forebrain is largely diencephalon, the midbrain is the site of a marked ventral bend, and the hindbrain comprises four rhombomeres. Some embryologists include much of this period within the embryonic period.

EMBRYONIC PERIOD
Most of this description, from the fourth week to the end of eighth week of gestation, is taken from O'Rahilly and Müller.[9] During this period, all main systems and body organs are laid down and major external body features are established. In early embryos, growth energy expenditure results in predominance of neural structures, contributing a large proportion to total embryonic weight. At about 22 days, the neural folds close in adjacent hindbrain and spinal regions, forming a tube. Two constrictions divide the tube's rostral end into

prosencephalon, mesencephalon, and rhombencephalon. The prosencephalic diencephalon consists of a future thalamic region and an optic portion; a chiasmatic plate connects the optic primordia. The rostral neuropore closes at about 24 days, when hypophyseal primordia appear. The caudal neuropore closes during stage 12 (about 26 days) at the future S2 vertebral level, and neural tube liquid is ependymal fluid. From stages 10 to 12, the rhombencephalon is the largest embryonic brain region, with the pontine flexure developing during stages 13 to 16. Cerebellar anlage emerge at stage 13. The rhombic lips (cerebellar precursors) develop and fuse rostrally and dorsally during stage 17 (about 41 days). The first cerebellar portion to become obvious is the flocculonodular lobe. In general, vermis and flocculonodular lobe fissures and lobules develop earlier than hemispheral fissures and lobules.[10] Hemispheric development is essentially complete at term.

Both neuropores have closed at stage 13 (about 28–32 days), and most cranial nerve ganglia are present. The future cerebral hemispheres begin to bulge from the diencephalic ventricle at stage 14 (approximately 32 days). In prosencephalon, the hypothalamic, amygdaloid, hippocampal, and olfactory regions are discernible. Both ganglionic eminences (medial and lateral) arise at stage 15 (approximately 33 days), and epithalamus, dorsal thalamus, ventral thalamus, and subthalamus are apparent. Spinal axodendritic synapses appear first in the cervical region (see Chapter 9). The neurohypophysis evaginates at stage 16 (approximately 37 days), and 4 days later olfactory bulb and first amygdaloid nuclei become evident and a deep longitudinal interhemispheric fissure is conspicuous. The future corpus striatum, inferior cerebellar peduncle, and dentate nucleus are evident at stage 18 (approximately 44 days). At stage 19, the fourth ventricular choroid plexuses appear and the lateral ventricular plexuses follow 3 days later (stage 20, 51 days). The cortical plate is visible in cerebral hemispheres at stage 21 (approximately 52 days) and 2 days later the internal capsule and olfactory tract appear. The embryonic period ends at approximately 57 days, with the cortical plate extending over most of cerebral surface.

FETAL PERIOD

This is the period from the third gestational month until birth. During this time, the body undergoes a rapid absolute increment in size rather than striking differentiation. Changes in external body form come about quite slowly because of slight differences in relative growth rates of various segments and body parts. Similarly, the brain increases mainly in size without major new differentiation of its parts. Neuroblasts, nonetheless, are still dividing in the hemispheric ventricular zone and new neurons continue forming until about week 18 of gestation.[11]

Growth functions

There are five different growth functions that have been used to model growth of various organs; all require age as the independent variable.

EXPONENTIAL GROWTH

A steadily increasing growth rate characterizes exponential growth, and therefore there is no inflection point. The exponential growth model assumes that no resource limitation constrains the 'intrinsic growth rate.'

SIGMOID GROWTH

An S-shaped curve with a decreasing growth rate following a period of increasing rate characterizes sigmoid growth. The point of inflection is the point where the curve turns from concave to convex and defines the age when the organ shows its fastest growth. Sigmoid growth functions arise from many natural processes.[12] Its relevance to biologic growth has been particularly fruitful. In describing *complex* (multiunit) growing systems, similar principles apply to mass and size increase, although it is generally not possible to infer mechanisms. Among the most complex growing units are the human embryo and fetus.

LOGISTIC GROWTH

This model, also sigmoid, incorporates a parameter to account for resource limitation. The initial stage of growth is approximately exponential, but subsequently there is a growth constraint with consequent slowing. The point of inflection is the midpoint of mature value.

GOMPERTZ GROWTH

The Gompertz growth curve is sigmoidal,[13] with the point of inflection always a fixed proportion of the mature value, usually 36.8%. The Gompertz function is applicable to sigmoid growth processes and is the most frequently used curve in growth mathematics (for instance see reference 14). Of fundamental importance to the historic use of sigmoid growth functions, predominantly the Gompertz and logistic, is Sewell Wright's[15] rationale for using the Gompertz rather than the logistic function for biologic growth. Wright noted, based on the classic paper by Minot,[16] that population growth often appears to follow the logistic curve quite well. For instance, a logistic curve describes the United States population growth from 1800 through 1920, although earlier predictions of growth limitation based on plateauing functions had not held up.[17] Growth of individual organisms, in contrast, usually shows a maximum growth rate (inflection point) earlier than the same organism in whole populations and is often about one-third of asymptotic growth. Laird and co-workers used the Gompertz function, in slightly altered form, as a growth model for human postnatal brain and body weight,[18] postnatal growth of birds and mammals,[19] and embryonic growth of various animals and birds,[20] as well as tumor growth,[21,22] as did others.[23]

BELL SHAPED

The bell-shaped growth function is appropriate to organs undergoing an involution, such as the germinal matrix lining the hemispheral ventricular wall or thymus.

Historic introduction to growth studies

Before 1921 there were about 500 reports of brain weight growth between the third fetal month and birth.[24] Much early work considered neural development, along with other organs, either as a proportion of final adult weight[25] or total body weight at any particular age[5] or as a ratio of brain weight to some other body structure such as crown–rump length, crown–heel length, fronto-occipital diameter, or temporal diameter. Age was not taken into account. Thus, these were relative growth functions.[7]

Age estimates for early human embryos have always been problematic. Until recently, with the increased prevalence of abortion, these specimens were sparse; therefore, well-preserved, often unique, embryos were studied in great detail in the early twentieth century.[26] The most commonly used morphometric time correlation was the embryonic or fetal crown–rump or crown–heel length at various estimated gestational ages. Embryo length depends on methods of tissue handling, fixation, and preservation. Gestational age estimated in the early weeks or months from the date of the last menstrual period has a possible error of at least 2 weeks. This uncertainty, reflected in wide-ranging observations, potentially yields a high percentage error because of the early gestational ages of these specimens. Total body weight is even less reliable as it normally varies considerably at any given age. In addition, a wide range in degree of development at each gestational age was recognized among human embryos.[27] Reflecting these difficulties with morphometric analysis, many systems of classification using morphologic criteria have arisen, such as those of Streeter[28] and later O'Rahilly and Müller.[8,9] In summation, gestational age cannot be calculated solely from body weight while simultaneously used to determine normal values of some other body parameter.[29]

These major obstacles in dating young specimens are magnified when obtaining quantitative organ data.[30] Of specific interest in this chapter is embryonic and fetal human brain weight and size. It appears that direct brain measurements are unreliable before 12 to 15 weeks' gestation; values in this period are suspect because of friability of these minute pieces of tissue and the rapid changes in water content during abortion, tissue extraction, and fixation. Additional complications arise when investigators adjust age estimates using other standards, such as clinical, sonographic, or biometrical criteria.[31] Thus, these studies do not necessarily reflect true growth rates.

Allometric relationships of brain weight to body parameters

Many existing brain growth studies are based on total body weight. Huxley[32] defined the well-known allometric relationship between growth of an organism and its parts; the logarithms of the mass or size of parts of an organism are linearly related to each other and to the whole organism. This relationship was extensively verified. All the same, because it does not require knowing the age of an organism, is difficult to obtain exactly, and needs estimation, the allometric law provides only relative information for comparing growing systems within an organism and does *not* generate a growth curve.[33] Laird et al[34] and Barton and Laird[35] showed that the allometric plot is an insensitive growth indicator. In contrast, Gompertz growth curves of individual parts provided a more accurate interpretation. Despite this obvious limitation, exhaustively detailed descriptions of weight relationships between the growing brain and body or body parts abound and are prevalent in general biology.[2,24,33,36–38]

On the other hand, several intriguing allometric observations have emerged over time. On average, tall people have heavier brains than short people.[1] The brain, like the liver, heart, and thyroid, has a constant ratio to body weight throughout fetal growth, unlike the thymus, adrenal, and spleen (gradually increasing ratio), kidney (increasing and then plateauing), or lung (increasing then decreasing).[37] Scammon and Calkin's remarkable observation[39] was the substantial variation in head circumference when compared with body length.

The skull and brain have parallel growth curves for the first 6 to 7 years of life, with the brain occupying 97.5% of cranial volume. After the age of 7 years, the brain occupies increasingly less skull volume—only 92.5% in adulthood.[2] Fronto-occipital circumference is often used as a surrogate for brain weight, but remarkably little quantitative work has been done on the relationship between these two variables. Cooke et al[40] found a linear relationship between $\log_{10}$ brain weight and $\log_{10}$ fronto-occipital circumference in stillborn infants and in infants who died in the first week of life. Winick and Rosso[41] showed a correlation between the fronto-occipital circumference and brain weight in infants who died during the first year of life. The caveat is that measured fronto-occipital circumference fluctuates with head shape, scalp edema, and hemorrhage. Head shape itself alters the relationship between the fronto-occipital diameter and intracranial volume.[42]

Differential growth of brain regions

The brainstem weighs approximately 5g at birth, the cerebellum 20g, and the cerebrum 325g.[2] Cerebral hemispheres at birth constitute 93% of brain weight, decreasing to 88% at the age of 2 years and remaining so throughout life. The cerebellum is 10% of total brain weight after the first year of life.[43]

DIENCEPHALON

Throughout the embryonic period, individual diencephalic parts do not develop at the same rate. The hypothalamus, epithalamus, and subthalamus lose their germinal layer much earlier than the thalamus proper; the thalamus primordium still contains three primitive layers at 9.5 weeks. Between 7.5 and 11 weeks, lateral thalamus cell grouping begins. The diencephalic germinal layer is depleted at 11 weeks. From 11 to 21 weeks, the internal medullary lamina is formed and at 21 weeks all thalamic nuclear groups are established. From midgestation to term, the anterior nuclear group differentiates into separate nuclei. The thalamus has a uniform cell distribution up to 4 or 5 fetal months, except for geniculate bodies, compared with well-defined cell groups present in other diencephalic regions, such as the subthalamus or hypothalamus, at around 46 days.[44,45] All thalamic subdivisions are present at term.

CEREBRAL HEMISPHERE

From midgestation to term, cerebral hemispheric growth outstrips diencephalic and basal ganglia growth.[46] During late embryonic and early fetal life, the cerebrum is small relative to the lateral ventricle. Lateral ventricular width is normally two-thirds of the cerebral width at 15 gestational weeks and decreases relatively with cerebral growth. (See Chapter 3 for details of ventricular size changes during gestation.)

INFRATENTORIAL AND SUPRATENTORIAL REGIONS

The infratentorial and supratentorial components grow at different rates.[47,48] The infratentorial growth curve accelerates at around 24 to 25 weeks of gestation, but the multiple criteria used to correct age limit this study.[31] The ratio of infratentorial brain weight to total brain weight decreases until 22 to 23 weeks of age and then increases after 28 weeks.

Cerebellum

On the basis of DNA-P studies, Dobbing and Sands[49] felt that cerebellar growth started later than cerebral growth but finished earlier, proceeding faster throughout its shorter growth period. Moreover, cerebellar cortical neuronal packing density is greater than in the cerebral cortex, thereby accounting for some differences in growth rates. Interestingly, from 26 to 40 weeks of gestational age, intrauterine growth retardation seems not to affect transverse cerebellar diameter.[50] The cerebellum is approximately 20g at birth (6% of total brain weight, increasing to 10% after the first year of life).[43]

Spinal cord growth and peripheral nervous system

Between 15 and 40 weeks, the spinal cord increases in volume 9.9-fold.[51] At birth, the spinal cord weighs about 2.5g and is one-third of the total body length.[52] Over the next 6 months, cord weight doubles; it has quadrupled at no later than 5 years, and at maturity is about 10 times that at birth.[53] The length increases 2.7-fold between birth and adulthood.

Given its size, there is remarkably little information about peripheral nervous system growth, including the autonomic nervous system. The peripheral nervous system is estimated to be 50% of total brain weight (or 175g) at birth compared with that of the adult, when it is approximately 72% of brain and cord weight[2] (although this paper provides no primary data).

Variations in weight of 'normal' organs at various ages

There are major weight variations in ostensibly normal organs, including the brain, at specific ages.[54–56] Brain weight varies as much as ±20% in early life and ±10% after the fifth year of life.[2]

Sex dimorphism

Females have sometimes been thought to have slightly smaller brains than males of the same age,[1,2] but when corrected for body mass or length, this difference disappears.[37,57,58]

Developing brain vulnerability

Growth spurts characterize mammalian brain growth. The increase in human brain weight is greatest during the third trimester to a few months after birth. The later stage in weight gain is due largely to glial proliferation and differentiation into astrocytes and oligodendroglia, axonal growth, myelin deposition, dendritic sprouting and synaptic elaboration, and connectivity as well as a marked vascular bed increase.

A distinct earlier cerebral growth spurt, occurring between 12 and 18 weeks of gestation, is responsible for the neuronal deposition, in contrast to the later growth advance.[59,60] Hypothetically, multiple environmental risk factors could interfere with this earlier stage, such as radiation, viral infections, chromosomal abnormalities, maternal medication, or other unknown causes.

In late gestation and early postnatal life, the fetal and neonatal brain is especially vulnerable because of a relatively high growth rate requiring increased nutritional needs that must be maternally met. Therefore, the growth of fetuses and infants at these ages is susceptible to factors that directly affect their growth capacity, as well as maternal capacity to provide sufficient nourishment. Undernutrition in children, associated with many other environmental influences, results in smaller brain weight and lower myelin lipids.[61] The cerebellum may be differentially affected. Marks and colleagues[62] demonstrated in living but unhealthy preterm-born infants that fetal brain growth, reflected in serial head circumference measurements, fell below the expected growth curve during the period of acute illness. During recovery, head growth paralleled normal fetal growth following a 'catch-up' growth in head circumference. Nevertheless, others have not confirmed these data.[1]

Cellularity and total cell number

Dobbing and Sands[49] used DNA-P as concentration/gram fresh weight or total DNA-P to esti-mate cellularity and total cell number in whole brain, forebrain, cerebellum, or brainstem. The total number of cells includes glial and vascular cells. With increasing age, cellularity (DNA/g tissue) decreases in whole brain, forebrain, and brainstem, but increases in cerebellum. The decrease occurs simultaneously with the rise in the total number of cells. Whole brain cellu-larity decreases because of quantitative forebrain dominance. Nonetheless, increased weight exceeds increased numbers of cells owing to more rapid expansion in cell size, axons, vas-cular beds, dendritic branching, and myelination. In contrast, cerebellar cellularity increases simultaneously with cerebral fall. This is presumably related to the rapid rate of cerebellar cell multiplication, and the late gestational and early postnatal production of external and internal granule cells. Total cell number is more important and it changes correspondingly to the total weight gain sigmoid curve.

The development of maximal neuronal cell numbers likely precedes the development of glial cell numbers, because even though these overlap somewhat, glial cell proliferation gen-erally follows neuronal proliferation.[63] Most human neurons are present by 16 to 18 weeks, whereas glial cell deposition and multiplication are mainly second-trimester events.[11] In all of their DNA studies on human fetal forebrain, Dobbing and Sands[49] found a clear change in curve angulation at 18 gestational weeks and suggested a separate earlier growth spurt for the cerebellum. This does not mean that adult numbers of neurons are completely present at 18 weeks, as cerebellar granular cells continue to be deposited throughout the last trimester and postnatally.

Prenatal brain growth model

THE GOMPERTZ FUNCTION AND HUMAN BRAIN WEIGHT

Gompertz and logistic sigmoid functions, as well as several other growth models, were inves-tigated for their ability to describe prenatal human brain growth.[7] One hundred and thirty-nine specimens (16–44 weeks, weighed without dura) were selected because their gestational age determination was believed to be sufficiently accurate and they lacked abnormality. These brains came from Children's Hospital Boston,[1] and the Yakovlev subset of National Collaborative Perinatal Project (NCPP) material[2] (mostly <30 gestational weeks).

The Gompertz function was superior to the logistic and also to several nonsigmoid func-tions, such as the generalized exponential and the polynomial, even though the latter has been considered important.[58] The first and second Gompertz function derivatives provided prenatal brain instantaneous and maximum growth rate and acceleration. The prenatal brain growth model was:

$$Y=1.190e^{-e^{(1.99-0.04375X)}}$$ (Equation 2.1)

where Y is brain weight in grams and X is gestational age in weeks (Fig. 2.1). Maximum growth acceleration occurred at 24.5 weeks and maximum growth rate occurred after term at 48.4 weeks.

NATIONAL COLLABORATIVE PERINATAL PROJECT GROWTH MODEL (PRENATAL)
Using the Gompertz model as the best functional form to express prenatal human brain growth, standard nonlinear statistical methods were similarly applied to the large heterogeneous National Institute of Neurological and Communicative Disorders and Stroke NCPP population of brains. As our primary concern was the brain, all available NCPP cases with recorded gestational and survival ages and fresh brain weights were coalesced into a data set totaling 1537 cases. Some cases were removed from this database because of impossible or highly unlikely values for age or brain weight, as, for instance, reversed recorded data. Removal criteria were conservative, as we felt that NCPP data heterogeneity should be reflected analytically. Cases were infrequent after the perinatal period; we therefore generated a prenatal growth model

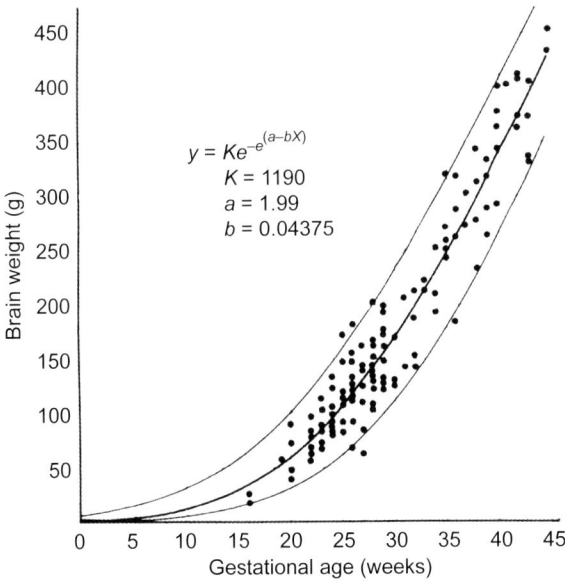

Fig. 2.1 Prenatal nonlinear Gompertz regression of brain weight (g) on gestational age (Children's Hospital Boston data). At the end of gestation, the brain is growing at the greatest rate. The inflection point is at the end of the second trimester, meaning brain weight accretion per week is maximally accelerating.

for the NCPP population that allowed extension (of this function) from 40 to 65 weeks' total age. An earlier normal prenatal model demonstrated that the function continued to follow true brain growth satisfactorily for several postnatal months.[7]

The edited NCPP population prenatal brain growth model, excluding cases older than 44 weeks, was:

$$Y=1.065e^{-e^{(2.108-0.04981X)}}$$ (Equation 2.2)

based on $n=1233$ cases. This curve is shown with data points and the 95% confidence band in Figure 2.2; included are data points for cases through 65 weeks total age, although the statistical regression did not use these additional cases beyond week 44. This NCPP model for prenatal brain growth provides a referent for epidemiologic events and conditions predisposing to grossly abnormal brain weight, as well as for subtle variations of subpopulations from the norm.

The inflection point and rates of maximal growth are similar to the original Gompertz model, namely the end of the second trimester and end of term gestation. Dobbing and Sands[49] found a similar change in rate of growth at the second trimester's end in 118 infants up to 14 postnatal months of age. Others found the inflection point occurring several weeks earlier; however, these authors 'corrected' fetal age estimates ultrasonographically or used

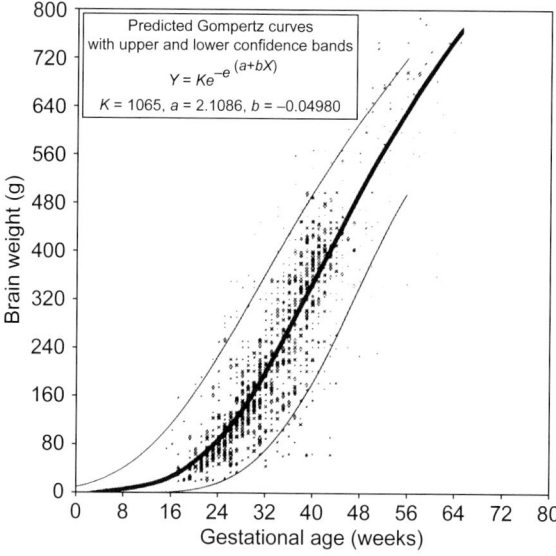

Fig. 2.2 Gompertz prediction (heavy line) and 95% confidence limits ($n=1233$) of edited National Collaborative Perinatal Project (NCPP) data covering 15 to 60 weeks. [Brain weight (g), gestational age (weeks), total age after term]. Data points through 65 weeks (total age) are included, although the statistical regression did not use cases beyond 44 weeks. Again the greatest rate of brain growth occurs at the end of gestation and the inflection point is at the end of the second trimester.

organ maturation estimates at autopsy.[64] The fetal brain undergoes a growth spurt, reflected in maximal brain weight acceleration at 24 to 25 weeks just before, and concomitant with, the greatest proliferation of sulci and gyri (see Chapter 5) that becomes apparent at 26 to 28 weeks. This finding disagrees with others who contend that brain growth, as reflected in brain weight, follows a smooth course until 33 weeks.[65]

AUTOPSY CHARACTERISTICS OF HUMAN FETAL NEURAL TISSUE

Four measurements were available for the Yakovlev subset of infants: head circumference, fresh brain weight, brain volume following fixation in 10% formalin, and brain volume following alcohol dehydration before celloidin embedding. For the purposes of this section, we have assumed that brain weight and volume are virtually interchangeable. We constructed simple regressions of fetal brain weight or volume on head circumference (Fig. 2.3).

The relationship of volume of formalin-fixed brains to fresh brain weight indicates that fetal brains enlarge considerably during fixation, particularly after 28 weeks of gestation—a frequent observation.[31,66–68] In fact, in infants with larger head sizes at the end of gestation, the brain weight–volume ratio is one-third higher than that of fresh brain. The regression of postalcohol dehydration on head circumference indicates that about half of postformalin fixation volume is lost during alcohol dehydration.

Brain weight changes post mortem and during fixation

Many conditions influence final autopsy brain weight. The volume of edema fluid and blood modifies brain weight,[3] as does cause of death and nutritional condition.[69] Weighing before or after fixation is an important factor[70] as fresh brain weight is less than fixed brain weight.[31] On average, there is an increase of 10% during formalin fixation. These changes modify head measurements.[39] Adult brain weight also varies depending on body size, age at death, sample

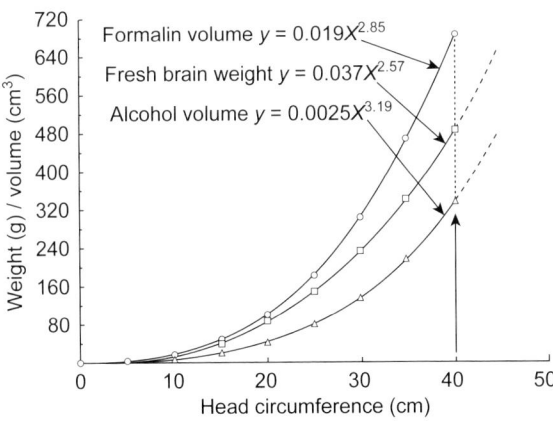

Fig. 2.3 Regressions of fresh brain weight (squares) after formalin fixation (circles) and following alcohol dehydration volume (triangles) on head circumference.

23

selection, sex, and lapse of time after death.[71] Infratentorial postfixation brain weight increases less than whole brain weight.[31]

Postnatal growth model

The postnatal brain weight growth curve was generated from 260 children who had survived birth, even though some were preterm and had survived only a few days. They ranged in age from 30 weeks of gestation to two postnatal years. A sigmoid growth curve was generated from birth to two postnatal years (Fig. 2.4) (McLennan and Gilles, 1983, unpublished data). The sigmoid curve models postnatal, but not prenatal, growth well. Postnatal brain growth in our model is similar to that of Dobbing and Sands,[72] although they had a small number of cases beyond 12 months. Again, there is a wide range in brain weight at each specific week.

    The significant implication is that most postnatal brain growth is completed within the first two postnatal years, similar to other reports.[1,73]

Conclusions

The derivation of prenatal and early childhood brain growth models based on extensive consideration of embryonic and fetal brain development as well as the history and prior application of growth functions to brain growth have been discussed. Unfortunately, we had too few preterm infants with a significant postnatal follow-up to study the effect of preterm birth on subsequent brain growth. The intent of this section has been to demonstrate the range of possibilities for similar studies. Once reference criteria are established, they are useful as comparisons for future cases involving individual and combined characteristics that alter brain weight.

    One common problem in developmental neuropathology is the differentiation between atrophy (loss of previously existing tissue) and failure of acquisition of fetal neural tissue (hypoplasia). The regression curve of fresh brain weight on head circumference allows a first approximation of whether atrophy or hypoplasia is present if three assumptions are accepted:

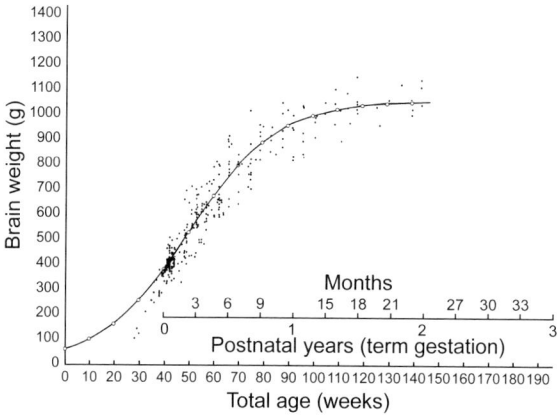

Fig. 2.4 Regression of postnatal brain weight (g) on total age. After birth, the rate of brain weight accretion slows particularly in the last half of the second postnatal year.

24

(1) brain and skull volume are closely related; (2) head circumference provides an accurate estimate of fetal cranial volume, but is a poor cranial volume estimator for the child and adult (McLennan and Gilles, unpublished data); and (3) skull size does not decrease following an insult to the developing brain. If cerebral atrophy is present, the head circumference is likely to indicate a brain weight greater than that actually found. If cerebral hypoplasia is present, the head circumference (while small for conceptional age) is likely to indicate a brain weight close to that actually found.

Dobbing and Sands[74] said it nicely: '… there exists a once-only opportunity to construct a complete brain, and that if this opportunity is missed it is not possible to remedy the situation later.'

REFERENCES

1. Voigt J, Pakkenberg H (1983) Brain weight of Danish children. A forensic material. *Acta Anat (Basel)* 116: 290–301.
2. Minckler TM, Boyd E (1968) Physical growth of nervous system. In: Minckler TM, editor. *Pathology of the Nervous System*. New York: McGraw-Hill, pp. 120–137.
3. Roessle R, Roulet F (1938) *Mass und Zahl in der Pathologie*. Berlin: Springer.
4. Kehrer M, Krageloh-Mann I, Goelz R, Schoning M (2003) The development of cerebral perfusion in healthy preterm and term neonates. *Neuropediatrics* 34: 281–286.
5. Donaldson HH (1896) *The Growth of the Brain*. London and New York: Walter Scott Ltd and Charles Scribner's Sons.
6. Bartley AJ, Jones DW, Weinberger DR (1997) Genetic variability of human brain size and cortical gyral patterns. *Brain* 120(Pt 2): 257–269.
7. McLennan JE, Gilles FH, Neff R (1983) A model of growth of the human fetal brain. In: Gilles FH, Leviton A, Dooling EC, editors. *The Developing Human Brain: Growth and Epidemiologic Neuropathology*. Boston: Wright-PSG, pp. 43–58.
8. O'Rahilly R, Müller F (1987) *Developmental Stages in Human Embryos*. Washington: Carnegie Institution of Washington.
9. O'Rahilly R, Müller F (1994) *The Embryonic Human Brain: An Atlas of Developmental Stages*. New York: Wiley-Liss.
10. Lemire RJ, Loeser JD, Leech RW, Alvord EC Jr. (1975) *Normal and Abnormal Development of the Human Nervous System*. Hagerstown, Maryland: Harper and Row.
11. Rakic P (1988) Specification of cerebral cortical areas. *Science* 241(4862): 170–176.
12. Gray J (1929) Kinetics of growth. *Br J Exp Biol* 6: 248–274.
13. Gompertz B (1825) On the nature of the function expressive of the law of human mortality, and on a new mode of determining the value of life contingencies. *Phil Trans Roy Soc* 36: 513–585.
14. Luecke RH, Wosilait WD, Young JF (1995) Mathematical representation of organ growth in the human embryo/fetus. *Int J Biomed Comput* 39: 337–347.
15. Wright S (1926) Reviews. *J Am Stat Assoc* 21: 493–497.
16. Minot C (1891) Senescence and rejuvenation. *J Physiol* 12: 97–153.
17. Pearl R, Reed L (1920) On the rate of growth of the population of the United States since 1790 and its mathematical representation. *Proc Natl Acad Sci USA* 6: 275–288.
18. Laird A (1967) Evolution of the human growth curve. *Growth* 31: 35–55.
19. Laird A (1966) Postnatal growth of birds and mammals. *Growth* 30: 349–363.
20. Laird A (1966) Dynamics of embryonic growth. *Growth* 30: 263–275.
21. Laird A (1964) Dynamics of tumor growth. *Br J Cancer* 13: 490–502.
22. Laird A (1965) Dynamics of tumour growth: Comparison of growth rates and extrapolation of growth curve to one cell. *Br J Cancer* 19: 278–291.
23. Burton A (1966) Rate of growth of solid tumours as a problem of diffusions. *Growth* 30: 157–176.

24. Dunn HL (1921) Growth of the central nervous system in the human fetus as expressed by graphic analysis and empirical formulae. *J Comp Neurol* 33: 405–491.
25. Scammon R (1923) A summary of the anatomy of the infant and child. In: Abt JA, editor. *Pediatrics*. Philadelphia: WB Saunders Co., pp. 257–444.
26. Mall FP (1910) Determination of the age of human embryos and fetuses. In: Keibel F, Mall FP, editors. *Human Embryology*. Philadelphia: JB Lippincott, pp. 202–242.
27. His W (1880–5) *Anatomie Menschlichen Embryonen*. Leipsig: F.C.W. Vogel.
28. Streeter GL (1920) Weight, sitting height, head size, foot length, and menstrual age of the human embryo. *Contrib Embryol (Carnegie Inst)* 11: 143–170.
29. Gruenwald P, Minh H (1960) Evaluation of body and organ weights in perinatal pathology. I. Normal standards derived from autopsies. *Am J Clin Path* 34: 247–253.
30. Jenkins G (1921) Relative weight and volume of the component parts of the brain of the human embryo at different stages of development. *Contri Embryol (Carnegie Inst)* 59: 41–60.
31. Guihard-Costa AM, Larroche JC (1990) Differential growth between the fetal brain and its infratentorial part. *Early Hum Dev* 23: 27–40.
32. Huxley JS (1932) *Problems of Relative Growth*. New York: Dial.
33. Shepard TH, Shi M, Fellingham GW, et al (1988) Organ weight standards for human fetuses. *Pediatr Pathol*. 8: 513–524.
34. Laird A, Barton A, Tyler S (1968) Growth and time: an interpretation of allometry. *Growth* 32: 347–354.
35. Barton A, Laird A (1969) Analysis of allometric and non-allometric differential growth. *Growth* 33: 1–16.
36. Count E (1947) Brain and body weight in man: their antecedents in growth and evolution; study in dynamic somatometry. *Ann NY Acad Sci* 46: 993–1122.
37. Tanimura T, Nelson T, Hollingsworth RR, Shepard TH (1971) Weight standards for organs from early human fetuses. *Anat Rec* 171: 227–236.
38. Marecki B (1989) Developmental relations between the weight of internal organs and somatic features of fetuses and newborns. *Z Morphol Anthropol* 78: 107–115.
39. Scammon R, Calkins L (1929) *The Development and Growth of the External Dimensions of the Human Body in the Fetal Period*. Minneapolis: University of Minnesota Press.
40. Cooke RW, Lucas A, Yudkin PL, Pryse-Davies J (1977) Head circumference as an index of brain weight in the fetus and newborn. *Early Hum Dev* 1: 145–149.
41. Winick M, Rosso P (1969) Head circumference and cellular growth of the brain in normal and marasmic children. *J Pediatr* 74: 774–748.
42. Buda B, Rabe E, Reed J (1975) Skull volume in infants, methodology, normal values and application. *Am J Dis Child* 129: 1171–1176.
43. Scammon R, Dunn HL (1924) On the growth of the human cerebellum in early life. *Proc Soc Exp Biol Med* 21: 217–221.
44. Dekaban AS (1953) Human thalamus. An anatomical, developmental and pathological study. I. Division of the human adult thalamus into nuclei by use of the cyto-myelo-architectonic method. *J Comp Neurol* 99: 639–683.
45. Dekaban AS (1954) Human thalamus. An anatomical, developmental and pathological study. II. Development of the human thalamic nuclei. *J Comp Neurol* 100: 63–97.
46. Siedler DE, Filly RA (1987) Relative growth of the higher fetal brain structures. *J Ultrasound Med* 6: 573–576.
47. Noback CR, Moss M (1956) Differential growth of the human brain. *J Comp Neurol* 105: 539–551.
48. Roessmann U (1974) Weight ratio between the infratentorial and supratentorial portions of the central nervous system. *J Neuropathol Exp Neurol* 33: 164–170.
49. Dobbing J, Sands J (1973) Quantitative growth and development of human brain. *Arch Dis Child* 48: 757–767.
50. Reece EA, Goldstein I, Pilu G, Hobbins JC (1987) Fetal cerebellar growth unaffected by intrauterine growth retardation: a new parameter for prenatal diagnosis. *Am J Obstet Gynecol* 157: 632–638.
51. Lassek A, Rasmussen G (1939) A regional volumetric study of the gray and white matter of the human prenatal spinal cord. *J Comp Neur* 70: 137–151.
52. Lassek A, Rasmussen G (1938) A quantitative study of the newborn and adult spinal cords of man. *J Comp Neurol* 69: 371–379.
53. Grenell R, Scammon R (1943) An iconometrographic representation of the growth of the central nervous system in man. *J Comp Neurol* 79: 329–354.

54. Jackson CM (1909) On the prenatal growth of the human body and the relative growth of the various organs and parts. *Am J Anat* 9: 119–165.
55. Dunn HL (1926) Variability in the growth of the fetal central nervous system as measured by biometric constants. *J Comp Neurol* 42: 165–209.
56. Boyd E (1935) A method of establishing the probable limits of normal variation in the weight of organs. *Anat Rec* 62: 1–6.
57. Ho KC, Roessmann U, Hause L, Monroe G (1981) Newborn brain weight in relation to maturity, sex, and race. *Ann Neurol* 10: 243–246.
58. Ho KC, Roessmann U, Hause L, Monroe G (1986) Correlation of perinatal brain growth with age, body size, sex, and race. *J Neuropathol Exp Neurol* 45: 179–188.
59. Winick M (1968) Changes in nucleic acid and protein content of the human brain during growth. *Pediatr Res* 2: 352–355.
60. Dobbing J, Sands J (1970) Timing of neuroblast multiplication in developing human brain. *Nature* 226(5246): 639–640.
61. Fishman MA, Prensky AL, Dodge PR (1969) Low content of cerebral lipids in infants suffering from malnutrition. *Nature* 221: 552.
62. Marks KH, Maisels MJ, Moore E, Gifford K, Friedman Z (1979) Head growth in sick premature infants–a longitudinal study. *J Pediatr* 94: 282–285.
63. Peters VB, Flexner LB (1950) Biochemical and physiological differentiation during morphogenesis. VIII Quantitative morphologic studies on the developing cerebral cortex of the fetal guinea pig. *Am J Anat* 86: 133–161.
64. Guihard-Costa AM, Menez F, Delezoide AL (2002) Organ weights in human fetuses after formalin fixation: standards by gestational age and body weight. *Pediatr Dev Pathol* 5: 559–578.
65. Fujimura M, Seryu JI (1977) Velocity of head growth during the perinatal period. *Arch Dis Child* 52: 105–112.
66. Appel FW, Appel E (1942) Intracranial variation in the weight of the human brain. *Hum Biol* 14: 48–68.
67. Appel FW, Appel E (1942) Intracranial variation in the weight of the human brain (concluded). *Hum Biol* 14: 235–250.
68. Larroche JC (1977) *Developmental Pathology of the Neonate*. Amsterdam: Excerpta Medica.
69. Brown RE (1965) Decreased brain weight in malnutrition and its implications. *E Afr Med J* 42: 584–595.
70. Schremmer CN (1967) Gewichtsänderungen verschiedener Gewebe nach Formalinfixierung. *Frankfurt Z Path* 77: 299–304.
71. Tobias PV (1970) Brain size, grey matter and race. Fact or fiction. *Am J Phys Anthrop* 32: 3–25.
72. Dobbing J, Sands J (1978) Head circumference, biparietal diameter and brain growth in fetal and postnatal life. *Early Hum Dev* 2: 81–87.
73. Coppoletta JM, Wolbach SB (1933) Body length and organ weights of infants and children: Study of body lengths and normal weights of more important vital organs of body between birth and 12 years of age. *Am J Pathol* 9: 55–70.
74. Dobbing J, Sands J (1971) Vulnerability of developing brain. IX. The effect of nutritional growth retardation on the timing of the brain growth spurt. *Biol Neonate* 19: 363–378.

3
FETAL VENTRICULAR SIZE, SURFACES, AND APPENDAGES

Introduction: the embryonic development of ventricles

Knowledge that the brain contains ventricles dates from the descriptions of Herophilus and Erasistratus in the third century BC. According to Galen, Herophilus recognized cerebral ventricles and Erasistratus described a ventricle in each cerebral hemisphere, a third ventricle and a foramen connecting the two, as well as a ventricle in the cerebellum.[1] The ventricular epithelial lining was recognized by Purkinje,[2] was subsequently quoted by Wislocki[3] and Valentin,[1,4] and confirmed 10 years later by Virchow in 1846.[5]

Lateral and third ventricular epithelial surface morphology changes during human embryonic and fetal brain development. The caudal neuropore closes at about postovulatory day 26, isolating ventricular fluid from amniotic fluid. Only primitive mesenchyme or menix exists external to the brain at this time, without any true subarachnoid space. Mesenchyme, condensed into a dense peripheral layer around the rostral neural tube, is the future chondrocranium and membranous bone site. Immediately subjacent is future pachymeninx; between it and looser arachnoidal villi, the arachnoid will form.[6] At about the seventh week, the future subarachnoid space appears as various-sized meshes containing fluid; a week later, subarachnoid cisterns arise. Arachnoid and subarachnoid spaces are visible ventrally, around the spinal cord and brain base, before dorsally. Pia mater develops on the neural surface just beneath primitive meningeal blood vessels. The ventricular system is continuous from the terminal ventricle (at and below conus medullaris), rostrally through ventricles of the spinal cord, rhombencephalon, mesencephalon, and diencephalon to lateral ventricles with their olfactory ventricles in embryo and fetus. The olfactory ventricle closes by gestational end. From birth and through adulthood, the spinal ventricle is closed in most humans and the central canal is discontinuous.[7] The embryonic diencephalic ventricle consists mostly of optic precursor at approximately postovulatory day 24. At around 30 postovulatory days, the midline telencephalic cavity is evident, and by 2 days later the cerebral hemispheral cavities and rhomboid fossa appear. At about 33 postovulatory days, medial and lateral ventricular (ganglionic) eminences indent the future ventrolateral ventricular floor, and, 10 days later, the olfactory ventricle and choroid plexus precursors emerge. At 48 postovulatory days, the midbrain mesocolic recess appears, and olfactory ventricle is present by 52 postovulatory days. Subsequently, the lateral ventricle becomes C-shaped. The optic, infundibular, and pineal outpouchings from the third ventricle develop in the embryonic period. The posterior lateral ventricular horns, suprapineal recess, aqueduct, and midline and fourth ventricular lateral foramina develop later during the fetal period.[8] All ventricular surface zones produce neuronal and glial precursors throughout embryonic and early fetal periods. Afterwards, ependymal cells replace the dividing ventricular zone cells at varying times during gestation.

This chapter stresses ependymal surface changes and, separately, relative ventricular size changes throughout gestation; pineal gland development, mesocoelic recess, and sub-commissural organ—ependymal specializations at the mesodiencephalic junction—follow. The differences between ventriculomegaly and hydrocephalus are examined independently in Chapter 15.

Developmental changes in ventricular epithelia

MATERIALS AND METHODS

A total of 111 serially sectioned fetal National Collaborative Perinatal Project (NCPP) brains from fetuses ranging in gestational age from 13 to 42 weeks and without gross defects or lesions were selected.[9] At least one coronally sectioned brain at each gestational week (except weeks 15 and 19) was examined. For two-thirds of the sampled ages, at least one brain was cut in either the horizontal or sagittal plane. Approximately one-third of brains were from stillborn infants; few neonates had survived more than 24 hours. Two neuropathologists simultane-ously reviewed every hematoxylin and eosin-stained section. Ependymal intactness, along the medial, dorsal, and lateral walls of the lateral ventricle, was recorded as preserved or inter-rupted. Interrupted ependyma was defined as the loss of several adjoining ependymal cells.

HISTOLOGIC FEATURES

Closely packed multilayered ependymal cells, distinct from the underlying densely cellular germinal matrix, lined the primitive ventricles in fetuses of less than 20 weeks' gestational age. Ependymal cells are glial fibrillary acidic protein-positive early in fetal development, and two types are present: epithelial and tanycytes. Immunostaining disappears with advanc-ing gestational age.[10] The histologic stains used in this study precluded evaluation of this phenomenon. Subsequently, this complex epithelium thins, becoming a single cuboidal layer. Different ventricular surface areas exhibited low cuboidal epithelium, while, simultaneously, particularly laterally over germinal epithelium of the ganglionic eminence subventricular zone, a complex multilayered epithelium remained.

Between 21 and 25 gestational weeks, the lateral occipital horn ependyma gradually atten-uates with loss of cuboidal or columnar appearance adjacent to intact ependymal cells. At 26 to 27 weeks, early degenerative changes of pyknosis, hyperchromatism, nuclear vesiculation, and occasionally cytoplasmic ballooning were seen in these cells. The dorsolateral occipital horn, caudal to the atrium, sometimes contained ependymal cell loss by 27 to 28 weeks' gestational age; multifocal losses, usually just anterior to the occipital tip, also occurred.

Ependymal defects, associated with reduced numbers or absence of underlying residual matrix cells, as well as ependymal tubules or rosettes in the subependymal zone, were frequent. In areas of ependymal loss, glial proliferation and hypercellularity were not pronounced. There was no 'granular ependymitis.' Additional changes in occipital horn ependyma were evident

29

TABLE 3.1

Distribution of focal ependymal changes in normal fetal brains

| | Percentage of brains showing ependymal loss | | | |
| | | | Occipital horns | |
Gestational age (weeks)	Frontal horns	Hippocampal CA$_2$	Medial	Lateral
<28 (*n*=31)	6	10	0	33
28–35 (*n*=49)	60	65	16	99
>35 (*n*=31)	85	85	65	100

after 32 weeks, consisting of irregular lining of the medial wall and extensive loss lining the lateral wall (Table 3.1).

Focal regions overlying hippocampal sector CA$_2$ underwent progressive thinning, blunting, and attenuation of ependyma after 28 weeks (Table 3.1), but was more extensive in most brains after 32 weeks when focal glial proliferation occasionally occurred. Generally, gliosis was not prominent in the denuded CA$_2$ sector subependymal zone. Temporal horn lining remained unbroken except for an occasional small focus of attenuated ependyma. Near the medial temporal horn angle and over Sommer's sector, the ependyma was always intact in these otherwise normal brains.

In the rostral ventricular system, patchy loss of ependyma along the ventral surface of corpus callosum and lateral walls of septum pellucidum occurred, occasionally seen at 25 weeks, but especially marked after 32 weeks. Dorsolateral and ventrolateral lateral ventricular angles often lack a continuous ependyma. Abrupt disruption of ependyma without any associated reactive change, such as cellular influx of macrophages or glia, and with underlying intact matrix, is usually distinguishable from ventricular angle blunting (associated with mild to moderate ventricular dilation), which is accompanied by ependymal loss and buried ependymal tubules. In the latter cases, it is common to find widespread ependymal loss at all lateral ventricular levels, both medially and laterally.

Third ventricular ependymal lining was continuous in all cases (except those with massive ventriculomegaly). Aqueductal ependyma was well preserved and highly specialized dorsally in the subcommissural region. Buried ependymal tubules, ependymal gaps, and subependymal gliosis were rare. Fourth ventricular ependymal lining, except overlying area postrema, remained unbroken.

SUMMARY

Occipital horn ependymal loss began toward the end of second trimester (28–35 weeks). This is a period of rapid fetal brain growth (see Chapter 2) and gyral and sulcal patterns become increasingly complex (see Chapter 5). Simultaneously, widespread loss was more evident at specific sites: along both occipital horn walls, over sector hippocampal CA$_2$, along lateral septum pellucidum walls, and on ventrorostral corpus callosum surface (Fig. 3.1). The denuded areas did not contain marked subependymal gliosis or other reactive changes.

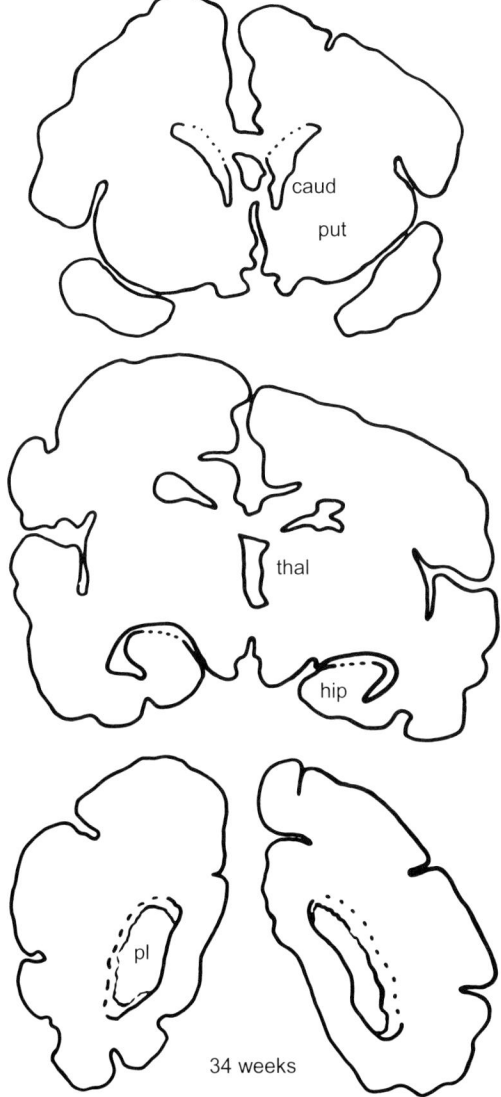

Fig. 3.1 Schematic drawing of areas of ependymal loss in a 34-week-old fetus. This example depicts ependymal loss (indicated by the dotted line) common in human fetuses. In the upper figure, an anterior coronal cut through the temporal tips, there is extensive ependymal loss on the ventricular corpus callosum surface. In the middle figure, a coronal cut through the midthalamus, there is extensive ependymal loss over the hippocampus. In the lower figure, a coronal cut through the occipital lobes, there is extensive ependymal loss over the lateral occipital horns. Caud, caudate; put, putamen; thal, thalamus; hip, hippocampus; pl, parieto-occipital lateral ventricle.

31

Relative ventricular sizes throughout gestation

FETAL VENTRICULAR SIZE CHANGES

After the first embryonic month and during early fetal life, the lateral ventricles are large relative to overall cerebral size. At 15 weeks, lateral ventricular width is normally two-thirds that of the cerebrum but decreases as the cerebrum grows. At 17 weeks, it is less than half that of the cerebrum, and at 20 weeks is approximately one-third of cerebral width.[11] Atrial diameter remains stable at 7.6 (SD 0.6) mm from 14 to 38 weeks.[12] The cerebrum grows around the lateral ventricles without ventricular enlargement. Fetuses with lateral ventricular widths more than 4 standard deviations above the mean (widths >10mm) are more likely to have malformations and higher mortality than their peers;[13] those without malformations have an increased risk of developmental delay after birth.[14]

Sonographers are especially interested in fetal lateral ventricular width in order to accurately diagnose fetal ventriculomegaly and hydrocephalus.[15] Bilateral occipital horn and trigonal dilation are the earliest signs of hydrocephalus.[16,17,18–22] Fetal ventriculomegaly can be isolated or associated with other anomalies or chromosomal disorders, and coronal cerebral mantle thickness is correlated with crown–rump length, foot length, and head circumference.[23] Lateral ventricle asymmetry is probably not abnormal.[24] In preterm newborns, a postnatal ventricular width of at least 15mm suggests the likelihood of requiring a ventricular shunt.[25]

CHANGES IN LATERAL VENTRICULAR SIZE FOLLOWING NORMAL VAGINAL DELIVERY

Compressed and slit-like neonatal lateral ventricles found in neonates with brain damage are often used prognostically as a marker of cerebral edema and in establishing the timing of neonatal brain injury.[26,27] We show in this section that the width of lateral ventricles after an uncomplicated delivery is normally slit-like.[28] Slit-like means that no cerebrospinal fluid (CSF) space is identified within lateral ventricles by cranial ultrasound in both coronal and sagittal planes; ependymal surfaces touch.

Materials and methods

A total of 143 newborn infants had videotaped cranial ultrasound examinations via the anterior fontanelle as soon as possible after birth [from 1h to 156h (mean 47h, median 40h)]. All births were from normal vaginal deliveries without complication, had Apgar scores of 9 or 10 at 5 and 10 minutes, had uncomplicated postnatal courses, and were discharged from the nursery within 48 hours. Most were first studied when they came for their first postnatal visit; 27% of neonates were studied for a second time at their normal newborn clinic visits (2–7 days after birth). Rarely, a third and sometimes fourth examination were performed on follow-up visits.

A single observer classified each lateral ventricle as completely closed (slit), partially open, or completely open (Fig. 3.2). A slit-like, completely closed lateral ventricle contained no definable CSF space. 'Partially open' was defined by finding an anechoic CSF space in any part of lateral ventricle. 'Completely open' was defined as the entire ventricle being filled with anechoic CSF and no ventricular walls touching. Incidental findings such as choroid plexus (five infants, less than 1cm) and retrocerebellar cysts (three infants) were recorded but did not disqualify the infant from the study.

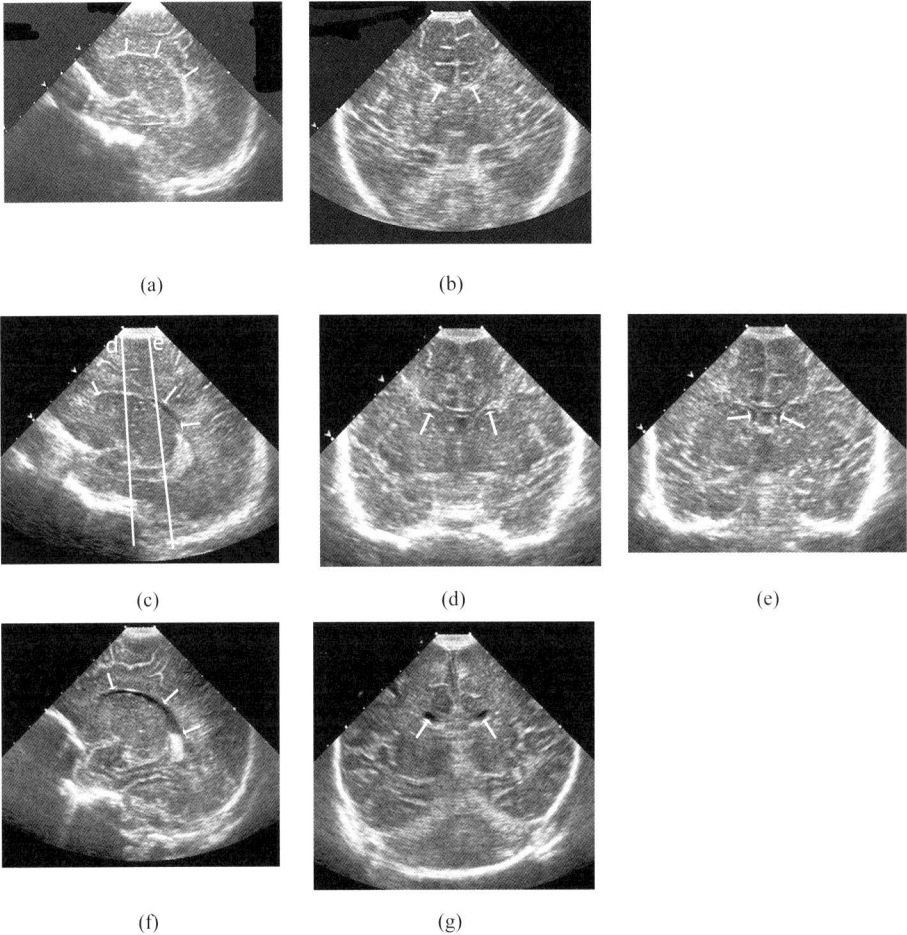

(a)   (b)

(c)   (d)   (e)

(f)   (g)

Fig. 3.2 Normal cranial ultrasounds in three different patients. Sagittal (a, c, f) and coronal (b, d, e, g) views through the lateral ventricle bodies. (a, b) Closed lateral ventricles. The walls touch each other and there is no identifiable cerebrospinal fluid collection within the ventricles (arrows indicate closed lateral ventricle). (c, d, e) Partially open lateral ventricle. The ventricle has expanded slightly in size with fluid now seen in the atria and posterior body. The anterior ventricle is still closed [arrows indicate partially open lateral ventricles; line **d** in (c) indicates the transducer plane angle in (d); line **e** in (c) indicates the transducer plane angle in (e)]. (f, g) Completely open lateral ventricles. The ventricular walls no longer touch each other in any ventricle portion (arrows indicate completely open lateral ventricles).

Statistical methods

We analyzed the data using three different methods: (1) estimating the percentage of slit, partially open, and open ventricles at different time points after delivery using the method of smoothed percentages; (2) constructing a life table in order to calculate the time after delivery of slit to partially open ventricles;[29] and (3) fitting a geometric distribution to the data estimating the median time to partially open ventricles. Geometric distributions are widely used to model waiting times.[30] In this case, the waiting time was the time from slit to partially open ventricles. For a geometric distribution with parameter q, expected waiting time to event is $1/(1-q)$; q was estimated by the method of maximum likelihood. We attempted to use methods 2 and 3 to estimate the mean time after delivery to fully open ventricles; however, by the end of the study period, only 18 infants (13%) had fully open ventricles. Consequently, a 'good' estimate of the time to open ventricles was not possible.

Results

The median time for the first ultrasound examination was 40 hours after birth (mean of 47h) (Table 3.2). The range was quite broad, with one examination at 6.5 days after birth. The median times for the second and third ultrasound examinations were less than 3.5 days after delivery (means of 84 and 78h, respectively)—still a wide range. Of 143 newborns given an initial ultrasound before discharge, 27% had a second, 13% a third, and 1.3% a fourth.

Using the method of overlapping intervals (smoothed percentages) to construct the approximate distributions of slit, partially open, and open ventricles, slit ventricles gradually decreased and partially open and fully open ventricles gradually increased following birth. Within 12 hours of delivery, an estimated 80% of neonates had slit ventricles and 19% had partially open ventricles. In only 1% were the ventricles of normal size within 12 hours of birth. The estimated median time from delivery to partially open ventricles was 36 to 60 hours (1.5–2.5 days). At 3.5 days after birth, the proportion of neonates with slit ventricles was 25%, and only in 12% were the ventricles fully open. Using the life table for slit ventricles, the estimated median time from delivery to partially open ventricles was 73.66 hours, or approximately 3 days (from the last column of Table 3.2; see also Fig. 3.3). Using the geometric model for waiting times, the maximum likelihood estimate of q was 0.984, resulting in an expected mean time from delivery to partially open ventricles of approximately 63 hours (about 2.5 days).

Summary

This study shows that slit lateral ventricles are normal in the majority of newborns following unremarkable vaginal delivery. During the first postnatal week, the lateral ventricles accumulate CSF, expanding their walls so they are no longer in contact. Using three models for this study population, the estimated median time to partially open ventricles is 1.5 to 3 days after delivery, with an estimated mean time of 2.5 days.

The postnatal process of expanding from slit to open ventricles induces speculation that normal forces of skull compression (molding) as the infant passes through the birth canal also expel CSF out of the lateral and third ventricles, possibly into the subarachnoid space around the spinal cord, implying that the thecal sac is distensible. Factors allowing the infant to compensate for the tight birth canal include skull bone mobility, as well as displacement of spinal fluid. It would be interesting to know when the ventricles open completely.

TABLE 3.2

Percentages of slit, partially open, and open ventricles for overlapping time intervals

Hours after delivery	Interval (hours after delivery)	Number of infants	Percentage slit	Percentage partially open	Percentage open
12	0–24	75	80	19	1
24	12–36	55	67	33	0
36	24–48	34	65	32	3
48	36–60	20	20	65	15
60	48–72	30	23	67	10
72	60–84	55	29	60	11
84	72–96	52	25	63	12
96	84–108	40	30	55	15
108	96–120	29	31	52	17

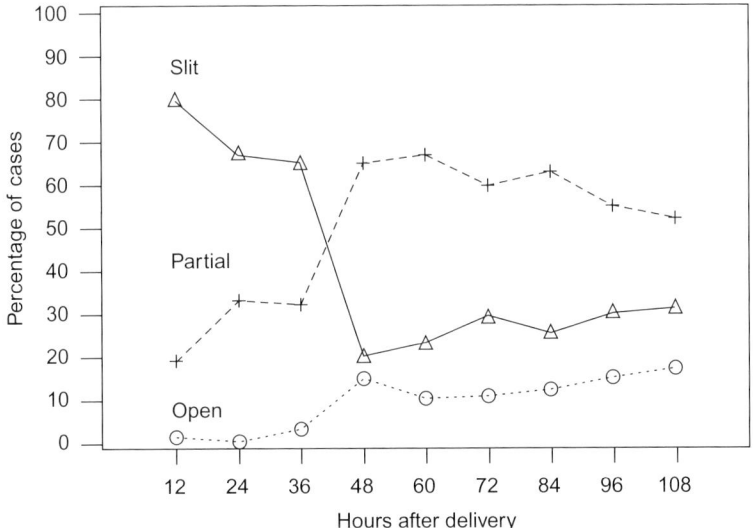

Fig. 3.3 The proportion of cases containing slit-like ventricles decreases with time after birth. There is a large drop within the first 48 hours and then the proportion is roughly steady until 4 days of age. There is a complementary increase in the proportion of cases over the first 2 days of life. The proportion of cases with fully open ventricles slowly increases over the first 4 postnatal days. Overall, it takes almost 4 days for slit-like ventricles to open following birth.

Dorsal mesodiencephalic junction: pineal, subcommissural organ, and mesocoelic recess

At the prosencephalic–mesencephalic junction there are three unique neural tube specializations—the pineal, subcommissural organ, and mesocoelic recess. During human pineal development, neuromelanin initially accumulates in, and then subsequently disappears from, fetal neuroepithelial cells. The subcommissural organ epithelium extends ventrally around the posterior commissure from the pineal recess to the retrocommissural mesocoelic recess. The mesocoelic recess is the final part of the embryonic mesencephalic ventricle to disappear; the specialized subcommissural organ epithelium is on its rostral surface.[31,32] In this section, we review pineal and subcommissural organ development and their relationships with the mesocoelic recess.

PINEAL

The pineal has long interested biologists and philosophers. The pineal contains pinealocytes, interstitial cells, and neurons, and receives sympathetic and parasympathetic innervation as well as fibers penetrating along the pineal stalk. The discovery of high concentrations of melatonin and serotonin in the pineal renewed interest in its significance as a neuroendocrine gland.[33–36] Melatonin secretion in humans was subsequently shown to follow a circadian rhythm. Another problem complicating pineal evaluation is that a large proportion of fetuses with other brain injury have pineals that are also injured.[37]

In a general review of both serially and nonserially sectioned brains of fetuses and infants, ranging from 10 to 44 weeks, pineal pigment deposits were noted in 90% of those cases, including pineal sections.[38] This observation prompted a description of developing pineal morphology and the consideration of the possible significance of pigment in pineal parenchymal cells.

Materials and methods

A total of 118 pineal glands collected from two sources were studied. Of 360 brains embedded in celloidin, serially sliced at 35μm and stained with hematoxylin and eosin—Nissl for cells, or Loyez for myelin—the pineal was identified in 72 brains (20%). In a group of 580 brains sectioned nonserially, according to a protocol, the pineal was identified in 46 (8%) cases. Percentages were low because the pineal is frequently torn out during brain separation from tentorial and vascular attachments at autopsy. Hematoxylin and eosin-stained sections were reviewed to determine cellular composition, amount of stroma, degree of vascularity, general arrangement of pineal structures, and amount and location of pineal pigment. Melanin, lipofuscin, and hemosiderin were identified or ruled out with appropriate stains.

Results

General histologic features

Pineal development begins as a small dorsal diencephalic ventricular diverticulum at 5 to 6 weeks,[39] but is actually seen earlier at 33 postovulatory days as a thickening in the diencephalic caudal end.[6] Between 10 and 15 gestational weeks, the structure increases in size and further growth occurs in six stages from 14 weeks to term. Local proliferation of primitive roof ependymal cells gives it a multilobulated appearance. At 14 weeks, loose mesenchyme surrounds parenchyma; subsequent epithelial and ependymal cell proliferation forms irregularly sized glands and tubules, which are usually lined by a single layer of large cuboidal cells and contain prominent vascular stroma. Many large and small glands appear between 16 and 23 weeks, with a basement membrane lining their empty lumens. More mature ependymal cells with cilia line the main diverticulum. Owing to its morphologic appearance at this gestational age, the pineal was designated a gland.

By 24 to 27 weeks, the variably sized tubular structures with empty central lumens become less prominent, remaining glands are uniform in size and appearance, and adjacent cell proliferation transforms some larger tubular structures into solid cords. Strands and nests of parenchymal cells are interspersed with glands. Glands with cellular pigment are most often found in the periphery, while pigmented parenchymal cells are diffusely dispersed. The admixture of parenchymal cell strands and moderately cellular and vascular stroma results in an alveolar pattern that persists through the early third trimester. The fibrovascular stroma occasionally produces discrete perivascular pseudorosette-like structures.

From 28 to 31 weeks, parenchymal cell nests enlarge, with a smooth expanding margin in a palisading fashion, and contain a recognizable basement membrane. Fewer glands with central lumens than at earlier ages exist, usually at the organ's periphery. The pigment granules become less conspicuous. Small stromal hyperchromatic cells with nuclei full of coarse chromatin and no distinct cell border are present. They are distinct from larger pineal parenchymal cells, with round or ovoid nuclei, moderate amounts of chromatin, identifiable nucleoli, and abundant cytoplasm. An occasional parenchymal cell mitosis is seen; this is also seen, less frequently, in stromal cells.

During the last 8 weeks (32–39 weeks), small hyperchromatic cells gradually increase, obscuring the parenchymal–stromal distinction. Basement membrane between parenchyma and stroma is less recognizable, and the tubular structures with central lumens are rare. Cells containing pigment granules are scattered infrequently throughout, and occasional glial cells are embedded in the parenchyma. Connective tissue septa are infrequent, even though collagen fibers are present in pineal connective tissue capsule at 36 to 39 weeks.

Term pineal glands are composed of large vesicular cells intermixed with small, hyperchromatic cells. The vesicular cells lie on a loose fibrovascular stroma, while the small cells are densely packed. Cords of small cells, separated from large cell synctia by connective tissue bands in some areas, give the pineal a mosaic appearance. Ependymal tubules are rarely present; pigment granules, seldom seen, are best recognized in parenchymal cell aggregates.

The morphologic features of more than one period are infrequently found in a pineal, illustrating overlap of developmental phases and architectural transition. Persistent glandular structures with heavily pigmented cells appear in close apposition to solid-appearing sheets of nonpigmented pineal cells. No mature ganglion cells are present in infant pineals under 40 weeks, but some silver-impregnated processes are present as early as 24 to 27 weeks.

Pigment

Throughout much of gestation, the fetal pineal contains rod- and needle-shaped refractile brown pigment. Ninety percent of human fetal pineal glands contain pigment granules, apparent as early as 14 weeks in the apices of primitive ependymal cells abutting the luminal end. Other epithelial cells with pigment are clustered and show no morphologic differences from adjacent nonpigmented cells.

In 16- to 19-week-old fetuses, pigment is prominently present in juxtaluminal location, in pinched-off glandular structures. It is located in both proper ependymal cells and in glandular parenchymal cells. Pigment is distributed more peripherally than centrally. At times, pigment granules are so densely packed that pigment-containing glands stand out at low magnification as dark garlands; many tubules resemble rosettes because dense pigment obscures the lumen.

With fetal maturation, pigment granules are less densely aggregated, occurring in solid, nonglandular areas by 24 to 27 weeks. This pigment dispersion is synchronous with the disappearance of tubular and glandular pineal structures.

As small glandular structures are not prominent after 31 weeks' gestation, pigment is usually present in random parenchymal cells. Although pigment density varies, generally it is very prominent in early gestation, and it gradually becomes less prominent to minimal by term with pigment in only a few pineal cells. Multiple cell processes of meningeal melanocytes, at term, have round-to-ovoid coarse brown cytoplasmic granules and are not found within the pineal gland proper. Pineal gland development is summarized in Table 3.3 and Figure 3.4.

Summary

The presence of melanin pigment granules in fetal pineal is interesting; it is maximally dense during the second trimester and decreases markedly by birth. Melanin has been found in embryonic or fetal pineal in sea squirt tadpole,[40] pig,[41] quail,[42] adult brown bat,[43] cat,[44] dog,[45] horse,[46] rat,[47] and cow.[48,49] Pigmented cells in the brain arise from differentiated neuroectoderm, either neuroepithelium or neural crest. In human pineal parenchyma, from at least 14 weeks and after, melanin pigment granules appear in typical (cuboidal or columnar) ciliated ependymal cells and glandular or epithelial cells—all cell types derived from neuroepithelium. Melanocytes derived from the neural crest, present in leptomeninges surrounding and invaginating the pineal, are sometimes seen in the mature infant.

A pineal or median eye, with the histologic components of a persistent lateral or paired eye, is present in a few reptiles (for instance, *Sphenodon punctatus*) and produces melatonin. If pigment in fetal pineal is an ontogenetic expression of pineal phylogenesis, its gradual diminution in human gland by term suggests that pigment is vestigial rather than functional. Another interpretation of pineal pigment notes that this pigment is associated with pineal neurosecretory granules. The pineal has a high diurnal concentration of serotonin and melatonin, supporting its neuroendocrine function. Small amounts of melanin pigment in adults possibly indicate that the pineal remains active postnatally.[50,51]

The pineal shows a definite pattern of growth and development (Fig. 3.4 and Table 3.3), providing clear criteria to assess pineal gestational age. For example, typical ependymal tubules with dense lining cell pigmentation at luminal poles are not seen after 30 weeks, a solid lymphoid appearance is usually not present before 25 weeks, and an alveolar pattern

TABLE 3.3

Human fetal pineal temporal development

Gestational age (weeks)	General appearance	Pineal parenchyma	Pineal stroma	Pineal pigment
12–15 (*n*=2)	Multiple lobules around a single large ependymal cavity	Prominent pineal diverticulum. Active radial proliferations of cells from the ependymal zone	Ingrowth of primitive vascular mesenchyme	Moderate amount in primitive ependymal lining cells and ependymal tubules
16–23 (*n*=11)	Typical alveolar pattern ('glandular' pineal)	Neuroepithelial cords. Numerous large and small ependymal tubules. Distinct inner and outer basement membrane	Loosely textured fibroblastic, vascular tissue	Marked amount, mostly in ependymal tubules
24–17 (*n*=24)	Typical alveolar pattern	Irregularly branched epithelial processes. Smaller and more uniform ependymal tubules. Perivascular pseudorosettes prominent	Dense and cellular fibrovascular stroma. Small, hyperchromic cells	Moderate amount in both tubules and nonglandular cells
28–31 (*n*=25)	Typical alveolar pattern	Reduced number of ependymal tubules. Nonglandular parenchyma prominent. Loss of outer basement membrane. Perivascular pseudorosettes	Relatively compact, less vascular stroma. Many small, hyperchromic cells. Occasional large, vesicular cells	Slight to moderate amount in peripheral tubules and scattered parenchymal cells
32–39 (*n*=34)	Less distinct alveolar pattern. Beginning mosaic pattern	Rare ependymal tubules. Prominent nonglandular component. More small cells	Increased small, hyperchromic cells. Large cells more vesicular. Less vascular stroma	Slight amount, mostly in diffusely scattered nonglandular cells
40 (*n*=11)	Mosaic pattern. Encapsulated	Very rare ependymal tubules. Large, vesicular cells distinct from small, hyperchromic cells	No clear distinction of parenchyma from stroma. Many large, vesicular cells intermixed with small, hyperchromic cells	Minimal amount only in solid, nonglandular part

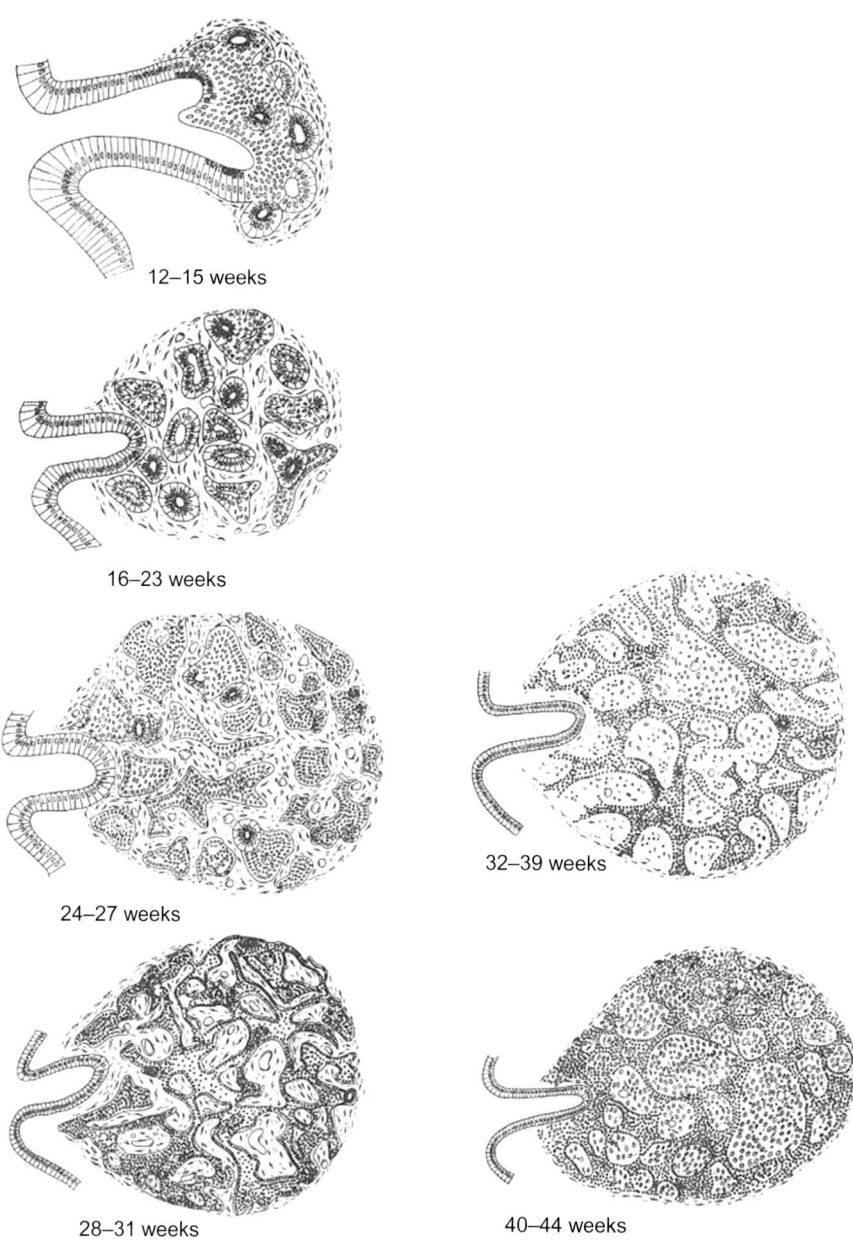

12–15 weeks

16–23 weeks

24–27 weeks

32–39 weeks

28–31 weeks

40–44 weeks

Fig. 3.4 Pineal development. Proliferating epithelial cells form irregular tubules separated by a loose mesenchyme. By 16 to 23 weeks, many large and small nests of epithelial cells are present, and at the end of the second trimester (24–27 weeks) the tubular structures are less prominent; many have been transformed into solid cords. At this age, melanin pigment granules are found in both the nests of parenchymal cells, particularly at the periphery, and individual pigmented parenchymal cells dispersed throughout the pineal. The gland retains its alveolar pattern into the first part of the third trimester (28–31 weeks).

characterizes pineal of infants at 20 to 30 weeks. Pineal morphologic features are not completely fixed at birth; histologic changes continue during the first postnatal year.[52] The pineal undergoes further changes including cyst formation, glial scarring, calcification, and fibrosis with advancing age, suggesting that continuing pineal morphologic remodeling is correlated with changing function. Some malformations and genetic abnormalities are associated with pineal agenesis.[53–55]

SUBCOMMISSURAL ORGAN AND MESOCOELIC RECESS

The subcommissural organ is wrapped around the rostral, ventral, and caudal surfaces of posterior commissure, and in the fetus it extends into the mesocoelic recess just behind the commissure. It is one of five circumventricular organs (organum vasculosum laminae terminalis, subfornical organ, subcommissural organ, tanycytes in third ventricular floor, and area postrema) lacking a blood–brain barrier (their capillaries have fenestrated endothelium). These are the only brain regions in which neurons are exposed to the systemic circulation and chemical environment. They contain different densities of serotonin fibers and are the sites of increased vascular permeability for peptides and other molecules that usually do not cross the blood–brain barrier. Dense aggregates of a diversity of peptidergic receptors are also present, suggesting involvement in circulatory and central nervous system communication.[56,57]

The subcommissural organ is a conserved brain gland, present throughout the vertebrate phylum, and, in the human, is morphologically evident at about 41 days.[8] The human fetal subcommissural organ shares the distinct subcommissural organ ultrastructural features of all other species, containing secretory granules but not secreting the glycoproteins necessary for Reisner's fiber found in some species, such as the rat.[58] This seems to be the only difference between the human subcommissural organ and other species. The mesocoelic recess, also found in all vertebrates, including the human fetus,[31,32] was first described early in the twentieth century.[59] It is composed of two bands of characteristically elongated columnar epithelium, uniting in the form of a groove, which becomes vestigial in adults. Gilbert, in 1960, found a secretory subcommissural organ in adult brains.[60] However, Rakic could not identify it beyond the second decade of life.[32] He postulated that its disappearance correlated with other regressive phenomena affecting the third ventricle and aqueduct epithelial lining.

Materials and methods

The subcommissural organ was identified and well preserved in 30 of 62 nonserially sectioned brains, hematoxylin and eosin stained, used to study pineal gland development.[61] The fetal gestational ages ranged from 12 to 44 weeks.

Simultaneously, the nests of parenchymal cells enlarge and the pigment granules become less conspicuous. From 32 to 39 weeks, an increase in small hyperchromic cells obscures the parenchymal–stromal distinction and the pigment granules are infrequent. The pineal gland of the term infant contains large vesicular cells mixed with packed small hyperchromic cells within a loose fibrovascular stroma. Pigment granules are rarely found in aggregates of parenchymal cells.

Results

The subcommissural organ occupies the posterior commissural ventricular surfaces and extends into the mesocoelic recess.[62,63] Its epithelium is arrayed on rostral and lateral, and to a lesser extent, caudal surfaces and overlies a condensation of cells, the hypendyma or subependymal zone. Histologic features vary at different gestational ages (Table 3.4). The organ is more prominent in early gestation, appearing to be a secretory structure, and gradually becomes less prominent by the end of gestation.

At approximately 20 weeks, tall, columnar epithelial cells with prominent apical cytoplasmic vacuoles and basal nuclei are pronounced. The specialized columnar cells are closely aligned on a basement membrane forming a single layer; their cytoplasm is abundant, eosinophilic, often vesicular or finely granular; their nuclei, with or without nucleoli, usually have distinct margins and finely dispersed chromatin granules. They are easily distinguished from typical pineal recess cuboidal epithelium. Cilia are usually absent during gestation, except in a few very young fetuses (12–16 weeks) in which cytoplasmic vacuoles are present. A fairly abrupt transition subsequently occurs yielding typical cuboidal ependymal cells with prominent cilia and densely stained basal nuclei without cytoplasmic granules or vacuoles. At 20 and 25 weeks, the subepithelial tissue consists of loose reticulum with many small vascular channels containing scattered immature cells. No definite neuronal or glial differentiation is present. The subependymal zone or hypendyma progressively thickens with increasing age. After 25 weeks, typical epithelial cells are cuboidal with vacuoles; subepithelial tissue becomes condensed, exhibiting less vascularity, denser cellularity, and glia-like cells. Between 33 weeks and term, the subcommissural organ is composed of very low cuboidal epithelial cells, the height of which is often lower than adjacent typical ependymal cells. Gaps between cells give a striking appearance of atrophy. The subepithelial tissue has many mature glial cells, often with fibrillary processes; occasional hypertrophic astrocytes are present. After 40 weeks, low or very much attenuated epithelial cells and subepithelial gliosis, no longer showing evidence of a secretory epithelium, characterize the subcommissual organ.

Summary

The developing subcommissural organ displays sequential changes indicating that this structure varies in prominence and morphology with gestational age. The histologic features reflecting a secretory structure were marked in the mesodiencephalic junction where modified roof ependymal cells invaginated posteriorly and anteriorly to form the mesocoelic and pineal recesses. Neurons, while found in the subcommissural organ in rabbit fetuses,[64] did not occur in the human subcommissural organ. Epithelial cells comprising the subcommissural organ lost their cilia before they became definitely secretory in all cases we studied. As the fetus approached term, the tall, columnar cells that looked secretory during early gestation became smaller and flattened with considerable reduction of cytoplasm. Also, the nuclei became smaller and hyperchromatic. In addition, it was not uncommon to see a focal loss of epithelial cells or a small gap between normal ependymal cells on the dorsal mesodiencephalic junction. The mesocoelic recess, which is so prominent during the early and midgestational periods, also became smaller and less distinct as the fetus approached term. All these changes suggest that the human subcommissural organ is vestigial after birth, as postulated by Rakic.[32]

TABLE 3.4

Human subcommissural organ development

Gestational age (weeks)	Ependyma	Hypendyma
12–16 (n=3)	Ciliated, pseudostratified columnar cells. Well-developed mesocoelic recess	Cells loose, reticular. Dense capillary network
17–24 (n=12)	Tall, columnar cells. Tiny granules in apical cytoplasm. Nuclei midposition	Increased density and thickness of cells. Less loose. Vascularity increased
25–32 (n=12)	Cuboidal, vacuolated cells. Cilia absent	Glial cells present. Compact. Less vascular
33–40 (n=10)	Low cuboidal or flat cells without cilia. Small ependymal gaps	Cellular. Mature glial cells. Occasional hypertrophic astrocytes. Occasional neurons

Nevertheless, whether atrophic changes after birth were associated with concomitant loss of function cannot be determined at this time. Subepithelial hypertrophic astrocytes suggest a degenerative process, but hypertrophic astrocytes and ependymal irregularity or discontinuity were found regularly around the ventricular walls, especially occipitally, and were interpreted by us as morphologic markers of physiologic remodeling consequent to brain maturation.

Discussion

Ependymal and choroid plexus cells, found in the CSF at various ages, are probably not related to improper handling of tissue.[65] Others, observing epithelial cells in CSF, commented on their high numbers in young infants (and particularly in children with hydrocephalus).[66] Thus, ependymal gaps probably reflect discrete desquamation during fetal life.

Friede noted ependymal defects near lateral ventricle corners and on the ventral callosal surface, without specifying fetal ages.[67] Although he identified either slight glial proliferation or matrix rarefaction, he did not feel that glial response became marked with increasing gestational age. Pedunculated transependymal excrescences of germinal matrix cells in the absence of ependymal gaps suggested to Friede a malformative or degenerative process, but we have found them after fetal viral infections, such as rubella. Other investigators have interpreted any ependymal loss as an abnormality. In a study of 80 cases of kernicterus and seven cases of posticteric encephalopathy, Haymaker et al[68] found, in 'occasional' cases, denudation of ependymal cells 'here and there,' with underlying sparse germinal cells. Among 51 infants (74% preterm) who had sustained severe 'anoxia,' Banker and Larroche[69] found that occipital horn lateral wall ependyma frequently disappeared when adjacent to zones of focal white matter necrosis. In more chronic cases, subependymal gliosis was present and medial ventricular wall ependymal lining was intact.

Ependymal defects in the fetal brain, occurring more frequently in the late second and early third trimester, stereotyped in location, and consistent in extent, probably result from a modeling process engendered by increasing size and growing brain complexity. Ventricular walls, subject to varying pulsatile hydrostatic pressure, have less support in regions adjacent to incompletely myelinated tracts, in contrast to frontal horns with nearby dense cellular neuronal aggregates, allowing the ependymal lining there to be more easily lost and explaining the predilection for occipital horn ependymal loss.

Conclusion

By the end of the first postovulatory month, the ventricular system is isolated from amniotic fluid and any fluid therein is considered of ventricular origin. Thereafter, lateral and third ventricular epithelial morphology changes during human embryonic and fetal growth and patches of ependymal loss are expected as a usual developmental event in several regions. At the same time, the pineal, subcommissural organ, and the mesocoelic recess form at the mesodiencephalic junction. Neuromelanin first accumulates in, and then subsequently disappears from, human fetal neuroepithelial cells. The pigment is maximally dense during the second trimester, tending to diminish markedly by birth. The functional significance of pineal pigment remains unclear, but it is unlikely that it is only vestigial. Small amounts of melanin pigment, lipofuscin, and variable amounts of calcium have been recognized in adult pineal.

Subcommissural organ prominence and morphology varies sequentially with gestational age. Its histologic features reflect a secretory structure, marked in the mesodiencephalic junction, with modified roof ependymal cells invaginated posteriorly and anteriorly forming the mesocoelic and pineal recesses. Progressive atrophy and loss of specialized epithelial cells, associated with subependymal gliosis, lead to a small, less distinct structure by the end of gestation.

As a solitary finding, slit lateral ventricles are normal in the newborn for the first postnatal week. To be considered abnormal, cranial ultrasound requires additional findings such as increased brain parenchyma echogenicity or subarachnoid space closure in the medial to temporal lobes or around the brainstem suggesting the presence of cerebral injury.

REFERENCES

1. Clarke E, O'Malley C (1996) *The Human Brain and Spinal Cord: A Historical Study Illustrated by Writings from Antiquity to the Twentieth Century*. San Francisco: Norman Publishing.
2. Purkinje JE (1836) Über Flimmerbewegungen im Gehirn. *Müller's Arch Anat Physiol* 3: 289–290.
3. Wislocki GB (1932) *The Cytology of the Cerebrospinal Pathway*. New York: Hoeber.
4. Valentin GG (1836) Über den Verlauf und die letzten Ende der Nerven. *Nova Acta Phys Med Acad* 18: 51–240.
5. Virchow R (1846) Über das granulirte Ansehen der Wanderungen der Gehirnventrikel. *Allg Z Psychiat* 3: 242–250.
6. O'Rahilly R, Müller F (1994) *The Embryonic Human Brain: An Atlas of Developmental Stages*. New York: Wiley-Liss.
7. Agduhr E (1932) *Choroid Plexus and Ependyma*. New York: Hoeber.
8. O'Rahilly R, Müller F (1990) Ventricular system and choroid plexuses of the human brain during the embryonic period proper. *Am J Anat* 189: 285–302.
9. Dooling EC, Chi JG, Gilles FH (1977) Ependymal changes in the human fetal brain. *Ann Neurol* 1: 535–541.
10. Roessmann U, Velasco ME, Sindely SD, Gambetti P (1980) Glial fibrillary acidic protein (GFAP) in ependymal cells during development. An immunocytochemical study. *Brain Res* 200: 13–21.

11. Campbell S, Thoms A (1977) The use of ultrasound in the antenatal diagnosis of neural tube defects. *Birth Defects Orig Artic Ser* 13(3D): 209–216.
12. Cardoza JD, Goldstein RB, Filly RA (1988) Exclusion of fetal ventriculomegaly with a single measurement: the width of the lateral ventricular atrium. *Radiology* 169: 711–714.
13. Goldstein RB, La Pidus AS, Filly RA, Cardoza J (1990) Mild lateral cerebral ventricular dilatation in utero: clinical significance and prognosis. *Radiology* 176: 237–242.
14. Bromley B, Frigoletto FD Jr., Benacerraf BR (1991) Mild fetal lateral cerebral ventriculomegaly: clinical course and outcome. *Am J Obstet Gynecol* 164: 863–867.
15. White DN (1992) The early development of neurosonology: II. Fetal and neonatal echoencephalography. *Ultrasound Med Biol* 18: 227–247.
16. Gilles FH, Kassirer M (1976) Hydrocephalus. *Hum Pathol* 7: 123–166.
17. Johnson ML, Dunne MG, Mack LA, Rashbaum CL (1980) Evaluation of fetal intracranial anatomy by static and real-time ultrasound. *J Clin Ultrasound* 8: 311–318.
18. Fiske CE, Filly RA, Callen PW (1981) Sonographic measurement of lateral ventricular width in early ventricular dilation. *J Clin Ultrasound* 9: 303–307.
19. Fiske CE, Filly RA (1982) Ultrasound evaluation of the normal and abnormal fetal neural axis. *Radiol Clin North Am* 20: 285–296.
20. Reeder JD, Kaude JV, Setzer ES (1983) The occipital horn of the lateral ventricles in premature infants. An ultrasonographic study. *Eur J Radiol* 3: 148–150.
21. Gilles FH, Gilles EE (1986) Pathological effects of hydrocephalus. In: Epstein F, editor. *Anomalies of the Developing Central Nervous System*. Ames, IA: Blackwell Scientific Publications, pp. 541–572.
22. Glonek M, Kedzia A, Derkowski W (2003) Prenatal assessment of ventriculomegaly: an anatomical study. *Med Sci Monit* 9: MT69–77.
23. Siebert JR, Nyberg DA, Kapur RP (1999) Cerebral mantle thickness: a measurement useful in anatomic diagnosis of fetal ventriculomegaly. *Pediatr Dev Pathol* 2: 168–175.
24. Achiron R, Yagel S, Rotstein Z, Inbar O, Mashiach S, Lipitz S (1997) Cerebral lateral ventricular asymmetry: is this a normal ultrasonographic finding in the fetal brain? *Obstet Gynecol* 89: 233–237.
25. Muller WD, Urlesberger B (1992) Correlation of ventricular size and head circumference after severe intra-periventricular haemorrhage in preterm infants. *Childs Nerv Syst* 8: 33–35.
26. Babcock DS, Ball W Jr. (1983) Postasphyxial encephalopathy in full-term infants: ultrasound diagnosis. *Radiology* 148: 417–423.
27. Siegel MJ, Shackelford GD, Perlman JM, Fulling KH (1984) Hypoxic–ischemic encephalopathy in term infants: diagnosis and prognosis evaluated by ultrasound. *Radiology* 152: 395–399.
28. Nelson MD Jr., Tavarè CJ, Petrus L, Kim P, Gilles FH (2003) Changes in the size of the lateral ventricles in the normal term newborn following vaginal delivery. *Pediatr Radiol* 33: 831–835.
29. Klein J, Moeschberger M (1997) *Survival Analysis: Techniques for Censored and Truncated Data*. New York: Springer-Verlag.
30. Mood A, Graybill F, Baes D (1974) *Introduction to the Theory of Statistics*. New York: McGraw Hill.
31. Olsson R (1961) Subcommissural ependyma and pineal organ development in human fetuses. *Gen Comp Endocr* 1: 117–123.
32. Rakic P (1965) Mesocoelic recess in the human brain. *Neurology* 15: 708–715.
33. Giarman N, Freedman D, Picard-Ami L (1960) Serotonin content of the pineal glands of man and monkey. *Nature* 186: 480–481.
34. Quay W (1974) *Pineal Chemistry in Cellular and Physiological Mechanisms*. Springfield, IL: Charles C. Thomas.
35. Vaughan G, Pelham R, Pang S, et al (1976) Nocturnal elevation of plasma melatonin and urinary 5-hydroxyindoleacetic acid in young men: attempts at modification by brief changes in environmental lighting and sleep and by autonomic drugs. *J Clin Endocrinol Metab* 42: 752–764.
36. Wurtman R, Axelrod J (1965) *The Formation, Metabolism and Physiologic Effects of Melatonin in Mammals*. Amsterdam: Elsevier.
37. Laure-Kamionowska M, Maslinska D, Deregowski K, Czichos E, Raczkowska B (2003) Morphology of pineal glands in human foetuses and infants with brain lesions. *Folia Neuropathol* 41: 209–215.
38. Dooling EC, Chi JG, Gilles FH (1977) Melanotic neuroectodermal tumor of infancy: its histological similarities to fetal pineal gland. *Cancer* 39: 1535–1541.
39. Patten B (1968) *Human Embryology*, 3rd edn. New York: Blakiston Division, McGraw-Hill.

40. Sato S, Yamamoto H (2001) Development of pigment cells in the brain of ascidian tadpole larvae: insights into the origins of vertebrate pigment cells. *Pigment Cell Res* 14: 428–436.
41. Regodon S, Franco AJ, Gazquez A, Redondo E (1998) Presence of pigment in the ovine pineal gland during embryonic development. *Histol Histopathol* 13: 147–154.
42. Ohshima K, Hiramatsu K (1993) Ultrastructural study of post-hatching development in the pineal gland of the Japanese quail. *J Vet Med Sci* 55: 945–950.
43. Bhatnagar KP, Hilton FK (1994) Observations on the pineal gland of the big brown bat, *Eptesicus fuscus*: possible correlation of melanin intensification with constant darkness. *Anat Rec* 240: 367–376.
44. Calvo JL, Boya J, Garcia-Maurino JE, Rancano D (1992) Presence of melanin in the cat pineal gland. *Acta Anat (Basel)* 145: 73–78.
45. Calvo J, Boya J, Garcia-Maurino JE, Lopez-Carbonell A (1988) Structure and ultrastructure of the pigmented cells in the adult pineal gland. *J Anat* 160: 67–73.
46. Cozzi B, Ferrandi B (1984) The pineal gland of the horse. Morphological and histochemical results (with notes on the donkey and mule pineal). *Basic Appl Histochem* 28: 81–90.
47. Kastin AJ, Kuzemchak B, Tompkins RG, Schally AV, Miller MC, 3rd (1976) Melanin in the rat brain. *Brain Res Bull* 1: 567–572.
48. Santamarina E (1958) Melanin pigmentation in bovine pineal gland and its possible correlation with gonadal function. *Can J Biochem Physiol* 36: 227–235.
49. Santamarina E, Meyer-Arendt J (1956) Identification of melanin in the bovine pineal gland. *Acta Histochem* 3(1–2): 1–5.
50. Rodin A (1961) The present state of the pineal gland. *Alberta Med Bull* 26: 2–7.
51. Tapp E, Huxley M (1972) The histological appearance of the human pineal gland from puberty to old age. *J Pathol* 108: 137–144.
52. Kerényi N, Sarkar K (1968) The postnatal transformation of the pineal gland. *Acta Morph Acad Sci Hung* 16: 223–236.
53. Mitchell TN, Free SL, Williamson KA, et al (2003) Polymicrogyria and absence of pineal gland due to *PAX6* mutation. *Ann Neurol* 53: 658–663.
54. Barth PG, Uylings HB, Stam FC (1984) Interhemispheral neuroepithelial (glio-ependymal) cysts, associated with agenesis of the corpus callosum and neocortical maldevelopment. A case study. *Childs Brain* 11: 312–319.
55. Rosser T (2003) Aicardi syndrome. *Arch Neurol* 60: 1471–1473.
56. Takeuchi Y, Sano Y (1983) Serotonin distribution in the circumventricular organs of the rat. An immunohistochemical study. *Anat Embryol (Berl)* 167: 311–319.
57. Ferguson AV, Bains JS (1996) Electrophysiology of the circumventricular organs. *Front Neuroendocrinol* 17: 440–475.
58. Rodriguez EM, Oksche A, Montecinos H (2001) Human subcommissural organ, with particular emphasis on its secretory activity during the fetal life. *Microsc Res Tech* 52: 573–590.
59. Dendy A, Nichols G (1910) On the occurrence of a mesocoelic recess in the human brain, and its relation to the sub-commissural organ of lower vertebrates; with special reference to the distribution of Reissner's fibre in the vertebrate series and its possible function. *Proc Roy Soc Lond* 82: 515–529.
60. Gilbert G (1960) The subcommissural organ. *Neurology* 10: 131–142.
61. Dooling EC, Chi JG, Gilles FH (1983) Developmental change in ventricular epithelia. In: Gilles FH, Leviton A, Dooling EC, editors. *The Developing Human Brain: Growth and Epidemiologic Neuropathology*. Boston: Wright-PSG, pp. 113–117.
62. Palkovits M (1965) Participation of the epithalamo–epiphyseal system in the regulation of water and electrolytes metabolism. *Prog Brain Res* 10: 627–634.
63. Mollgard K (1972) Histochemical investigations on the human foetal subcommissural organ. I Carbohydrates and mucosubstances, proteins and nucleoproteins, esterase, acid and alkaline phosphatase. *Histochemie* 32: 31–48.
64. Kimble JE, Mollgard K (1975) Subcommissural organ-associated neurons in fetal and neonatal rabbit. *Cell Tissue Res* 159: 195–204.
65. Shuangshoti S, Netsky MG (1970) Human choroid plexus: morphologic and histochemical alterations with age. *Am J Anat* 128: 73–95.
66. Wilkins RH, Odom GL (1966) Cytological changes in cerebrospinal fluid associated with resections of intracranial neoplasms. *J Neurosurg* 25: 24–34.
67. Friede RL (1989) *Developmental Neuropathology*, 2nd edn. New York: Springer-Verlag.

68. Haymaker W, Margoles C, Pentschew A, et al (1961) Pathology of kernicterus and posticterus encephalopathy. In: Thomas CA, editor. *Kernicterus and its Importance in Cerebral Palsy*. Springfield, IL: Charles C. Thomas, pp. 21–228.

69. Banker BQ, Larroche JC (1962) Periventricular leukomalacia of infancy. A form of neonatal anoxic encephalopathy. *Arch Neurol* 7: 386–410.

4
GERMINAL TISSUE (SUBVENTRICULAR ZONE)

Germinal matrix lining all ventricles

VENTRICULAR AND SUBVENTRICULAR ZONES

Transient structures in human embryonic and fetal brain include the ventricular germinal zone, subplate, thalamic reticular complex, and ganglionic eminence (described by many early investigators; for a recent description see reference 1). The embryonic central nervous system arises as an epithelium that folds in on itself to form a tube. Its inner surface, the germinal layer, is where all neuronal and glial precursors proliferate, whether located in the lateral, third, aqueduct, fourth, olfactory, spinal, or terminal ventricle.[2,3] Historically, telencephalic germinal tissue names included germinal matrix, ganglionic eminence, medial and lateral ventricular eminences, and medial and lateral striatal ridges. At midgestation, human germinal tissue is a thin covering of diencephalic and caudal structures. It is somewhat thicker over many lateral ventricular surfaces, particularly overlying the caudate nucleus head ('ganglionic eminence' or medial and lateral ventricular eminences) and continues as a smaller bulge over caudate body and tail. The caudate head ganglionic eminence lies largely anterior to the interventricular foramen and striothalamic sulcus, bulging into the frontal horn. The caudate body and tail germinal tissue lies largely lateral to the striothalamic sulcus, which extends posteriorly from the interventricular foramen and contains the terminal vein. Subependymal veins lie between germinal matrix tissue and the caudate.[4,5] The ganglionic eminence, as well as germinal tissue lining the remaining lateral ventricle, attains its maximum volume at the end of the second trimester, rapidly disappearing over the next few weeks.[6,7]

Neuronal or glial precursors arising within the germinal layer must move away from the ventricular wall to another central nervous system location. Germinal matrix production of neuronal or glial precursors is activated at differing times during gestation. Despite its widespread embryonic nervous system distribution, most human germinal matrix studies in the literature were done on ganglionic eminence tissue.

Ventricular and subventricular zone development

After neural tube closure, at about postovulatory day 30, neural tissue surrounding the central nervous system consists largely of the ventricular zone. Originally, the Boulder Committee[8] developed nomenclature for four basic developmental zones: ventricular, subventricular,

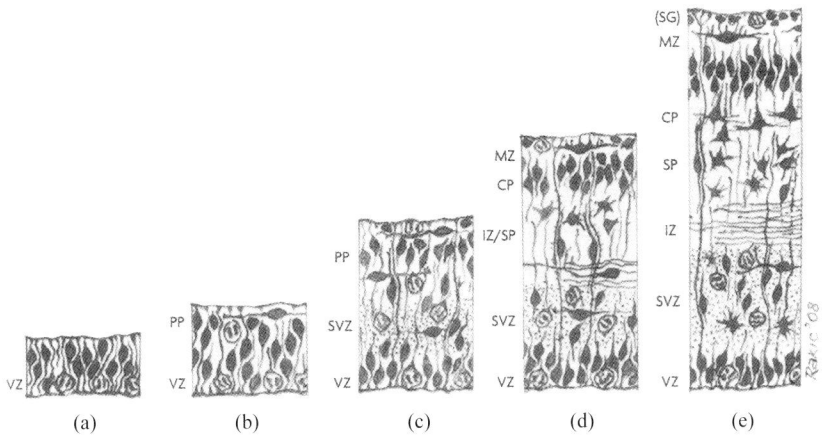

Fig. 4.1 Cerebral cortex development. The Boulder Committee provided a schematic model of human isocortical development in 1970. Subsequently, Rakic and several others modified it to include the preplate, intermediate, and subplate zones. (a) Embryonic day (E) 30; (b) E31–32; (c) E45; (d) E55; (e) gestational week 14. CP, cortical plate; IZ, intermediate zone; MZ, marginal zone; SVZ, subventricular zone; SG, subpial granular layer (part of MZ); VZ, ventricular zone. These times are only best estimates of an idealized cortex; they vary somewhat as cortices vary in their time of development. Reproduced with permission from Nature Publishing Group from Bystron et al.[9]

intermediate, and marginal, with the cortical plate interposed between the marginal and intermediate layers. All other central nervous system regions contain the four basic zones. None directly corresponds to any adult component. Subsequently, Rakic and others[9] modified the nomenclature to include the preplate, intermediate, and subplate zones (Fig. 4.1).

Radial glial development

All central nervous system regions contain ventricular and marginal zones. The subventricular zone has been recognized in the telencephalon, diencephalon, and rhombencephalon, but not in the spinal cord.[10] Although the ventricular zone antedates the subventricular zone in having a large proportion of cells undergoing mitosis, the subventricular zone is important in both cell development and replacement throughout gestation. Subventricular mitoses numerically increase until about the fourth month of gestation, when they outnumber ventricular zone mitoses (Fig. 4.2).[11] Ventricular zone epithelial cells extend processes across adjacent neural tissue to future pial surface; their nuclei undergo intermitotic movements depending on cell cycle stage.[12,13] Ventricular zone cells differentiate into radial glia, neurons, and a subset of astrocytes. Ventricular zone daughter cells (neuronal precursors), and particularly projection neurons, migrate toward the future pial surface using radial glia as guides.[14] Radial glia daughter cells span the neural tube, divide, and produce both neurons and astrocytes, and thus satisfy some criteria of bipotential stem cells.[15–19] Several investigators recognized epithelial cell transneural processes at the end of the nineteenth century, and these studies are nicely summarized and depicted in Cajal's 1899 masterpiece[20] (new translation). Neurons born earlier

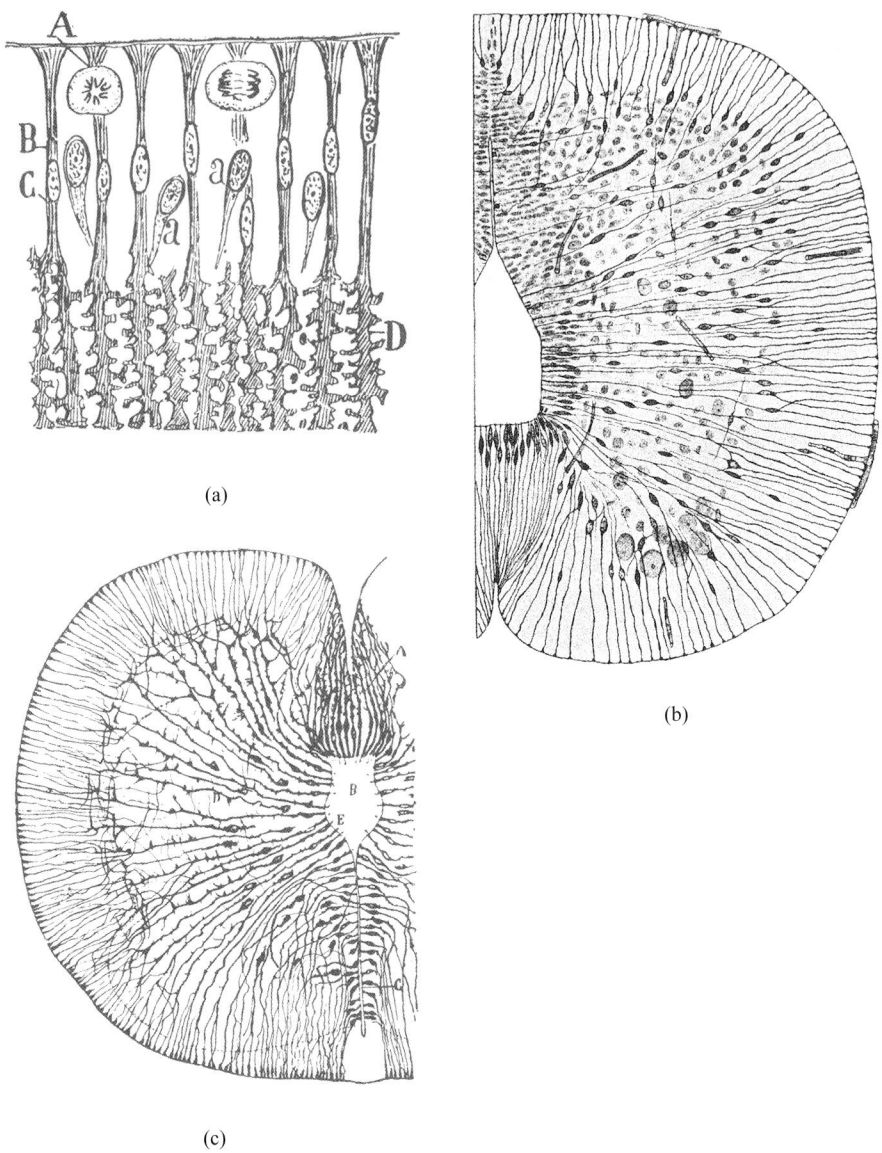

(a)

(b)

(c)

Fig. 4.2 (a) Schematic section through the wall of the spinal groove (after His) A, germinal cells; B, epithelium; C, nucleus of a primary epithelial cell; D, outer process of an epithelial cell; a, neuroblast. It is clear from this drawing that the concept of a transmural radial cell was established by the beginning of the twentieth century. Three of four neuroblasts have an intimate relationship with one of these radial cells. Reproduced with permission of Oxford University Press from Cajal.[20] (b) Drawing of spinal cord of an 8-week-old embryo showing distribution and character of transmural spongioblasts. While Kershman called these radial glia spongioblasts, he clearly recognized that they spanned the entire neural wall. Reproduced with permission of the American Medical Association from Kershman.[11] Copyright © 1938 American Medical Association. All rights reserved. (c) Ependymal cells in lumbar region of a 44-mm

50

at the ventricular end terminate in deep cortical layers, whereas later-born neurons settle in more superficial layers. The ganglionic eminence gives origin to most cortical interneurons.[21]

The ganglionic eminence (largely in the subventricular zone), a transient yet conspicuous developing forebrain structure, is divided into medial and lateral masses. The medial and lateral ganglionic eminences vary regionally in neuronal types and glia generated, as well as in the embryonic and fetal brain regions they will populate. Although this work is based mainly on mouse embryos, we should be able to extrapolate findings to other mammals, including humans. Both medial and lateral ganglionic eminences furnish cells to the striatum, thalamus, septum, and olfactory bulb (Fig. 4.3). The medial ganglionic eminence contributes cells to the hippocampus and diencephalic structures as well as the globus pallidus.[22] The lateral ganglionic eminence is an intermediate target for axons growing toward the cerebral cortex.[23] Ganglionic eminence in ventricular and subventricular zones persists to the end of the second trimester and, to a lesser extent, to the beginning of the third trimester. The ganglionic matrix (ganglionic eminence) subventricular zone provides neuroblasts to subcortical neuronal aggregates (basal ganglia) and to the ventrolateral hemispheral cortical plate (insula and orbital cortex); the extraganglionic matrix subventricular zone contributes neuroblasts exclusively to the dorsolateral and medial hemispheral isocortical plate.[24–26]

The subventricular zone appears later and persists longer than the ventricular zone. At the border between the ventricular and the cell-sparse intermediate zone, the subventricular zone expands markedly during the last third of prenatal development (mouse). Ventricular and subventricular zones differ in cellular morphology. The subventricular zone is a dense aggregate of matrix cells with a rich microvasculature and sparse intercellular supporting tissues. The number of cells is thought to peak at about 35 weeks (human),[11,27] although our studies place the peak at about 10 weeks earlier (see below). A residual subventricular zone persists into adulthood in some cerebral regions. The subventricular zone produces oligodendroglia, among other cells. Basal telencephalic radial glia are the source of only a few basal ganglia neurons.[19]

At 19 weeks, the lateral ventricle ganglionic eminence contains glial fibrillary acidic protein (GFAP) positivity in the ventricular zone, and, at around 21 weeks, a few glial fibrils in the subventricular zone. At around 27 to 28 weeks, there is only a sparse glial network composed of astrocytic and tanycytic fibers. On the other hand, radial glia (vimentin-positive cells) are present in ganglionic eminence ventricular and subventricular zones until the end of the second trimester.[28] These cells form the basis for neuronal migration from the subventricular zones into the cortex and also provide guiding cues for growing axons.[29,30] Germinal layer glial fibrils gradually increase throughout, particularly posteriorly.[31]

Ciliated ependymal cells and tanycytes, which gradually replace the ventricular zone,[32,33] are transiently positive for GFAP. For descriptive purposes, tanycytes contain a soma, neck, and tail portion. The somatic portion is in the ependymal layer; the neck, originating from

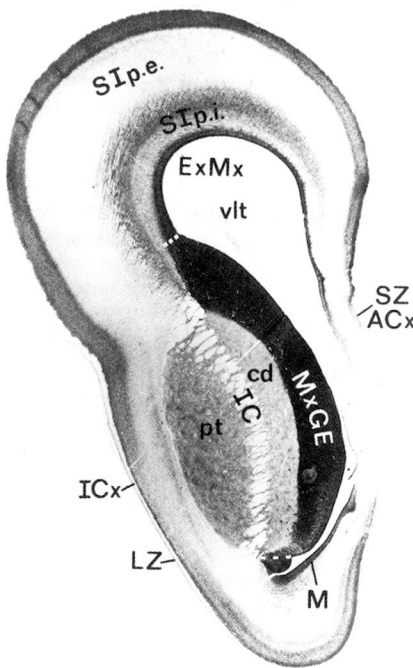

Fig. 4.3 The ganglionic matrix (MxGE) is the thick layer of germinal tissue overlying the caudate (cd) and the extraganglionic matrix (M and ExMx) lines the remainder of the hemispheral ventricle (about 16 weeks). ICx, isocortex; LZ, lamina zonalis; IC, internal capsule, anterior limb; SZ, stratum zonale; vlt, telencephalic lateral ventricle; SIp.e. and SIp.i., external and internal portions of the intermediate stria; Acx, allocortex (the anatomic nomenclature is that of reference 26). From Gilles et al.[73]

the soma, extends into the subependymal region. Both the soma and neck have fine radiating processes. The tail terminates as small bulbous swellings either on a vessel or at the pial surface. Spinal cord tanycytes radiate from central canal ependyma into surrounding gray matter. Important morphologic differences that distinguish simple ependymal cells from tanycytes include the end-feet shape, numbers of apical microvilli and cilia, cytoplasmic processes, and intercellular junctions. Simple ependymal cells have numerous cilia and few microvilli on their ventricular surface; tanycytes possess few cilia and numerous microvilli.[34] Other differences include nuclear shape and cytoplasmic contents. Tanycytes have more irregularly shaped nuclei than ordinary ependymal cells and do not possess the perinuclear swirling filament bundles, but rather contain more intracytoplasmic microtubules. However, both cell types are immunoreactive to antibodies for GFAP.

    Tanycytes have intricate relationships with blood vessels. The tail forms multiple contacts as it crosses superficial blood vessels before its termination as a foot-like expansion in apposition to a deeply placed blood vessel. Numerous foot processes converge onto a single capillary or a larger spinal cord blood vessel. A basal lamina separates the peripheral processes of tanycytes, forming end-feet at vascular surfaces, from the vessel endothelium.

Germinal matrix vessels

Vascular networks within the ventricular and subventricular zones of fetuses from 10 to 22 weeks share regional networks (see Chapter 8). Thin-walled capillaries are uniformly distributed throughout germinal tissue.[4,5,35] At 10 to 12 weeks, basal lamina is present between opposing endothelial, pericytic, and glial surfaces, but is discontinuous. Nearby astroglial processes do not form complete perivascular astrocytic investments. Between 15 and 17 weeks, endothelial and perithelial cells develop complex interdigitations, basal laminae thicken with only occasional discontinuities, and astrocytic end-feet more completely cover the capillary wall. By 22 weeks, basal laminae are well developed and continuous and the gliovascular relationship more closely resembles the adult configuration. Astrocytic end-foot vascular coverage develops more slowly in germinal tissue than in the cortex or white matter.[36] Germinal matrix vessel and lumen areas may be significantly greater than cortical vessels at the same gestational age.[37] Morphologically, germinal matrix capillaries are otherwise similar to cortical and cord capillaries at equivalent ages. Tight junction molecules develop at comparable rates in the fetal cortex, white matter, and germinal tissue.[38] New barrier strap junctions develop in germinal matrix vessels.[39] With advancing gestation there is a gradual increase in vessel density, particularly of capillaries. This is not a uniform process. Capillary plexuses are prominent immediately beneath the ependyma while the more central germinal matrix contains fewer, but often of larger diameter, vessels.[40] Type VI collagen is widely distributed throughout the body's connective tissues, including meninges and central nervous system vessels. In fetuses, neonates, and children, type VI collagen is found in meningeal arteries and veins, large striatal vessels at the end of the second trimester, and cortical and white matter vessels in the middle to the end of the third trimester, but not in germinal layer vessels.[41] Others have found that germinal matrix vessels were immunoreactive for collagens I, III, and IV.[42]

Ganglionic eminence—plasminogen activator

Fibrinolytic activity in the brain, choroid plexus, leptomeninges, and spinal fluid of older individuals increases with age, does not vary significantly with brain region, and is believed to be associated with vascular endothelium.[43-45] Fibrinolytic activity is present in brain tumors,[46] multiple sclerosis plaques,[47] and mature astrocytes.[48] Germinal tissue masses of other organs elaborate enzymes with proteolytic activity as well as specific inhibitors.[49] The purpose of this section is to describe regional variation of fibrinolytic activity with special emphasis on the ganglionic eminence.

Homogenates of ganglionic eminence, white matter, thalamus, and putamen from 10 fresh unfixed brains (22–40 weeks), when applied to commercial bovine fibrinogen plates of standard thickness, lyse the plate; the size of the resultant lysed area gives an estimate of fibrinolytic activity.[50] Tranexamic acid (predominantly an inhibitor of plasminogen activator) and prior heating of fibrinogen plates (presumably destroying heat-labile plasminogen) inhibits ganglionic eminence fibrinolytic activity. The ganglionic eminence and white matter have greater fibrinolytic activity earlier rather than later in gestation. Homogenate fibrinolytic activity varies with age, being greater from 22 to 30 than from 31 to 40 weeks, with the ganglionic eminence from the youngest infant (estimated at 22 weeks) yielding the greatest fibrinolytic activity. From 28 to 31 weeks, ganglionic eminence fibrinolytic activity exceeds white matter as well as that in the thalamus and putamen. Fibrinolytic activity decreases as gestational age increases, being apparent in white matter at an earlier gestational age than in ganglionic eminence.

It is possible that ganglionic eminence fibrinolytic activity arises from either the matrix cell or the plasminogen activator-laden endothelial cell.[51] Usually, astrocytes regulate brain capillary endothelial expression of tissue plasminogen activator and its inhibitor, plasminogen activator inhibitor-1,[52] but whether this has any role in brain development is unknown. The ganglionic eminence vasculature, especially in its medial two-thirds, consists of capillaries and venules that are similar in density and microscopic characteristics to the nearby comparable vessels in the caudate and surrounding white matter. During ganglionic eminence involution, this vasculature gradually disappears.

Interleukin receptor development

Interleukin-6 receptor (IL-6R) is a multifunctional inflammatory cytokine. It promotes survival and differentiation of specific nerve cell groups.[53] Between 22 and 28 weeks, IL-6R is highly expressed in human fetal ganglionic eminence cells and is less expressed in adjacent caudate and white matter, and progressively decreases from 32 to 36 weeks.[54] IL-6R may activate immature IL-5-positive cells to secrete a protease likely involved in germinal matrix involution.

Ganglionic eminence—antigen development

BrdU and Musashi1 are highly conserved potential stem cell markers.[55] Musashi1 colocalizes with nestin and Ki-67 in immature cells; its expression correlates in time and proximity with the transient fetal lateral ventricular germinal matrix before ependymal formation. This expression maximizes at around 27 weeks, gradually diminishing by term.

In beagle puppies, there is no difference in the vessel density of the germinal matrix, deep white matter, and cortex except for decreasing density in the germinal matrix as the matrix size decreases.[56] Matrix vessels stain for many factors: α_2-macroglobulin, collagen V, endothelin, factor VIII-related antigen, glial fibrillary acidic protein, laminin, and vimentin, but not for α-smooth muscle antigen. Concurrently, there is a significant increase in laminin concentration and a smaller increase in collagen V concentration.

Ganglionic eminence—growth factors

Various growth factors are expressed in human ganglionic eminence in the last half of gestation. They are grouped into those associated with germinal cells themselves, with fine fibrillary matrix, and with microvasculature. Some are significant for neuronal or glial development: nerve growth factor and its receptor, platelet-derived growth factors and their receptors, epidermal growth factor receptor and one of its ligands, fibroblast growth factor and its receptors, and insulin-like growth factors and receptors. Others are important for microvasculature growth and maintenance, such as vascular endothelial growth factor, and for extracellular matrix components laminin, collagen type IV, fibronectin, and vitronectin.[57]

Ganglionic eminence—synaptogyrin development

Synaptogyrin is a synaptic vesicle protein uniformly distributed throughout the nervous system. The ganglionic eminence is transiently involved in the development of cortical connections. Ulfig and collaborators[58] demonstrated that synaptogyrin is maximal in human ganglionic eminence between 12 and 20 weeks, sharply declining thereafter.

Growth and loss of lateral ventricle germinal tissue

As previously mentioned, the ventricular and subventricular zones of germinal tissue line prospective lateral ventricles from their origin at 4 to 5 weeks of fetal life. At about the same time, the medial ganglionic eminence arises just lateral to the prospective interventricular foramen (Fig. 4.4).[22] Magnetic resonance imaging (MRI) of ganglionic eminence of 13 fixed, but not processed, fetal heads ranging in age from 7 to 28 weeks revealed a maximum absolute volume at 23 weeks.[7]

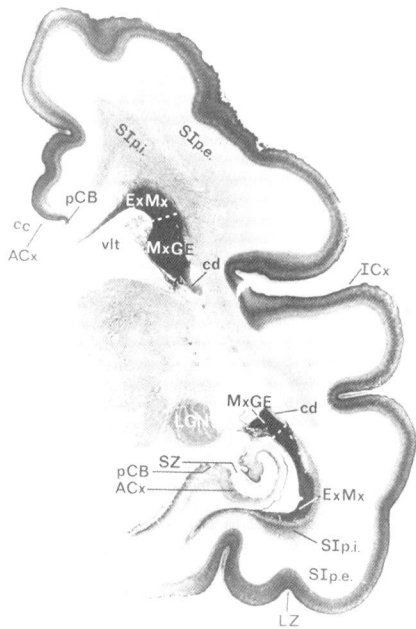

Fig. 4.4 The differences between ganglionic and extraganglionic matrix are seen in this coronal section at the lateral geniculate nucleus level (LGN) (about 28 weeks). The abbreviations are the same as the previous figure except for: cc, corpus callosum; pCB, parahippocampal clinoid border; Acx, allocortex. From Gilles et al.[73]

When cerebral lateral ventricular matrix layer volume is measured, specifically ganglionic eminence matrix over the striatum, separately from extraganglionic matrix (the remaining dorsolateral and medial wall matrix), both ganglionic and extraganglionic matrix sectors have equivalent volumes at 13 weeks. Total matrix volume increases between 13 and 26 weeks (Fig. 4.5). From 21 to 26 weeks the two sectors increase at different rates, in favor of extraganglionic matrix, and by 26 weeks the extraganglionic matrix volume is about double that of the ganglionic matrix. Matrix volume then declines rapidly from 26 to 28 weeks, falling to about half, and gradually regresses thereafter. Extraganglionic matrix persisted longest in the ventromedial angle of the temporal horn.

Other embryonic ventricles

Even before the rostral neuropore has closed, the forebrain and hindbrain ventricles contain local, segmentally arranged, transverse bulges in their walls marking the sites of proliferative activity (an old observation, but repeatedly confirmed).[22,59] Important nervous system components arise from these bulges.

At 22 days, before anterior neuropore closure, major brain divisions are apparent. The diencephalon contains two bulges: the rostral bulge containing optic evagination primordia and chiasmatic plate; and at 33 days, the more caudal bulge contains primordia of adenohypophysis, hypothalamus, ventral thalamus, dorsal thalamus, and epithalamus.[22] The hypothalamus undergoes early differentiation. The ventral thalamus, which develops early, decreases in

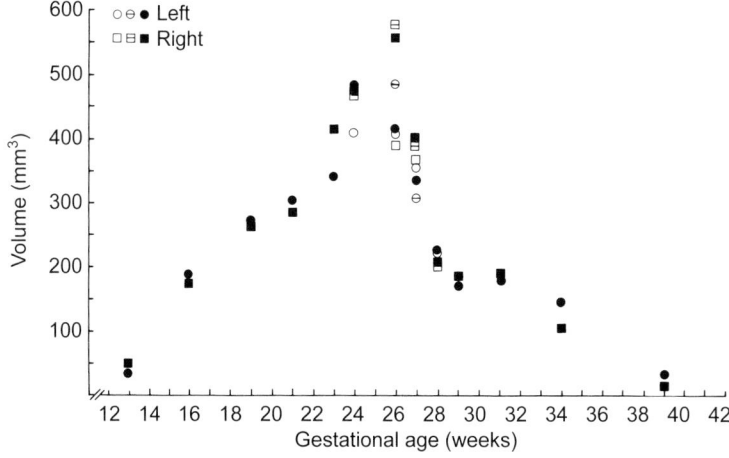

Fig. 4.5 The volume (mm³) of the entire germinal layer of each cerebral half (telocele) is plotted against gestational age. The germinal layer grows rapidly until the end of the second trimester. Thereafter it decays rapidly, losing half of its volume between 26 and 28 gestational weeks, during the period that inherent plasminogen activator is maximal. From Gilles et al.[73]

relative size late in development to become the subthalamus; the dorsal thalamus develops into the complex sensory nuclei of the adult thalamus.[60] Not all diencephalic parts differentiate at the same rate as the leading hypothalamus, epithalamus, and subthalamus.[61] The thalamus preserves its germinal layer far longer in development than other diencephalic regions. Thalamic organization into nuclear aggregates occurs while the telencephalic ganglionic eminence reaches maximal absolute size shortly after midgestation. In many thalamic neuronal aggregates, appreciably sized neurons emerge.

AQUEDUCT

Galen, in the second century AD, first described a connection between the third and fourth ventricles. Aranzi, in 1587, called this the 'aqueduct,' even though this name was later ascribed to Sylvius (1633).[62] At about 22 days, before neural tube closure, three major neural tube divisions are present—prosencephalon, mesencephalon, and rhombencephalon. The mesencephalon develops a prominent ventral bend, bringing the head to the chest. When the neural tube closes 4 days later, the mesencephalon exhibits two lateral bulges.[22] At the end of the embryonic period, at 54 to 57 days, the mesencephalic ventricle is still ballooned over the rhombencephalon.[63] The midbrain tectum differentiates dorsal to the aqueduct and tegmentum, and the cerebral peduncles differentiate ventrally.

FOURTH VENTRICLE

At about day 24, the rhombencephalon occupies approximately three-quarters of the embryo's length. The fourth ventricle is the residual rhombencephalic cavity. Unlike other nervous system regions, the rhombencephalic roof becomes attenuated, increases in width, separating the alar plates, and ends up dorsolaterally relative to the basal plate, instead of the more usual nervous system dorsal location. This happens concurrently with pontine flexure development, widening the floor into a rhomboid shape. The lateral recesses develop laterally at the widest ventricular portion. The pons and cerebellum develop rostrally, and the medulla caudally, in the rhombencephalon. Thus, the alar ventricular and subventricular germinal layers as well as their derivatives are moved sideways to occupy relatively different positions than in other neural segments.

OLFACTORY VENTRICLE

The olfactory placodes, on each side of the embryo's rostrum (Fig. 4.6), are critical to olfactocerebral bulge (outpouching) formation and subsequent cerebral development. Olfactocerebral outpouching parallels olfactory placode differentiation before the connection between these basic structures. Olfactory bulbs do not appear on the telencephalic base until after a few olfactory nerves (fila olfactoria) from peripheral olfactory placodes penetrate the anterior basal olfactocerebral outpouching. Meanwhile, differentiation of the hippocampal primordia, olfactory tubercle, and amygdala is completed,[64] and the inward growing nerve fibers from the olfactory placode migrate to the site between the olfactory tubercle primordia and hippocampal formation. Olfactory placodes are epithelial thickenings bilaterally above the stomodeum at about 30 days; a shallow olfactory ventricle is present at about 6 weeks.[65] Olfactory pits are located bilaterally between the optic vesicle and the most rostral tip of the primordial single

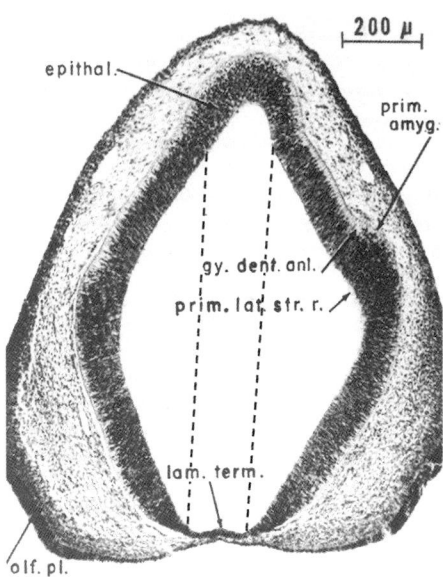

Fig. 4.6 This section of prosencephalic ventricle (~5 gestational weeks) is cut at a coronal angle through the prospective interventricular foramina (indicated by the dotted lines). The lamina terminalis (lam. term.) is rostral. The epithalamus is antebasal (epithal.). The olfactory placodes (olf. pl.) are laterally placed on the head. The caudal end of the lateral striatal ridge (prim. lat. str. r.), the amygdala primordium, and the hippocampal formation caudal termination (gy. dent. anl.) adjacent to the amygdala are indicated. Reproduced with permission of John Wiley and Sons from Humphrey.[74]

midline prosencephalic endbrain vesicle, and are still present at about 43 days. During this period, the surrounding ectoderm gradually overgrows the two olfactory placodes (medial and lateral nasal folds) owing to proliferation and condensation of adjacent mesenchyme. The olfactory pit is gradually buried; the lateral fold separates the olfactory pit from the eye. At approximately the same age, two forehead bulges above the nasal apparatus overlie the two primordial olfactocerebral outpouching. The eye is still located laterally and caudally to the nose. No olfactory bulb is as yet present at the hemispheral outpouching base.[66]

As the olfactory bulb begins to separate from the basal olfactocerebral outpouching by the second month, it points laterally and caudally toward the olfactory placode and the incoming fibers from the placode. The bulb is capped with penetrating olfactory nerves. The terminal nerve enters more posteriorly and medially and the vomeronasal nerve enters the accessory olfactory bulb on its upper medial border. On the telencephalic undersurface, the olfactory bulb appears to incorporate the sharp basal ventricular angle. The connection between the olfactory ventricle and the frontal horn descends basally and caudally through the rostral olfactory tubercle.[64] The remaining caudal medial cerebral surface, rostral to the lamina terminalis and commissural plate, contains the rostral septal nuclei anlage[67] and the rostral hippocampal formation.

On the external basal surface, the olfactory bulb is directed caudally past the olfactory tubercle toward the optic chiasm from 8 to 10 weeks, then basally at 10 weeks, and then curves in on itself with its tip directed rostrally and medially toward the rapidly developing future face by 10.5 weeks (Fig. 4.7). The olfactory cortex starts lamination at about 56 to 57 days, the end of the embryonic period.[65] Thus, the final configuration of the olfactory bulb and its ventricle is a U-shaped loop with its base directed toward the chiasmatic plate. This shape is basically retained even after islands of ependymal cells largely close the olfactory ventricle at the end of gestation. Olfactory ventricle closure starts during the end of the first trimester. Medial to the greatly modified basal frontal horn angle, the olfactory ventricle root is subjacent to the septal region and nucleus accumbens septi. Subsequently, the olfactory ventricle is gradually obliterated, leaving scattered islands of ependymal tubules and germinal cells along the olfactory bulb length. These islands extend medial to the striatum to the frontal horn base.

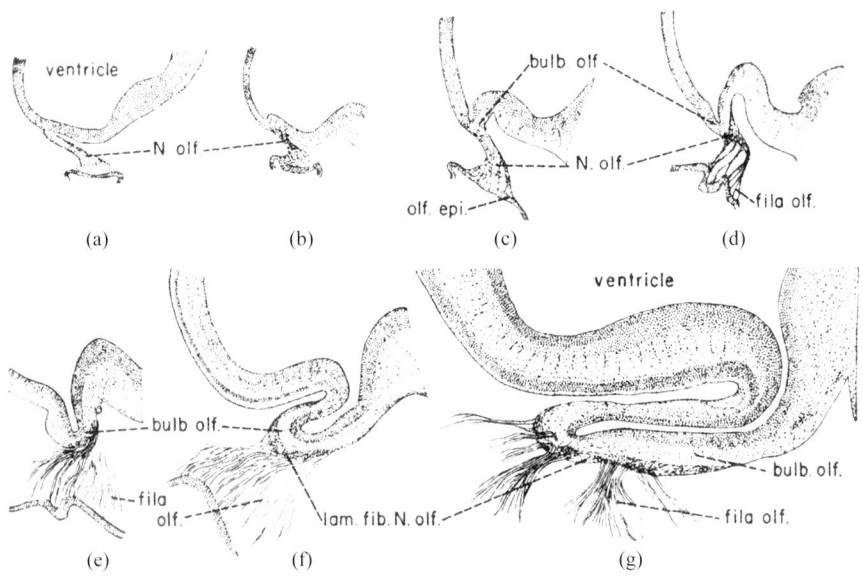

Fig. 4.7 Olfactory ventricle. Olfactory nerves (N. olf.) originate in the olfactory epithelium (olf. epi.) and pass as the fila (fila olf.) through the prospective cribriform plate to contact the undersurface of the telencephalic outpouching (a,b) before olfactory bulb evagination (bulb olf.). In this figure of successive developmental stages of the olfactory outpouching from the basal surface of the right telencephalon it is clear that the olfactory bulge first points caudally (d) toward the chiasmatic plate (to the right) and then swings rostrally (to the left) with basicranial growth at later gestational ages. In some fetuses, the caudal outpouching is more extensive than indicated in this figure. The olfactory ventricle is continuous with the lateral ventricle and is lined by the same germinal epithelium as found elsewhere within the telencephalon. Reproduced with permission of John Wiley and Sons from Pearson.[66]

SPINAL CORD

The spinal central canal is formed from the embryonic neural plate closure and the central canal extends from the conus medullaris to the fourth ventricular caudal angle. Ventricular zone vimentin is present at 7 weeks; glial fibrillary protein positive cells are evident at 9 weeks in the spinal cord and at 15 weeks in the cerebrum.[68] Initially (age less than 1 year), the spinal cord central canal is patent, but thereafter it progressively closes in an increasing proportion of cases.[69,70] When over the age of 10 years, it is occluded at many levels with local proliferation of astrocytes and ependymal cells, and eventually at all levels.[71]

TERMINAL VENTRICLE

The terminal ventricle is an ependymal cavity in caudal conus medullaris, normally present as a virtual cavity or a mere rostral filum terminale ependymal residue. The filum terminale continues caudally to the sacrum, where it penetrates the midline dura and eventually attaches to the periosteum of the first coccygeal vertebral body. In addition to ependymal cells and tubules, the intradural filum contains bundles of glial fibers, scattered neurons and segments of peripheral nerve, blood vessels, fibrous connective tissue, and, sometimes, fat. Filum glial cell clusters, varying from 5 to 100 cell layers thick, constitute its bulk.[72] An opening from the central canal is sometimes found in human filum terminale with the ependymal lining of this terminal ventricle directly contacting pia.[71]

Sonographic and fetal magnetic resonance images of normal germinal matrix

The densely cellular germinal matrix has the imaging characteristics of gray matter by ultrasound, computed tomography, and MRI. On ultrasound, the bulging ganglionic eminence of the germinal matrix over the head of the caudate nucleus and anterior to the caudothalamic groove can be appreciated in preterm infants of less than 32 weeks' gestation (Fig. 4.8a,b). The thin band of germinal matrix lining the ventricular system is otherwise not appreciated by ultrasound. However, using MRI, the matrix appears as a band of low signal on fast spin-echo T2-weighted images (Fig. 4.9).

Conclusion

Ventricular epithelium undergoes great changes during the embryonic and fetal periods. Ependymal cells replace germinal epithelium, initially the source of all neural and glial cells, at differing rates in different nervous system regions. Early in germinal epithelial development, transneural glial fibers act as cables for migrating neuronal precursors and, later, developing axons. Every ventricular region appears to direct where its neuronal precursors will terminate, whether in the cortex or any other nervous system location. In the ventrolateral lateral ventricular wall, large masses of ventricular and subventricular germinal cells persist longer than in germinal tissue caudal to the telencephalon. Although large and impressive in midgestation fetal brain, their volume is only about one-half of the germinal tissue lining the remaining lateral ventricular wall. During dissolution of ganglionic eminences, at the end of the second trimester, large amounts of plasminogen activator are released locally. Fetal ventricles change in shape and size throughout gestation, with some ventricles losing their central cavity and some changing shape dramatically. One of the most striking changes in lateral ventricular

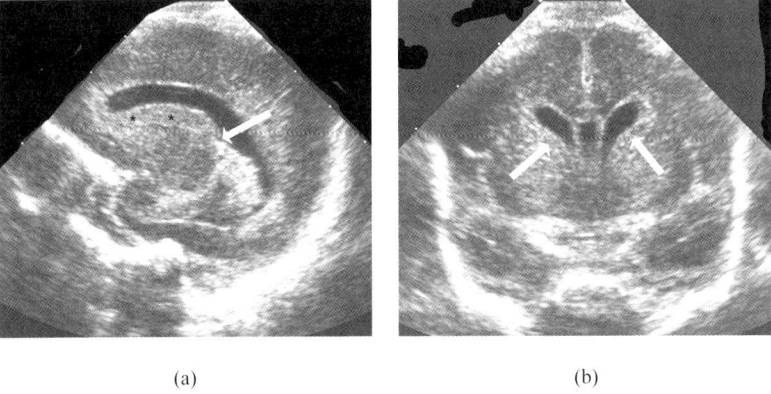

(a)   (b)

Fig. 4.8 Cranial ultrasound of a 27-week premature infant imaged through the anterior fontanelle. (a) Oblique sagittal image. (b) Coronal image through the head of the caudate nuclei. (a) This oblique sagittal image shows the sausage-shaped ganglionic eminence of the germinal matrix (asterisks) over the head of the caudate nucleus and anterior to the caudothalamic groove (arrow). (b) The coronal image shows the ganglionic eminence of the germinal matrix (arrows) having similar echogenicity to the cortical gray matter.

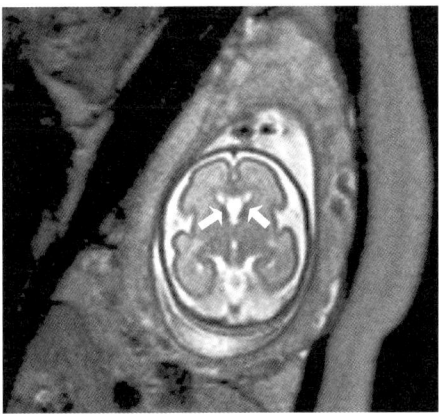

Fig. 4.9 Fetal magnetic resonance image of an infant of 26 weeks' postconceptual age. Fast spin-echo T2-weighted coronal image of the brain in utero. The densely cellular germinal matrix appears as a zone of low signal intensity (black) over the head of the caudate nuclei (arrows). Note the prominent cavum septi pellucidi.

shape occurs with an uncomplicated vaginal delivery. The ventricular wall is the source of several major structures, including the circumventricular organs [subcommissural organ and pineal, and transient ventricular outpouchings (mesocoelic recess) and tanycytes in the third ventricular floor and anterior wall].

REFERENCES

1. Ulfig N, Neudorfer F, Bohl J (2000) Transient structures of the human fetal brain: subplate, thalamic reticular complex, ganglionic eminence. *Histol Histopathol* 15: 771–790.
2. Choi BH (1986) Glial fibrillary acidic protein in radial glia of early human fetal cerebrum: a light and electron microscopic immunoperoxidase study. *J Neuropathol Exp Neurol* 45: 408–418.
3. Choi BH (1985) On the origin of oligodendrocytes. *Yonsei Med J* 26: 143–149.
4. Kuban KCK, Gilles FH (1985) Human telencephalic angiogenesis. *Ann Neurol* 17: 539–548.
5. Nelson MD, Gonzalez-Gomez I, Gilles FH (1991) The search for human telencephalic ventriculofugal arteries. *Am J Neuroradiol* 12: 215–222.
6. Jammes JL, Gilles FH (1983) Telencephalic development: matrix volume and isocortex and allocortex surface areas. In: Gilles FH, Leviton A, Dooling EC, editors. *The Developing Human Brain Growth and Epidemiologic Neuropathology*. Littleton: John Wright – PSG, Inc, pp. 87–93.
7. Kinoshita Y, Okudera T, Tsuru E, Yokota A (2001) Volumetric analysis of the germinal matrix and lateral ventricles performed using MR images of postmortem fetuses. *AJNR Am J Neuroradiol* 22: 382–388.
8. The Boulder Committee (1970) Embryonic vertebrate central nervous system: revised terminology. The Boulder Committee. *Anat Rec* 166: 257–261.
9. Bystron I, Blakemore C, Rakic P (2008) Development of the human cerebral cortex: Boulder Committee revisited. *Nat Rev Neurosci* 9: 110–122.
10. Brazel CY, Romanko MJ, Rothstein RP, Levison SW (2003) Roles of the mammalian subventricular zone in brain development. *Prog Neurobiol* 69: 49–69.
11. Kershman J (1938) The medulloblast and the medulloblastoma—a study of human embryos. *Arch Neurol Psychiat* 40: 937–967.
12. Sauer FC (1935) Mitosis in the neural tube. *J Comp Neurol* 62: 377–405.
13. Sauer FC (1936) The interkinetic migration of embryonic epithelial nuclei. *J Morphology* 60: 1–11.
14. Rakic P (1971) Neuron–glia relationship during granule cell migration in the developing cerebellar cortex: a Golgi and electronmicroscopic study in Macacus Rhesus. *J Comp Neurol* 141: 283–312.
15. Malatesta P, Hartfuss E, Gotz M (2000) Isolation of radial glial cells by fluorescent-activated cell sorting reveals a neuronal lineage. *Development* 127: 5253–5263.
16. Noctor SC, Flint AC, Weissman TA, Dammerman RS, Kriegstein AR (2001) Neurons derived from radial glial cells establish radial units in neocortex. *Nature* 409(6821): 714–720.
17. Hartfuss E, Galli R, Heins N, Gotz M (2001) Characterization of CNS precursor subtypes and radial glia. *Dev Biol* 229: 15–30.
18. Noctor SC, Flint AC, Weissman TA, Wong WS, Clinton BK, Kriegstein AR (2002) Dividing precursor cells of the embryonic cortical ventricular zone have morphological and molecular characteristics of radial glia. *J Neurosci* 22: 3161–3173.
19. Malatesta P, Hack MA, Hartfuss E, et al (2003) Neuronal or glial progeny: regional differences in radial glia fate. *Neuron* 37: 751–764.
20. Cajal SR (1995) *Histology of the Nervous System of Man and Vertebrates*. Translated by Swanson N and Swanson LW. New York: Oxford University Press.
21. Marin O, Rubenstein JL (2001) A long, remarkable journey: tangential migration in the telencephalon. *Nat Rev Neurosci* 2: 780–790.
22. O'Rahilly R, Müller F (1994) *The Embryonic Human Brain: An Atlas of Developmental Stages*. New York: Wiley-Liss.
23. Ulfig N, Chan WY (2004) Expression patterns of PSA-NCAM in the human ganglionic eminence and its vicinity: role of PSA-NCAM in neuronal migration and axonal growth? *Cells Tissues Organs* 177: 229–236.
24. Ulfig N (2002) Ganglionic eminence of the human fetal brain—new vistas. *Anat Rec* 267: 191–195.
25. Filimonov IN (1947) Rational subdivision of the cerebral cortex. *Arch Neurol Psychiatry* 58: 296–311.
26. Filimonov IN (1949) Cytoarchitectonics. General ideas. Classifications of the architectonic formations. In: Sarkisov S, Filimonov IN, Preobrazenskaya NS, editors. *Cytoarchitectonic of the Cerebral Cortex in Man*. Moscow: Medgiz, pp. 11–32.
27. Globus JH, Kuhlenbeck H (1944) Subependymal cell plate (matrix) and its relationship to brain tumors of ependymal type. *J Neuropathol Exp Neurol* 3: 1–35.
28. Ulfig N, Neudorfer F, Bohl J (1999) Distribution patterns of vimentin-immunoreactive structures in the human prosencephalon during the second half of gestation. *J Anat* 195(Pt 1): 87–100.

29. Norris CR, Kalil K (1991) Guidance of callosal axons by radial glia in the developing cerebral cortex. *J Neurosci* 11: 3481–3492.
30. Rakic P (1995) Radial versus tangential migration of neuronal clones in the developing cerebral cortex. *Proc Natl Acad Sci USA* 92: 11323–11327.
31. Gould SJ, Howard S (1988) Glial differentiation in the germinal layer of fetal and preterm infant brain: an immunocytochemical study. *Pediatr Pathol* 8: 25–36.
32. Roessmann U, Velasco ME, Sindely SD, Gambetti P (1980) Glial fibrillary acidic protein (GFAP) in ependymal cells during development. An immunocytochemical study. *Brain Res* 200: 13–21.
33. Gould SJ, Howard S (1987) An immunohistochemical study of the germinal layer in the late gestation human fetal brain. *Neuropathol Appl Neurobiol* 13: 421–437.
34. Horstmann E (1954) Die Faserglia des Selachiergehirns. *Z Zellforsch* 39: 588–617.
35. Povlishock JT, Martinez AJ, Moossy J (1977) The fine structure of blood vessels of the telencephalic germinal matrix in the human fetus. *Am J Anat* 149: 439–452.
36. El-Khoury N, Braun A, Hu F, et al (2006) Astrocyte end-feet in germinal matrix, cerebral cortex, and white matter in developing infants. *Pediatr Res* 59: 673–679.
37. Grunnet ML (1989) Morphometry of blood vessels in the cortex and germinal plate of premature neonates. *Pediatr Neurol* 5: 12–16.
38. Ballabh P, Hu F, Kumarasiri M, Braun A, Nedergaard M (2005) Development of tight junction molecules in blood vessels of germinal matrix, cerebral cortex, and white matter. *Pediatr Res* 58: 791–798.
39. Møllgård K, Saunders NR (1986) The development of the human blood–brain and blood–CSF barriers. *Neuropathol Appl Neurobiol* 12: 337–358.
40. Gould SJ, Howard S (1988) An immunocytochemical study of the germinal layer vasculature in the developing fetal brain using Ulex europaeus 1 lectin. *J Pathol* 156: 129–135.
41. Kamei A, Houdou S, Mito T, Konomi H, Takashima S (1992) Developmental change in type VI collagen in human cerebral vessels. *Pediatr Neurol* 8: 183–186.
42. Anstrom JA, Thore CR, Moody DM, Challa VR, Block SM, Brown WR (2005) Morphometric assessment of collagen accumulation in germinal matrix vessels of premature human neonates. *Neuropathol Appl Neurobiol* 31: 181–190.
43. Porter JM, Acinapura AJ, Kapp JP, Silver D (1966) Fibrinolytic activity of the spinal fluid and meninges. *Surg Forum* 17: 425–427.
44. Takashima S, Koga M, Tanaka K (1969) Fibrinolytic activity of human brain and cerebrospinal fluid. *Br J Exp Pathol* 50: 533–539.
45. Tovi D (1973) Fibrinolytic activity of human brain. A histochemical study. *Acta Neurol Scand* 49: 152–162.
46. Tucker WS, Kirsch WM, Martinez-Hernandez A, Fink LM (1978) In vitro plasminogen activator activity in human brain tumors. *Cancer Res* 38: 297–302.
47. Hirsch HE, Blanco CE, Parks ME (1981) Fibrinolytic activity of plaques and white matter in multiple sclerosis. *J Neuropathol Exp Neurol* 40: 271–280.
48. Toshniwal PK, Firestone SL, Barlow GH, Tiku ML (1987) Characterization of astrocyte plasminogen activator. *J Neurol Sci* 80(2–3): 277–287.
49. Blackwood CE, Hosannah Y, Mandl I (1968) Proteolytic enzyme systems in developing rat tissues. *J Reprod Fertil* 17: 19–33.
50. Gilles FH, Price RA, Kevy SV, Berenberg W (1971) Fibrinolytic activity in the ganglionic eminence of the premature human brain. *Biol Neonate* 18: 426–432.
51. Todd AS (1961) Tissue activator of plasminogen and thrombosis. In: Walker W, editor. *Thrombosis and Anticoagulant Therapy*. London: Livingstone, pp. 30–31.
52. Kim JA, Tran ND, Wang SJ, Fisher MJ (2003) Astrocyte regulation of human brain capillary endothelial fibrinolysis. *Thromb Res* 112: 159–165.
53. Zhao B, Schwartz JP (1998) Involvement of cytokines in normal CNS development and neurological diseases: recent progress and perspectives. *J Neurosci Res* 52: 7–16.
54. Ulfig N, Friese K (1999) Interleukin-6 receptor is highly expressed in the ganglionic eminence of the human fetal brain. *Biol Neonate* 76: 320–324.
55. Chan C, Moore BE, Cotman CW, et al (2006) Musashi1 antigen expression in human fetal germinal matrix development. *Exp Neurol* 201: 515–518.
56. Ment LR, Stewart WB, Ardito TA, Madri JA (1991) Beagle pup germinal matrix maturation studies. *Stroke* 22: 390–395.

57. Nakamura Y, Yamamoto M, Itoh S, Haratake A, Nakano Y, Hashimoto T (1998) Growth factors in infant germinal matrix: relationship to extracellular matrix and cell adhesion molecules. *J Neuropathol Exp Neurol* 57: 858–865.

58. Ulfig N, Feldhaus C, Bohl J (2000) Transient expression of synaptogyrin in the ganglionic eminence of the human fetal brain. *Ann Anat* 182: 505–508.

59. von Baer KE (1828) *Uber Entwicklungsgeschichte der Thiere: Beobachtung und Reflexion*. Königsberg: Bornträger.

60. Gilbert MS (1935) The early development of the human diencephalon. *J Comp Neurol* 62: 81–115.

61. Dekaban AS (1954) Human thalamus. An anatomical, developmental and pathological study. II. Development of the human thalamic nuclei. *J Comp Neurol* 100: 63–97.

62. Clarke E, O'Malley C (1996) *The Human Brain and Spinal Cord; A Historical Study Illustrated by Writings from Antiquity to the Twentieth Century*. San Francisco: Norman Publishing.

63. Bartelmez GW, Dekaban AS (1962) The early development of the human brain. *Contr Embryol Carnegie Instn* 37: 13–32.

64. Humphrey T (1966) Correlations between the development of the hippocampus. *Alabama J Med Sci* 3: 235–269.

65. Müller F, O'Rahilly R (2004) Olfactory structures in staged human embryos. *Cells Tissues Organs* 178: 93–116.

66. Pearson A (1941) The development of the olfactory nerve in man. *J Comp Neurol* 75: 199–217.

67. Hines M (1922) Studies in the growth and differentiation of the telencephalon in man; the fissura hippocampi. *J Comp Neurol* 34: 73–171.

68. Sasaki A, Hirato J, Nakazato Y, Ishida Y (1988) Immunohistochemical study of the early human fetal brain. *Acta Neuropathol* 76: 128–134.

69. Agduhr E (1932) *Choroid Plexus and Ependyma*. New York: Hoeber.

70. Yasui K, Hashizume Y, Yoshida M, Kameyama T, Sobue G (1999) Age-related morphologic changes of the central canal of the human spinal cord. *Acta Neuropathol* 97: 253–259.

71. Sakata M, Yashika K, Hashimoto PH (1993) Caudal aperture of the central canal at the filum terminale in primates. *Kaibogaku Zasshi* 68: 213–219.

72. Choi BH, Kim RC, Suzuki M, Choe W (1992) The ventriculus terminalis and filum terminale of the human spinal cord. *Hum Pathol* 23: 916–920.

73. Gilles FH, Leviton A, Dooling EC (1983) *Developing Human Brain: Growth and Epidemiologic Neuropathology*. Boston: John Wright-PSG Publishing Co.

74. Humphrey T (1968) The development of the human amygdala during embryonic life. *J Comp Neurol* 132: 135–165.

5
SURFACE CONFIGURATION—GYRAL PATTERN DEVELOPMENT

Introduction

Mammalian isocortical (basic six-layered cortex of cerebrum) surface area varies considerably among species; however, organization into vertical columns and horizontal laminae is consistent. Isocortical expansion and complex gyral patterns differ among human and other mammalian brains.[1] The smooth-surfaced fetal human brain develops curvilinear elevations, creating complex gyral patterns, which are probably unique for each individual and for each hemisphere. Gyral elevations from the brain surface expand at dissimilar rates in different regions. Some gyri completely cover others. Eventually, regional subdivision into smaller secondary and tertiary gyri occurs. The distinctive variability and complexity of individual cortical gyral patterns has required imaging investigators to develop algorithms for comparisons of individual functional imaging results in order to ensure that such equivalence is functionally relevant. Occasionally it is advantageous to eliminate gyri altogether and merely study sulcal configurations and depth. For gyral and sulcal reference points throughout this chapter, we have inserted some of the original idealized drawings from Ecker[2] (Figs. 5.1–5.4).

All cortical neurons arise outside the cortex. According to the radial unit hypothesis, cortical neurons arise from progenitor cells in specific locations in lateral ventricle ventricular and subventricular zones and end in specific cytoarchitectonic cortical regions.[3] The latter have distinct cellular and biochemical features, receptor densities,[1] and probably unique connections with other cortical and brain areas. Future cortical neurons, following radial glial guides from specific ventricular wall locations, migrate to future cerebral cortex regions predetermined by their ventricular wall locations. Therefore, the basic gyral and intervening sulcal pattern is likely to be genetically determined. Other lateral ventricular wall regions (the ganglionic eminences) supply additional neurons that migrate to the cortex and continue migrating tangentially. Golgi and Magini[4,5] were probably the first to detect radial glia in the spinal cord and cortex (see Chapter 3). Magini, noting varicosities along the radial glia, described cells currently considered to be migrating neuroblasts along the glial fibrils. Afferent input can modify the size of some cortical areas.

Human cortical neurons are most likely generated between 6 and 19 gestational weeks and migrate to the future cortex, thereafter following radial glial guides from specific ventricular zone sites to specific cortical locations (Fig. 5.5).[3] The first gyri formed on the external cerebral surface, between 20 and 22 weeks, are the pre- and postcentral gyri. Cortical growth is

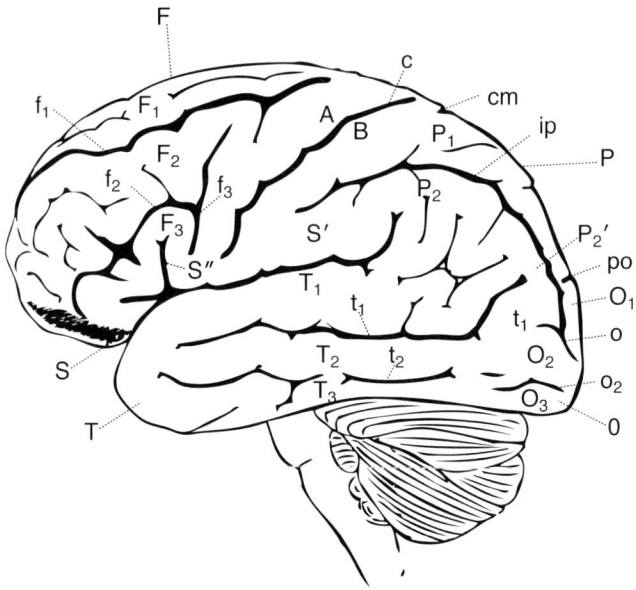

Fig. 5.1 Idealized gyri and sulci, lateral surface. These drawings were assembled in 1873 by Ecker and represent the conceptual framework of gyral configuration held by many over the last century. Heavy drawing lines and lowercase labels indicate the primary sulci except for S, S', and S'', the lateral sulcus with its horizontal and ascending branches; uppercase labels indicate the lobes, frontal, parietal, occipital, and temporal, and the primary gyri (A, precentral gyrus; B, postcentral gyrus; F_1, F_2, and F_3, superior, middle, and inferior frontal gyri or first, second, and third frontal gyri; P_1 and P_2, the superior and inferior parietal lobules; T_1, T_2, and T_3, superior, middle, and temporal gyri; O_1, O_2, and O_3, occipital gyri); lowercase labels the primary sulci [f_1, superior frontal or first frontal sulcus; f_2, inferior frontal or second frontal sulcus; t_1 and t_2, superior and inferior temporal sulci; c, central sulcus; o and o_1 and o_2 occipital sulci; ip, interparietal sulcus (the inferior part of the interparietal sulcus merges with the postcentral sulcus between p_1 and p_2 (unlabeled); po, parieto-occipital sulcus]. From Ecker.[2]

probably maximal along the sides and tops of gyri and minimal around the depths, as gyri enlarge away from the ventricular wall, leaving sulcal trenches, which remain at relatively constant distances from the ventricular wall. In fact, the pre- and postcentral gyri are so prominent as they transform the smooth fetal cortical surface that they form a prominence, once called Ecker's lobule.[6]

The upper surfaces and sides of the gyri develop additional crops of smaller gyri and sulci, producing a complex superficial pattern. Some gyri grow faster than others, distorting or overgrowing adjacent gyri, and thereby further complicating the superficial gyral and sulcal pattern. So-called primary sulci form long trenches between adjacent gyri and are called sulcal fundi (the deepest sulcal regions) (Fig. 5.6). These fundi form earliest in the least variable locations among individuals; their location is likely to be under genetic control, and the deepest portions, the pits, may be encoded in the Rakic protomap in the ventricular wall germinal matrix.[7]

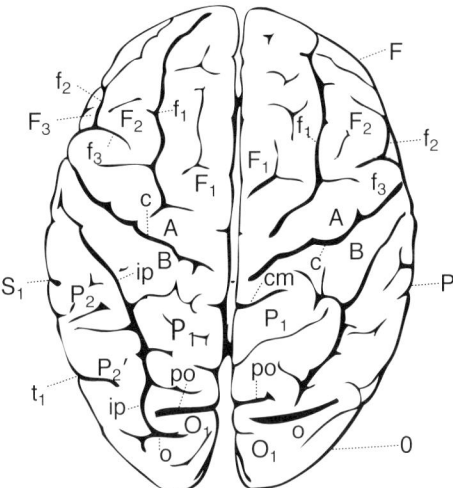

Fig. 5.2 Idealized gyri and sulci, dorsal surface. Heavy lines and lowercase labels indicate the primary sulci; uppercase labels indicate the lobes, frontal, parietal, occipital, and temporal and the primary gyri [A, precentral gyrus; B, postcentral gyrus; f_1, superior frontal or first frontal sulcus; f_2, inferior frontal or second frontal sulcus; c, central sulcus; o and o_1 and o_2 occipital sulci; ip, interparietal sulcus; po, parieto-occipital sulcus; F_1, F_2, and F_3, superior, middle, and inferior frontal gyri or first, second, and third frontal gyri; P_1 and P_2, the superior and inferior parietal lobules; O_1, O_2, and O_3, occipital gyri]. From Ecker.[2]

The processes of human fetal brain expansion, lobation, gyral development, and opercu-lation transform an initially smooth embryonic and early fetal brain into a large convoluted brain. During the first trimester, as the brain is slowly expanding, rudimentary hemispheral lobes become apparent; by midgestation the lobes are more prominent; and at the end of the second trimester, gyral formation accelerates simultaneously with maximally accelerating brain weight accretion (see Chapter 2). Localized cortical regions differentiate, expand, and grow outward from the brain surface more rapidly than adjacent regions. Similarly, rapidly expanding gyri grow laterally, covering or pushing aside more slowly growing adjacent gyri, and give rise to opercula. Lobes become more prominent occipitally, laterally, and frontally.

In this chapter, we examine surface area development of human fetal cerebral hemisphere; time development of human fetal gyri; gyral and sulcal variability, particularly secondary and tertiary gyri, across human populations, both fetal and more mature; and some gyral development theories.

Cortical surface area development: isocortex and allocortex

Isocortical surface growth rate is biphasic with growth acceleration occurring between 21 and 26 weeks (Fig. 5.7). A distinctly faster rate occurs from 26 to 42 weeks, when dorsolateral, parieto-occipital, temporal, and medial hemispheral surfaces expand. The increase in surface area growth rate parallels accelerating brain weight accretion (see Chapter 2), and there are no consistent differences in surface area gains and growth rate between the left and right

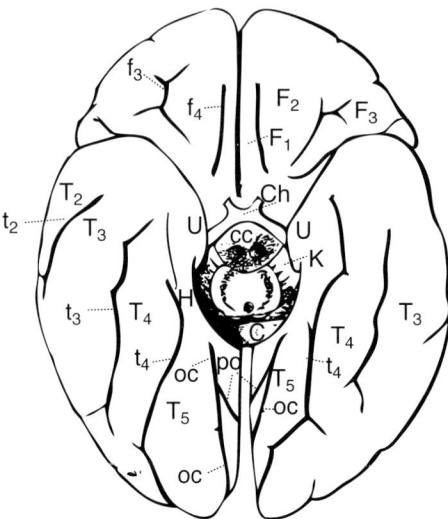

Fig. 5.3 Idealized gyri and sulci, basal surface. F_1, gyrus rectus; F_2, middle orbital gyrus; F_3, inferior frontal gyrus; f_4, olfactory sulcus; f_5, orbital sulcus; U, uncus; T_2, second or middle temporal gyrus; T_3, third temporal gyrus or inferior temporosphenoidal gyrus; T_4, lateral occipitotemporal gyrus (fusiform lobule); and T_5, medial occipitotemporal gyrus; t_2 and t_3, inferior and middle temporosphenoidal sulci; t_4, inferior occipitotemporal sulcus; po, parieto-occipital sulcus; oc, calcarine sulcus; H, parahippocampal gyrus; Ch, optic chiasm; K, crura cerebri; and cc, tuber cinereum. From Ecker.[2]

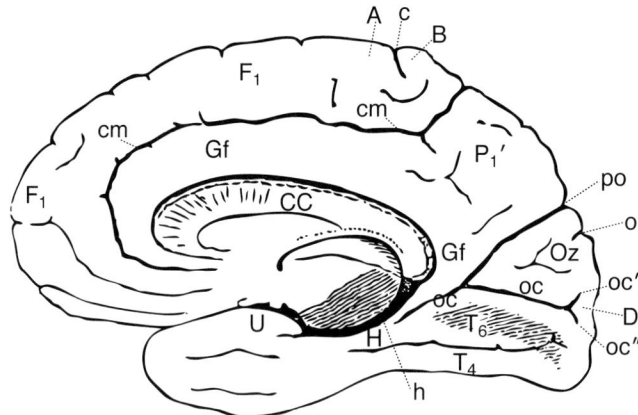

Fig. 5.4 Idealized gyri and sulci, medial surface of right hemisphere. CC, corpus callosum; Gf, gyrus cinguli; H, parahippocampal gyrus; h, choroidal fissure; U, uncus; cm, callosomarginal sulcus; F_1, medial aspect of first frontal gyrus; c, terminal portion of central sulcus; A and B, pre- and postcentral gyri; P_1', precuneus; Oz, Cuneus; po, parieto-occipital sulcus; o, transverse occipital sulcus; oc, calcarine sulcus; oc', superior ramus of calcarine sulcus; oc", inferior ramus of calcarine sulcus; T_4, lateral occipitotemporal gyrus (fusiform lobule); T_5, medial occipitotemporal gyrus (lingual lobule). From Ecker.[2]

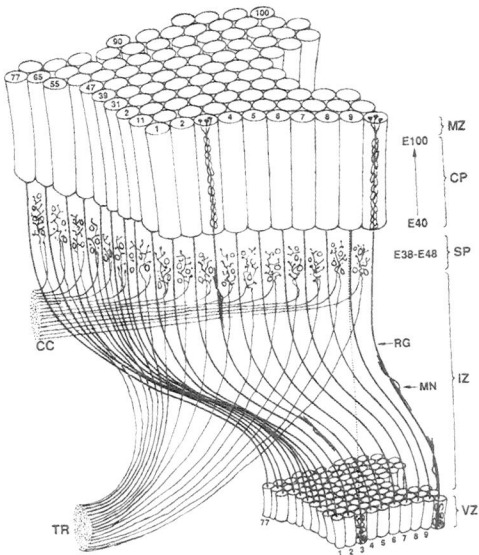

Fig. 5.5 Rakic's radial unit hypothesis. The relation between a small patch of the proliferative ventricular zone (VZ) and its corresponding cortical plate (CP) area in the developing cerebrum. Although the cerebral surface in primates expands and shifts during prenatal development, ontogenetic columns (represented by VZ columns 1 … 100 and corresponding CP columns 1 … 100) remain attached to the corresponding proliferative units by the grid of radial glial fibers. Neurons produced between embryonic day 40 and embryonic day 100 by a given proliferative unit migrate in succession along the same radial glial guides (RG) and stack up in reverse order of arrival within the same ontogenetic column. Each migrating neuron (MN) first traverses to the intermediate zone (IZ) and then the subplate (SP) that contains interstitial cells and 'waiting' afferents from the thalamic radiation (TR) and ipsilateral and contralateral corticocortical connections (CC). After entering the cortical plate, each neuron bypasses earlier generated neurons and settles at the interface between the CP and marginal zone (MZ). As a result, proliferative units 1 to 100 produce ontogenetic columns 1 to 100 in the same relative position to each other without a lateral mismatch (for example, between proliferative unit 3 and ontogenetic column 9, indicated by a dashed line). Thus, the specification of cytoarchitectonic areas and topographic maps depends on the spatial distribution of their ancestors in the proliferative units, whereas the laminar position and phenotype of neurons within ontogenetic columns depends on the time of their origin. Reproduced with permission of the American Association for the Advancement of Science from Rakic.[3]

hemispheres. These estimates of surface area are smaller than those previously obtained,[8] probably because of marked methodologic differences.

The total allocortical surface area (olfactory lobes, hippocampal rudiment, and Ammon's horn) grows at a regular rate between 13 and 31 weeks, after which it plateaus.[9] There is no hemispheral difference in allocortical surface area growth. Isocortex (six-layered) and allocortex (less than six layers such as the hippocampus, olfactory lobes, septal area) are separated by three topographic boundaries: (1) pronounced isocortical plate cell layer attenuation as it approaches allocortex, (2) isocortical overriding of allocortex at this juncture, and (3) stepwise isocortical molecular layer widening into the wide plexiform allocortical layer

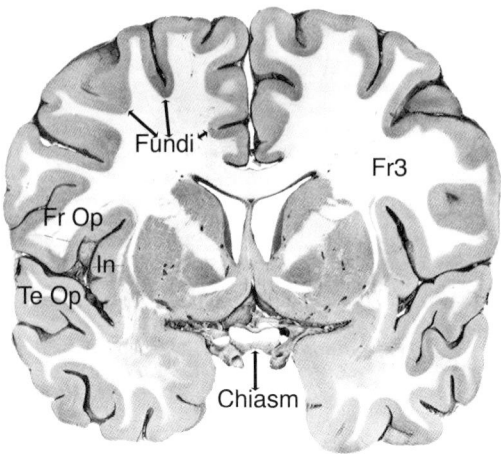

Fig. 5.6 This image of a mature brain slice demonstrates two points. Gyri wander and sometimes over-grow (form opercula) adjacent gyri (for instance, the frontal and temporal opercula). Some opercula are common from brain to brain such as the frontal, parietal, and temporal opercula covering the insula. Some vary considerably amongst most brains. The second point is that sulci fundi are the deepest sulcal portions between adjacent gyri (sometimes called 'pits'). Because of great gyral pattern variation from brain to brain, some have used the fundi as they are relatively standard from brain to brain. Fundi, the deepest sulci; Fr Op, frontal operculum; In, insula; Te Op, temporal operculum; Fr3, the gyral white matter core of the right third frontal gyrus; chiasm, optic chiasm. Reproduced with permission of Lippincott Williams & Wilkins from Roberts and Hanaway.[83]

in older fetuses[10–12] (Fig. 5.8). These landmarks are found along the hippocampal subiculum, callosal sulcus, and olfactory bud, and are distinct at first appearance of the isocortical cell plate during the eighth week. The boundary between the allocortex and diencephalon is arbitrarily defined as the sulcus between the telencephalon and diencephalon containing the optic tract, back to the lateral geniculate body, or the point at which the allocortex ends in the choroidal fissure. The allocortex of supracallosal hippocampal rudiment (longitudinal striae Lancisii and induseum griseum) was measured where nerve cells were present. Isocortical cell plate surface was measured separately in each hemisphere. The allocortex was considered as a median telencephalic formation containing septal area, olfactory tubercle, diagonal band, lateral and medial olfactory gyri, and subcallosal gyri anteroventrally; and dorsomedially containing induseum griseum and the paired Ammon's horns with the fascia dentate. Their measurements were summed.

Timing of gyration: changing gyral patterns related to gestational age
Regional gyral development, when described by its relation to brain weight,[13] broad gestational periods,[14] restricted periods of embryogenesis,[15] or maturation of other fetal organs,[16] provides conflicting information. The development of gyri, sulci, and fissures was estimated

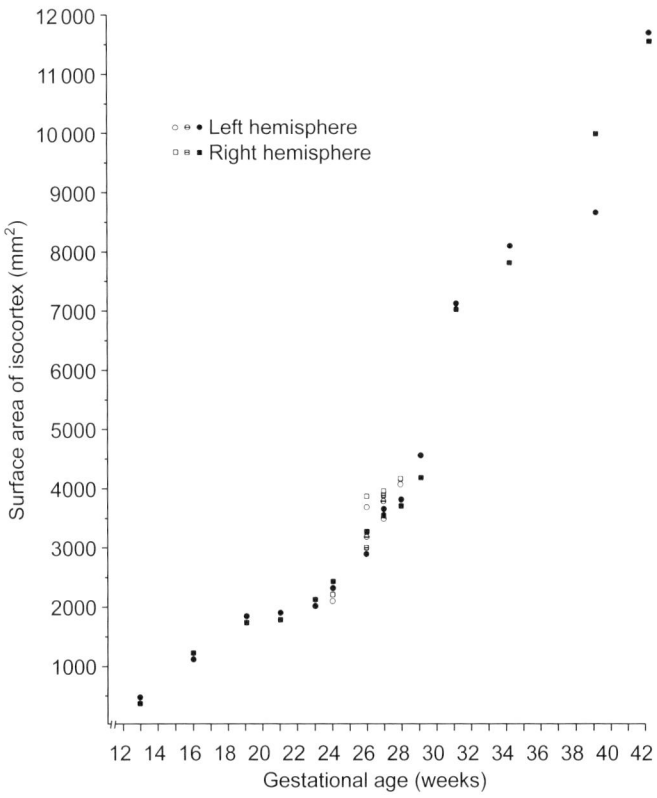

Fig. 5.7 The isocortical surface area (mm²) of each hemisphere is plotted against gestational age. Both hemispheres have roughly the same total surface area despite asymmetry in secondary and tertiary gyri and prominent asymmetry in the planum temporale. Note the bimodal growth with the change in rate at the end of the second trimester. From Gilles et al.[81]

using mothers' estimates of gestational age in 207 serially sectioned National Collaborative Perinatal Project (NCPP) embryonic and fetal brains and photographs of 300 nonserially sectioned NCPP brains[17] (Fig. 5.9).

A gyrus is the tissue lying between two sulci. The gestational and regional development of gyri and sulci shown in Tables 5.1 and 5.2 indicates the gestational age at which 25% to 50% of brains contain the structure: in age groups with fewer than five specimens this figure was arbitrarily set at 25%, and in age groups with more than five specimens at 50%. Generally, an interval of about 2 weeks occurred between the earliest gyral or sulcal manifestation in any one brain and its appearance in 75% to 100% of brains, a variation attributable to the effect of diverse biologic forces on brain maturation or errors in estimated gestational ages.

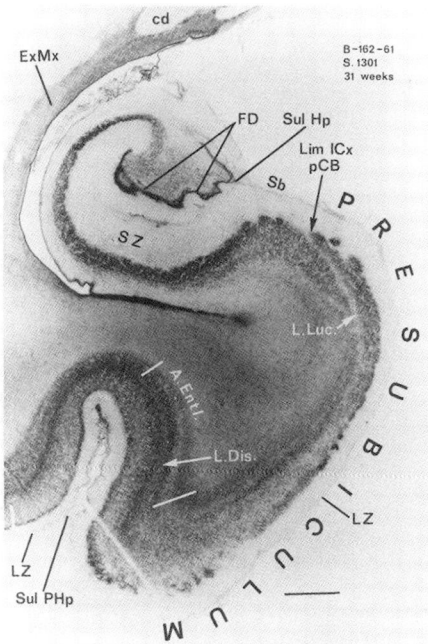

Fig. 5.8 Isocortex changes to allocortex in the presubiculum (about 31 weeks). At the label Lim ICx pCB, the terminal superficial lamina of the isocortex overrides the allocortex. The stratum zonale (SZ) is wider than the lamina zonale (LZ). cd, caudate; ExMx, extraganglionic matrix; FD, fascia dentata; Sul Hp, sulcus hippocampi; Sb, subiculum; L. Dis, lamina dissicans; A. Entl, entorhinal area; Sul PHp, parahippocampal sulcus. From Gilles et al.[81]

The primary gyri, sulci, and fissures
As gyri extend away from brain surface, either relative to ventricular walls or to sulcal fundi, it is simpler to describe gyral development in terms of the intervening sulci. Growth of gyri, sulci, and fissures during gestation is outlined in Table 5.1.

Interhemispheric fissure (longitudinal fissure)
The interhemispheric fissure (Figs. 5.2, 5.3, 5.6, and 5.9), the first primary fissure to emerge, is recognizable at 8 weeks. Originating rostrally, during week 10 it extends as the telencephalic vesicle expands and becomes a distinct longitudinal fissure, separating the hemispheres.

Transverse fissure
During the ninth or tenth week, the transverse fissure (separating cerebellum from diencephalon and cerebrum) emerges as a wide furrow, appearing at about the same time as the interhemispheric fissure, and forms its base before the corpus callosum appears. With increasing gestational age, it narrows to a transverse slit between the corpus callosum and the third ventricle roof. The choroidal fissure was not studied.

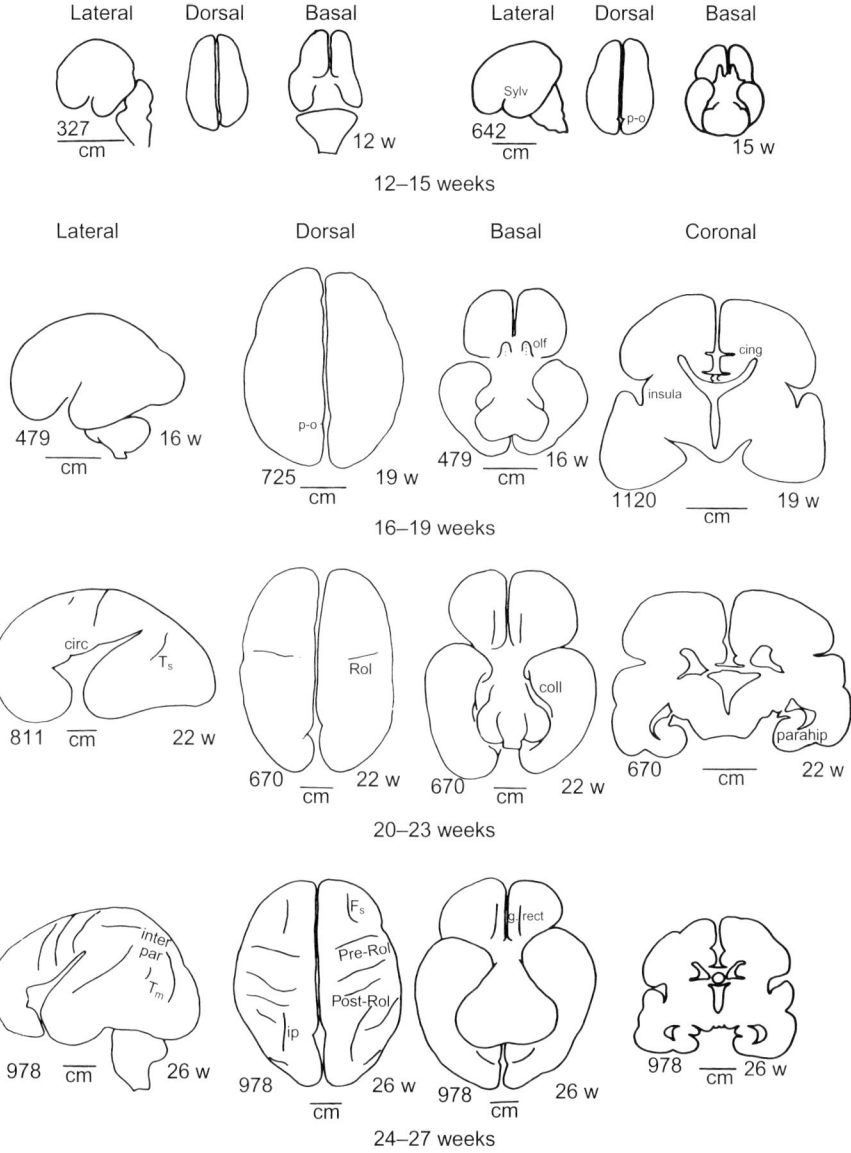

Fig. 5.9 Schematic drawings from brain photographs of serially numbered sections show progressive gyral and sulcal development. (continued overleaf)

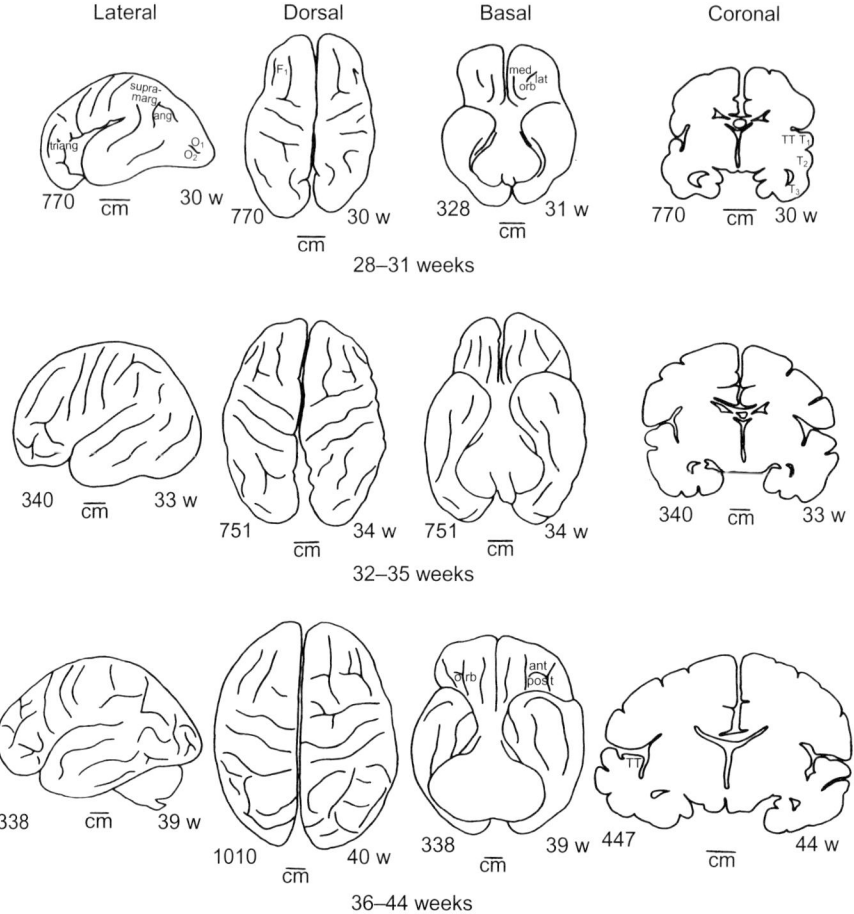

Lateral	Dorsal	Basal	Coronal

28–31 weeks

32–35 weeks

36–44 weeks

Fig. 5.9 (continued) The lateral hemispheral surface remains essentially smooth throughout the first gestational half with the exception of the lateral sulcus and beginning insula. Early in the second half of gestation, the pre- and postcentral gyri appear and by the end of the second trimester almost all primary gyri are in place. Primary gyri are distorted by secondary and tertiary gyri during the third trimester, giving each hemisphere, and each brain, a unique gyral pattern. ang, angular gyrus; ant/post, anterior and posterior orbital gyri; cing, cingulate sulcus; circ, circular sulcus; coll, collateral sulcus; F_1, superior frontal gyrus; F_s, superior frontal sulcus; g. rect, gyrus rectus; ip or interpar, interparietal sulcus; med/lat orb, medial and lateral orbital gyri; O_1, superior occipital gyrus; O_2, inferior occipital gyrus; olf (dotted lines to indicate sulci are underneath the olfactory bulbs), olfactory sulcus; parahip, parahippocampal gyrus; p-o, parieto-occipital sulcus; post-Rol, postcentral sulcus; pre-Rol, precentral sulcus; Rol, central sulcus; T_1, superior temporal gyrus; T_2, middle temporal gyrus; T_3, inferior temporal gyrus; T_m, middle temporal sulcus; triang, triangular gyrus; T_s, superior temporal sulcus; TT, transverse temporal gyrus. Reproduced with permission of John Wiley & Sons from Chi et al.[17]

TABLE 5.1

Cerebral hemispheral gyral and sulcal development

Postovulatory age (weeks)	Gyri	Sulci and fissures
10–15	–	Longitudinal cerebral fissure
	–	Transverse cerebral fissure
	–	Hippocampal sulcus
	–	Lateral sulcus
	–	Callosal sulcus
16–19	–	Parieto-occipital sulcus
	Gyrus rectus	Olfactory sulcus
	–	Circular sulcus of insula
	Cingulate gyrus	Cingulate sulcus
	Cuneus	Calcarine sulcus
20–23	–	Central sulcus
	Superior temporal gyrus	Superior temporal sulcus
	Parahippocampal gyrus	Collateral sulcus
24–27	Precentral gyrus	Precentral sulcus
	Middle temporal gyrus	Inferior temporal sulcus
	Inferior temporal gyrus	–
	Lingual gyrus	–
	Fusiform gyrus	–
	Postcentral gyrus	Postcentral sulcus
	Superior frontal gyrus	Superior frontal sulcus
	Superior parietal lobule	Interparietal sulcus
	Inferior parietal lobule	–
	Precuneus	–
	Superior occipital gyrus	Lunate sulcus
	Inferior occipital gyrus	–
28–31	Middle frontal gyrus	Inferior frontal sulcus
	Inferior frontal gyrus	–
	Triangular gyrus	–
	Orbital gyri	Orbital sulci
	Transverse temporal gyrus	–
	Angular gyrus	–
	Supramarginal gyrus	–

TABLE 5.1 (continued)

Postovulatory age (weeks)	Gyri	Sulci and fissures
32–35	Paracentral lobule	Cingulate sulcus, marginal
	–	Secondary superior, middle, inferior frontal
	–	Secondary superior and middle temporal
	–	Superior and inferior parietal
	–	Pre- and postcentral sulci
36–39	–	Secondary transverse temporal
	–	Secondary inferior temporal
	–	Secondary cingulate
	–	Tertiary inferior temporal
	–	Tertiary superior, inferior occipital
	–	Tertiary inferior frontal
	–	Tertiary superior parietal
40–44	Short insular gyri	Insular sulci
	Long insular gyri	–
	–	Secondary orbital
	–	Tertiary inferior temporal
	–	Tertiary superior and inferior occipital

Hippocampal sulcus

This sulcus emerges very early, at 10 weeks, along with the interhemispheric and transverse fissures. As the medial temporal lobe develops, the sulcus narrows.

Lateral sulcus (Sylvian fissure, Sylvian fossa) and insula

At 14 weeks, the lateral sulcus appears as a shallow depression, or fossa, on the lateral hemispheral surface between future orbitofrontal and temporal lobes (Fig. 5.9). Subsequently, it deepens owing to rapid growth of surrounding frontal, parietal, and temporal areas. The fossa base can be designated as insula by week 19 (Fig. 5.10). At 39 weeks, the superior insular border is the circular sulcus and the inferior border is the lateral sulcus proper. The circular sulcus first extends rostrally, then curves posteriorly to form a circle and is joined by the posterior lateral sulcus. The circular sulcus remains distinct until full maturation of the triangular gyrus and frontal and parietal opercula. With development of the frontal operculum, the circular sulcus gradually loses its circular shape and merges with the lateral sulcus.

Two buried lateral sulcal structures of considerable importance to the developing human are the insula and transverse temporal gyri (of Heschl) dorsally on the superior temporal gyrus (Fig. 5.11). The first is important because oral and gastrointestinal function is likely to find insular representation and the second because the transverse temporal gyri are primary

TABLE 5.2
Cerebral hemisphere regional development

Lobe	Gyri	Gestational age (weeks)	Fissures and sulci	Gestational age (weeks)
Frontal	Gyrus rectus	16	Interhemispheric fissure	10
	Insula	18	Transverse cerebral fissure	10
	Cingulate gyrus	18	Hippocampal sulcus	10
	Central gyrus	24	Callosal sulcus	14
	Superior frontal gyrus	25	Sylvian fissure	14
	Middle frontal gyrus	27	Olfactory sulcus	16
	Triangular gyrus	28	Circular sulcus	18
	Medial and lateral orbital gyri	28	Cingulate sulcus	18
	Callosomarginal gyrus	28	Central sulcus	20
	Anterior and posterior orbital gyri	36	Central sulcus	24
	–		Superior frontal sulcus	25
	–		Inferior frontal sulcus	28
Parietal	Cingulate gyrus	18	Interhemispheric fissure	10
	Central gyrus	25	Transverse cerebral fissure	10
	Superior parietal lobule	26	Sylvian fissure	14
	Inferior parietal lobule	26	Parieto-occipital sulcus	16
	Angular gyrus	28	Central sulcus	20
	Supramarginal gyrus	28	Central sulcus	25
	Paracentral gyri	35	Interparietal sulcus	26
Temporal	Superior temporal gyrus	23	Sylvian fissure	14
	Parahippocampal gyrus	23	Superior temporal sulcus	23
	Middle temporal gyrus	26	Collateral sulcus	23
	Fusiform gyrus	27	Middle temporal sulcus	26
	External occipitotemporal gyrus	30	Inferior temporal sulcus	30
	Transverse temporal gyrus	30	–	
Occipital	Superior occipital gyri	27	Interhemispheric fissure	10
	Inferior occipital gyri	27	Calcarine sulcus	16
	Cuneus	27	Parieto-occipital sulcus	16
	Lingual gyrus	27	Collateral sulcus	23
	External occipitotemporal gyrus	30	Lateral occipital sulcus	27

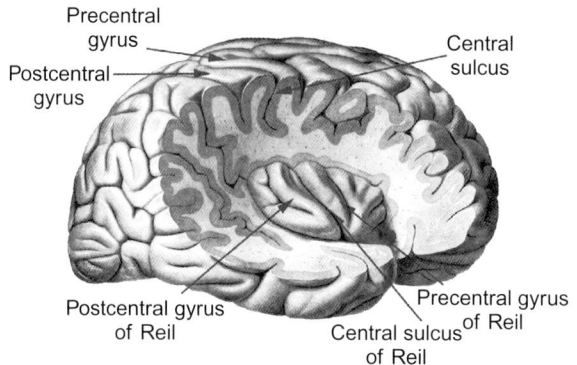

Precentral gyrus

Postcentral gyrus

Central sulcus

Postcentral gyrus of Reil

Precentral gyrus of Reil

Central sulcus of Reil

Fig. 5.10 Insula and central sulcus drawing. The insula is separated from the surrounding brain by the circular sulcus. Above, on the brain convexity, the central sulcus, as well as the pre- and postcentral gyri, are indicated. Within the insula, the central insular sulcus (central culcus of Reil) is indicated as well as the pre- and postcentral insular gyri. Notice how the insular central sulcus is roughly aligned with the plane of the central sulcus. Reproduced with permission of Elsevier GmbH from Putz and Pabst.[84] © Elsevier GmbH, Urban & Fischer Verlag Munich.

auditory sensory areas. The transverse temporal gyri will be discussed later in this chapter (right–left asymmetries).

Insular gyral development

Because it is so well hidden, insular development attracted little attention during the last century.[18,19] Temporoparietal and frontal opercula progressively cover the insula, causing its apparent sinking below the surface. The insula is the first isocortex to differentiate, and development begins from 6 weeks.[20] Eberstaller[21] identified an insular sulcus, with the same plane and orientation as the central sulcus, dividing the insula into an anterior and posterior part; he suggested that this should be called the sulcus centralis Reilii, with an additional sulcus in front and behind, called the sulcus precentralis Reilii and sulcus postcentralis Reilii (Fig. 5.10). The insular region and Sylvian fossa are first macroscopically obvious at 18 weeks owing to a shallow peri-insular sulcal depression and developing adjacent structures. Before the fifth month the insula is smooth; during the fifth month the three sulci Reilii emerge. Remaining insular gyri exhibit great diversity.[19] The central sulcus continues onto the posterior insular surface along with precentral and postcentral gyri. Development on the right leads the left. More recently, duplications and other variations in and around Heschl's gyrus were reported.[22]

Callosal sulcus

The callosal sulcus separates the corpus callosum from the dorsal overlying cingulate gyrus. It emerges at week 14, concomitantly with the corpus callosum and the developing cingulate gyrus (Fig. 5.9). There is little variation in the time of its first appearance.

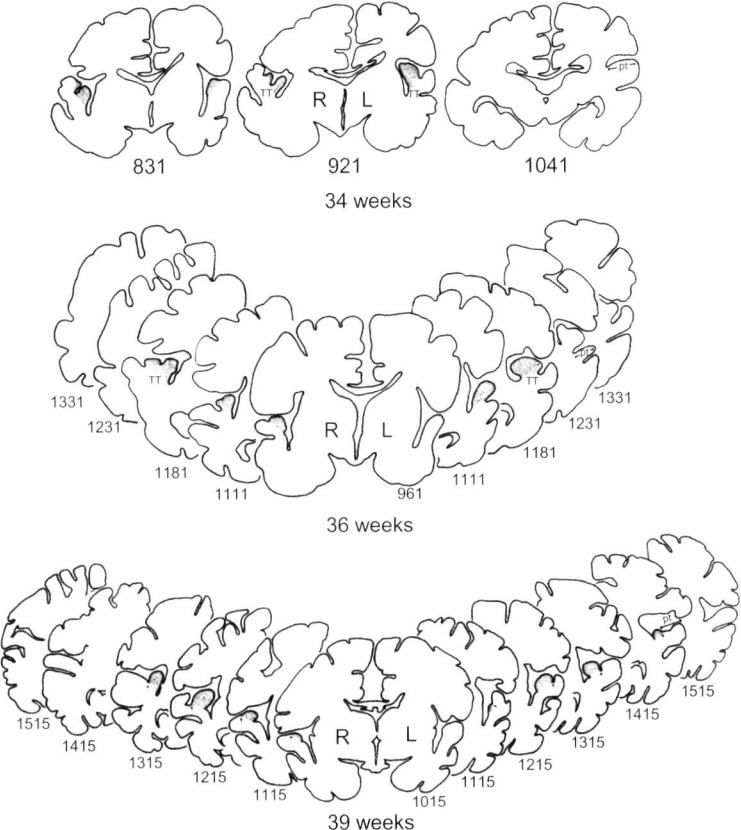

Fig. 5.11 Tracings of photographs of serially numbered sections in the coronal plane of representative fetal brains of different gestational ages. 34 weeks—top, most rostral section on left; most caudal on right. 36 and 39 weeks—most rostral sections located in center. Note double transverse temporal (TT) or Heschl's gyri on right side in top and center tracings, and greater surface areas are in bottom tracing. The temporal plane (pt), the surface behind the transverse temporal gyrus or gyri, which terminates at the lateral sulcus posterior boundary, is longer in extent in sections of the left hemisphere. Reproduced with permission of the American Medical Association from Chi et al.[85] Copyright © 1977 American Medical Association. All rights reserved.

Olfactory sulcus

The olfactory sulcus starts during week 16 as a shallow depression along the medial orbital surface and runs parallel to the interhemispheric fissure, subjacent to the olfactory bulb and tract (Fig. 5.9). It extends anteriorly and delineates the gyrus rectus medially. The sulcal groove gradually deepens and is distinct by week 25.

The olfactory sulcus in the frontal orbital isocortex is unique in some respects. It is juxtaposed to a nonisocortical structure, the olfactory bulb and tract, separated only by a double layer of leptomeninges. The arachnoidal barrier layer (most adjacent to the dura) bridges the olfactory sulcus external to the olfactory bulb and tract. It is constant in all human brains containing bulb and tract, foreshortened when bulb and tract are hypoplastic, and absent when bulb and tract are absent.

Parieto-occipital sulcus

Present on the medial cerebral surface, this sulcus usually appears during week 16, separating occipital and parietal lobes [Figs. 5.4 and 5.9 (po)]. Even before the sulcus emerges, the isocortical molecular layer at the sulcus site has a distinctive layer of cells, which is carried down in the sulcal walls during development, and eventually disappears (Fig. 5.12). The sulcus starts as a prominent groove dorsomedially, and remains a distinct furrow but becomes tortuous because of subsequent secondary occipital lobe gyri and parietal precuneus (isocortex between parieto-occipital and central sulci) growth. Secondary occipital gyri emerge at 34 weeks, with tertiary gyri noted medially and laterally 6 to 8 weeks later. Thus, the parieto-occipital sulcus seems unique in that the underlying isocortex develops differently than other isocortices. This transient layer disappears by the end of gestation.

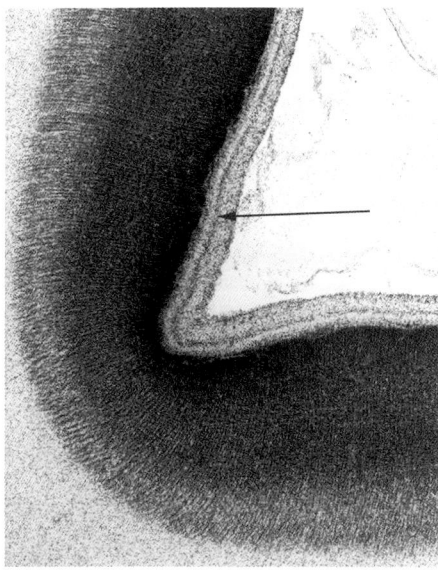

Fig. 5.12 The parieto-occipital sulcus at the beginning of its formation. There is a distinctive layer of cells midway in the molecular layer (arrow), which is transient in fetal life. Fetal leptomeninges fill the sulcus. The radial columns of isocortical neurons are particularly well seen in the lower laminae. From Gilles et al.[81]

Calcarine sulcus

This sulcus is definite by week 16, joining the parieto-occipital sulcus rostrally [Fig. 5.4 (oc)]. The right calcarine sulcus usually appears earlier than the left (cf. central sulcus). At about 27 weeks, parieto-occipital and calcarine sulci deepen because of adjacent cuneus and lingual gyral growth, and the cortex around the calcarine sulcus indents the lateral ventricular occipital horn.

Central sulcus

The central sulcus emerges as a distinct groove between precentral and postcentral gyri at 20 to 22 weeks [Figs. 5.1 (c), 5.2 (c), 5.4 (c), and 5.9 (rol)]; the right central sulcus is rarely visualized earlier than 17 weeks. The sulcus extends parasagitally over the convexity, downward, and forward (oblique to the interhemispheric fissure) creating a distinct linear sulcus by 22 to 23 weeks.

LOBAR DEVELOPMENT

Cerebral hemispheral regional development is detailed in Table 5.2.

Frontal lobe

The gyrus rectus is the first orbital frontal gyrus to emerge at 16 weeks, separating the olfactory sulcus from the adjacent smooth orbital surface (Fig. 5.9). Twelve weeks later, at the end of the second trimester, the medial and lateral orbital gyri are distinguishable, and finally, at 36 weeks, the anterior and posterior orbital gyri become prominent.

The gyrus cinguli separates from the hemispheral medial surface, leaving the cingulate sulcus, parallel to the callosal sulcus, recognizable at 18 weeks, its anterior part emerging first [Figs. 5.4 (Gf) and 5.9 (cing)]. No right–left asymmetry in the gestational time of development of this sulcus is observed. The gyrus dorsal to the cinglate gyrus, called the 'callosomarginal' gyrus, becomes apparent at 29 weeks (Fig. 5.9 (cing)).

The precentral gyrus emerges at approximately 24 weeks (Fig. 5.9), when the precentral sulcus is distinguished as a shallow groove anterior to the central sulcus.

The insula (island of Reil) first emerges as a conical, smooth-surfaced area delineated by the circular and lateral sulci at 18 weeks (Fig. 5.9). It remains smooth until 28 to 29 weeks, when the frontal, temporal, and parietal operculae begin to conceal it, and the longitudinal sulcus, a deep oblique furrow, becomes obvious. By 34 to 35 weeks, three or four insular gyri are present; those on the right usually develop earlier (Fig. 5.10).

The first, or superior, frontal gyrus generally is identifiable by the 25th week, earlier on the right than the left (Fig. 5.9). Simultaneously, the superior frontal sulcus, a longitudinal middle-to-posterior frontal lobe furrow, emerges. By 32 weeks, the superior frontal gyrus shows secondary sulcation.

The middle and inferior frontal gyri are separated by the inferior frontal sulcus by 28 weeks, less than a month later than the superior frontal sulcus (Fig. 5.9). The triangular gyrus and frontal operculum, visible by 28 weeks, evolve rapidly. At approximately 32 weeks, secondary sulcation in middle and inferior frontal gyri become distinct, concomitant with that in the superior frontal gyrus. Tertiary frontal gyri are recognizable by 40 weeks.

81

Parietal lobe

Medially, the cingulate gyrus and sulcus mostly emerge at 18 weeks, earlier precentrally than postcentrally (Fig. 5.9). Secondary gyri appear at 29 to 30 weeks. The callosomarginal gyrus becomes prominent at 29 to 30 weeks, gradually differentiating into complex gyri, later comprising the paracentral lobule. The paracentral lobule and marginal sulcus are evident by 34 to 35 weeks (Fig. 5.4).

The lateral parietal lobe remains smooth until the postcentral gyrus and sulcus arise at 25 weeks, about a week later than the precentral gyrus and sulcus. The interparietal sulcus, between superior and inferior parietal lobules, first shows at 26 weeks, followed by rapid parietal gyral and sulcal formation [Figs. 5.2 (ip) and 5.9]. By 28 weeks, supramarginal and angular gyri are distinguishable, earlier on the right than the left, and become convoluted concurrently with posterior superior and middle temporal gyri. By 33 weeks, secondary gyri are obvious in both superior and inferior parietal lobules; by 39 weeks, tertiary gyri are seen.

Temporal lobe

The lateral temporal lobe, bounded anteriorly by the dorsolateral lateral sulcus and posteriorly by the preoccipital notch, remains smooth-surfaced until 23 weeks when the superior temporal gyrus, in its mid to posterior parts, is delimited by an initial superior temporal sulcus [Figs. 5.1 (T_1) and 5.9]. Again, this is discernible earlier on the right. At 26 weeks, the middle temporal gyrus, delineated by the middle temporal sulcus, appears (Fig. 5.9). Two months later, at 34 to 35 weeks, secondary sulcation and gyration in the superior and middle temporal gyri occur. The inferior temporal gyrus and sulcus are perceptible at 30 weeks, with secondary sulcation and gyration not happening until the last month. By 23 weeks the collateral sulcus is visible on the basal hemispheral surface, delimiting parahippocampal and fusiform gyri (Fig. 5.9). Further demarcation between fusiform gyrus and external occipitotemporal gyrus develops at 27 weeks. The external occipitotemporal and inferior temporal gyri are distinct by week 30 [Fig. 5.3 (T_4 and T_5)].

Occipital lobe

The calcarine and parieto-occipital sulci, seen on the medial occipital lobe at 18 weeks [Fig. 5.4 (oc and po)], delineate the cuneus (dorsal to calcarine sulcus) and lingual gyri (ventral to calcarine sulcus); the lateral and inferior gyral surfaces remain smooth until 27 weeks. The medial and external occipitotemporal gyri do not visibly extend posteriorly until 30 weeks.

RIGHT–LEFT ASYMMETRIES

An observable developmental right–left lateral sulcal asymmetry affects the transverse temporal gyri (the gyri, or gyrus, medial to a distinct furrow on the dorsal and medial surfaces of superior temporal gyrus) [Fig. 5.11 (TT)]. The furrow extends posteriorly and medially until its terminal junction with the posterior insula. The transverse temporal gyrus, arising at 31 weeks, is notably asymmetric in its development. Transverse temporal gyri are evident 1 to 2 weeks earlier on the right in any plane of section in about two-thirds of cases, and simultaneously bilaterally in most brains; only a few brains show earlier manifestation on the left. In addition to these differences in development, this gyrus varies in expanse bilaterally; extending more rostrally on the right and more caudally on the left. Furthermore, there is a disparity in gyral angulation with reference to the interhemispheric fissure. The left transverse temporal gyrus is shorter in height, with a more obtuse angle to the cerebral anterior–posterior axis. Related to the longer anterior–posterior length of the left lateral sulcus, the planum temporale [the superior temporal surface area posterior to the first (or second) transverse temporal gyrus on each side, located anterior to the lateral sulcus termination] is also more extensive on the left. The discrepancy in planum temporale length becomes more striking with advancing gestation.

After 36 weeks, secondary transverse temporal gyri appear. In 54% of brains, two transverse temporal gyri are present on the right and only one on the left; in 18%, the findings are reversed, with two left transverse temporal gyri and one on the right. An equal number on each side are present in the remaining 28%. No sex-dependent variations in gyral development were noted among brains at any given age, specifically in the number of transverse temporal gyri or in the planum temporale area. The number of male and female brains was about equal.

FETAL SECONDARY AND TERTIARY GYRAL FORMATION
While the formation of primary gyri and sulci is fairly consistent among fetuses at the end of the second trimester, secondary and tertiary gyral development on primary gyral surfaces complicate late fetal brain appearance; by the end of gestation, multiple smaller gyri, visible on the cerebral surface, seem unique to each fetus and to each hemisphere. The primary gyri affected by this process are superior, middle, and inferior frontal gyri (32 weeks); superior and inferior parietal lobules (secondary 33 weeks; tertiary 39 weeks), superior and middle temporal gyri (34 to 35 weeks); transverse temporal gyri (36 weeks); inferior temporal gyrus and sulcus (39 weeks); and occipital gyri (secondary 34 weeks, tertiary 39 weeks).

Human gyrus formation
There is little time disparity in gyral development among the different cerebral lobes (Table 5.1). Many primary gyri become well defined within a short period of time between 26 and 28 weeks; secondary and tertiary gyri cluster later in gestation, with the orbital and occipital gyri becoming increasingly complex a few weeks after frontal and temporal gyri. During the last trimester, previously formed gyri become more prominent, with subsequent development of secondary and tertiary gyri at 40 to 44 weeks. Inferior frontal gyrus, particularly opercular and triangular parts, develop about a month earlier than inferior and transverse temporal gyri; some orbital gyri develop complex gyral patterns only late in gestation.

Our observations differ from observations of other investigators on time of first appearance of the superior frontal, superior temporal, and central sulci. Our studies place these events 2 to 3 weeks earlier than other descriptions. According to Larroche,[23] the superior temporal sulcus appears at 28 weeks, but we identified a definitive first temporal sulcus as early as 23 weeks and found it present at 26 weeks in 80% of brains. This disparity is likely to be based on methodologic differences or in our specific populations of brains. Early indications of sulci and gyri are sometimes difficult to determine by gross inspection alone without the availability of serial sections.

Of special interest is the developmental left–right asymmetry of several hemispheral areas. The superior frontal and superior temporal gyri are visualized 1 to 2 weeks earlier on the right. Secondary gyri also emerge earlier in these same areas. Asymmetry in transverse temporal gyri has interested various investigators;[24–26] temporal plane measurements, the area behind these gyri, in infant and adult brains may indicate an anatomical substrate for right–left hemispheral functional differences, particularly in speech, language, and nonverbal skills. We found more complex transverse temporal gyri on the right with a larger left temporal plane in 54%; and more complex transverse temporal gyri on the left in 18%. There was no gyral asymmetry or temporal plane areal difference in 28%. These proportions are consistent with those found by Bossy et al[27] in 20 fetal brains.

GYRAL DEVELOPMENT

A century of descriptive gyral and sulcal morphology has focused on sulcal patterns rather than on the functional tissue, the gyri. Gyral cortical thickness and columnar and laminar architecture differ relatively little in different mammals, but the cortical surface area varies extensively, with marked discrepancies in gyral development. In some sulci, for instance the central sulcus, cortical lamination differs on the two sulcal sides; in most sulci, such lamination does not change at sulcal bottom.[28] Gyri vary in height, width, length, and shape. Opercula grow over adjacent gyri, sometimes leaving buried gyri within sulci. Secondary and tertiary cortical sulci exhibit various forms in adult brains with unclear meaning.

Theories

Several late fetal and childhood brain observations require explanation:

1   The isocortex around the sulcal fundi is much thinner than the isocortex over gyral crests.
2   During development, primary sulcal fundi maintain approximately the same distance from the nearest ventricular wall.
3   Primary sulci are at similar relative positions in different brains during fetal development, whereas secondary and tertiary sulci are not.
4   The outer arachnoidal membrane bridges sulci.

These observations have generated three theories partially accounting for gyral formation: Gyri grow outward from the cerebral surface, leaving sulcal bottoms (fundi) behind;[28–31] brain surface passively crinkles;[32,33] and axonal tension causes gyri to form.[34]

Welker

Welker,[28,29] relying on his own work and many earlier investigators, particularly that of Smart and McSherry,[30,31] summarized the literature and his own investigations of gyral development and concluded that the distance between sulcal fundi and either ventricular surface or deep subcortical plate edge remained constant as gyri grew from the cortical surface. Thus, gyral formation results from cortical tissue expansion between sulci. In ferrets and raccoons, the sulcal fundi divide the somatosensory cortex into specific body regions, such as head from trunk and trunk from extremities, and thus predict a strong correspondence of functional area borders with sulci. This hypothesis satisfies several histologic findings in gyral growth:

1   Gyral crown neuronal differentiation and dendrogenesis is greater than in sulcal fundi.
2   Cortical neuronal orientation differs at crown rather than at sulcal fundi.
3   Thalamocortical afferents are more profuse in gyral crowns than in sulcal fundi; and
4   Synaptogenesis is apparently more profuse in crowns than in sulcal walls.

Human gyri and sulcal fundi are not specifically related to functional regions with a few major exceptions.

Van Essen

The cortex folds in a characteristic pattern due to tension along white matter axons according to the tension-based theory of gyral morphogenesis, predicting that functional zones with strong connections should co-vary with sulcal pits such that the aggregate axonal length is minimized.[34,35] Although primary sulci have a more consistent spatial relationship with neighboring functional areas, this does not hold true for secondary and tertiary sulci. There was no strict correspondence between gyral crowns and functional area centers or between sulci and functional borders.[36]

Richman

Additional cortex is achieved by simple mechanical surface buckling into sulci in evolving functionally more complex mammals. Specific sulci grow inward from the cerebral surface[32,33,37] and develop because of simple random buckling from greater tangential growth rates in superficial cortical layers. This concept has never been critically examined and would not account for those observations needing explanation mentioned above.

Sulcal fundi, roots, pits, and annectant gyri

Sulcal fundi extend along the sulcal length, sulcal roots or pits being the deepest parts (Figs. 5.1–5.4). There is more than one sulcal root for major sulci. For instance, the central sulcus [Figs. 5.1, 5.2, 5.4 (c), and 5.9 (Rol)] has two roots, the first frontal sulcus [Fig. 5.2 (f_1)] has three or four roots, and the superior temporal sulcus [Fig. 5.1 (T_1)] usually has four roots and four annectant gyri.[38] There is a general correspondence between the depth of a furrow and its time of origin. The earlier a furrow makes its appearance in fetal brain, the deeper and more stable it will be in the adult brain.[7,39,40] Sulci have fewer deeper level branches and their pattern becomes more consistent across individuals. Agreement between nomenclatures exists only for main sulci.

GYRAL AND SULCAL VARIABILITY FROM SIDE TO SIDE AND HEMISPHERE TO HEMISPHERE

The marked gyral asymmetry and variability exhibited in the human brain was recognized by Ecker in 1873:[2] 'The difficulties which stand in the way of a solution of this problem are numberless, not the least of these being one which is inherent in the very study of the convolutions, viz. the difficulty of recognizing a constant unity of form which underlies the multiplicity of individual variations.'

Lateral sulcal asymmetry was identified during development.[18] The right insula generally develops before the left. Secondary and tertiary gyri and sulci, together constituting a large portion of cortex, create a topography so variable that it seems impossible to establish anatomical correspondence among individuals, and this is reflected in the lack of well-defined neuroanatomic names for some gyri and sulci.[41] In fact, probability maps have been suggested for gyri, sulci, and gyral white matter, even though these would sacrifice interindividual variability information.[42] Quantitative studies of interindividual variation reveal more consistent sulcal patterns at increasing depths below the surface, particularly in monozygotic twins, indicating an increasing genetic influence with increasing sulcal depth (Fig. 5.13).[43] Second, the deepest parts of the sulci form early and retain their identity during development; more complex (and variable) superficial gyri form later.[29-31] We would expect the fundi to have a more consistent relationship to cytoarchitectonic areas than is generally found in sulcal fundi, even though the relationships between sulcal features and cytoarchitectonic areas, being distorted during the process of gyral growth, are difficult to discern in adult brains.[44] Among children, association cortices mature only after somatosensory and visual cortices.[45] Spatial relationships between sulcal landmarks and the underlying functional and architectonic maps are questionable.[1,46] Reliable and precise correspondences for gyral and sulcal subdivisions across different brains are often difficult to establish among individuals because of a lack of clear homologies.[1]

One phenomenon distorting gyral and sulcal relationships is operculation, a growth phenomenon related to the annectant gyrus concept (Fig. 5.6, temporal and frontal opercula). An operculum is a covering or a lid. Operculation occurs when more actively developing cortical regions grow outward or sideways faster than adjacent cortex, which lags behind at sulcal fundi as, for instance, lateral sulcus formation induced by more rapid growth of temporal and frontal lobe operculae. Primary gyri are sometimes indented from side to side, displacing secondary and tertiary sulci out of recognizable position. Another phenomenon distorting gyral and sulcal relationships is buried, or annectant, gyri.[47] According to Cunningham,[47] Gratiolet in 1854 described small gyri buried in main sulcal depths and called them *plis de passage* or crossing gyri. Cunningham called them annectant gyri. An annectant gyrus is a bridging or connecting gyrus deep in the sulcus between two gyri, crossing the sulcal fundus. Near the end of the fifth month, the central sulcus appears in two separate portions. The lower two-thirds appears in the form of a shallow oblique groove. During this period, the posterior annectant gyrus is visible and always superficial. The middle sulcal root becomes visible around the seventh month, anteriorly limiting the intermediate annectant gyrus. Thus, two central sulcus roots divide the fetal central sulcus. Usually, annectant gyri are buried, but in some brains these gyri are externally visible, leading to an interrupted central sulcus. Lastly, in the more consistent sulci and gyri, comparable among individuals, their locations, which can be typically expressed in coordinates based on the anterior and posterior commissures, show high interindividual variation (a range of ±10mm for central and calcarine sulci).[41]

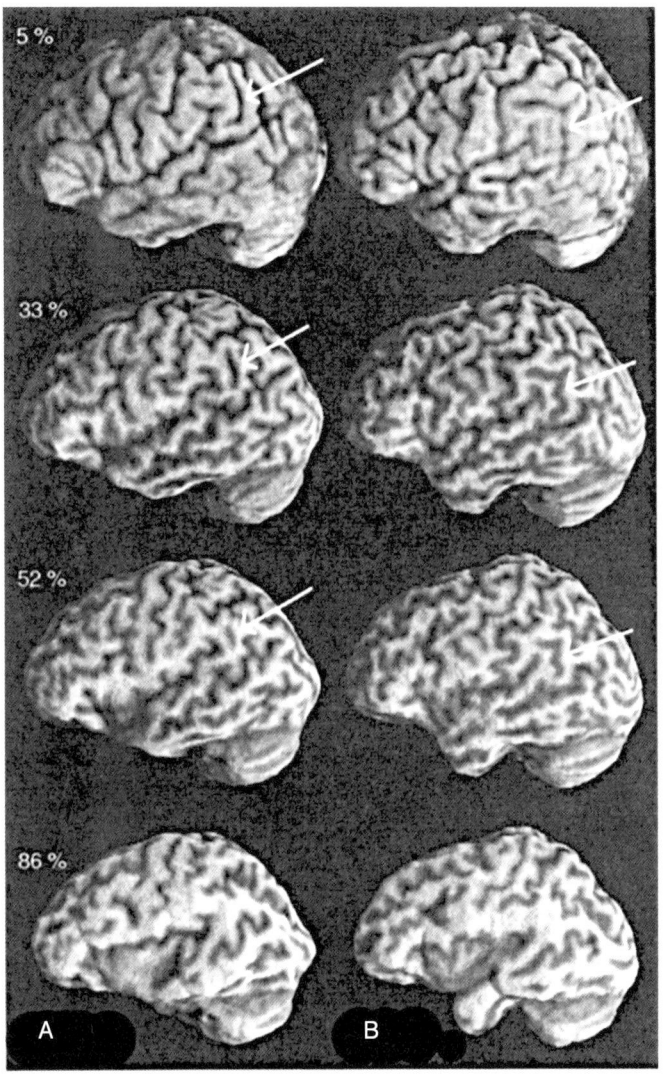

Fig. 5.13 Complexity of sulcal pattern decreases with depth. This image shows the sulcal patterns of two individuals at four different levels of depth. Note the sulcus within the angular gyrus marked by the arrow. The marked sulcus in subject A could be called 'primary intermediate sulcus' as it is a side branch of the intraparietal sulcus, whereas the marked sulcus in subject B is the 'angular sulcus' as it is a branch of the superior temporal sulcus. However, at the innermost depth, it is clear that the two sulci have a common sulcal pit, suggesting they are morphologically homologous. In the lowest pair of images, the insula is well depicted, particularly in subject A. Reproduced with permission of Oxford University Press from Lohmann et al.[7]

87

Gyri, cortical thickness, neuronal maxima, and synapses

Cortical layer thickness increases linearly with age and cortical neuronal density reaches a maximum at 20 to 28 weeks and then declines by about 70%,[48] with additional decreases during adolescence.[49] The human infant's cerebral cortex at term has a gyral pattern similar to the adult cortex, but has only one-third of the total surface area. The gyral pattern is probably unique for each hemisphere and for each individual. Postnatal cortical expansion varies considerably from lobe to lobe and with lobes: regions of lateral temporal, parietal, and frontal cortex expand nearly twice as much as locations in insular and medial occipital cortex.[50,81,82] Within the cerebral cortex, homotypical association cortices mature only after heterotypical agranular somatic motor and granular sensory and visual cortices are developed, and phylogenetically older brain areas mature earlier than newer ones.[45] Thus, primary sensory and motor areas generally attain peak cortical thickness before adjacent secondary areas, and before other polymodal association areas. Specifically, in the brain behind the central sulcus, the first region to reach peak thickness is the granular somatic sensory cortex (8 years), followed by the calcarine cortex, containing striate granular primary visual area (7 years on the left and 8 years on the right), and then the remaining homotypical parieto-occipital cortex, with polymodal regions (such as the posterior parietal cortex) reaching peak thickness later (9–10 years). In the frontal cortex, the primary agranular motor cortex attains peak cortical thickness early (9 years), followed by the supplementary motor areas (10 years) and most of the frontal pole (10 years). High-order cortical areas, such as the dorsolateral homotypical frontal cortex and cingulate cortex, reach peak thickness later (10 years 6 months). The anterior insular transition cortex reaches its maximum thickness at 18 years. In the medial views, the occipital and frontal poles attain peak thickness early, and then a wave sweeps from these areas, with the medial frontal and cingulate cortex attaining peak thickness last. There is also a marked dorsal to ventral progression of development.[51]

Studies in nonhuman animals suggest that cortical dimensions during critical periods for the development of cognitive functions reflect experience-dependent molding of the architecture of cortical columns along with dendritic spine and axonal remodeling.[52–55] Such morphologic events are likely to contribute to the childhood phase of increase in cortical thickness, which occurs in regions with either a cubic or quadratic trajectory. The phase of cortical thinning, dominating adolescence, is likely to reflect the use-dependent selective elimination of synapses that could refine neural circuits, including those supporting cognitive abilities.[51,52,56,57]

Functionally, the posterior medial orbitofrontal areas have been linked with the limbic system and autonomic nervous system control. These areas are thought to monitor the outcomes associated with behavior, particularly punishment or reward[58,59]—cognitive functions so fundamental that they are unlikely to undergo prolonged development. In contrast, isocortical regions often support more complex psychologic functions, which show clear developmental gradients, characterized by rapid development during critical periods. The delineation of critical periods for human skill development is complex, but late childhood is a period of particularly rapid development of executive skills of planning, working memory, and cognitive flexibility, an age period which coincides with an increase in cortical thickness in the lateral frontal cortex.[60] In contrast, the critical period for certain visual functions (such as letter acuity and global motion detection) has been estimated as ending in middle childhood (age 6 or 7 years).[61] Likewise, the period of increase in cortical thickness in the visual cortex also ends around this time (approximately ages 7–8 years).

The fate of all cerebral cortical cells is tied to the cortical vasculature, which supplies oxygen and nutrients, maintains homeostasis, and removes metabolic waste. Considering the increasing surface area of neuronal soma, dendrites, and axons that accompany brain enlargement, it has been estimated that each human neocortical neuron consumes 3.3 times more adenosine triphosphate to fire a single spike than in rats, and 2.6 times more energy to maintain resting potentials.[62]

ISOCORTEX DEVELOPMENT

What distinguishes the cerebral cortex from other brain regions is its remarkable diversity of cellular subtypes arrayed in a stereotyped laminar and radial organization. Six layers, which are generated in an orderly sequence during development, characterize the adult human isocortex of specialized neurons with specific phenotypes and synaptic connections. Cortical neurons generally belong to either of two fundamental classes: projection neurons or interneurons that regulate cortical function through local circuits. Projection neurons have long axons that extend to different cortical areas or to subcortical structures, use the excitatory neurotransmitter glutamate, and usually have a pyramidal morphology. In contrast, interneurons have short axons that arborize locally, use the inhibitory neurotransmitter gamma-aminobutyric acid, and have several morphologies.[63,64] During development of the isocortex, the marginal zone (layer I) and the subplate are the first layers to form subjacent to pia. The cortical plate (layers II–VI) is subsequently established between these superficial and deep components. Neurons in the early zones are thought to play important roles in the formation of the cortex: the marginal zone Cajal–Retzius cells are instrumental in neuronal migration and laminar formation, and subplate cells are involved in cortical connection formation. A substantial proportion of marginal zone neurons, and of the subplate and lower intermediate zone, is not born in the ventricular zone but instead originates in the medial ganglionic eminence (see Chapter 4).[64,65] Each successive generation of migrating neurons passes through the previously born cells before arriving at the final destination at the interface between the cortical plate and the marginal zone. Neurons use a transient population of radial glial cells during migration. According to the radial unit hypothesis of cortical development, the horizontal location of cortical neuron is determined by the position of its precursor cells in the proliferative ventricular zone, while its depth results from its birth order. Disruptions of neuronal migration have been found in several developmental disorders, such as lissencephaly.

SYNAPTIC MAXIMA

There is regional dendritic variation in neonatal human isocortex.[66] Synaptogenesis occurs concurrently with dendritic and axonal growth and with subcortical white matter myelination. Postnatal synaptic density rises after birth, reaches a plateau in childhood, and then decreases to adult levels by late adolescence. In macaque monkeys, subsets of terminal synapses, as well as a subset of en passant synapses, appear and disappear each week with no net change in overall density, suggesting ongoing processes of synaptogenesis and elimination.[66] Huttenlocher and Dabhokar's[56] examination of visual cortex synapse number and density in brain tissue of deceased infants, children, and adults shows an exuberant growth of number and density of synapses from a neonatal level of about 30% to 40% of the adult level to about 80% above the adult level at 6 to 8 months followed by a gradual decline to the norm, an approximate plateau from adolescent to adult age. Synapse formation in granular auditory cortex and homotypical middle frontal gyrus begins before 27 weeks' conceptual age, and reaches a maximum before 1 year of age in primary auditory and visual cortices, and at approximately 3 years and 6 months of age in the middle frontal gyrus. Interestingly, whereas in the human auditory cortex synaptic elimination is complete by 12 years of age, pruning continues until midadolescence in the middle frontal gyrus. The frontal cortex develops somewhat more slowly and declines somewhat later. Further, in human brains there is a separation in time of a few years between peaks in visual cortex synapse density and metabolic rate.[67]

Effects of preterm birth on gyral development
The fetus enters the second half of gestation with a smooth brain. By 22 weeks precentral and postcentral gyri push out from the brain surface, and by the end of the second trimester primary gyri are in place. Should the fetus be delivered at this time, it is likely to have less cortical surface area and less gyral complexity than infants imaged at term, and this is true even in the absence of intraventricular hemorrhage and white matter damage.[68,69] Regional brain volume reductions persist into childhood.[70,71]

Conclusion
Despite approximately equal hemispheral surface areas, the cerebral cortex grows from a smooth surface to a complex convoluted surface, possibly unique for each individual and for each hemisphere. The deepest cortical parts form early and, despite much operculation, are retained during development. Brain expansion (as in the frontal lobe, see reference 72), lobation, gyral growth, and operculation modify the earliest formed gyri. Maximal gyral appearance and development occurs concomitantly with the late second-trimester major brain weight acceleration. In normal fetuses, the sulcation landmarks emerge on magnetic resonance images, in the same order predicted by anatomic studies, as long as the same defining features are used, in contrast to the 0- to 8-week lag in imaging visualization of sulci reported elsewhere.[73]

Although asymmetry of gyral patterns has been recognized since the late nineteenth century,[18,47] the extent of interindividual and interhemispheric variation in gyral pattern, caused by secondary and tertiary gyration, continues to annoy neuroanatomists and neuroradiologists. For instance, the positions and extent of striate and extrastriate cortex (Brodmann's areas 17 and 18) have major interhemispheric and interindividual differences;[44,74] both areas reached significantly more caudal and medial positions on the left. Similarly, central sulcus sensory motor variations[75,76] and parasylvian differences between children and adults indicate dramatic changes into young adulthood.[77] To further complicate gyral pattern recognition, major sex differences exist in the human olfactory system.[78] There are marked increases in morphologic complexity of secondary and tertiary sulci in frontal and postcentral areas[79] and for multiple sulci during childhood, as well as asymmetry of lateral, superior temporal, inferior frontal, inferior temporal, occipitotemporal, and interparietal sulci.[46] These changes are reflected dramatically in appropriate callosal regions in children who are repeatedly scanned over time.[80] All of this happens in both hemispheres with about the same surface area throughout the fetal period.

REFERENCES

1. Zilles K, Schlaug G, Matelli M, et al (1995) Mapping of human and macaque sensorimotor areas by integrating architectonic, transmitter receptor, MRI and PET data. *J Anat* 187: 515–537.
2. Ecker A (1873) *On the Convolutions of the Human Brain*. London: Smith, Elder & Co.
3. Rakic P (1988) Specification of cerebral cortical areas. *Science* 241(4862): 170–176.
4. Golgi C (1873) Sulla struttura della sostanza grigia del cervello. *Gazzetta Medica Italiana, Lombardia* 33: 244–246.
5. Magini J (1888) Sur la névroglie et les cellules céré chez le fetus. *Arch Ital Biol* 9: 59–60.
6. Ecker A (1868) Zur Entwicklungsgeschichte der Furchen und Windungen der Grosshirnhemisphären im Fetus des Menschen. *Arch f Anthrop* 3: 203–224.
7. Lohmann G, von Cramon DY, Colchester AC (2008) Deep sulcal landmarks provide an organizing framework for human cortical folding. *Cereb Cortex* 18: 1415–1420.
8. Hesdorffer MB, Scammon RE (1935) Growth of human nervous system; growth of cerebral surface. *Proc Soc Exper Biol Med* 33: 415–418.
9. Jammes JL, Gilles FH (1983) Telencephalic development: matrix volume and isocortex and allocortex surface areas. In: Gilles FH, Leviton A, Dooling EC, editors. *The Developing Human Brain Growth and Epidemiologic Neuropathology*. Littleton: John Wright – PSG, Inc, pp. 87–93.
10. Vogt C, Vogt O (1919) Allegemeinere ergebnisse unserer hirnforschung. *J Psychol u Neurol* 25: 279–462.
11. Filimonov IN (1947) Rational subdivision of the cerebral cortex. *Arch Neurol Psychiatry* 58: 296–311.
12. Yakovlev P (1967) Telencephalon 'impar', 'semipar', and 'totopar' (morphologic, tectogenetic and architectonic definitions). *Int J Neurol* 6: 245–265.
13. Rorke L, Riggs H (1969) *Myelination of the Brain in the Newborn*. Philadelphia: JB Lippincott.
14. Retzius G (1896) *Das Menschenhirn. Studien in der Makroskopischen Morphologie*. Stockholm: P.A. Norstedt & Söner.
15. Hochstetter F (1929) *Beitrage zur Entwicklungsgeschichte des Menschlichen Gehirns*. Vienna and Leipzig: Deuticke.
16. Dorovini-Zis K, Dolman CL (1977) Gestational development of brain. *Arch Pathol Lab Med* 101: 192–195.
17. Chi JG, Dooling EC, Gilles FH (1977) Gyral development of the human brain. *Ann Neurol* 1: 86–93.
18. Cunningham D (1891) The development of the gyri and sulci on the surface of the island of Reil of the brain. *J Anat Physiol* 25: 338–348.
19. Afif A, Bouvier R, Buenerd A, Trouillas J, Mertens P (2007) Development of the human fetal insular cortex: study of the gyration from 13 to 28 gestational weeks. *Brain Struct Funct* 212: 335–346.
20. Streeter GL (1912) The development of the nervous system. In: Keibal F, Mall FP, editors. *Manual of Human Embryology*. Philadelphia: Lippincott, pp. 1–156.
21. Eberstaller O (1887) Zur Anatomie und Morphologie der Insula Reilii. *Anat Anz* 24: 739–760.
22. Leonard CM, Puranik C, Kuldau JM, Lombardino LJ (1998) Normal variation in the frequency and location of human auditory cortex landmarks. Heschl's gyrus: where is it? *Cereb Cortex* 8: 397–406.
23. Larroche J (1966) The development of the central nervous system during intrauterine life. In: Falkner F, editor. *Human Development*. Philadelphia: WB Saunders, pp. 257–276.
24. Geschwind N, Levitsky W (1968) Human brain: left–right asymmetries in temporal speech region. *Science* 161: 186–187.
25. Witelson S, Pallie W (1973) Left hemisphere specialization for language in the newborn. Neuroanatomical evidence of asymmetry. *Brain* 96: 641–646.
26. Wada J, Clarke R, Hamm A (1975) Cerebral hemispheric asymmetry in humans. Cortical speech zones in 100 adult and 100 infant brains. *Arch Neurol* 32: 239–246.
27. Bossy J, Godlewski G, Maurel JC (1976) [Study of right–left asymmetry of the temporal planum in the fetus]. *Bull Assoc Anat (Nancy)* 60(169): 253–258.

28. Welker WI, Campos GB (1963) Physiological significance of sulci in somatic sensory cerebral cortex in mammals of the family procyonidae. *J Comp Neurol* 120: 19–36.
29. Welker W (1990) Why does the cerebral cortex fissure and fold? In: Peters A, Jones EG, editors. *Cerebral Cortex*. New York: Plenum Press, pp. 1–135.
30. Smart IH, McSherry GM (1986) Gyrus formation in the cerebral cortex in the ferret. I. Description of the external changes. *J Anat* 146: 141–152.
31. Smart IH, McSherry GM (1986) Gyrus formation in the cerebral cortex of the ferret. II. Description of the internal histological changes. *J Anat* 147: 27–43.
32. Clark WEL (1945) Deformation patterns in the cerebral cortex. In: Le Gros Clark WE, Medawar PB, editors. *Essays on Growth and Form Presented to D'Arcy Wentworth Thompson*. Oxford: Clarendon Press, pp. 1–22.
33. Richman DP, Stewart RM, Caviness VS Jr. (1974) Cerebral microgyria in a 27-week fetus: an architectonic and topographic analysis. *J Neuropathol Exp Neurol* 33: 374–384.
34. Van Essen DC (1997) A tension-based theory of morphogenesis and compact wiring in the central nervous system. *Nature* 385(6614): 313–318.
35. Hilgetag CC, Barbas H (2006) Role of mechanical factors in the morphology of the primate cerebral cortex. *PLoS Comput Biol* 2: e22.
36. Hasnain MK, Fox PT, Woldorff MG (2006) Hemispheric asymmetry of sulcus-function correspondence: quantization and developmental implications. *Hum Brain Mapp* 27: 277–287.
37. Jerison HJ (1973) *Evolution of the Brain and Intelligence*. New York: Academic Press.
38. Mangin JF, Riviere D, Cachia A, et al (2004) A framework to study the cortical folding patterns. *Neuroimage* 23(Suppl 1): S129–13.
39. Pansch A (1877) Einige sätze über die grosshirnfaltungen. *Centralblatt für die Medicinischen* (36).
40. Regis J, Mangin JF, Ochiai T, et al (2005) 'Sulcal root' generic model: a hypothesis to overcome the variability of the human cortex folding patterns. *Neurol Med Chir (Tokyo)* 45: 1–17.
41. Ono M, Kubik S, Abernathey C (1990) *Atlas of the Cerebral Sulci*. Stuttgart: Thieme.
42. Tzourio-Mazoyer N, Herve PY, Mazoyer B (2007) Neuroanatomy: tool for functional localization, key to brain organization. *Neuroimage* 37: 1059–1060; discussion 66–68.
43. Lohmann G, von Cramon DY, Steinmetz H (1999) Sulcal variability of twins. *Cereb Cortex* 9: 754–763.
44. Amunts K, Malikovic A, Mohlberg H, Schormann T, Zilles K (2000) Brodmann's areas 17 and 18 brought into stereotaxic space—where and how variable? *Neuroimage* 11: 66–84.
45. Gogtay N, Giedd JN, Lusk L, et al (2004) Dynamic mapping of human cortical development during childhood through early adulthood. *Proc Natl Acad Sci USA* 101: 8174–8179.
46. Blanton RE, Levitt JG, Thompson PM, et al (2001) Mapping cortical asymmetry and complexity patterns in normal children. *Psychiatry Res* 107: 29–43.
47. Cunningham D (1892) *Surface Anatomy of the Cerebral Hemispheres*. Dublin: Academy House.
48. Rabinowicz T, de Courten-Myers GM, Petetot JM, Xi G, de los Reyes E (1996) Human cortex development: estimates of neuronal numbers indicate major loss late during gestation. *J Neuropathol Exp Neurol* 55: 320–328.
49. Rabinowicz T, Petetot JM, Khoury JC, de Courten-Myers GM (2009) Neocortical maturation during adolescence: change in neuronal soma dimension. *Brain Cogn* 69: 328–336.
50. Hill J, Inder T, Neil J, Dierker D, Harwell J, Van Essen D (2010) Similar patterns of cortical expansion during human development and evolution. *Proc Natl Acad Sci USA* 107: 13135–13140.
51. Shaw P, Kabani NJ, Lerch JP, et al (2008) Neurodevelopmental trajectories of the human cerebral cortex. *J Neurosci* 28: 3586–3594.
52. Mataga N, Mizuguchi Y, Hensch TK (2004) Experience-dependent pruning of dendritic spines in visual cortex by tissue plasminogen activator. *Neuron* 44: 1031–1041.
53. Chklovskii DB (2004) Exact solution for the optimal neuronal layout problem. *Neural Comput* 16: 2067–2078.
54. Chklovskii DB (2004) Synaptic connectivity and neuronal morphology: two sides of the same coin. *Neuron* 43: 609–617.
55. Hensch TK (2005) Critical period plasticity in local cortical circuits. *Nat Rev Neurosci* 6: 877–888.
56. Huttenlocher PR, Dabholkar AS (1997) Regional differences in synaptogenesis in human cerebral cortex. *J Comp Neurol* 387: 167–178.
57. Fagiolini M, Fritschy JM, Low K, Mohler H, Rudolph U, Hensch TK (2004) Specific GABAA circuits for visual cortical plasticity. *Science* 303(5664): 1681–1683.

58. Rolls ET (2004) The functions of the orbitofrontal cortex. *Brain Cogn* 55: 11–29.
59. Kennerley SW, Walton ME, Behrens TE, Buckley MJ, Rushworth MF (2006) Optimal decision making and the anterior cingulate cortex. *Nat Neurosci* 9: 940–947.
60. Burton H, Snyder AZ, Diamond JB, Raichle ME (2002) Adaptive changes in early and late blind: a FMRI study of verb generation to heard nouns. *J Neurophysiol* 88: 3359–3371.
61. MacKay TL, Jakobson LS, Ellemberg D, Lewis TL, Maurer D, Casiro O (2005) Deficits in the processing of local and global motion in very low birthweight children. *Neuropsychologia* 43: 1738–1748.
62. Sherwood CC, Stimpson CD, Raghanti MA, et al (2006) Evolution of increased glia–neuron ratios in the human frontal cortex. *Proc Natl Acad Sci USA* 103: 13606–13611.
63. Anderson SA, Eisenstat DD, Shi L, Rubenstein JL (1997) Interneuron migration from basal forebrain to neocortex: dependence on *Dlx* genes. *Science* 278(5337): 474–476.
64. Lavdas AA, Grigoriou M, Pachnis V, Parnavelas JG (1999) The medial ganglionic eminence gives rise to a population of early neurons in the developing cerebral cortex. *J Neurosci* 19: 7881–7888.
65. Parnavelas JG, Anderson SA, Lavdas AA, Grigoriou M, Pachnis V, Rubenstein JL (2000) The contribution of the ganglionic eminence to the neuronal cell types of the cerebral cortex. *Novartis Found Symp* 228: 129–139; discussion 39–47.
66. Travis K, Ford K, Jacobs B (2005) Regional dendritic variation in neonatal human cortex: a quantitative Golgi study. *Dev Neurosci* 27: 277–287.
67. Chugani HT (1998) A critical period of brain development: studies of cerebral glucose utilization with PET. *Prev Med* 27: 184–188.
68. Ajayi-Obe M, Saeed N, Cowan FM, Rutherford MA, Edwards AD (2000) Reduced development of cerebral cortex in extremely preterm infants. *Lancet* 356(9236): 1162–1163.
69. Inder TE, Warfield SK, Wang H, Huppi PS, Volpe JJ (2005) Abnormal cerebral structure is present at term in premature infants. *Pediatrics* 115: 286–294.
70. Peterson BS, Vohr B, Kane MJ, et al (2002) A functional magnetic resonance imaging study of language processing and its cognitive correlates in prematurely born children. *Pediatrics* 110: 1153–1162.
71. Soria-Pastor S, Padilla N, Zubiaurre-Elorza L, et al (2009) Decreased regional brain volume and cognitive impairment in preterm children at low risk. *Pediatrics* 124: e1161–1170.
72. Sowell ER, Thompson PM, Holmes CJ, Jernigan TL, Toga AW (1999) In vivo evidence for post-adolescent brain maturation in frontal and striatal regions. *Nat Neurosci* 2: 859–861.
73. Levine D, Barnes PD (1999) Cortical maturation in normal and abnormal fetuses as assessed with prenatal MR imaging. *Radiology* 210: 751–758.
74. Filimonoff IN (1932) Über die Variabilität der Großhirnrindenstruktur. Mitteilung II Regio occipitalis beim erwachsenen Menschen. *J Psychol u Neurol* 45: 65–137.
75. White LE, Andrews TJ, Hulette C, et al (1997) Structure of the human sensorimotor system. I: Morphology and cytoarchitecture of the central sulcus. *Cereb Cortex* 7: 18–30.
76. White LE, Andrews TJ, Hulette C, et al (1997) Structure of the human sensorimotor system. II: Lateral symmetry. *Cereb Cortex* 7: 31–47.
77. Sowell ER, Thompson PM, Rex D, et al (2002) Mapping sulcal pattern asymmetry and local cortical surface gray matter distribution in vivo: maturation in perisylvian cortices. *Cereb Cortex* 12: 17–26.
78. Garcia-Falgueras A, Junque C, Gimenez M, Caldu X, Segovia S, Guillamon A (2006) Sex differences in the human olfactory system. *Brain Res* 1116: 103–111.
79. Turner O (1948) Growth and development of the cerebral pattern in man. *Arch Neurol Psychiatry* 59: 1–12.
80. Thompson PM, Giedd JN, Woods RP, MacDonald D, Evans AC, Toga AW (2000) Growth patterns in the developing brain detected by using continuum mechanical tensor maps. *Nature* 404(6774): 190–193.
81. Gilles FH, Leviton A, Dooling EC (1983) *The Developing Human Brain: Growth and Epidemiologic Neuropathology*. Boston: Wright-PSG.
82. Dooling EC, Chi J, Gilles FH (1983) Telencephalic development: changing gyral patterns. In: Gilles FH, Leviton A, Dooling EC, editors. *The Developing Human Brain: Growth and Epidemiologic Neuropathology*. Boston: Wright-PSG, pp. 94–104.
83. Roberts M, Hanaway J (1987) *Atlas of the Human Brain in Section*, 2nd edn. Philadelphia: Lea & Febiger.
84. Putz R, Pabst R, editors (2006) *Sobotta Atlas der Anatomie des Menschen*, 22nd edn. Munich: Urban & Fischer.
85. Chi J, Dooling EC, Gilles FH (1977). Left–right asymmetries of the temporal speech areas of the human fetus. *Arch Neurol* 34: 346–348.

6
MYELINATED TRACTS: GROWTH PATTERNS

Introduction

HISTORY

The freshly cut adult brain has two basic components, gray matter and white matter, a distinction recognized in the sixteenth century. While not describing the difference between gray and white matter, Vesalius[1] drew a separate cortex and underlying white matter. It took another 30 years before Colter (1572) and Piccolomini (1586) described the distinction between white and gray matter (quoted from ref. 2).[3] Another 230 years passed before Tiedemann (1816) recognized that there was no distinction between white and gray matter in the freshly cut fetal or neonatal brain.[4] In Tiedemann's time there was no achromatic microscope, which did not become available until 1830, nor were there adequate microtomes, or cell or myelin stains until the 1870s. Leeuwenhoek probably saw myelin (from Greek *myelos*, marrow) around the axon. However, still thinking under the Galenic dogma that nerves were fine tubes through which a liquid flowed, in a 1717 letter he described and drew minute tubules containing a 'central cavity.' In his figure, the 'central cavity' looks like the axon.[3]

After Tiedemann, apparently little was done on fetal or infantile myelination until Paul Flechsig took up this issue in 1872, making a detailed study of human tract myelination.[5,6] Flechsig recognized that myelin is deposited at diverse and relatively specific developmental times in selected dorsal or ventral roots, specific tracts, and in differing parts of an individual axon.[7] Cranial and spinal nerve root motor fibers myelinate slightly before sensory fibers, except for the vestibular portion of the acoustic nerve that myelinates simultaneously with other cranial motor fibers. Myelination continues throughout childhood and much of adolescence,[8] and possibly into adulthood.[9] He showed that cerebral cortex regions myelinate at dissimilar times and subdivided the cortex into 40 or 50 regions on the basis of myelination time. Myelin accumulation contributes a major portion of brain growth late in gestation and postnatally; in late fetal brain, myelinated pathways constitute a dramatic and prominent feature. Recent reviews have extensively summarized myelination, biochemistry, and ultrastructure,[10,11] so only a few salient points will be repeated.

This chapter demonstrates the sequence of myelination during the time period of most dramatic myelination, using (1) a sample of fetuses and (2) a separate sample of infants from birth through the second postnatal year. Both studies assessed myelination in all autopsied fetuses or infants, irrespective of disease entities, except those well substantiated to adversely affect myelination or myelin staining. We also use selected images from the literature as well as selected magnetic resonance images of fetuses and infants to explicate the development of white matter in the human. Finally, we explicate the effects of delayed myelination and hypoplastic white matter on the neonate.

HISTOLOGIC CHANGES

For each myelinating tract, there is a difference in the time when prospective white matter is penetrated by axons and the later time when myelinogenesis begins, the latter marked by the appearance of a local glial cell population increase. For instance, medial longitudinal fasciculus axons are present by 4 to 5 weeks,[12] but its myelination begins early in the second half of gestation. Cerebral, brainstem, and spinal cord white matter contain axons during the first half of gestation, few of which are myelinated, although aversive responses occur to lip stimulation (see Chapter 9). Later in gestation, at a site about to myelinate, glial cells change dramatically just before and during myelin sheath deposition. This process, unfortunately designated 'myelination gliosis',[13] implies similarity to the commonly used term 'astrogliosis.' However, glial cells undergoing myelination-associated changes do not have the cytoplasmic eosinophilia of hypertrophic astrocytes or the glial fibrils of fibrillary astrocytosis during myelination. A subset of glial cells develops large nuclei (up to 15 μm in diameter), pale, and vesicular with fine chromatin stippling. These large nuclei seem 'naked'.[14–16] The nucleoli enlarge and become prominent, and cytoplasm accumulates premyelin lipids, in part as sterol esters, that contribute to marked cellular sudanophilia. These histologic events, demonstrated in the human, pig, lagomorph, monkey, ruminant, and carnivore,[17–19] are easily confused with glial fatty metamorphosis[20,21] (see Chapter 11). Virchow (1867)[22] identified these sudanophilic cells and considered them abnormal. Parrot (1868)[23] confirmed their presence. Jastrowitz[24–26] thought that these cells were part of myelination, but as a byproduct. Others generally agreed that lipids, stored in glial cells, were used for myelin sheath formation. Flechsig[6] found a connection between the number of fat-containing glial cells and the myelination process intensity in different spinal cord regions. Most authors agree that the majority of neonates have fat-containing glia,[14] that the regions of fat-containing glia are not necrotic, and fat-filled macrophages differ from fat-containing glia. Most also agree that the cellular populations of unmyelinated, myelinating, and previously myelinated regions of hemispheral white matter are distinct. The fat-surrounded glial cells have long expansions in many directions. Nerve fibers are normal even in fat-surrounded fibers.[14,16] After birth, the fat-containing glial cells disappear at about 8 months of age.[27] It appears that the earliest axons to myelinate are the largest.[28]

In the forebrain, after neurons migrate from the ventricular wall to form the cerebral cortex, axons, to and from the cortex, elongate and extend to intracortical and subcortical targets. These axonal changes start during migration, gradually unfolding until well after completion of migration. In human parietal lobe cortex, neurofilaments are found only after midgestation. Molecular and genetic markers of axonal growth and elongation have high levels of expression after 21 postconceptional weeks and lower levels beyond 17 postnatal months. Markers of myelination, such as myelin basic protein expression, are found in the parietal lobe during the middle of the first postnatal year, reaching adult levels early in the second postnatal year,[29] but this author does not mention which parietal lobe myelinating axonal systems were used.

The first peripheral nerve to exhibit loose myelin is the trigeminal in its ganglion when the first Schwann cell revolutions occur during the twelfth week. Three weeks later, the trigeminal myelin sheath increases in thickness and becomes a compact, laminated structure.[30]

Myelin appears first in ventral roots between 17 and 18 postconceptional weeks at C8-Th1; in the lumbosacral cord between 25 and 34 weeks; and, to a lesser extent, in dorsal roots at the same spinal level and location.[31] However, Keene and Hewer[32] detected myelination of a few posterior root fibers and the cuneate fasciculus by 14 weeks, but did not mention the specific spinal level. Sciatic nerve myelination begins between the sixteenth and eighteenth week, and the number of myelinated fibers increases with advancing age.[33] At 15 weeks, the phrenic nerve is composed mainly of large bundles of axons surrounded by one or two Schwann cell layers. Eight weeks later, it contains many axons with thick compact myelin sheaths as well as fibers in early-stage myelin formation.[34] Sural nerve myelination occurs between 21 and 36 weeks.[35]

BIOCHEMICAL EVENTS ASSOCIATED WITH MYELINATION

The accumulation of central nervous system myelin lipid components has been demonstrated biochemically or histochemically in several species, including the human.[17,18,31,36–45] Cerebroside (and probably sulfatide) appears concurrently with first stainability of the myelin sheath. A local increase in activity of several enzymes (particularly oxidative enzymes) accompanies the local increased numbers of glial cells during myelination.[46] Simultaneously, esterified lipids decrease and white matter histochemical characteristics change as mature myelin accumulates. Glial cell density diminishes as enlarging myelin sheaths displace glial nuclei[47], and glial cells gradually acquire the form of mature oligodendroglia.

During proliferation of glial cells, many myelin lipid constituents accumulate in prospective white matter before myelin deposition. Biochemical sequences of myelin-associated lipids and myelin-specific proteins closely follow previously described anatomic sequences temporally, and are identical in all sites sampled; sphingomyelin is followed simultaneously by cerebrosides, myelin basic protein, proteolipid protein, and nonhydroxy-sulfatide, followed by hydroxy-sulfatide. The expression, onset, and tempo of individual constituents were quite variable among sites. Cholesterol ester was transiently elevated during late gestation and early infancy when cerebrosides, sulfatides, proteolipid protein, and myelin basic protein were being deposited.[11]

Myelin basic protein was the first oligodendrocyte marker detected in the spinal cord, present at 10 weeks at more rostral levels. Proteolipid protein and myelin-associated glycoprotein were detected 2 to 4 weeks later. By the late second trimester, expression of all three was noted in spinal white matter in all locations except the corticospinal tract. Expression of myelin-associated glycoprotein was particularly marked at the posterior root entry zone and propriospinal tracts.[48]

The morphologic events leading to myelin sheath deposition are transient. Thus, it would be expected that tracts containing fibers that myelinate simultaneously and rapidly (for instance, with a short 'myelinogenetic cycle',[9] such as the medial longitudinal fasciculus) would have little mix of sudanophilic material among myelinated axons. Conversely, telencephalic white matter, with wave after wave of different systems myelinating over prolonged periods of time, is expected to contain mixtures of variably myelinated fibers and sudanophilic material (a marker of sterol esters) for the process duration.

There is agreement that myelination of multiple brain-connecting systems takes place at varying times in development;[4,8] one cannot speak correctly of 'myelination' as a single event occurring at a specific developmental time.[11] Myelination tempo differs among tracts, and there is marked, easily recognizable temporal diversity in topographic myelination patterns throughout the last half of gestation and first postnatal year. In humans, the process of myelination is almost completed within the lengthy period from beginning medial longitudinal fasciculus myelin deposition near the end of the first half of gestation (in some fetuses) to the second postnatal year. Moreover, some authors report myelination in a few systems in the isocortex some decades later.[9] Therefore, a sample of white matter containing several tracts is likely to look entirely different from a comparable sample from the same region at another developmental time or from another region at the same time.

SITE-SPECIFIC GESTATIONAL BIOLOGIC VARIATION IN TIME OF MYELINATION

There are several ways to approach the questions of when a specific tract myelinates and the sequence in which it myelinates. It is not possible to find the precise gestational age of myelin deposition onset at any site for the human; specimens are limited to brains obtained at different gestational or postnatal ages (from the random processes contributing to death and who gets autopsied). Myelin presence at any degree of intensity at each specific site can be related to a real time measure of development (for example, gestational age) or to a stage of development as estimated by some body measurement (for example, body length or weight). Often authors using these strategies apparently assumed that myelin emerges at each site at a specific time or stage in development,[6,8,32] and therefore ignored the realities of normal biologic variation, and, more importantly, the effect of adverse fetal environmental circumstances (which may have contributed to the fetus's death) on times of myelin deposition at each site.

Nevertheless, as with all biologic systems, there is predictable variation in myelination degree at any given site with respect to estimated gestational age, body length, and body weight.[49] Rorke and Riggs[49] found that, using body measurements for grouping, the proportions of fetuses in each group displayed a standard pattern of myelinated pathways. Concomitantly, they recognized a retarded set of brains in each group, and thus were the first authors to recognize morphologically delayed myelination. In this chapter, formal measures of biologic variation and degree of myelination at each specific myelinating site are provided. Unfortunately, ranges and confidence intervals for each gestational age are sufficiently wide, a result of small sample sizes, to sometimes obscure the details of specific myelination sequences.

Any level, degree, or intensity of myelination can be used as an end point as long as the parameter is clear. Even ultrastructural first myelin lamellae detection has been proposed as the marker of myelination onset.[50] For instance, the first turns of Schwann cell processes around peripheral trigeminal ganglion axons occur in the twelfth week.[30] Beginning phrenic nerve myelination is later at 15 weeks.[34] However, the problems of sampling sites and preserving tissue for adequate ultrastructural examination seem almost insurmountable for efficient application to a large number of sites in many fetal brains, particularly in view of the large number of cases necessary to ascertain simultaneously normal biologic variation. Other authors used microscopic and gross levels of myelination for ascertainment. Immature white matter grossly looks gelatinous gray and is barely distinguishable from adjacent gray matter except by location. Creamy white myelinating systems stand out in prominent relief against this translucent background, allowing a first gross assessment of myelination degree.

Several limitations and assumptions weaken previous myelination human fetal brain studies. The first limitation is a small number or, even, single cases at each gestational age. Second is the assumption of a fixed fetal age of myelin deposition at each specific brain site.[6,8,9,32] For instance, Keene and Hewer[32] used nine fetuses (ranging in age from 14 to 36 weeks; two were less than 20 weeks), four term neonates, and three infants (3–9 months). These two limitations lessen recognition of the wide range in myelin deposition times at any specific site. As will be seen later in this chapter, the idea of a broad time range for myelin deposition and rate of development at each specific site in fetal brain is important in myelination assessment. The third limitation of previous studies is the lack of a formal myelination degree ranking system. For instance, several studies never state whether the authors used gross or microscopic slide inspection to assess myelination degree. This accounts for conflicting literature statements as to when a tract 'first appears' or 'first commences.' To evaluate a brain for possible effects of an adverse maternal or fetal environment on myelin accumulation, comparisons of myelination degree must be as specific as possible, and a reference population must be available.

The following studies attempted to minimize these limitations by using (1) a large number of cases, (2) a formal system ranking myelin amount or degree at each site, and (3) by using several analyses, each with different assumptions, to provide multiple viewpoints of sequential patterns of developing system tract myelination.

Materials and methods

TWO DATA SETS: PRENATAL AND POSTNATAL
Our material for prenatal myelination consisted of myelin-stained, serially sectioned National Institute of Neurological and Communicative Disorders and Stroke fetal brains of 20 to 40 weeks.[51] The material for postnatal myelination consisted of myelin-stained random sections of 'least abnormal' brains ranging in age from 37 gestational weeks to 24 postnatal months.[52] The use of two data sets (each with its own collection criteria, section thickness, and histologic stain) probably induced the discrepancies noted between prenatal and postnatal timing for some tracts.

Prenatal data set

The National Collaborative Perinatal Project (NCPP) data consisted of information about the degree of myelination at 53 sites in 323 serially sectioned human fetal brains from the last half of gestation. The spinal cord was included in about one-third of cases. Brains with marked hemorrhagic disruption or malformation, inadequate staining, and those greater than one postnatal month in age were excluded. The remaining cases were included without a priori judgment of whether or not the amount of myelin was 'normal'. The NCPP utilized celloidin-embedded, Loyez-stained sections 20μm thick. The myelination assessment sites were chosen for three reasons: first, the site had to be easily found in the absence of nearby myelinated landmarks; second, most sites had to be large enough to assess with the unaided eye (in the majority of cases older than 20 weeks); third, while all tracts in the central nervous system could not be evaluated, those chosen would complete a large portion of myelination during gestation and others, with either slow or rapid myelination, that would begin myelination during the second half of gestation.

Postnatal data set

For the study of postnatal myelination, we added several additional tracts, particularly in the brainstem and forebrain, which included 62 tracts in 162 postnatal infants from the first 2 years of life [term newborn infants (≥37 weeks' gestation) to 33 months postconception]. Preterm infants who lived at least 1 month and attained a postconceptional age of more than 260 days were included. Newborns with a gestational age of less than 37 weeks and a birthweight of less than 2500g were classified as preterm. From this entire pool, cases were randomly drawn for study to obtain a minimum of five or a maximum of 10 cases at each postconceptional month. Cases excluded from evaluation were those with (1) severe central nervous system malformations precluding clear identification of white matter sites; (2) leukodystrophies, for instance Alexander or Krabbe disease; (3) widespread pannecrosis involving gray and white matter altering myelin-stain tinctorial properties (so-called 'respirator brain'); and (4) those with infarcts or hemorrhages. The 10-μm sections were stained with hematoxylin, eosin, and luxol fast blue. The thinner sections probably decreased the possibility of finding microscopic myelin tubules, the earliest indicator of myelination in both the NCPP and the postnatal studies.

METHODS

For each case, a myelination check-off sheet was filled out. For the prenatal cases, every hundredth Loyez-stained serial section was inspected; if a tract was not identified in that section, additional intervening sections were examined. For the postnatal cases, all slides were inspected. We used an internal standard tract in each case for myelin staining variability, a tract that had been exposed to the same premorbid and processing conditions as all other tracts in that case; the medial longitudinal fasciculus for prenatal cases and inferior cerebellar peduncle for postnatal cases. For further details, see the original publications.[51,52]

Case handling
After randomization, two observers reviewed the slides simultaneously with discussion to agree on myelination degree without knowledge of estimated gestational age or clinical history. This tactic is helpful in reducing observer variation.[53]

Myelin ranking

Prenatal myelination
The degree of myelination of each tract was ranked on an ordinal scale: 3, grossly visible myelin or the intensity of myelin staining approaching that of a mature brain or, operationally, the intensity of medullary medial longitudinal fasciculus staining of a late gestational or postnatal fetus; 2, myelin staining just perceived by the unaided eye (see below); 1, myelin visible microscopically, but not as above (2 or 3); 0, no myelin seen microscopically.

These four degrees of myelin intensity are not to be construed as equal steps in tract myelination. Thus, the increment of myelin represented in the change from degree 1 to degree 2 is not necessarily equal to the increment of myelin represented in the change from degree 2 to degree 3. This system of evaluating intensity is merely a ranking system.

Postnatal myelination
Postnatal myelination required a grading system modification. Because the inferior cerebellar peduncle (ICP) reaches an advanced degree of myelination early in the third trimester, it was used as an internal standard of comparison. If this structure was grossly visible with a distinctive blue, the case was considered technically adequate and that intensity of blue given a grade of degree 3. The remaining tracts were then ranked on an ordinal scale as follows: 0, no tubules visible at ×400 microscopic magnification; 1, at least one well-defined myelin tubule visible at ×400; 2, a blue color visible to the unaided eye but less intense than the ICP, with well-defined myelin tubules visible at ×400; 3, a grossly visible intensity equal to the ICP; and 4, a deep 'electric' blue intensity greater than the ICP. Occasionally, luxol fast blue lightly stained precursor lipid constituents that accumulate before formation of myelin lamellae; therefore, definite myelin tubules, not background particulate staining, had to be visible at ×400 for a tract to warrant degree 2. For very small tracts, such as stria medullaris thalami and lateral olfactory stria, sharpness of outline proved helpful in distinguishing degree 2 from degree 3.

Statistics

Prenatal myelination
Recording the proportion of encounters of myelin at any degree in each tract demonstrates an age-free myelination progression (Table 6.1). The advantage of this approach is that sequence and myelination direction information is free of limitations of gestational age estimates and/or measures of other body parameters. Thus, the tracts with high percentages of encounters (for instance, the medial longitudinal fasciculus) are expected to start myelination much earlier than tracts with low percentages of encounters (for instance, the optic radiation). Otherwise, for the remainder of this chapter the gestational age at which 50% of cases contained grossly

TABLE 6.1

Progression of fetal myelination by degree 1, 2, or 3 [the percentages of encounters reflect the gestational length over which each site contained any amount (degree 1, 2, or 3) of myelin]

%	Tract
98	Medial longitudinal fasciculus, medulla
97	Medial longitudinal fasciculus, pons
96	Medial longitudinal fasciculus, mesencephalon
96	Fasciculus gracilis, thoracic
96	Fasciculus proprius, lumbar
95	Fasciculus proprius, thoracic
95	Lateral spinothalamic tract, thoracic
95	Fasciculus gracilis, lumbar
94	Fasciculus gracilis, cervical
94	Lateral spinothalamic tract, lumbar
94	Lateral spinothalamic tract, cervical
93	Fasciculus proprius, cervical
92	Dorsal spinocerebellar tract, thoracic
92	Dorsal spinocerebellar tract, cervical
91	Fasciculus cuneatus
91	Medial lemniscus, medulla
90	Inferior cerebellar peduncle
90	Trapezoid body
89	Medial lemniscus, pons
89	Spinal trigeminal tract
88	Lateral lemniscus, pons
85	Lateral lemniscus, mesencephalon
83	Medial lemniscus, mesencephalon
76	Superior cerebellar peduncle, pons
75	Cerebellum, parasagittal
75	Superior cerebellar peduncle, mesencephalon
72	Ansa lenticularis
66	Amiculum, olive
64	Habenulointerpeduncular tract
56	Capsule, red nucleus
53	Optic tract
50	Internal capsule, posterior limb
43	Optic chiasm
41	Middle cerebellar peduncle
40	Corticospinal tract, mesencephalon

TABLE 6.1 (continued)

%	Tract
39	Corticospinal tract, pons
37	Corona radiata, central
37	Transpontine
36	Pyramid
34	Corticospinal tract, cervical
31	Corticospinal tract, thoracic
29	Optic radiation, rostral
29	Cerebellum, hemisphere
25	Internal capsule, anterior limb
25	Corticospinal tract, lumbar
21	Mesencephalic peduncle, lateral
20	Cingulum
19	Optic radiation, occipital
17	Fornix
9	Corpus callosum
5	Mesencephalic peduncle, medial
4	Anterior commissure
1	Mammillothalamic tract

visible myelin (degree 3) is used for comparisons of prenatal and postnatal myelination. For the interested reader, the original publication contains several other ways of presenting data for degrees 1 and 2.[51]

Postnatal myelination

The Ayer method for time-censored (incomplete) data[54,55] provides estimates of postnatal myelination timing. Time-censored data are data where the exact time that an event occurs, such as myelination, cannot be observed directly. For example, at autopsy, a given tract in an infant's brain contains myelin degree 1; it is unknown at what point before the infant's death that degree was attained (left censored). Similarly, if a given tract is not yet myelinated, one needs to assume that the infant would have attained a degree of 2 or 3 at some unknown future time had he lived (right censored). Thus, the Ayer estimate utilizes information obtained from all study age groups to calculate the maximum likelihood estimate of the percentage of infants that will have a specific myelination degree for each age group, and presents it as an expected overall population percentage. In this way, the Ayer estimate differs from a standard percentile. The following tables present the sequence in which at least 50% of cases reached

TABLE 6.2

TABLE 6.2

Grossly visible myelin within spinal cord (percentage of cases containing grossly visible myelin) (degree 3)

Myelinating tract	Prenatal (gross myelination) weeks		
	10%	50%	90%
Proprius, lumbar	<20	35	>40
Proprius, thoracic	<20	37	>40
Proprius, cervical	29	37	>40

No data for postnatal myelination.

degree 3 according to the Ayer estimates. The original publications provide additional data.[52,56] Myelination is organized by functional and anatomic systems.

Sequence of myelination

In biologic groups, if the data values are approximately normally distributed, the median is a statistic such that 50% of data will have values greater than the median, and 50% lower. Ages when 50% of each group had reached grossly visible myelination are most important. When myelination using other than degree 3 (grossly apparent) is described, the appropriate degree is mentioned.

SPINAL CORD

Fasciculus proprius (propriospinal)

Spinospinal fiber systems, lying close to the spinal cord gray matter, are ascending and descending, crossed and uncrossed, and begin and end in the spinal cord (Table 6.2); they support local spinal reflexes (Fig. 6.1).

The spinospinal systems enter the second half of gestation with one-quarter to one-third of cases containing microscopic myelin (degree 1). Cervical fasciculus proprius myelination follows lumbar by about 2 weeks. By gestational end, only about three-quarters of cases have attained degree 3 myelination at all cord levels. For the most part, the growth curves in lumbar, thoracic, and cervical levels are similar.

AFFERENT TO BRAINSTEM AND/OR FOREBRAIN

Spinal

The distal dorsal root ganglionic processes receive impulses from encapsulated somatic receptors such as neuromuscular spindles; neurotendinous organs; touch and pressure receptors of subcutaneous Pacinian or Meissner's corpuscles on joint capsules; muscle surfaces of lower thoracic, lumbar, and sacral regions and pelvis, legs, and toes (supplying the gracile tract);

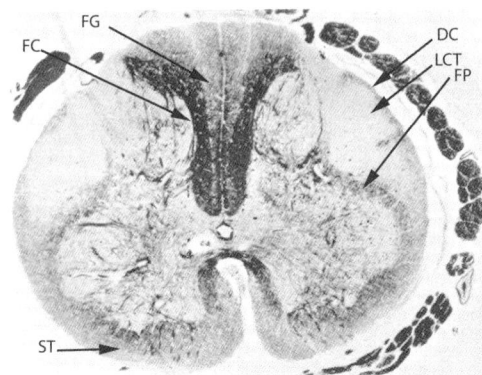

Fig. 6.1 Cervical spinal cord, 25 fetal weeks. Anterior is down. The anterior horn is relatively large, indicating that the section lies between C5 and T1. The fasciculus proprius (FP) is the myelinated (black) band surrounding the anterior horn. The fasciculus cuneatus (FC) (dorsal root fibers from the shoulder girdle, arm, and hand) is considerably more myelinated than the fasciculus gracilis (FG) (dorsal root fibers from the pelvic girdle, leg, foot, and thorax). The lateral corticospinal tract (LCT) is not myelinated. External to the lateral corticospinal tract are the dorsal (posterior) (DC) and ventral (anterior) spinocerebellar tracts. The spinothalamic tract (ST) (external to the fasciculus proprius) is not well myelinated. Well-stained dorsal and ventral roots lie external to the cord. Weigert–Pal myelin stain. Reproduced with permission of John Wiley & Sons, Inc. from Keene and Hewer.[32]

and the shoulders, arms, and hands [supplying the cuneate tract (Fig. 6.1)]. The lower six thoracic and all lumbosacral dorsal root ganglia send long ascending branches up the gracile tracts (located dorsally near the spinal cord midline) to synapse in the medullary gracile nucleus. The cuneate tracts are composed of similar, upper six thoracic and cervical ganglia branches, and lie lateral to the posterior intermediate septum. Thus, some dorsal root ganglia neurons (whose distal processes innervate the foot and toes and whose proximal processes end in medulla) comprise the longest and largest body cells. Both gracile and cuneate tracts carry tactile and kinesthetic sense. The cervical cuneate tract fibers ascend to low medullary levels and terminate somatotopically in the medial cuneate nucleus. Fibers from the lateral cuneate nucleus travel to the forelimb regions of the cerebellar anterior lobe, pyramis, and paramedian cerebellar lobes. Early cuneate tract myelination is likely to be related to these anatomic connections.

Gracile tract (fasciculus gracilis)
The lumbar fasciculus gracilis (Figs. 6.1 and 6.2) enters the second half of gestation with at least 10% of cases containing grossly visible myelin (degree 3) (Table 6.3). Two weeks later, 10% of cases have grossly visible thoracic gracilis myelin, but it takes until 29 weeks to find grossly visible cervical gracilis myelin. In any case, 50% of cases contain grossly visible myelin in lumbar and thoracic gracilis by the end of the second trimester and 90% by 34 weeks. The cervical gracilis is slower by about 5 to 6 weeks and does not reach grossly visible

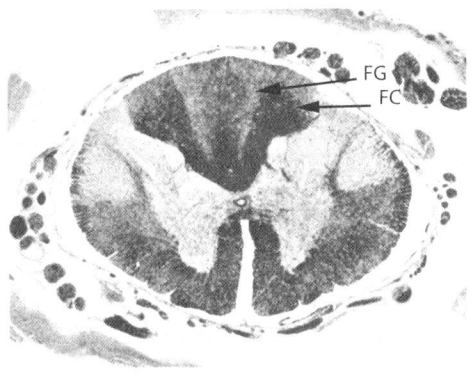

Fig. 6.2 Cervical spinal cord, 36 fetal weeks. Anterior is down. The anterior horn is relatively small, indicating that the section lies between C1 and C4. The anterior and lateral spinothalmic tracts are well myelinated. The fasciculus cuneatus (FC) is more abundant. The fasciculus gracilis (FG) is wider but still not fully myelinated. The anterior and posterior spinocerebellar tracts (external to the unmyelinated lateral corticospinal tract) are more fully stained. Weigert–Pal myelin stain. Reproduced with permission of John Wiley & Sons, Inc. from Keene and Hewer.[32]

myelin in 90% of cases until term. These findings are consistent with caudal–rostral gracile tract myelination, with most fibers gathering their myelin simultaneously at levels of tract origination (largely lumbar and lower thoracic spinal cord) and then myelinating rostrally.

Cuneate tract (fasciculus cuneatus)

While the fasciculus cuneatus (Figs. 6.1 and 6.2) enters midgestation with 10% of cases myelinated, it myelinates more rapidly than the cervical gracilis, with 50% of cases myelinated at the end of the second trimester and 90% of cases at 37 weeks. This is 4 weeks earlier than cervical gracilis myelination, and thus follows a myelination pattern unlike any other spinal cord system (Table 6.3). The contrast between cuneate and gracile tract myelination is reflected in gracile tract pallor and striking myelin staining of fasciculus cuneatus usually seen in third-trimester fetal brains[8,32,49] (Fig. 6.2). The rapidity of cuneate myelination is rivaled only by medullary medial longitudinal fasciculus myelination, although slightly behind the latter, and, like the latter, eclipses medial and lateral lemnisci and trapezoid body myelination. By term, most cases contain intensely stained fasciculus cuneatus myelin.

Dorsal spinocerebellar tract

Afferent fibers arising in the lower thoracic and upper lumbosacral posterior roots synapse in the ipsilateral dorsal nucleus of Clarke, giving rise to the dorsal spinocerebellar tract, supplying cerebellar vermis. Fibers from lower levels lie medial to those from higher levels. Cervical and upper thoracic spinal muscle afferent fibers do not terminate in the dorsal nucleus of Clarke. The thoracic dorsal spinocerebellar tract appears in the second half of gestation, with

TABLE 6.3

Afferents to brainstem and/or forebrain (percentage of cases containing grossly visible myelin, degree 3)

Myelinating tract	Prenatal (gross myelination) weeks			Postnatal (gross myelination) months		
	10%	50%	90%	10%	50%	90%
Spinal cord						
Fasciculus gracilis, lumbar	20	27	34	M	M	M
Fasciculus gracilis, thoracic	22	28	34	M	M	M
Fasciculus gracilis, cervical	29	34	41	M	M	M
Fasciculus cuneatus	20	27	37	M	M	M
Spinocerebellar, thoracic	20	30	>40	ND	ND	ND
Spinocerebellar, cervical	25	32	>40	ND	ND	ND
Spinothalamic, lumbar	<20	35	>40	ND	ND	ND
Spinothalamic, thoracic	<20	35	>40	ND	ND	ND
Spinothalamic, cervical	29	38	>40	ND	ND	ND
Brainstem						
Medial lemniscus, medulla	23	27	34	ND	ND	ND
Medial lemniscus pons	25	30	35	ND	ND	ND
Medial lemniscus, midbrain	25	32	36	ND	ND	ND
Spinal trigeminal	24	29	35	ND	ND	ND
Auditory						
Trapezoid body	23	28	34	ND	ND	ND
Lateral lemniscus, pons	25	29	35	ND	ND	ND
Lateral lemniscus, midbrain	26	30	35	ND	ND	ND
Brachium, inferior colliculus	NM	NM	NM	4	24	>24
Auditory radiation, proximal	NM	NM	NM	2	7	26
Transverse gyrus	NM	NM	NM	<10% until 11 months	12	24

M, myelinated; NM, no myelin; ND, not done.

10% of cases grossly myelinated (degree 3) (Table 6.3). The cervical dorsal spinocerebellar tract (Figs. 6.1 and 6.2) reaches this level about a month later; by early third trimester, 50% of cases are grossly myelinated (degree 3 or fully myelinated). Despite this rapid myelination at the end of the second trimester, many cases are still not fully myelinated at term.

Lateral spinothalamic tract

The lateral spinothalamic tract (Fig. 6.2) originates in spinal posterior horn gray matter after receiving synapses from dorsal root fibers conveying pain, itch, coarse touch, pressure, and thermal sense. In the cord, it lies lateral to the ventral spinocerebellar tract and projects largely to the contralateral ventral posteriolateral thalamic nucleus, where the body surface is represented in an orderly, distorted, somatotopic fashion.

The lateral spinothalamic tract appears in the second half of gestation, with 20% to 30% of cases containing microscopic myelin (degree 1); transitions to degree 2 and degree 3 occur at the end of the second trimester and in the mid-third trimester, with the rostral end beginning slightly later than the caudal. The pattern of lateral spinothalamic tract myelination is similar to the fasciculus proprius. By term, only 60% to 70% of cases have attained degree 3 myelination (Table 6.3).

Brainstem

Medial lemniscus (medulla, pons, midbrain)

Fasciculi gracilis and cuneatus fibers, topographically organized in the spinal cord, synapse in medullary gracile and cuneate nuclei (Fig. 6.3) and give origin to the medial lemniscus while retaining the topographic organization. These fibers cross the midline ventrally and form the contralateral medial lemniscus, terminating topographically on the thalamic ventral posteriolateral nucleus.

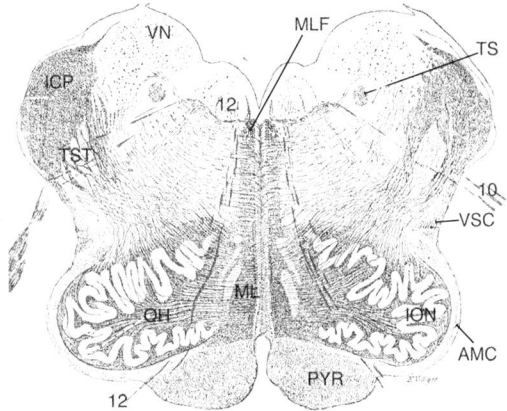

Fig. 6.3 Horizontal section medulla, caudal to lateral recess, adult. Down is toward face. TS, solitary tract (surrounded by a clear space representing the solitary tract nucleus); MLF, medial longitudinal fasciculus; VSC, ventral spinocerebellar tract; AMC, amiculum; ION, inferior olivary nucleus; PYR, pyramid or corticospinal tract; 12, hypoglossal nerve and nucleus; 10, vagus nerve; VN, medial vestibular nucleus; ICP, inferior cerebellar peduncle; TST, trigeminal spinal tract; OH, hilus of olivary nucleus; ML, medial lemniscus. Weigert–Pal myelin stain. From Rasmussen.[138]

Similar to the medial longitudinal fasciculus (Table 6.4 and Fig. 6.3), the medullary medial lemniscus enters the second half of gestation with few cases containing any myelin; 10% of cases contain grossly visible myelin at 23 weeks, 50% at 27 weeks, and 90% at 34 weeks. Both the medial longitudinal fasciculus and medullary medial lemniscus have a very large proportion (95%) of cases containing intensely stained myelin sheaths by term (Table 6.3). Pontine and midbrain medial lemnisci are delayed by 1 or 2 weeks, supporting the idea that myelination progresses in the direction of information flow along the axon.

Trigeminal spinal tract
The trigeminal spinal tract (Fig. 6.3) constitutes the central processes of Gasserian ganglion dorsal root cells and contains fibers activated by pain, thermal, and tactile receptors from the face, lips, and mouth, and is the earliest sensory pathway to develop in the human fetus (see Chapter 9).[57] Trigeminal spinal tract myelination follows a pattern very similar to the medial lemniscus, with 10%, 50%, and 90% of cases containing grossly visible myelin at 24, 29, and 35 weeks (Table 6.3). The rate and timing of trigeminal spinal tract myelination lags far behind (about 10 gestational weeks) the appearance of trigeminal spinal tract upper cervical cord axons and the development of human fetal withdrawal reflexes during the embryonic period at 5 to 9 weeks[58–60] (see Chapter 9).

Auditory

Trapezoid body
Trapezoid body fibers (Fig. 6.4 and Table 6.3) arise mainly from the ventral cochlear nucleus, cross to the opposite side, and turn abruptly rostral to ascend as the lateral lemniscus, the principal ascending auditory pathway. The lateral lemniscus (Figs. 6.4 and 6.5) synapses in the inferior colliculus, which gives origin to the inferior colliculus brachium (lying laterally on the midbrain tegmentum) and ends in the medial geniculate body. The medial geniculate body in turn gives origin to the auditory radiation supplying primary auditory cortex or transverse gyrus of Heschl (Fig. 6.6, Q) on the first temporal gyrus. The proximal auditory radiation lies on the lateral geniculate body as it swings laterally.

The trapezoid body myelinates similarly to the medial lemniscus at each brainstem level (Table 6.3). Early in the second half of gestation, only a small proportion of cases contain myelin; by the third trimester the trapezoid body is densely myelinated, with 10%, 50%, and 90% of cases containing gross myelination at 23, 28, and 34 weeks.

Lateral lemniscus, pons, and midbrain
Pontine lateral lemniscus carries auditory fibers to the inferior colliculus (Figs. 6.4 and 6.5). The pontine lateral lemniscus contains gross myelin in 10%, 50% and 90% of cases at 25, 29, and 35 weeks; the midbrain lateral lemniscus contains gross myelin in 10%, 50% and 90% of cases at 26, 30, and 35 weeks (Table 6.3). By term, 98% of fetuses contain intensely stained myelin in all lower brainstem auditory pathways. In many respects, auditory pathway myelination is similar to, but later than, medial longitudinal fasciculus myelination.

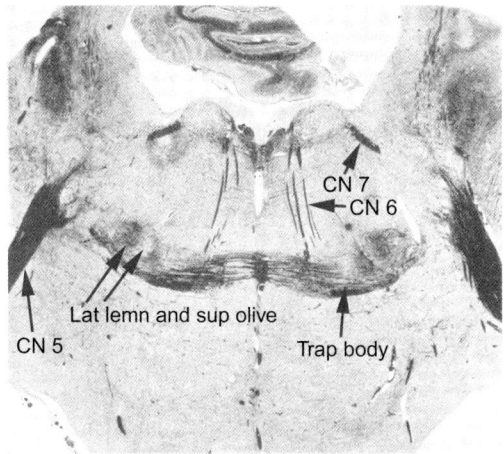

Fig. 6.4 Horizontal section pons, rostral to medullary–pontine junction, term. Down is toward face. The myelinated intramedullary cranial nerves (CN 5, trigeminal nerve; CN 6, abducens nerve; CN 7, facial nerve) are indicated. On the medial proximal end are the trigeminal sensory nuclei from which the spinal trigeminal nucleus and tract originate. The middle cerebellar peduncle lies lateral to the myelinated trigeminal nerve roots on either side. Unmyelinated transpontine fibers lie in the basis pontis. Trap body, trapezoid body; Lat lemn and sup olive, lateral lemniscus (black) and superior olive (light). Weigert–Pal myelin stain. Reproduced with permission of John Wiley & Sons, Inc. from Keene and Hewer.[32]

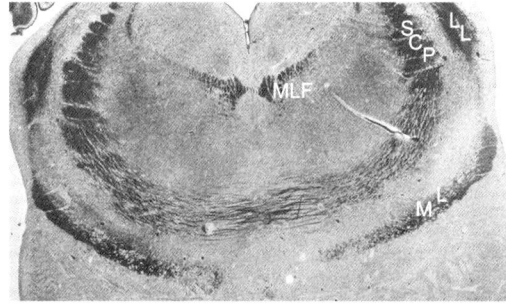

Fig. 6.5 Horizontal section upper pontine tegmentum near lower midbrain, term. Down is toward face. The lateral lemniscus (LL) is located on the side at the level of the upper fourth ventricle. The medial lemniscus (ML) separates tegmentum from basis pontis. The medial longitudinal fasciculus (MLF) lies on either side of the midline. The superior cerebellar peduncle (SCP) occupies much of the tegmentum curving from behind forward and just beginning the lower edge of the decussation. The central tegmental tract is the faintly myelinated tract lying between the SCP and MLF. Weigert–Pal myelin stain. Reproduced with permission of John Wiley & Sons, Inc. from Keene and Hewer.[32]

109

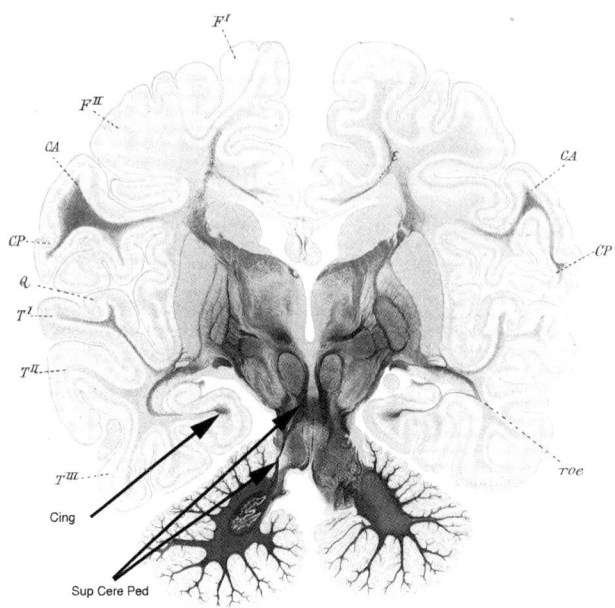

Fig. 6.6 Coronal section through basal ganglia, red nucleus, and cerebellum, 7 postnatal weeks. Down is inferior or toward feet. Early auditory radiation myelination occupies the superior temporal gyrus (T^I) subjacent to the transverse gyrus (Q). Sup Cere Ped, superior cerebellar peduncle. As the superior cerebellar peduncle enters the midbrain, it encompasses the red nucleus. Early optic radiation myelination (roe) shows the optic radiation as it curves around the temporal lateral ventricular horn. T^I, T^{II}, and T^{III} indicate the first, second, and third temporal gyri. The T^I marker points to the myelinated auditory radiation. Cing, cingulum; e, cingulum myelin in gyrus cinguli; F^I and F^{II} indicate the first and second frontal gyri; CA and CP, pre- and postcentral gyri. This coronal section angle is tipped forward at the top sufficiently to include the face area of the central sulcus. The sulcus appears minute because of a large annectant gyrus crossing the central sulcus. Myelin stain. The myelin in the pre- (CA) and postcentral (CP) gyri constitutes the distal corona radiata. Weigert–Pal myelin stain. The cingulum, optic radiation (roe), and auditory radiation [myelin in transverse temporal gyrus (Q)] are partially myelinated. The superior cerebellar peduncle is well myelinated and forms a capsule around the red nucleus (the large oval structure above the arrowhead). Modified from Flechsig.[6] A color version of this figure is available in the color plate section in the back of the book.

Inferior colliculus brachium (lateral to superior colliculus)

The inferior colliculus brachium, carrying auditory fibers to the medial geniculate body, myelinates largely postnatally with 10%, 50%, and 90% of cases containing grossly visible myelin at 4, 24, and >24 months (Table 6.3). Thus, the brachium continues myelination after the second year.

Auditory radiation, proximal

The auditory radiation, linking the medial geniculate body to the superior temporal cortex, Heschl's transverse temporal gyrus, myelinates largely postnatally; 10%, 50%, and 90% of cases were grossly myelinated at 2, 7, and 26 months (Fig. 6.6 and Table 6.3).

Heschl's transverse temporal gyrus

Transverse temporal gyrus white matter (primary auditory cortex) failed to show much myelination until the very end of the first year when half of all cases contained grossly visible myelin (Fig. 6.6 and Table 6.3). One year later, 90% of cases contained grossly visible myelin.

Thus, while auditory fibers in the trapezoid body and lateral lemniscus had attained degree 3 myelination by gestational end, auditory fibers in the inferior colliculus and medial geniculate fibers in auditory radiation going to primary auditory cortex white matter myelinated at a much later developmental time.

INTRABRAINSTEM

Medial longitudinal fasciculus

The medial longitudinal fasciculus (MLF) contains ascending and descending fibers, both crossed and uncrossed, from all vestibular nuclei (Figs. 6.3 and 6.5 and Table 6.4). Descending vestibular fibers from the medial vestibular nucleus project to ipsilateral spinal levels via the anterior funiculus of cervical and upper thoracic spinal cord; ascending MLF fibers project to extraocular nuclei, bringing their muscular innervation under vestibular influence. The MLF also carries descending pontine reticular formation fibers.

Medial longitudinal fasciculus, medulla

The medullary MLF enters the second half of gestation with 67% of cases containing microscopically visible myelin; 10%, 50%, and 90% of cases contain grossly visible myelin at 22, 25, and 33 weeks (Table 6.4). The medullary MLF is striking in its myelination rate and its early gestational age of onset; by 36 weeks, 99% of cases contain grossly visible myelin.

Medial longitudinal fasciculus, pons

The pontine MLF enters the second half of gestation with 60% of cases containing microscopically visible myelin; 10%, 50%, and 90% of cases contain grossly visible myelin at 22, 26, and 33 weeks (Table 6.4). At 36 weeks, 99% of cases contain grossly visible myelin.

Medial longitudinal fasciculus, midbrain

The midbrain MLF enters the second half of gestation with 53% of cases containing microscopically visible myelin; 10%, 50%, and 90% of cases contain grossly visible myelin at 22, 26, and 33 weeks (Table 6.4). At 36 weeks, 97% of cases contain grossly visible myelin.

The MLF, with its early myelination onset and rapid development of intense myelin staining, surpasses the process in the medial lemniscus, trapezoid body, and lateral lemniscus,[8] and therefore is a useful reference point for evaluating myelination degree.

TABLE 6.4

Intrabrainstem (percentage of cases containing grossly visible myelin, degree 3)

Myelinating tract	Prenatal (gross myelination) weeks			Postnatal (gross myelination) months		
	10%	50%	90%	10%	50%	90%
Medial longitudinal fasciculus, medulla	22	25	33	M	M	M
Medial longitudinal fasciculus, pons	22	26	33	M	M	M
Medial longitudinal fasciculus, midbrain	22	26	33	M	M	M
Central tegmental tract	NM	NM	NM	18	>24	>24
Solitary tract	ND	ND	ND	1	>24	>24
Inferior olivary nucleus, hilus	ND	ND	ND	Birth	1	23
Inferior olivary nucleus, amiculum	31	38	>40	Birth	1	>24

M, myelinated; NM, no myelin; ND, not done.

Central tegmental tract (pons)
The central tegmental tract consists of descending midbrain fibers, largely from red nucleus, that project to the inferior olivary nucleus. It was barely identifiable in myelin stains in fetal brain (Table 6.4 and Fig. 6.5). Ten percent of cases contain grossly visible myelin at 18 months and it is still myelinating at the end of the second year.

Solitary tract (tractus solitarius)
Vagus, glossopharyngeal, and facial cranial nerves contribute visceral afferent fibers to this tract (Fig. 6.3). Dealing primarily with taste and other visceral afferent fibers, its nucleus also has a role in providing central pattern generators for swallowing, visceral, cardiovascular, and respiratory functions. This tract is rarely identified in myelin-stained fetal brains. It has grossly visible myelin in only 10% of cases throughout the first 2 years, with continued myelination subsequently (Table 6.4). These observations stand in distinct contrast to Keene and Hewer's observation of myelin in the solitary tract of one fetus said to be at 28 weeks' gestation.[32]

Inferior olivary nucleus, hilus
Emerging fibers from inferior olivary neurons collect in the hilus and cross the midline to enter the inferior cerebellar peduncle, projecting fibers to the contralateral cerebellar hemisphere (Fig. 6.3). These olivocerebellar fibers end as climbing fibers, ascending to Purkinje cell dendrites. At birth, about 10% of cases have grossly visible hilar myelin; this quickly rises to 50% within a month, and further to 90% toward the end of the second year (Table 6.4).

Inferior olivary nucleus amiculum
The amiculum (Fig. 6.3), a dense band of myelinated fibers surrounding the principal inferior olivary nucleus, is composed of descending fibers from the cerebral cortex, red nucleus, and

periaqueductal gray. There are many brainstem projections to the inferior olivary complex, including vestibular nuclei, caudal trigeminal spinal tract, and dorsal column nuclei. These are probably the source of amiculum regions myelinating during the latter half of gestation. The inferior olivary complex is the largest medullary cerebellar relay nucleus; its output is largely to the inferior cerebellar peduncle. Finally, spino-olivary fibers terminate largely on the medial and dorsal accessory olivary nuclei.

The amiculum myelinates far more slowly than many other brainstem tracts, with 10%, 50%, and 90% of cases containing grossly visible myelin at 31, 38, and >40 weeks (Table 6.4). Postnatally, the myelination pattern was much like that of the inferior olivary hilus, with 10% of cases containing visible myelin at birth, rising to 50% within a month, and further to 90% toward the end of the second year. The discrepancy across birth reflects the differences between the prenatal and postnatal cases.

CEREBELLUM

Afferent

Inferior cerebellar peduncle
The inferior cerebellar peduncle (Fig. 6.3), a major cerebellar afferent input, carries many, mostly peripheral, fiber systems to the cerebellum, including vestibulocerebellar, spinocer-ebellar, reticulocerebellar, and olivocerebellar fibers; among these, the dorsal spinocerebellar tract and cuneocerebellar fibers are major contributors. Inferior cerebellar peduncle myelina-tion follows dorsal spinocerebellar myelination, consistent with a myelination pattern occur-ring distal from the column of Clarke neurons (Table 6.5). Although the dorsal spinocerebellar tract is similar to the inferior cerebellar peduncle, it does not end gestation with such a high proportion of cases containing intensely stained myelin. The pattern of inferior cerebellar peduncle myelination almost replicates that of the spinal trigeminal tract, with both tracts having comparable entry percentages of myelinated cases at midgestation, slopes for each of the three degrees, transitions, and a very high proportion of cases containing intensely stained fibers at term. The inferior cerebellar peduncle contains grossly visible myelin in 0%, 50%, and 90% of cases at 23, 29, and 35 weeks (Table 6.5).

Corticopontine systems, general comments
The corticopontine systems consist of fibers from all cerebral isocortical regions to the basis pontis. These fibers synapse in pontine nuclei and then send fibers across the pons to the opposite middle cerebellar peduncle to form the largest cerebellar isocortical input. The midbrain cerebral peduncle white matter can be divided roughly into thirds (Fig. 6.7). The portion adjacent to the interpeduncular fossa is designated the medial third [Fig. 6.7(A)]; that in the middle, the middle third [Fig. 6.7(P)]; and that lateral, the lateral third [Fig. 6.7(T)]. Corticopontine frontal lobe fibers traverse the internal capsule anterior limb and form the medial cerebral peduncle (most anterior limb fibers are either thalamocortical or cortico-pontine and not corticospinal); fibers from the remaining cerebrum (parietal, occipital, and

TABLE 6.5

Cerebellar afferent and efferent tracts (percentage of cases containing grossly visible myelin, degree 3)

Myelinating tract	Prenatal (gross myelination) weeks			Postnatal (gross myelination) months		
	10%	50%	90%	10%	50%	90%
Inferior cerebellar peduncle	23	29	35	ND	ND	ND
Lateral crus pedunculi	>41	>41	>41	6	17	>24
Medial crus pedunculi	>41	>41	>41	17	25	>24
Transpontine pontocerebellar fibers	>41	>41	>41	2.5	8	>24
Middle cerebellar peduncle	39	>41	>41	2.5	4	>24
Parasagittal/peridentate	29	34	41	1	3	11
Cerebellar hemisphere	39	>41	>41	3	12	>24
Dentate, hilus	ND	ND	ND	<1	8	24
Superior cerebellar peduncle, pons	28	33	36	M	M	M
Superior cerebellar peduncle, midbrain	26	34	38	M	M	M
Capsule, red nucleus	35	40	>41	1	2.5	24

M, myelinated; ND, not done.

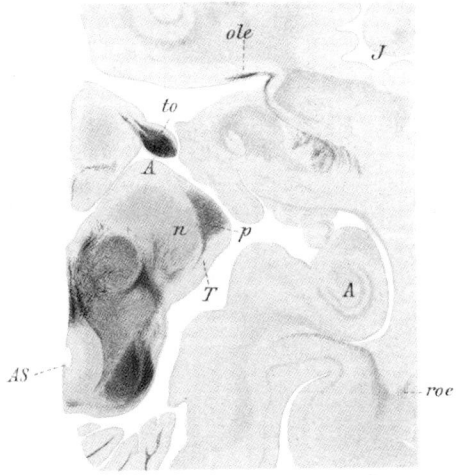

Fig. 6.7 Horizontal section through midbrain, 8-month fetus. The direction toward the face is to the top in the image. The only myelinated fibers in the cerebral peduncle are the corticospinal fibers (p). The frontopontine (left A) and the parieto-occipital-temporal (T) fibers are unmyelinated. The mammillary body lies to the left of A. AS, aqueduct; n, substantia nigra; to, optic tract; ole, lateral olfactory tract; right A, Ammon's horn or hippocampus; J, insula; roe, a portion of optic radiation. Modified from Flechsig.[6] A color version of this figure is available in the color plate section in the back of the book.

temporal lobes) come together in the posterior limb and form the lateral cerebral peduncle. Frontopontine fibers terminate on the rostral pontine neurons; those from the temporal lobe terminate on the caudal pontine neurons.

Cerebral peduncle, lateral (parietal, occipital, and temporal corticopontine fibers)
This was a late-myelinating system with grossly visible myelin present in a substantial number of cases after term; microscopically visible myelin, in the lateral third of the cerebral peduncle, is present in only 10% of cases at 34 weeks and in 50% at term [Fig. 6.7 (T) and Table 6.5]. 10%, 50%, and 90% of cases contain grossly visible myelin at 7 and 17 months postnatally, with subsequent myelination continuing in a significant proportion of cases after the second year.

Cerebral peduncle, medial
Medial cerebral peduncle myelination (medial to the corticospinal tract) has only microscopically visible myelin in 16% of cases at term, long after the development of lateral cerebral peduncle myelin, following the general pattern that the frontal lobe develops later than remaining cerebral lobes [Fig. 6.7(a) and Table 6.5]. Thus, prenatally, the medial cerebral peduncle myelinates later than the lateral cerebral peduncle and even after birth continues to myelinate more slowly than the lateral cerebral peduncle. Grossly visible myelin is present in 10% of cases at 17 months and in 50% at 25 months. Frontopontine fibers in the cerebral peduncle continue to myelinate after the second year.

Middle cerebellar peduncle
The middle cerebellar peduncle is the major isocortical cerebellar afferent input, arising from basis pontis nuclei (Fig. 6.4). Its myelination is in distinct contrast to that of the inferior cerebellar peduncle (myelinating earlier in the second half of gestation) and the superior cerebellar peduncle (slightly after the inferior cerebellar peduncle). The middle cerebellar peduncle has a myelination pattern similar to transpontine fibers, except that it occurs slightly earlier; however, it does not reach 10% of cases containing grossly visible myelin until 39 weeks (Table 6.5). After birth, at least 2.5 months elapse before 10% of cases develop grossly visible myelin, and it is another 1.5 months before 50% of cases are myelinated, with a considerable proportion of cases still myelinating after the second year.

Transpontine fibers
Transpontine fibers arise in basis pontis neurons, cross the midline, and enter the middle cerebellar peduncle (Fig. 6.4). They were slow to myelinate and significant proportions of cases do not show microscopic myelin until the third trimester. At 37 weeks, 44% of cases have only microscopic myelin and no grossly visible myelin; postnatally, 10% and 50% of cases contain grossly visible myelin at 2.5 and 8 months, with myelination continuing after the second year (Table 6.5).

Intracerebellum

Cerebellum, parasagittal (peridentate)
The cerebellar vermal, parasagittal (peridentate), and oculomotor (vestibular) regions are involved in mechanisms modifying voluntary eye movements such as saccades and smooth pursuit. Paravermal spinocerebellum, somatotopically organized, controls axial and girdle muscles. Myelination of parasagittal cerebellar white matter considerably precedes cerebellar hemispheral myelination. At midgestation, only a small number of parasagittal cases contain microscopic myelin; by 29, 34, and 41 weeks, 10%, 50%, and 90% of cases, respectively, contain grossly visible myelin (Table 6.5). Postnatally, 10%, 50%, and 90% of cases contain grossly visible myelin at 1, 3, and 11 months, respectively.

Cerebellum, hemisphere
The cerebellar hemispheres coordinate ipsilateral appendicular somatic motor activity. Myelination occurs much later than the vermis, with only a small proportion of cases containing microscopic myelin by the beginning of third trimester. In the last month of the third trimester, 10% of cases contain grossly visible myelin; postnatally, 10% and 50% of cases contain grossly visible myelin at 3 and 12 months, respectively, and myelination continues after the second year (Table 6.5). In many respects, cerebellar hemispheral myelination parallels that of middle cerebellar peduncle.

Efferent

Dentate, hilus
Dentate nucleus and other cerebellar roof nuclei fibers join together in the dentate nucleus hilus and continue as the superior cerebellar peduncle, a major cerebellar efferent system. Myelination was evaluated only in postnatal brains, in which 10% of cases have grossly visible myelin at the beginning of postnatal life, 50% are myelinated 8 months later, and 90% of cases are myelinated at 23 months (Table 6.5).

Superior cerebellar peduncle, pons
The superior cerebellar peduncle (SCP) pons is the largest cerebellar efferent bundle. In the lower midbrain, it crosses the midline, enters and surrounds the red nucleus, as its capsule, and continues rostrally to the subthalamus and thalamic ventrolateral nucleus [Figs. 6.5 (SCP) and 6.6]. SCP myelination in the pons starts slowly, with 10%, 50%, and 90% of cases containing grossly visible myelin at 28, 33, and 36 weeks (Table 6.5). Its pattern of myelination is similar to the parasagittal cerebellum. Further myelination postnatally in the SCP pons was not studied; however, the red nucleus capsule was a surrogate.

Superior cerebellar peduncle, midbrain
Midbrain SCP myelination is similar to that of the pons, with 10%, 50%, and 90% of cases containing grossly visible myelin at 26, 34, and 38 weeks.

Red nucleus capsule

The SCP forms the red nucleus capsule on its way to the ventral lateral thalamic nucleus (Fig. 6.6), which in turn projects in a topologic fashion to the motor cortex. Ten percent of cases contain grossly visible capsular myelin at 35 weeks and 50% at 40 weeks, but less than 90% of cases are myelinated at 41 weeks. Postnatally, 10%, 50%, and 90% of cases contain grossly visible myelin at 1, 2.5, and 24 months, respectively (Table 6.5).

The pattern of SCP myelination is similar to, but slower than, several other brainstem tracts; however, in contrast to the SCP, red nucleus capsule myelination is even slower.

INTERNAL CAPSULE (CORTICOTHALAMIC, THALAMOCORTICAL, CORTICOPONTINE, CORTICOBULBAR, AND CORTICOSPINAL TRACTS)

General comments

The internal capsule, lying between the thalamus, striatum, and globus pallidus, is composed of fibers in transit to and from the cortex (Figs. 6.6 and 6.8a,c–e). It is a system of mixed ascending incoming fibers from the brainstem and thalamus to the cortex and descending corticopontine, corticobulbar, and corticospinal fibers. In the fetal brain, a clear separation was not always possible. The posterior limb of the internal capsule adjacent to the thalamus (parathalamic; excluding the rim of external medullary thalamic fibers, at midthalamic level) myelinates first, and was used for evaluating the prenatal degree of myelination. More lateral portions of the posterior limb adjacent to the striatum (parastriatal) contain corticopontine, corticobulbar, and corticospinal fibers from precentral and postcentral gyri (motor and sensory cortices of Brodmann areas 4, 3, 1, and 2), and fibers from parietal, occipital, and temporal cortices. Postnatal myelination was evaluated at midthalamic levels using this parastriatal portion.

Posterior limb, parathalamic

The internal capsule parathalamic fibers in the posterior limb are largely ascending sensory thalamocortical fibers (Figs. 6.6 and 6.8a,c–e). These fibers provide sensory information to the postcentral and precentral gyri (sensorimotor cortex). In the parathalamic posterior limb, 10% and 50% of cases contain grossly visible myelin at 32 and 37 weeks. Ten percent, 50%, and 90% of cases contain grossly visible myelin at <1, 1, and 16 months, respectively (Table 6.6), with myelination continuing after 2 years.

Posterior limb, parastriatal

Postnatally, 10%, 50%, and 90% of cases contain grossly visible myelin at birth, 1 month, and 13 months, respectively (Table 6.6).

Anterior limb, internal capsule

The medial anterior limb contains thalamocortical fibers and the paraputaminal portions largely contain frontal corticopontine fibers [Fig. 6.8a,c (ci)]. The internal capsule anterior limb between the caudate and putamen, rostral to the genu and globus pallidus, was evaluated; in neither location could thalamocortical and corticothalamic fibers from corticopontine fibers be separated with certainty. Anterior limb myelination begins late in the third trimester, similar

117

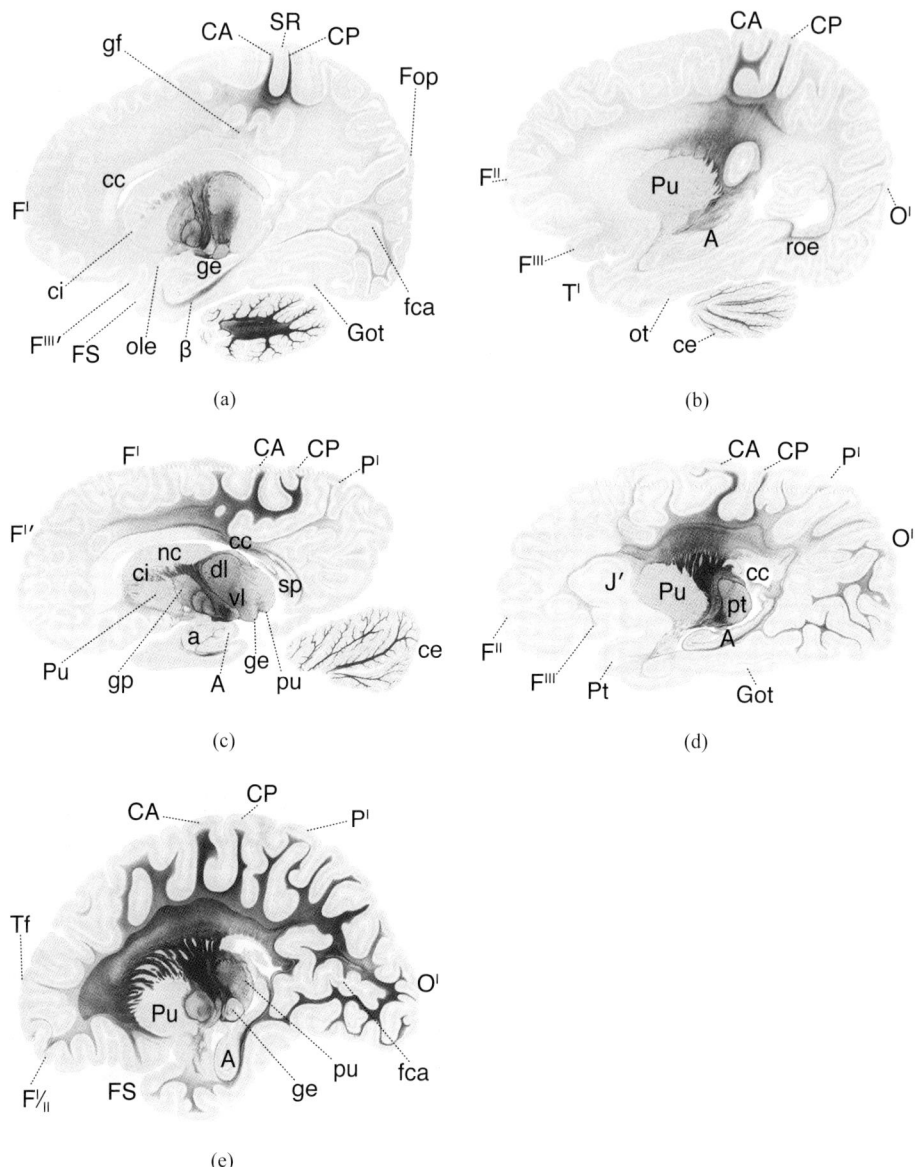

Fig. 6.8 (a) Sagittal section through lateral geniculate body, term brain. Anterior or nose to the left. Myelinated thalamocortical and corticospinal fibers are present in the internal capsule between the thalamus and globus pallidus. These same fibers are seen myelinated in the distal corona radiata inferior to the central sulcus and pre- and postcentral gyri. (b) Sagittal section through lateral putamen, term brain. The black myelinated fibers of the corona radiata sweep past the putamen in the internal capsule. (c) Sagittal section, term brain + 9 weeks postnatal age. In the interval since the above photographs, the amount of myelin in the corona radiata has increased considerably. The corpus callosum (cc) subjacent to the central sulcus is partially myelinated. The anterior limb of the internal capsule is partially myelinated. (d) Sagittal section, term + 9 weeks postnatal age. More laterally, the continuity between the internal

TABLE 6.6

Internal capsule—corticothalamic, thalamocortical, corticopontine, and corticospinal (percentage of cases containing grossly visible myelin, degree 3)

Myelinating tract	Prenatal (gross myelination) weeks			Postnatal (gross myelination) months		
	10%	50%	90%	10%	50%	90%
Posterior limb (parathalamic)	32	37	>41	<1	1	16
Anterior limb	>41	>41	>41	3	12	24
Posterior limb, parastriatal	ND	ND	ND	<1	1	13
Corticospinal, midbrain	36	40	>41	1	3	7
Corticospinal, pons	37	>41	>41	2	5	13
Corticospinal, medulla (pyramid)	36	>41	>41	8	16	>24
Lateral corticospinal, cervical	>41	>41	>41	3	21	>24
Lateral corticospinal, thoracic	>41	>41	>41	2	21	>24
Lateral corticospinal, lumbar	>41	>41	>41	18	25	>24

ND, not done.

to the fornix and cingulum, with a little less than half of cases containing microscopic myelin at term. Thus, anterior limb myelination was well behind that of the posterior limb in the term fetus, again perhaps reflecting later frontal lobe development. Postnatally, the anterior limb reaches grossly visible myelination in 10% of cases at 3 months, 50% at 1 year, and 90% at the end of the second year (Table 6.6).

---

capsule (between putamen and pulvinar) and the corona radiata below the pre and postcentral gyri is seen. (e) Sagittal section. Term + 4.5 months. In the few months between the above images and this one, the amount of hemispheral myelin has increased markedly. Note that occipital, parietal, posterior frontal, and posterior temporal myelination exceeds that in the anterior temporal and frontal lobes considerably. The most intense myelin staining is in the internal capsule (between Pu and pu), the corona radiata [particularly well seen in the pre- and postcentral gyral white matter cores (CA and CP)] and the optic radiation (particularly well seen below the calcarine sulcus fca). A, Ammon's horn; β, cingulum; CA and CP, pre- and postcentral gyri; cc, corpus callosum; ce, cerebellum; ci, internal capsule, anterior limb; dl, thalamus, dorsolateral nucleus; F^I and $F^{I'}$, first or superior frontal gyrus; $F^{I/II}$, superior and middle (first and second) frontal gyri; F^{II}, middle frontal gyrus; F^{III}, inferior or third frontal gyrus; $F^{III'}$, inferior frontal gyrus; fca, calcarine sulcus; Fop, occipito-parietal sulcus; FS, lateral sulcus; ge, lateral geniculate body; gf, gyrus cinguli; Got, occipitotemporal gyrus; gp, globus pallidus; J', insula; nc, caudate nucleus; O^I, first occipital gyrus; ole, lateral olfactory stria; ot, occipitotemporal gyrus; PI, superior parietal gyrus; Pt, temporal pole; Pu, putamen; pu, pulvinar; roe, external optic radiation; sp, splenium; SR, central sulcus; T^I, superior temporal gyrus; Tf, frontal pole; vl, thalamus, ventrolateral nucleus. Modified from Flechsig.[6] A color version of this figure is available in the color plate section at the back of the book.

Corticospinal

General comments
The corticospinal system is elongated, extending, in part, from the cortex to the spinal cord. Some corticospinal neurons are the longest in the body, with the exception of lumbosacral dorsal root ganglion cells supplying legs. Corticospinal myelination is well developed by the end of gestation in about 70% of cases. Corona radiata to and from precentral and postcentral gyri, by contrast, has less myelin at term. This may be because fetal posterior limb has concentrated ascending and descending fibers, while in the corona, fibers are more widely dispersed throughout hemispheral white matter with many intervening unmyelinated fibers.

Internal capsule, posterior limb, parastriatal
Both parastriatal and parathalamic portions are grossly myelinated at birth in about 10% of cases and 50% a little over a month later. The parastriatal portions reach 90% of cases myelinated at 13 months and the parathalamic portions reach the same level at 16 months (Table 6.6 and Fig. 6.8c).

Corticospinal tract, midbrain
Ten percent of cases attain grossly visible myelin in the middle third of the midbrain cerebral peduncle at 36 weeks and 50% of cases at 40 weeks (Fig. 6.7). Postnatally, 10%, 50%, and 90% of cases contain grossly visible myelin at 1, 3, and 7 months, respectively (Table 6.6). As most corticospinal tract fibers lie in the middle third of the peduncle, this suggests that many fibers in the posterior limb are descending corticospinal fibers.

Corticospinal tract, pons
Pontine corticospinal tract myelination lags behind midbrain myelination, with only 37% of cases containing microscopic myelin at term. Ten percent of cases contain grossly visible myelin at 37 weeks. Postnatally, 10% of cases are well myelinated at 2 months, 50% at 5 months, and 90% at 13 months (Table 6.6).

Corticospinal tract, medulla
Pyramidal, or medullary corticospinal tract, myelination (Fig. 6.3) occurs later than in the midbrain, similar to the pons, with 10% of cases containing grossly visible myelin at 36 weeks. Postnatally, 10% and 50% of cases contain grossly visible myelin at 8 and 16 months (Table 6.6). Myelination continues after the second year.

Lateral corticospinal tract, spinal cord
Spinal cord corticospinal tract myelination is well behind that of the brainstem and posterior limb, suggesting that the corticospinal tract myelinates from cerebral neurons distally, along the axon, to the spinal cord. Spinal cord corticospinal tract myelination lags in degree of myelination even though it started at about the same time in the early third trimester (Figs. 6.1 and 6.2). The preponderant degree of myelination is microscopic only at all spinal cord levels through to term.

Lateral corticospinal, cervical
Postnatally, 10% and 50% of cases contain grossly visible myelin at 3 and 21 months, respectively, with myelination continuing after the second year (Table 6.6).

Lateral corticospinal, thoracic
Postnatally, 10% and 50% of cases contain grossly visible myelin at 2 and 21 months, respectively, with myelination continuing after the second year.

Lateral corticospinal, lumbar
Lumbar postnatal myelination, in distinct contrast to the upper cord, is present in 10% of cases (degree 3) at 18 months and 50% at 25 months, with myelination continuing after the second year.

VISUAL SYSTEM

Optic chiasm
Retinal ganglion cell axons pass through the optic nerve, some cross in the chiasm and continue via the optic tract to the lateral geniculate body and the superior colliculus. Prenatal myelination of optic chiasm and tract is similar, with grossly visible myelin present in 10% and 50% of cases at 34 and 39 weeks (Table 6.7). Postnatally, optic chiasm myelination proceeds rapidly, with 10% of cases grossly myelinated within the first month, 50% at 2 months, and 90% at 4 months.

Optic tract
Prenatally, optic tract myelin deposition has a pattern similar to that of the optic chiasm [Fig. 6.7 (to)]. Postnatally, tract myelination is considerably different: 10% of cases are grossly myelinated within the first month, 50% at the end of the first month, and 90% at 11 months.

Optic radiation (geniculocalcarine tract), rostral
The rostral optic radiation, lateral to the lateral geniculate nucleus, arches anteriorly around the lateral ventricle atrium to reach temporal, parietal, and occipital deep white matter [Figs. 6.6, 6.7 and 6.8b (roe) and Table 6.7]. Still lateral to the ventricle, it continues as the external sagittal stratum for the remainder of its course to the striate, parastriate, and peristriate cortices (Brodmann areas 17, 18, and 19). The rostral radiation attains grossly visible myelin in 10% of cases at term; postnatally, myelination proceeds rapidly, with 10% of cases grossly myelinated at 2 months, 50% at 3 months, and 90% at 11 months.

Optic radiation, occipital
Distal optic radiation myelination, sampled lateral to the occipital horn (well behind the atrium), follows a pattern similar to that of rostral radiation, attaining grossly visible myelin in 10% of cases at term. Postnatally, myelination proceeds rapidly, with 10% of cases grossly myelinated at 2 months, 50% at 3 months, and 90% at 8 months.

TABLE 6.7

TABLE 6.7

Visual system (percentage of cases containing grossly visible myelin, degree 3)

Myelinating tract	Prenatal (gross myelination) weeks			Postnatal (gross myelination) months		
	10%	50%	90%	10%	50%	90%
Optic chiasm	34	39	>41	<1	2	4
Optic tract	34	39	>41	<1	1	11
Optic radiation, rostral	42	>41	>41	2	3	11
Optic radiation, occipital	<41	>41	>41	2	3	8
Stripe of Gennari	ND	ND	ND	>31	ND	ND

ND, not done.

Stripe of Gennari (myelinated fibers in calcarine cortical layer IV)
These fibers start myelinating well beyond the second year. Other cases, in our experience, started myelinating at around month 31.

BASAL GANGLIA

Putaminal pencils
The caudate and putamen receive afferent fibers from all cortical regions (Fig. 6.6). Efferent myelinated tracts within the putamen form myelinated white matter 'pencils,' which are largely directed to globus pallidus, and substantia nigra (Fig. 6.9). Postnatally, these tracts myelinate slowly, with only 10% of cases containing grossly visible myelin at 10 months and 50% at 26 months (Table 6.8). Putaminal pencil myelination continues beyond the second year.

Globus pallidus
Pallidal efferent fibers constitute a main corpus striatum (caudate and putamen) outflow, directed to the ventrolateral thalamus and substantia nigra (Figs. 6.6 and 6.8a,c,e). They appear as myelinated bands traversing the globus pallidus internal segment. Two groups of pallidal fibers, sampled in coronal sections at or posterior to the interventricular foramen, are those internally traversing the inner pallidal segment and those bundled at the base as the ansa lenticularis. Postnatally, inner segment fiber myelination is similar to that of putaminal pencil in that 10% of cases contain grossly visible myelin at 10 months and 50% at 26 months, and myelination also continues beyond the second year (Table 6.8).

Ansa lenticularis
The ansa lenticularis arises largely from the globus pallidus and is a major basal ganglionic output to ventrolateral thalamus (Fig. 6.9). It is an early forebrain tract to myelinate, with

TABLE 6.8

Basal ganglia (percentage of cases containing grossly visible myelin, degree 3)

Myelinating tract	Prenatal (gross myelination) weeks			Postnatal (gross myelination) months		
	10%	**50%**	**90%**	**10%**	**50%**	**90%**
Putaminal pencils	NM	NM	NM	10	26	>24
Globus pallidus	NM	NM	NM	10	26	>24
Ansa lenticularis	30	35	>41	<1	11	26

NM, no myelin.

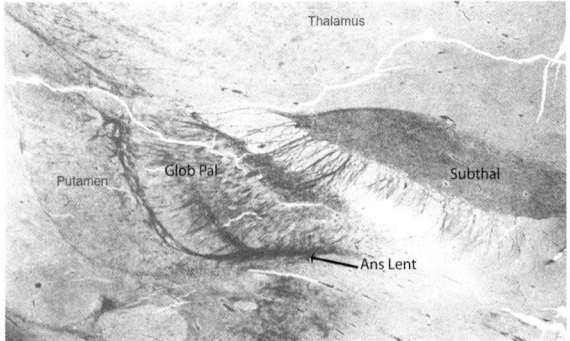

Fig. 6.9 Coronal section through ansa lenticularis, 28 fetal weeks. Down is inferior or toward feet. The thalamus, subthalamic nucleus (Subthal), globus pallidus (Glob Pal), and putamen are indicated. The parathalamic and paraputaminal portions of internal capsule occur in the unmyelinated band lying between the subthalamic nucleus and the globus pallidus. Myelinated pathways (subthalamic fasciculus) emerging from the globus pallidus and connecting with the subthalamic nucleus cross the unmyelinated internal capsule. The ansa lenticularis (Ans Lent) emerges as two fiber bundles from the globus pallidus and runs as a single bundle under the lateral and medial globus pallidus segments on its way to the thalamus. Weigert–Pal myelin stain. Reproduced with permission of John Wiley & Sons, Inc. from Keene and Hewer.[32]

10% of cases containing grossly visible myelin at 30 weeks and 50% at 35 weeks prenatally (Table 6.8). Postnatally, 10%, 50%, and 90% of cases contain grossly visible myelin at birth, 11 months, and 26 months.

OLFACTION

Olfaction is a unique sensory system in that it bypasses the thalamus on its way to the prepyriform cortex and to the corticoamygdaloid nucleus in the inferior anterior medial temporal lobe, near the anterior perforated substance, via the lateral olfactory stria.

TABLE 6.9

Olfaction (percentage of cases containing grossly visible myelin, degree 3)

Myelinating tract	Prenatal (gross myelination) weeks			Postnatal (gross myelination) months		
	10%	50%	90%	10%	50%	90%
Lateral olfactory tract	NM	NM	NM	2	20	26

NM, no myelin.

Lateral olfactory stria

Lateral olfactory tract myelination is a long, drawn-out process during the first two postnatal years, with 10% of cases containing grossly visible myelin at 2 months of age, 50% at 20 months, and 90% at 2 years [Table 6.9 and Fig. 6.8a (ole)].

LIMBIC SYSTEM

The limbic lobe is a conceptual construct consisting of multiple gyri surrounding the rostral brainstem and forming the medial hemispheral edge. Including the cingulate, subcallosal, para-hippocampal, dentate, hippocampal gyri, and the amygdala, it surrounds the interhemispheric commissures.[61] Prominent white matter tracts, connecting these various parts, form some of its input and output. It has an intimate association with the hypothalamus and upper midbrain. Limbic system components have major associations with the cortex and with autonomic and endocrine systems, and have a direct link to emotion.

The fornix is a band of fibers constituting a main hippocampal efferent and afferent system. It passes along the ventromedial edge of the temporal horn adjacent to the hippocampus as the alveus; continues occipitally as the fimbria; and, posteriorly at the hippocampal end, rises and arches dorsally under the splenium to course forward to the interventricular foramen (Fig. 6.6), where it forms the rostral edge. Above the anterior commissure, it divides into small precommissural and large postcommissural fornix bundles. The latter burrow into the third ventricular wall, dividing the hypothalamus into medial and lateral halves, before ending in the mammillary bodies. As the fornix descends through the hypothalamus, its fibers project to the anterior thalamic nucleus, hypothalamus, and midbrain. The cingulum extends from the septum as a large fiber bundle paralleling the corpus callosum in the gyrus cinguli and enters the parahippocampal gyrus [Figs. 6.6 (Cing) and 6.8a (b)], where it extends to the uncus. The mammillothalamic tract is a major mammillary body outflow, carrying fibers to the anterior thalamic nucleus, which in turn projects to the cingulate gyrus. Thus, the main cortical hippocampus projection is to cingulate gyrus via the mammillary body and anterior thalamic nucleus.

Myelination of the alveus, fimbria, fornix, mammillothalamic tract, and cingulum is largely a postnatal event, even though fornix and hippocampal anlage are the first to develop at the medial cerebral edge (Table 6.10).[62]

TABLE 6.10
Limbic system (percentage of cases containing grossly visible myelin, degree 3)

Myelinating tract	Prenatal (gross myelination) weeks			Postnatal (gross myelination) months		
	10%	50%	90%	10%	50%	90%
Alveus	NM	NM	NM	10	26	>24
Fimbria	NM	NM	NM	20	26	>24
Fornix, medial	>41	>41	>41	13	>24	>24
Fornix, lateral	>41	>41	>41	21	>24	>24
Mammillothalamic tract	>41	>41	>41	3	25	>24
Cingulum	>41	>41	>41	2	10	>24

NM, no myelin.

Alveus

Ten percent of cases contain grossly visible myelin at 10 months and 50% at the end of the second year. Thus, alveus myelination continues beyond the second year.

Fimbria

Fimbrial myelination is delayed until 20 months postnatally, when 10% of cases are myelinated (degree 3); 50% are myelinated by the end of the second year.

Fornix

Medial half

Few cases contain microscopic myelin until the last gestational month, when the proportion abruptly increases; almost half of cases at 40 weeks contain microscopic myelin. No significant proportions of cases reach grossly visible myelin by term. Postnatally, 10% of cases are myelinated at 13 months and most cases continue myelinating beyond the second year. This is in contrast to the magnetic resonance findings in T1-weighted images that the body and columns are myelinated at around 7 to 8 months.

Lateral half

The lateral fornix half is slower to myelinate than the medial half, with 10% of cases containing grossly visible myelin at 21 months.

Mammillothalamic tract

Mammillothalamic tract myelination is largely a postnatal event; 10% of cases contain grossly visible myelin at 3 months and 50% at the end of the second year.

Cingulum

Cingulum, sampled in deep parahippocampal gyrus white matter at midthalamic levels, is similar to other limbic system components, myelinating largely postnatally. Ten percent of cases are grossly myelinated at 2 postnatal months and 50% at 10 months. Myelination continues beyond the second year.

DEEP CEREBRAL WHITE MATTER

Deep cerebral hemispheral white matter contains three groups of intermingled fibers in massive quantities: projection fibers conveying impulses to and from the cortex to distant points; association fibers connecting various hemispheral cortical regions; and commissural fibers connecting homotopic or heterotopic regions between the two hemispheres.

Central corona radiata

The corona radiata extends from the frontal to the occipital lobe and carries thalamocortical, corticothalamic, and corticospinal fibers entering the parathalamic and parastriatal posterior limb. The central corona radiata, sampled midway between the midthalamus and central sulcus, between precentral and postcentral gyri, begins myelination late in gestation, with 10% of cases containing grossly visible myelin at 36 weeks; at term only 44% of cases contain grossly visible myelin (Table 6.11). Postnatally, myelination proceeds more rapidly, with 10%, 50%, and 90% of cases containing grossly visible myelin at 2, 3, and 10 months.

Distal radiation to precentral gyrus

In white matter, sampled deep to precentral gyrus, postnatal myelination proceeds slowly, with 10% and 50% of cases containing grossly visible myelin at 4 and 8 months, with the remaining cases continuing myelination after the second year (Fig. 6.8a–e).

Posterior frontal

In deep frontal white matter, sampled slightly anterior to the midthalamic level, excluding the distal radiation to precentral gyrus, postnatal myelination proceeds at a slow pace, with 10% and 50% of cases containing grossly visible myelin at 4 and 10 months and the remaining cases continuing myelination after the second year (Fig. 6.8e).

Posterior parietal

In deep parietal white matter, sampled at the level of the lateral ventricular atrium, lateral to optic radiation, postnatal myelination proceeds more rapidly, with 10%, 50%, and 90% of cases containing grossly visible myelin at 6, 15, and 24 months of age (Fig. 6.8e).

Temporal lobe

In deep temporal white matter, sampled at lateral geniculate nucleus level, 10%, 50%, and 90% of cases contain grossly visible myelin at 12, 20, and 23 months (Fig. 6.8e).

TABLE 6.11

TABLE 6.11

Deep cerebral white matter (percentage of cases containing grossly visible myelin, degree 3)

Myelinating tract	Prenatal (gross myelination) weeks			Postnatal (gross myelination) months		
	10%	50%	90%	10%	50%	90%
Corona radiata	36	>40	<40	2	3	10
Distal radiation to precentral gyrus	NM	NM	NM	4	8	>24
Posterior frontal	NM	NM	NM	4	10	>24
Posterior parietal	NM	NM	NM	6	15	24
Temporal lobe	NM	NM	NM	12	20	23
Temporal pole	NM	NM	NM	17	21	>24
Frontal pole	NM	NM	NM	7	20	>24
Occipital pole	NM	NM	NM	6	12	21
External capsule	NM	NM	NM	7	17	>24
Extreme capsule	NM	NM	NM	21	>24	>24

NM, no myelin.

Temporal pole
Deep temporal pole white matter, sampled anterior to amygdala, is a late myelinating site, with 10% and 50% of cases containing grossly visible myelin at 17 and 21 months (Fig. 6.8e). Myelination continues after the second year.

Frontal pole
Deep frontal pole white matter, sampled anterior to the lateral ventricle frontal horn, was a slowly myelinating site, with 10% and 50% of cases containing grossly visible myelin at 7 and 20 months (Fig. 6.8e). Myelination continued after the second year.

Occipital pole
Deep occipital pole white matter, sampled external to the sagittal strata at, or posterior to, the posterior tip of occipital horn (Fig. 6.8d,e). Myelination of this region occurs over the first 2 years of postnatal life, with 10%, 50%, and 90% of cases containing grossly visible myelin at 6, 12, and 21 months.

External capsule
The external capsule is a prominent white matter sheet lateral to the putamen, just medial to claustrum. It contains thalamic, anterior commissure, and subthalamic fibers. The dorsal half was sampled at, or rostral to, the subthalamic level. It is a slowly myelinating site, with 10% and 50% of cases containing grossly visible myelin at 7 and 17 months. Myelination continues after the second year.

Extreme capsule

The extreme capsule is a thin sheet of myelinated fibers lying external (lateral) to the claustrum, just inside the insular cortex. It probably contains fibers running between the claustrum and insular cortex and also fibers from frontal to parieto-occipital cortex and superior temporal lobe, as well as temporofrontal fibers. The dorsal half, sampled at or rostral to the subthalamic level, is a late myelinating system, with 10% of cases containing grossly visible myelin at 21 months. Myelination continues after the second year.

SUBCORTICAL ASSOCIATION FIBERS

The superficial cerebral white matter consists of a rim of fibers directly adjacent to, and within, the deepest portion of cortical layer VI of any gyrus (except the precentral gyrus); it contains short corticocortical fibers connecting adjacent cortical regions or adjacent gyri.

Frontal pole

Frontal pole subcortical association fibers, sampled anterior to the frontal horn, are a late myelinating system, with 10% and 50% of cases containing grossly visible myelin at 20 and 21 months (Fig. 6.8d,e). Once started, these fibers then myelinate rapidly (Table 6.12).

Temporal pole

Temporal pole subcortical association fibers, sampled anterior to the amygdala, are a curious system, with almost no cases containing grossly visible myelin until 21 months in only 50% of cases (Fig. 6.8e). Myelination continues after the second year.

Midtemporal

Temporal lobe subcortical association fibers, sampled at midthalamic levels excluding Heschl's gyrus auditory cortex, contain grossly visible myelin in 10% and 50% of cases at 18 and 25 months (Fig. 6.6), with myelination continuing after the second year.

Occipital pole

Occipital pole subcortical association fibers, sampled in any occipital gyrus except the calcarine cortex, contain grossly visible myelin at 12 and 21 months in 10% and 50% of cases, with myelination continuing after the second year.

Posterior parietal

Posterior parietal subcortical association fibers at atrial levels are myelinated (degree 3) in 10%, 50%, and 90% of cases at 9, 14, and 25 months (Fig. 6.8c–e).

Posterior frontal

Posterior frontal subcortical association fibers at midthalamic levels (except for precentral gyrus) are myelinated (degree 3) in 10% and 50% of cases at 8 and 20 months, with myelination continuing after the second year (Fig. 6.8e).

TABLE 6.12

**Superficial cerebral white matter—subcortical association fibers
(percentage of cases containing grossly visible myelin, degree 3)**

Myelinating tract	Postnatal (gross myelination) months		
	10%	50%	90%
Frontal pole	20	21	>24
Temporal pole	–	21	>24
Temporal, mid	18	25	>24
Occipital pole	12	21	>24
Posterior parietal	9	24	25
Posterior frontal	8	20	>24
Subcalcarine	6	8	>24

No myelin detected prenatally.

Subcalcarine cortex

Subcalcarine subcortical association fibers, adjacent to the calcarine visual cortex, myelinate during the first two postnatal years. Ten percent of cases contain grossly visible myelin at 6 postnatal months and and 50% at 8 postnatal months, with myelination continuing after the second year.

COMMISSURES

Anterior commissure, outer

The anterior commissure crosses the third ventricle midline in the lamina terminalis, immediately anterior to and below the anterior columns of the fornix. It forms a complicated axial curve, with its rostral portion in the anteriormost third ventral and its caudal portion far posterior under the globus pallidus. Its rostral surface contains olfactory fibers on its front, rostral, and inferior aspects as well as fibers from the pyriform areas and amygdalae; its caudal fibers connect with the external capsule and temporal lobe, including the parahippocampal gyrus. The olfactory fibers, sampled on its rostral surface, contain microscopic myelin in only about 10% of cases at term.

Anterior commissure, inner

The caudal anterior commissure fibers tend to lie deep and posteriorly. The inner anterior commissure fibers, sampled medial to or under the globus pallidus, start myelinating somewhat later in postnatal life, with 10% and 50% of cases containing grossly visible myelin at 12 and 25 months, with myelination continuing after the second year (Table 6.13 and Fig. 6.8c).

TABLE 6.13

Commissures (percentage of cases containing grossly visible myelin, degree 3)

Myelinating tract	Prenatal (gross myelination) weeks			Postnatal (gross myelination) months		
	10%	50%	90%	10%	50%	90%
Anterior commissure, outer	>41	>41	>41	5	>24	>24
Anterior commissure, inner	NM	NM	NM	12	25	>24
Corpus callosum, rostrum	NM	NM	NM	8	12	>24
Corpus callosum, body	>41	>41	>41	–	5	13
Splenium	NM	NM	NM	4	6	21

NM, no myelin.

Corpus callosum, rostrum

The corpus callosum is a large commissure connecting the two cerebral hemispheres and roofing the lateral ventricles. The anterior end under the genu bends inferiorly and posteriorly, as the rostrum, and connects with the dorsal lamina terminalis. It carries fibers connecting the orbital frontal lobes. The rostrum, sampled at or anterior to the caudate nucleus head, myelinates later than other callosal regions in postnatal life, with 10% and 50% of cases containing grossly visible myelin at 8 and 12 months, and myelination continuing after the second year.

Corpus callosum, body

Corpus callosum body fibers connect midportions of posterior frontal and parietal lobes (Figs. 6.6 and 6.8a,c,d). The corpus callosum body (posterior to foramen of Monro) begins myelinating prenatally, with about one-quarter of cases containing microscopic myelination at term. Postnatally, little myelination occurs until abruptly at 5 months of age, when 50% of cases contain grossly visible myelin, rising to 90% at 13 months.

Splenium

Fibers traversing the splenium connect regions of temporal and occipital lobes (Fig. 6.8c). Those fibers that form a sheet on the lateral occipital horn and separate optic radiation from ventricle are largely visual fibers traversing splenium from one calcarine cortex to the other. Splenial myelin appears before the rostral corpus callosum, with 10%, 50%, and 90% of cases containing grossly visible myelin at 4, 6, and 21 months, respectively.

HYPOTHALAMUS TO BRAINSTEM

Stria medullaris thalami

The stria medullaris thalami is a complex tract that contains fibers from septal nuclei, lateral anterior hypothalamus, anterior thalamic nuclei, hippocampus, amygdala, and globus pallidus and conveys impulses of limbic pathways to the rostral midbrain. This tract lies in the

TABLE 6.14

Hypothalamus to brainstem (percentage of cases containing grossly visible myelin, degree 3)

Myelinating tract	Prenatal (gross myelination) weeks			Postnatal (gross myelination) months		
	10%	50%	90%	10%	50%	90%
Stria medullaris thalami	ND	ND	ND	4	16	26
Habenulointerpeduncular tract	27	34	>41	ND	ND	ND

ND, not done.

lateral third ventricular roof, on the dorsomedial thalamic edge, and extends posteriorly to habenular nuclei. Ten percent, 50%, and 90% of cases contain grossly visible myelin at 4, 16, and 26 months.

Habenulointerpeduncular tract
The epithalamic habenular nuclei, at the juncture of caudal diencephalon and midbrain, receive stria medullaris thalami fibers and give origin to the habenulointerpeduncular tract, ending in the midbrain interpeduncular nucleus (Table 6.14). At 27 weeks, the habenulointerpeduncular tract has only 10% of cases containing grossly visible myelin and 50% at 34 weeks, with completion of myelination postnatally.

Discussion
The precise gestational age at which myelin deposition begins in any specific human fetal nervous system tract is indeterminable, as the event cannot be observed directly. These studies indicate gestational times and brain locations where myelination is important.

RANGE IN AGES OF MYELINATION AT EACH SPECIFIC SITE
One striking finding is the wide range of postconceptional/postnatal ages over which specific tracts become myelinated. They range in length (time to advance from 10% to 90% of cases with grossly visible myelin) from 8 weeks to over 2 years. In general, short times are found in a few sites dealing with vestibular (medial longitudinal fasciculus, 11 weeks); auditory (trapezoid body, 11 weeks; pontine lateral lemniscus, 10 weeks; midbrain lateral lemniscus, 9 weeks); facial, neck, and truncal sensory (medial lemniscus medulla, pons, and midbrain, 10–11 weeks); and spinal trigeminal input (11 weeks) to the brainstem. The briefest time range is 8 weeks for the pontine superior cerebellar peduncle, the major cerebellar outflow tract. The inferior cerebellar peduncle, a major inflow tract to the cerebellum, takes 12 weeks. Several tracts take the second half of gestation to reach 90% of cases with grossly visible myelin: intraspinal fasciculus proprius, spinothalamic, and fasciculus cuneatus.

There is both fetal and infantile fluctuation in myelin acquisition. The broad range in gestational ages of myelin deposition at different sites is consistent with considerable myelination lability. It remains to be shown which environmental agents contribute to this inconsistency and to discover when in gestation this influence occurs. A large number of potential ante-cedents are conceivable as contributory to this fetal brain developmental vulnerability; the worldwide distribution of malnutrition, to cite only one, suggests that evaluation of myelin deposition is of considerable social importance. Our study also confirms the findings of Rorke and Riggs[49] in that the ranges over which fetal brain myelin emerges at specific sites are extremely wide. These extensive ranges and the wide 95% confidence bounds for each fetal site have presumably contributed to some timing discrepancies in the literature.

SEQUENCE OF MYELINATION BY ANATOMIC SITES

Microscopic myelin (degree 1) emerges in different tracts at different times. By 18 post-conceptional months, myelination has begun in all telencephalic sites sampled except the stripe of Gennari (calcarine cortex), in which microscopic myelin is not evident until 31 months. Myelination proceeds at different rates among and within neuronal systems over time. Additionally, there are variable and often far-ranging degrees of myelination within any site at all ages. At the end of the second postnatal year (33 postconceptional months), myelination is notably still incomplete in many locations: medullary and spinal corticospinal tract; brainstem central tegmental and solitary tracts; forebrain fornix and fimbria; inferior olivary nucleus and amiculum; medial and lateral crus pedunculi; transpontine pontocerebel-lar fibers; middle cerebellar peduncle; cerebellar hemisphere and dentate hilus; red nucleus capsule; putamen; globus pallidus and ansa lenticularis; anterior commissure and corpus callosum rostrum; the limbic system; distal corona radiata to precentral gyrus; deep white matter of posterior frontal, temporal, and frontal poles; all subcortical association fibers; and external and extreme capsules.

GROUPS OF MYELINATING TRACTS

The medial longitudinal fasciculus contrasts starkly with other myelinating spinal cord and brainstem tracts at midgestation. Myelination of rostral medial longitudinal fasciculus lags somewhat behind rhombencephalic portions. The parallel early development of caudal medial longitudinal fasciculus and fasciculus cuneatus evokes speculation that those events are related to early maturing vestibular and cervical sensory mechanisms, which underlie head and neck reflexes. The eighth cranial nerve vestibular component is the earliest to myelinate;[8,63] semicircular canal myelinated fibers are evident at 14 weeks.[64]

END OF SECOND TRIMESTER AND EARLY THIRD TRIMESTER

In autopsy material, tracts in which 50% of cases contain grossly visible myelin included; medial longitudinal fasciculus, fasciculus gracilis, fasciculus cuneatus, trapezoid body, and inferior cerebellar peduncle.

Unless otherwise indicated, all of the following magnetic resonance images in this chapter were performed on a 3T Philips System (Philips Healthcare, Bothell, WA, USA) using the appropriately sized head coil. The sequence used was a T1-weighted fluid-attenuated inversion recovery (FLAIR) sequence, with 2mm-thick slides. Using this sequence the cerebrospinal fluid is black and myelin is hyperintense (white).

At 25 weeks, we see magnetic resonance myelin in the chiasm and in the superior cerebellar peduncle decussation (Figs. 6.10a, 6.11a, and 6.12a). At 36 weeks, brainstem magnetic resonance myelin is seen in the midbrain, medulla, and vermal cerebellum. In the prosencephalon magnetic resonance myelin is present in the posterior limb of the internal capsule (Figs. 6.10b and 6.11b).

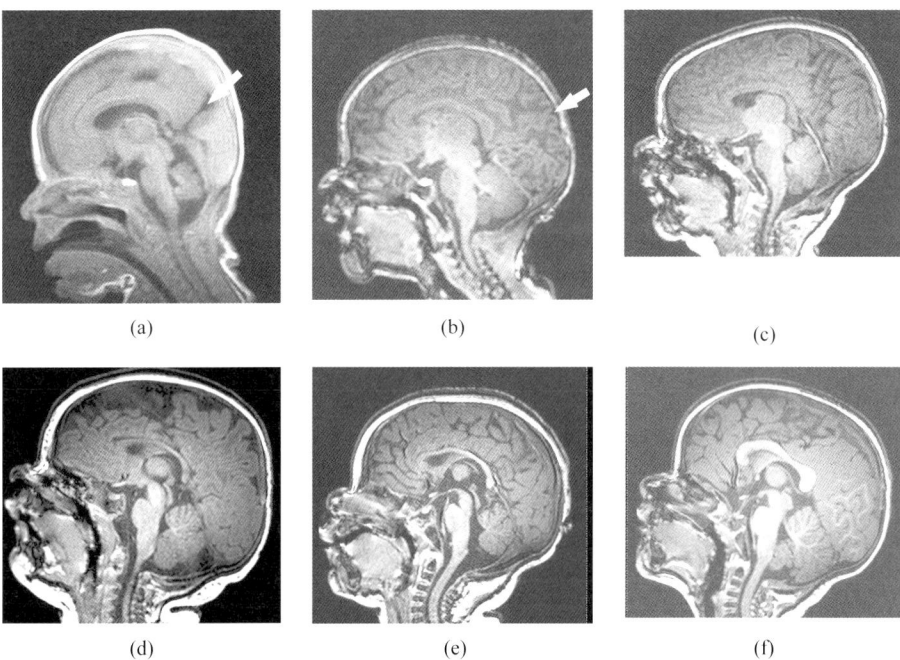

(a)　　　　　　　　　(b)　　　　　　　　　(c)

(d)　　　　　　　　　(e)　　　　　　　　　(f)

Fig. 6.10 T1-weighted fluid-attenuated inversion recovery magnetic resonance images, sagittal, midline. (a) Preterm, 25 weeks (1.5T). There is no apparent magnetic resonance myelination within the brain at this age. While the medial longitudinal fasciculus is expected to be well myelinated, it is too small to be visualized. The callosomarginal and calcarine sulci are apparent. The black indentation between the parietal and occipital lobes is the parieto-occipital sulcus (arrow). The cerebellum is small in a spacious retrocerebellar cavity. The entire pituitary gland is hyperintense (bright). (b) Preterm, 36 weeks. Near midline. The sulcal pattern is far more complex. The parieto-occipital sulcus (arrow) is distinct. The inferior cerebellar and superior cerebellar peduncles are myelinated, as are the trapezoid body, inferior colliculus, optic tracts, and optic chiasm. More myelin is present in the chiasm, midbrain, inferior colliculus, medulla, and vermal cerebellum. (c) Newborn. Near midline. Chiasmal myelin is seen, as is myelin in the superior cerebellar peduncle decussation. The corpus callosum, fornix, and occipital lobe are not myelinated. (d) Four and a half months. Parieto-occipital and calcarine sulci are distinct. The chiasma and mesencephalic tegmentum are myelinated. The posterior corpus callosum body and splenium show beginning myelination. Vermal myelination is more advanced. (e) Seven months. The posterior corpus callosum and splenium is more myelinated. The fornix is beginning to myelinate. The chiasm and decussation of the superior cerebellar peduncle are myelinated. Vermal myelination has extended into folial white matter cores. (f) One year. The corpus callosum is wider and is myelinated from the rostrum to the splenium. The fornix is partially myelinated, as is the anterior commissure. The chiasm, midbrain tegmentum, basis pontis, and cerebellar vermal white matter are myelinated. The vermis is brightly myelinated, as are the medial portions of the occipital lobe. A small amount of myelin is present just rostral to the prominent parieto-occipital sulcus.

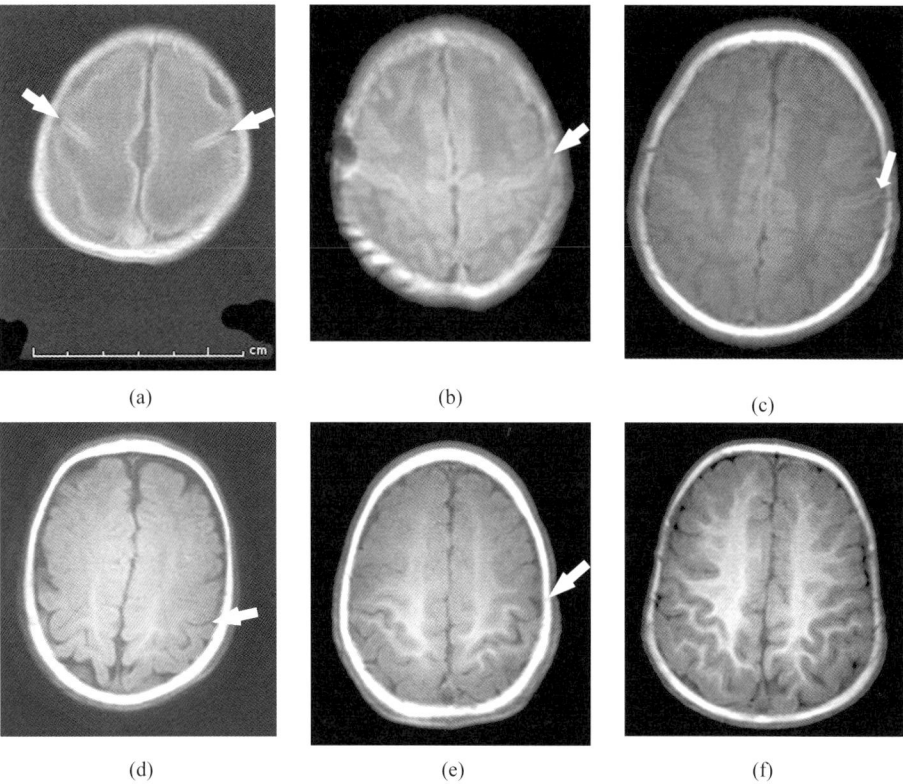

(a)   (b)   (c)

(d)   (e)   (f)

Fig. 6.11 T1-weighted fluid-attenuated inversion recovery magnetic resonance images, axial, high. (a) Preterm, 25 weeks (1.5T). There is no myelin in this high axial cut. The pre- and postcentral gyri bordering the central sulcus (arrows) are beginning to grow away from the smooth-surfaced midgestational brain. (b) Thirty-six weeks. The gyral pattern is far more complicated; the central sulcus is indicated (arrow). (c) Newborn. The gyral pattern is far more complicated, but there is no myelin at this level. The central sulcus lies posterior (arrow). (d) Four and a half months. The occipital and high parietal lobes contain early myelin. (e) Seven months. The myelin in the pre- and postcentral white matter is increased. The central sulcus lies posterior (arrow). (f) Twelve months. There has been a dramatic increase in the amount of myelin throughout the upper cerebrum.

AT BIRTH

In autopsy material from term infants, the following tracts have 50% of cases with grossly visible myelin: proprius, spinocerebellar, spinothalamic, medial lemniscus, spinal trigeminal, lateral lemniscus, parathalamic posterior limb, parasagittal cerebellum, superior cerebellar peduncle, red nucleus capsule, optic chiasm, optic tract, ansa lenticularis, inferior olivary nucleus amiculum, and habenulointerpeduncular tract.

In magnetic resonance images, early myelination is seen in the posterior corpus callosum body and splenium; optic nerves, chiasm, tracts, and radiations; superior cerebellar peduncle decussation; superior cerebellar peduncle; corona radiata of the posterior limb; and the inferior colliculus (Figs. 6.10c, 6.11c, 6.12.b, 6.13a, 6.14a, and 6.15a).

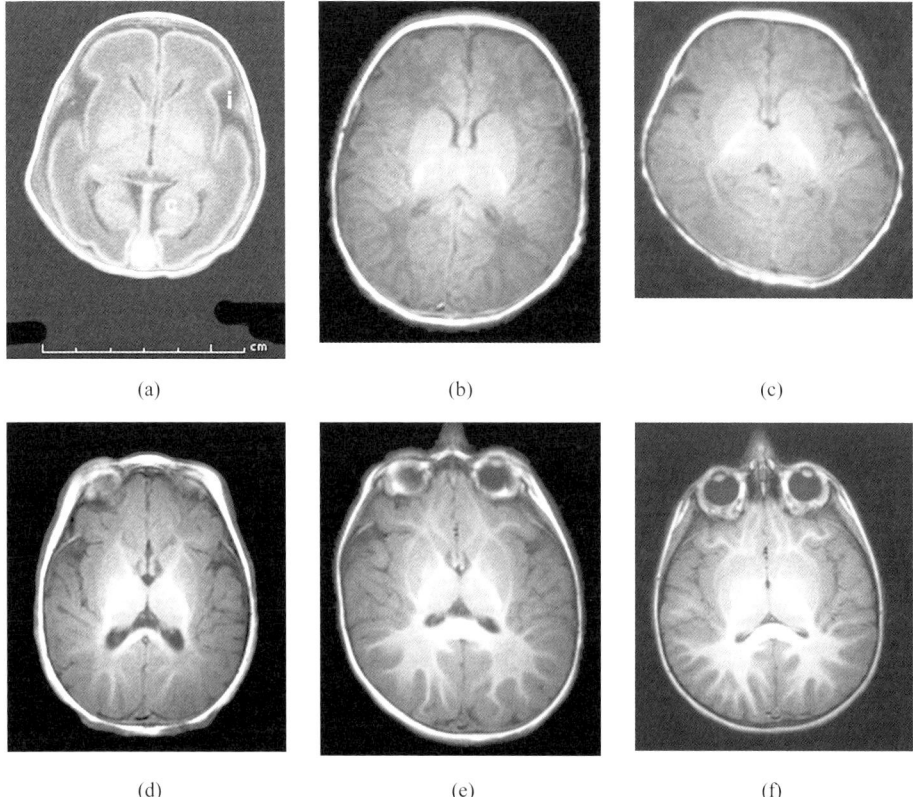

(a) (b) (c)

(d) (e) (f)

Fig. 6.12 T1-weighted fluid-attenuated inversion recovery magnetic resonance images, axial, midthalamus. (a) Twenty-five weeks (1.5T). The frontal and occipital horns, as well as third ventricle, are well visualized. The insula (i) is well developed in the bottom of the lateral sulcus. The posterior limb of the internal capsule separates basal ganglia from thalamus. Occipitally, the calcarine sulcus (c) indents medial occipital horn. There is no appreciable cerebral myelin. (b) Newborn. The insular fossa is almost covered. The gyral pattern is far more complicated. Myelin is present in the posterior limb. (c) Two months. Myelination is advanced in posterior limb and, to a lesser extent, in optic radiation. The insular fossa remains partially open. (d) Seven months. Posterior and anterior limbs are myelinated, as is the splenium. Occipital myelination is more advanced than frontal or temporal. The external capsule is well seen anteriorly. The insular fossa is still partially open. (e) Twelve months. Occipital myelination is more advanced than frontal or temporal. The fornix is myelinated, as is the mammillothalamic tract. The external capsule is well seen. Insular fossa is nearly closed. (f) Two years. The splenium is wider and is well myelinated. The temporal and frontal lobes are well myelinated. The extreme capsule (right) is myelinated. The fornix and mammillothalamic tracts are well myelinated.

At 1 year

The tracts in which 50% of cases contain grossly visible myelin include the hilus inferior olivary nucleus, auditory radiation, transverse gyrus of Heschl, transpontine, middle cerebellar peduncle, cerebellar hemisphere, dentate hilus, pontine corticospinal, occipital optic radiation, cingulum, corona radiata, distal radiation to precentral gyrus, posterior frontal, occipital pole, calcarine subcortical association fibers, and body, splenium, and rostrum of corpus callosum.

135

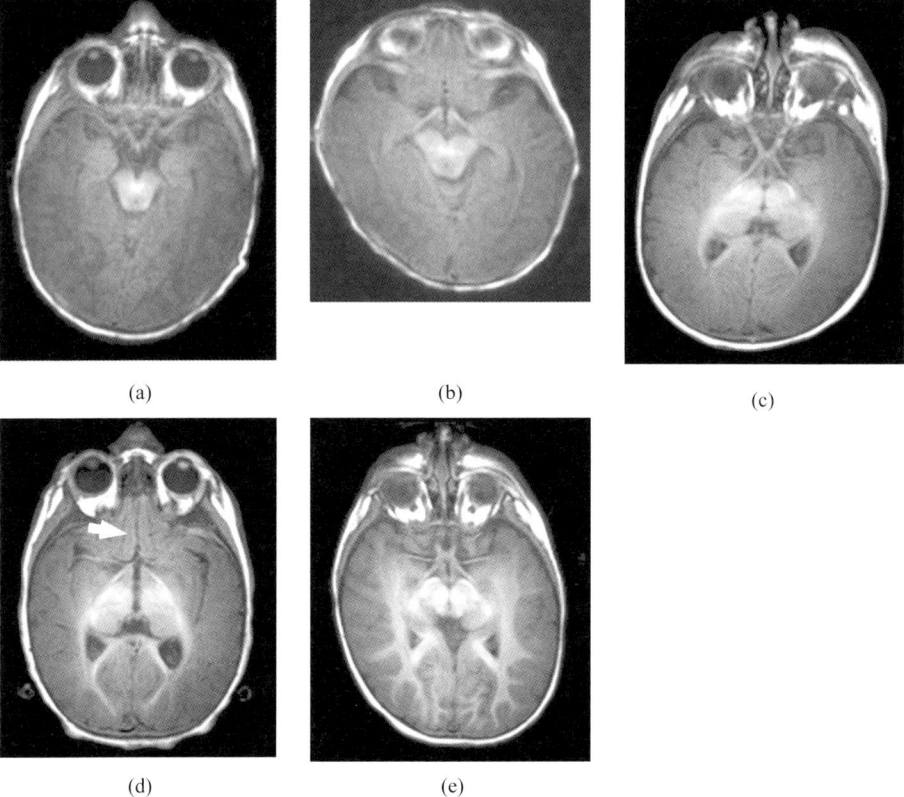

(a)   (b)   (c)

(d)   (e)

Fig. 6.13 T1-weighted fluid-attenuated inversion recovery magnetic resonance images, axial, optic nerves. (a) Newborn. The optic nerves and chiasm are well seen. The superior cerebellar peduncle decussation is seen in the midbrain. There is no myelin in the midbrain corticospinal tract. Myelin is not seen in temporal or occipital lobes. (b) Two months. The optic tracts and radiations are well seen. Corticospinal tracts in the midbrain show beginning myelination. Superior cerebellar peduncle and inferior colliculi are well myelinated. Remaining portions of temporal and occipital lobes are not myelinated. (c) Four and a half months. More myelin is present in midbrain corticospinal tracts. Transcallosal fibers lying on the atrial medial surfaces are myelinated. (d) Seven months. Optic tracts are well myelinated, as is the posterior limb. Optic radiation is well myelinated, as are the transcallosal fibers forming the tapetum wrapped around the calcarine cortex. There is no myelin in the temporal or basal frontal lobes. The gyrus rectus is prominent (arrow). (e) Twelve months. There is considerable myelin in the temporal and occipital lobes. The entire midbrain crus pedunculi is myelinated (corticospinal, frontopontine, and parietal, temporal, and occipital pontine fibers).

In magnetic resonance images at 1 year, myelin is present in the genu and the anterior limb, in addition to the posterior limb, occipital deep white matter, external capsule, anterior commissure, fornix, and mammillothalamic tract (Figs. 6.10f, 6.11f, 6.12e, 6.13e, 6.14e, and 6.15e).

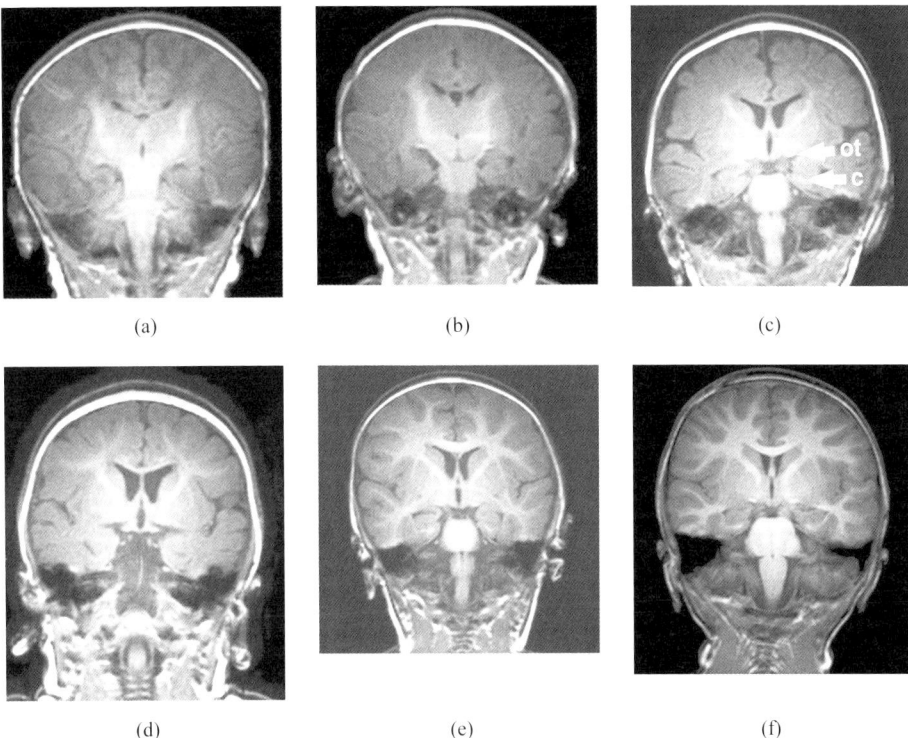

Fig. 6.14 T1-weighted fluid-attenuated inversion recovery magnetic resonance images, coronal, anterior third ventricle. (a) Newborn. Superior cerebellar peduncle, posterior limbs of the internal capsule, and optic tracts are myelinated. (b) Two months. Optic tracts, posterior limbs of the internal capsule, corticospinal tracts in midbrain, and pons contain myelin. Corona radiata shows beginning myelination. (c) Four and a half months. The cingulum (c) is well myelinated in the parahippocampal gyrus, as is the optic tract (ot). (d) Seven months. The frontal corona radiata, anterior limb, and corpus callosum body are all myelinated, as is the external capsule upper anterior end. (e) Twelve months. Temporal and frontal lobes are myelinated, as are anterior commissure and optic tract. Corticospinal tract in the pons and medulla is myelinated. (f) Two years. The medullary lamina between the putamen and globus pallidus is myelinated, as is the entire parahippocampal gyrus.

AT 2 YEARS

Similarly, the following are tracts in which 50% of cases contained grossly visible myelin at 2 years: inferior colliculus brachium; lateral crus pedunculi; midbrain, cervical, and thoracic corticospinal; lateral olfactory stria; deep white matter in posterior parietal, temporal, and frontal pole; external capsule; subcortical association fibers in frontal, temporal, and occipital poles, parietal, and posterior frontal; and stria medullaris thalami.

The myelinated tracts added during the second year include the upper cerebrum, splenium, deep temporal and frontal lobes, internal medullary lamina between the putamen and globus pallidus, entire parahippocampal gyrus, posterior portions of extreme capsule, and transverse temporal gyrus (Figs. 6.12f and 6.14f).

137

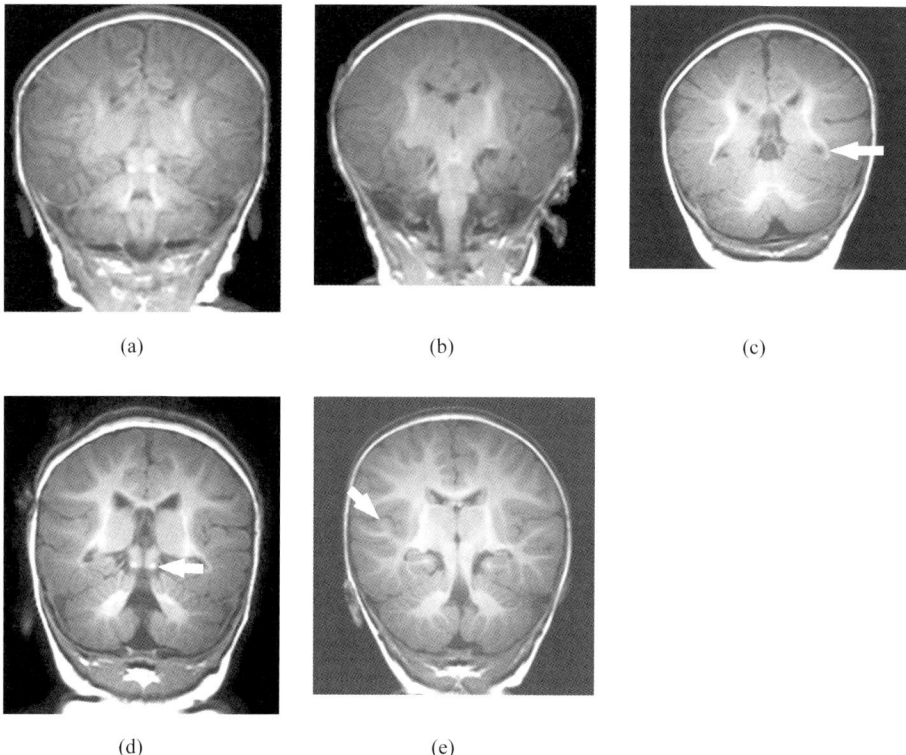

(a)   (b)   (c)

(d)   (e)

Fig. 6.15 T1-weighted fluid-attenuated inversion recovery magnetic resonance images, coronal, posterior thalamus. (a) Newborn. Behind splenium. The corona radiata of the posterior limb is myelinated, as is the inferior colliculus. The superior cerebellar peduncle is myelinated. (b) Two months. The corona radiata and optic radiations around the temporal horn are myelinated. The middle cerebellar peduncle is myelinated. (c) Four and a half months. Much posterior frontal and parietal white matter is myelinated. The posterior corpus callosum and optic radiation (arrow) are myelinated. Cerebellar hemispheral white matter is myelinated out to the folial white matter cores. (d) Seven months. Much posterior frontal and parietal white matter is myelinated out to gyral white matter cores. Much of temporal white matter, while showing some myelin, is not myelinated out the gyral white matter cores. The inferior colliculus (arrow) is myelinated. (e) Twelve months. Temporal white matter is myelinated, as are the posterior portions of extreme capsule, Heschl's transverse auditory gyrus on the right (arrow), posterior limb of internal capsule, and fornix.

GREATER THAN 2 YEARS

Late or slowly myelinating tracts included the central tegmental, solitary, medial crus pedunculi, lumbar corticospinal, putamen, globus pallidus, alveus, fimbria, fornix, extreme capsule, temporal subcortical association fibers, and anterior commissure (outer slightly before inner).

Finally, one feature needing re-emphasis is the largely postnatal myelination of fornix, cingulum, and anterior commissure. Prominently noted before, it is quite striking as these ancient telencephalic parts, important and recognizable at the point when telencephalic outpouching first evaginates, do not undergo myelination until much later in development, late in the second year and beyond.

DIRECTION OF MYELINATION

Cajal[65] viewed myelin formation as a result of axonal activity, beginning centrally (presumably at the neuron) and extending peripherally. Keene and Hewer[32] supported Cajal's concept and added the idea that, within related systems, myelin deposition progresses from the neuron along the axon in the direction of information flow. From our data, the oft-repeated idea that myelination occurs in a caudal–rostral direction is correct only in a very limited sense. While myelin does emerge in the spinal cord and brainstem before the forebrain, there were, within the spinal cord and brainstem, systems that myelinated slowly, for instance the fasciculus proprius.

Cajal's idea gains support in a few tracts, in which their distal ends not only start to myelinate later, but also at a slower rate. In the systems (e.g., fasciculus gracilis or corticospinal tract) where the same axons were supposedly sampled at multiple levels, myelin appears sequentially or simultaneously in caudal to rostral tract regions (e.g., fasciculus gracilis at lumbar, thoracic, and cervical levels). The only exception to this generalization is the curious relationship of optic tract and chiasm myelination. Chiasm myelination appears to follow tract and therefore seems consistent with previous observations of optic nerve direction of myelination toward the globe.[63] This myelinating system is likely to be unique.

The second aspect of directional information is the myelination of related systems. It seems, again with one exception, that myelination occurs in the direction of major information flow (fasciculus gracilis before medial lemniscus; dorsal spinocerebellar tract before inferior cerebellar peduncle before parasagittal cerebellum and superior cerebellar peduncle). The exception is that myelination of transpontine fibers and middle cerebellar peduncle antedates corticopontine fiber myelination in the mesencephalic cerebral peduncle. An apparent discrepancy in the relationship between the internal capsule posterior limb and the central corona radiata is accounted for by different systems myelinating in different directions in the posterior limb. As many long tract systems have caudally located neurons of origin in the nervous system (fasciculus gracilis, medial lemniscus), the idea of caudal–rostral progression is likely to support the directional flow of myelin deposition concept.

COMPARISONS WITH OTHER STUDIES

In Table 6.15, the timing of myelination in selected tracts is compared in four studies. Langworthy[8] used a small number of cases and Larroche[63] used a larger number of sites. While no other studies cited the wide range in gestational ages of myelination, the differences among them presumably reflect the factors mentioned above. The median ages for the NCPP population microscopic myelination are the same as or lower than the ages provided by other studies, suggesting that microscopic examinations were not done and/or that the earliest recorded ages (possibly outliers) were not used (in Table 6.15, all figures are in weeks of gestational age, gestational age plus survival age, or postnatal age, as each author indicated).

When myelination sequence standards, established in this study, are compared with those determined in previous studies, occasional significant discrepancies are revealed. For example, Yakovlev and Lecours[9] report that the corpus callosum body stains lighter in the brain of a 4-year-old child than in the single adult comparison brain, therefore concluding that the corpus callosum had a very long myelogenetic cycle. From our study, based on 101

139

TABLE 6.15

Comparison of several estimates of age at onset of human fetal nervous system myelination

	NCPP (microscopic myelin)	Yakovlev and Lecours[9]	Larroche[63]	Langworthy[8]
Spinal cord				
Fasciculus gracilis	<20	–	28	28
Dorsal spinocerebellar	<20	–	26	20
Spinothalamic	<20	–	26	28
Brainstem				
Medial longitudinal fasciculus	<20	20–22	24	20
Medial lemniscus	23–25	24	26–28	28 and 36
Acoustic	23–24	20–24	24–28	38
Inferior cerebellar peduncle	24	24	28	–
Superior cerebellar peduncle	26	32	32	28
Corticospinal	32–35	38	28–36	4 PN
Transpontine	35	4 PN	–	–
Middle cerebellar peduncle	35	8 PN	PN	4 PN
Cerebellum				
Parasagittal	27	–	32	–
Hemispheral	38	PN	40	–
Prosencephalon				
Habenulointerpeduncular	28	28	34	28
Ansa lenticularis	28	28	26	–
Optic chiasm	32	–	32	–
Optic tract	29	36	32	36
Optic radiation	38–39	38–40	38	–
Internal capsule, posterior limb	32	36	36	–
Corona radiata	34	30	–	–
Corticopontine				
Lateral Ped.	38	8 PN	–	8 PN
Medial Ped.	46	8 PN	–	8 PN
Cingulum	38	8 PN	–	–
Fornix	39	16 PN	PN	8 PN
Callosum	46	12 PN	PN	4 PN
Anterior commissure	46	12 PN	–	–
Mammillothalamic	48	36	–	8 PN

All figures are in gestational weeks or postnatal (PN) age as indicated by each author. The National Collaborative Perinatal Project (NCPP) figures are found earlier in this chapter.

cases between 11 and 33 postconceptional months, the central corpus callosum myelinated rapidly in the first 2 years; by 11 postconceptional months at least 50% of cases had myelin degree 3 or 4, and by 21 postconceptional months at least 90% had degree 3 or 4. Moreover, only 1 of 36 cases over the age of 21 postconceptional months had a grade less than degree 3. Yakovlev and Lecours relied upon the few cases they had available from the first decade of life, which very likely had variable staining characteristics. We believe that their prolonged myelination estimates, as in the corpus callosum and also in cerebral hemispheric white matter, although conceptually satisfying, are partially due to the small sample size and lack of an internal standard. Despite these variances, our estimates of earliest myelination are quite close to those of Yakovlev and Lecours.

Previous investigators attempted to choose 'normal' brains to use as their study population.[9] We maintain that this approach introduces the investigators' individual biases about normality, which are likely to be incorrect, and also neglects potentially important information. For example, sudden infant death syndrome brains had been used as 'normal' in myelination studies, but morphologic and neurochemical abnormalities of central nervous system white matter in sudden infant death syndrome brains question the validity of this assumption.[66] Clinicoanatomic reports have claimed delayed myelination in a few pediatric disorders,[67–71] and neurochemical studies, often contradictory, have reported white matter abnormalities in several others.[45,72,73] Although substantially aberrant central nervous system myelination is undeniable in certain cases, in most instances abnormal myelination must be defined in the light of data describing wide biologic variation. Entities associated with delayed myelination were not present in our autopsy sample. Nevertheless, some brains with aberrant myelination were possibly included in our population and, consequently, limit the data from accurately reflecting the sequence of myelination in normal living infants. Our inability to identify these aberrant brains based upon present knowledge justifies our approach to case selection. We strongly caution that the data presented in this report should not be interpreted as 'normative standards,' but should be compared with myelination data obtained in a different fashion, such as from neuroimaging studies.

DELAYED MYELINATION

Delayed myelination is easily recognized in that specific myelinating tracts are not keeping up with the schedule expected for an infant's age. This phenomenon is readily recognized on a magnetic resonance scan (Fig. 6.16). Spinal cord and brainstem tracts are difficult to visualize on magnetic resonance scans; however, hemispheral white matter is readily visualized. In the cerebrum, the best sites to visualize are the posterior and anterior internal capsule limbs, optic radiation, anterior commissure, and superficial and deep white matter in frontal, parietal, temporal, and occipital lobes.

Delayed myelination significance

The brain is potentially vulnerable to external forces during its myelination period, which occurs simultaneously with its major growth period during the second gestational half and the first 2 years of life (see Chapter 2). Myelin deposition quantitatively constitutes a major part of brain growth once the basic brain plan is established early in gestation. Factors such as

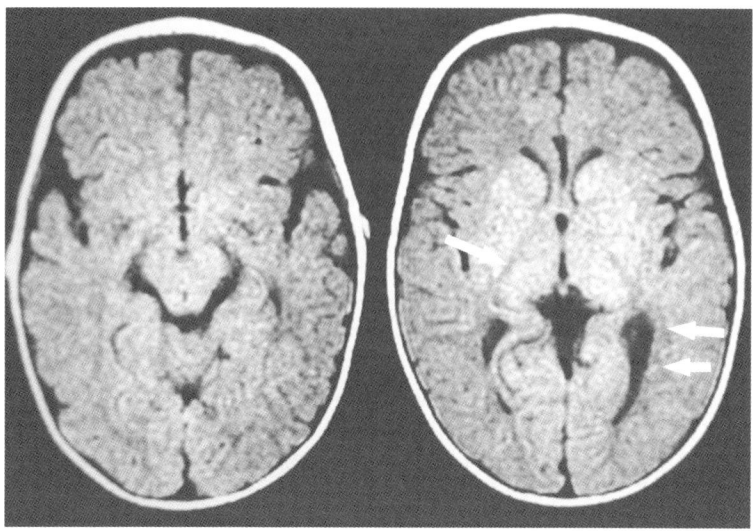

Fig. 6.16 T1-weighted spin-echo magnetic resonance images. Four-month-old with delayed development. There is no brain myelin deposition. At this age, the posterior limbs of the internal capsule (arrow) and optic radiations (two arrows) should be white (hyperintense) on this sequence. Compare with Figs. 6.10 to 6.15 of a typical infant at this age.

undernutrition, also associated with temporary reduced body growth, potentially reduce myelin precursor delivery to the developing brain.[74] Myelin previously laid down is unlikely to be reduced, but the myelination rate may be delayed.[75] A large body of data supports the hypothesis that the myelinating brain is vulnerable to the same factors that retard growth of other organs.[76–78] Conditions as diverse as twinning, sudden infant death syndrome, methylmalonic acidemia, 3-phosphoglycerate dehydrogenase deficiency, Tay syndrome (trichothiodystrophy or sulfur-deficient brittle hair disease), Larsson syndrome,[79–82] maternal phenylketonuria, iron deficiency, and several varieties of congenital muscular dystrophy[80,83–91] are associated with delayed myelination. Its most common clinical association is developmental delay.[92]

Delayed myelination risk factors
A myelination score, calculated for each infant from the sum of scores for each of 12 tracts, was the primary data collected for this chapter. Tracts were chosen on the basis of myelination timing (to ensure that the scoring procedure was appropriate for all gestational ages) and identification ease.[93] Adding the score for all 12 tracts allowed us to appreciate diffuse as well as localized delayed myelination.

In each of eight gestational age groups, approximately 15% of newborns with the lowest myelination scores were defined as having delayed myelination. A delay in myelination of at least several weeks was necessary for a newborn to qualify as having delayed myelination. As most newborns in this sample died during the first few postnatal days, postnatal events were unlikely to have contributed appreciably to a delay in myelination. For this reason, confounding postnatal events were excluded from the multivariate analysis.

'Seizures in siblings' had the risk ratio with the largest point estimate. 'Smoking at least one pack of cigarettes per day' had the next largest risk ratio. Low birthweight was associated with an increased risk of delayed myelination. Delayed myelination risk increased in older gestational age neonates, particularly over 36 weeks. Women who had third-trimester uterine bleeding were at an increased risk of their infant having delayed myelination, as were women whose lowest hematocrit during pregnancy was less than 35%. Maternal smoking during pregnancy increased the risk of fetal growth retardation, perinatal death, and lower Apgar score, based on a previous observation[94] and an observation subsequently confirmed.[95] Infants who died a few weeks after the first ultrasonographic expression of focal necroses had evidence of 'markedly depressed rates of white-matter growth'.[96]

CENTRAL HYPOMYELINATION OR DELAYED MYELINATION DISCUSSION
Central hypomyelination or delayed myelination in infants and children without a leuko-encephalopathy, signs of demyelination, or a metabolic abnormality, with or without hypoplasia of white matter, was probably first recognized experimentally in laboratory animals[97,98] and was then found in a variety of human diseases (for instance, some cases of Cockayne syndrome and Menkes disease),[99–102] neonatal hypothyroidism,[103] and in those with increased intracranial pressure in infantile hydrocephalus.[104] Hypomyelination sometimes accompanies atrophy of basal ganglia and cerebellum in children.[105,106]

Other environmental factors potentially affect human brain myelinogenesis. Essential fatty acid deficiency has been well studied for the important role of C22:6 in visual system myelinogenesis. The observation that dietary fatty acids sometimes affect membrane composition led to the use of modified diets in some central nervous system pathologic conditions. For example, preterm infants characterized by low levels of C22:6 who were fed with diets enriched in this fatty acid showed a recovery of visual function.[107] Myelination is delayed in cerebro-oculofacio-skeletal syndrome[108] and Salla disease.[109] Hypomyelination with white matter cysts occurs in pyruvate carboxylase deficiency.[110] In Pelizaeus–Merzbacher disease, the gene coding for myelin proteolipid protein is deficient and is associated with premature death of oligodendroglia.[111]

White matter hypoplasia

In older children past the myelination period, delayed myelination is far more difficult to recognize, either on magnetic resonance scans or at autopsy. The process then expresses itself as hypoplastic white matter. In infants in the second year of life, both delayed myelination and hypoplastic cerebral white matter are recognizable. The several abnormalities in hypoplastic white matter brains, besides the overall white matter paucity, include diffuse gliosis,[112,113] astrocytosis, and microgliosis;[114–116] however, the gliosis, rarely, may be absent.[117] Residual scars of old focal necrosis cavities do not account for the widely spread white matter astrocytosis. Oligodendroglia number may be depleted.[118] Children (especially those born preterm) sometimes have, in addition to focal necroses, paucity of white matter and corpus callosum thinning.[119–124] Hypoplastic white matter is found in several conditions, such as cytomegalo-virus infection,[125] maternal varicella,[126] Apert syndrome,[127] and epidermal nevus syndrome.[128] It is also found in several genetic abnormalities,[129,130] as well as in many conditions in which the primary abnormality is unknown.

Morgagni recognized ventriculomegaly without head enlargement.[131] In patients with normal or small head circumferences, Cruveilhier (early nineteenth century)[132] recognized ventriculomegaly accompanying gray and white matter damage and loss. Ventriculomegaly accompanying white matter damage only with relatively normal gray matter was recognized in the twentieth century when McClelland[133] demonstrated a case (case 6) with 'hydromicro-cephaly.' The child had died at age 11 months with ventriculomegaly and a 'normal' cortex, basal ganglia, and thalami. Subsequently, Benda[134,135] recognized that ventriculomegaly, white matter cysts, and preserved gray matter not only occurred together, but accompanied devel-opmental and myelination hemispheral white matter failure (Fig. 6.17). In 1954, Crome[112] reported an additional seven cases with white matter hypoplasia and ventriculomegaly and added the observation that there was white matter 'fibrillary gliosis' in most cases. Finally, in 1969, the association between white matter hypoplasia and a previous perinatal telencephalic leukoencephalopathy was suggested.[117,136]

Delayed myelination and white matter hypoplasia represent the ends of a continuum starting during the myelination period, and in many cases the causes are unknown. Some cases of delayed myelination are found in infants with perfectly normal white matter volume. Other cases occur with ventriculomegaly resulting from white matter loss but with adequate myelination of remaining white matter. Finally, many cases occur with both delayed myelina-tion and white matter hypoplasia.

Conclusion

Working with two data sets (different populations, section thickness, and staining techniques) led to a few major discrepancies in myelination timing. At a few sites, there was a discrepancy between the data sets of two or more months for the time at which 50% of cases contained grossly visible myelin. These were parasagittal cerebellum and red nucleus capsule with 3-month discrepancies, and ansa lenticularis with an 11-month discrepancy.

All ascending systems evaluated entered the second half of gestation with a small propor-tion of cases containing some myelin, and by term many peripheral sensory systems were at least partially myelinated, particularly the upper cervical cord fibers coming from the shoulders, arms, hands, and neck. The brainstem showed a similar myelination pattern for the major sensory systems, including facial, vestibular, auditory (at least to the inferior colliculus and medial lemniscus, with the exception of the solitary tract). Thus, incoming sensory input from the body to the thalamic ventrolateral posterior nucleus, via the medial lemniscus and spinothalamic tract, is well myelinated at term. Myelination of thalamocortical fibers, on the other hand (while starting prenatally), largely occurs postnatally.

We remind the reader that we have not implied a relationship between neurologic func-tion and myelination. Function occurs in unmyelinated systems. Functional acquisition is not dependent upon myelination in all systems, although the ability of the kitten's pyramidal tract to conduct rapid, repetitive stimuli occurs after myelin sheath development.[137] Axonal

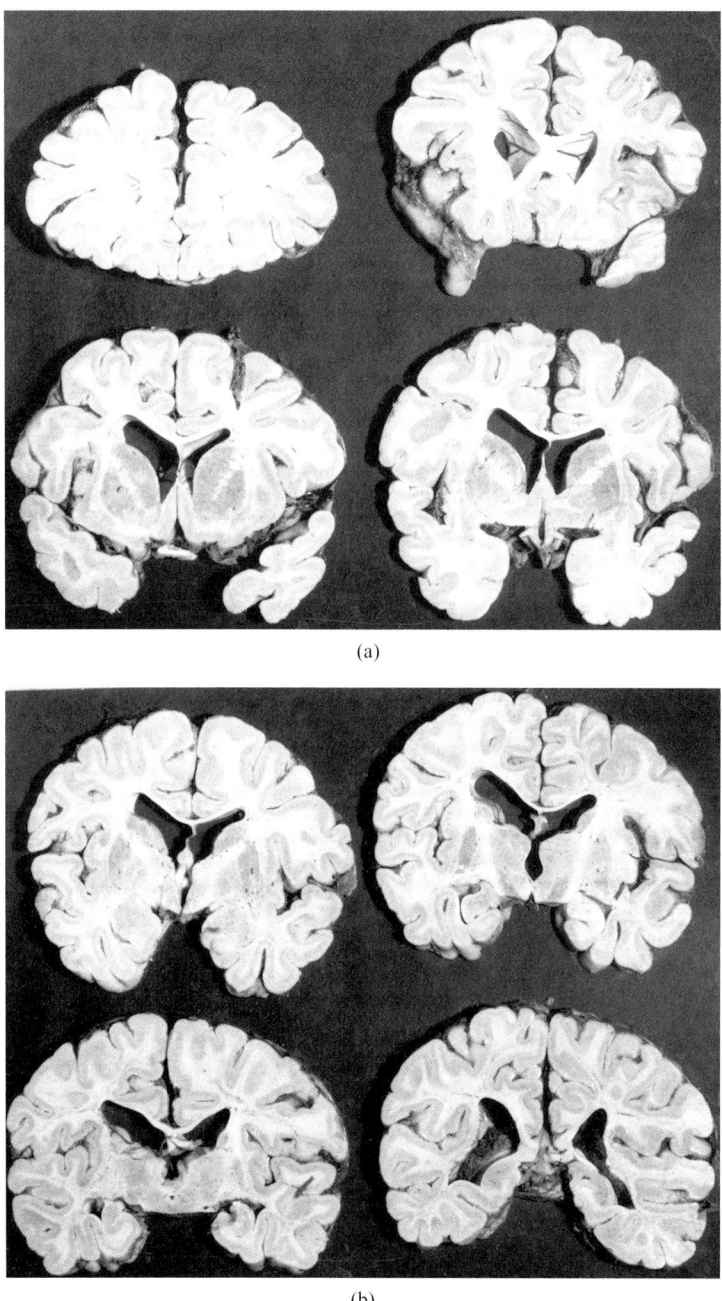

(a)

(b)

Fig. 6.17 Coronal sections demonstrating hypoplastic white matter. (a) Frontal. (b) Parietal and occipital. There is a gross disproportion between the amount of gray matter and the amount of white matter. Lateral ventricles are enlarged. Thalamus is of normal bulk. The corpus callosum is thin, including the splenium. Histologically there was a diffuse astrocytosis of white matter.

coating with myelin is an obvious developmental process, with the differences in myelination timing at various sites probably reflecting the interaction of a number of forces (such as phylogenetic, genetic, functional), and adverse environmental agents. The tracts selected in these studies represent the entire second half of gestation and first two postnatal years, with the goal that this important developmental myelination could be examined over an extended developmental period. Identifying myelinating sites with long or late-gestational myelinative phases should help to identify some of the influences to which myelination is vulnerable. Finally, these data also represent important guidelines for myelination assessment in living infants by high-resolution imaging techniques.

At the autopsy table in general pediatric hospitals and in hospitals serving individuals with severe brain damage, the most prevalent brain abnormalities are hypomyelination and hypoplastic white matter. In fact, these two abnormalities constitute a major societal outlay, as the resources required to support these people are considerable.

REFERENCES

1. Vesalius A (1543) *De humani corporis fabrica*. Basel.
2. Piccolomini A (1586) *Anatomicae praelectiones...explicantes mirificam corporis humani fabricam.* Rome: Bonfadinus.
3. Clarke E, O'Malley C (1996) *The Human Brain and Spinal Cord; A Historical Study Illustrated by Writings from Antiquity to the Twentieth Century*. San Francisco: Norman Publishing.
4. Tiedemann F (1826) *The Anatomy of the Foetal Brain*. Edinburgh: John Carfrae & Son.
5. Flechsig P (1901) Developmental (myelogenetic) localization of the cerebral cortex in the human subject. *Lancet* 2: 1027–1029.
6. Flechsig P (1920) *Anatomie des menschlichen Gehirns und Ruchenmarks*. Leipzig: Georg Thieme.
7. Flechsig P (1877) Über 'Systemerkrankungen' im Rückenmark. *Arch Heilk* 18: 101–141, 289–343, 461–483.
8. Langworthy O (1933) Development of behavior patterns and myelinization of the nervous system in the human fetus and infant. *Contr Embryology (Carnegie Institution of Washington)* 24: 1–57.
9. Yakovlev PI, Lecours AR (1967) The myelogenetic cycles of regional maturation of the brain. In: Minkowski A, editor. *Regional Development of the Brain in Early Life*. Oxford: Blackwell, pp. 3–70.
10. Richardson EP (1981) Myelination in the human central nervous system. In: Haymaker W, Adams R, editors. *Histology and Histopathology of the Nervous System*. Springfield, IL: Charles C. Thomas, pp. 146–173.
11. Kinney HC, Karthigasan J, Borenshteyn NI, Flax JD, Kirschner DA (1994) Myelination in the developing human brain: biochemical correlates. *Neurochem Res* 19: 983–996.
12. Müller F, O'Rahilly R (1988) The first appearance of the future cerebral hemispheres in the human embryo at stage 14. *Anat Embryol (Berl)* 177: 495–511.
13. Roback HN, Scherer HJ (1935) Über die feinere Morphologie des frünkindlichen Gehirns unter besonderer Berücksichtigung der Gliaentwicklung. *Virchows Arch Path Anat* 294: 365–413.
14. Rydberg E (1932) Cerebral injury in newborn children consequent on birth trauma; with an inquiry into the normal and pathological anatomy of the neuroglia. *Acta Pathol Microbiol Scand* Suppl. X.
15. Kershman J (1938) The medulloblast and the medulloblastoma—A study of human embryos. *Arch Neurol Psychiat* 40: 937–967.
16. Tuthill CR (1938) Fat in the infant brain in relation to myelin, blood vessels, and glia. *Arch Path* 25: 336–346.
17. Mickel HS, Gilles FH (1970) Changes in glial cells during human telencephalic myelinogenesis. *Brain* 93: 337–346.
18. Chi J, Gilles F, Kerr C, Hare C (1976) Sudanophilic material in the developing nervous system. *J Neuropathol Exp Neurol* 35: 119–120.

19. Meier C (1976) Some observations on early myelination in the human spinal cord. Light and electron microscope study. *Brain Res* 104: 21–32.
20. Leech RW, Alvord EC (1974) Glial fatty metamorphosis: an abnormal response of premyelin glia frequently accompanying periventricular leukomalacia. *Am J Pathol* 1974: 603–612.
21. Sumi S (1974) Periventricular leukoencephalopathy in the monkey. A search for the 'normal control' and the 'early lesion.' *Arch Neurol* 31: 38–44.
22. Virchow R (1867) Zur pathologischen anatomie des gehirns: I Congenitale encephalitis und myelitis. *Virch Arch* 38: 129–138.
23. Parrot MJ (1868) Etude sur la stèatose interstitielle diffuse de l'encèphale chez le nouveau-nè. *Arch Physiol Norm Patholol (Paris)* 1: 530–550, 622–642, 706–715.
24. Jastrowitz M (1870) Encephalitis und Myelitis des ersten Kindesalters 1. *Arch Psych Nervenkr* 2: 389–414.
25. Jastrowitz M (1872) Encephalitis und Myelitis des ersten Kindesalters. 2. *Arch Psych Nervenkr* 3: 162.
26. Jastrowitz M (1883) Encephalitis und Myelitis des ersten Kindesalters. 3. *Berl Klin Wschr* 30: 46.
27. Guillery H (1923) Entwicklungsgeschichtliche untersuchungun als Beitrag zur Frage der encephalitis interstitialis neonatorum (Virchow). *Zeitschr f Neurol u Psych* 84: 205–256.
28. Okado N (1982) Early myelin formation and glial cell development in the human spinal cord. *Anat Rec* 202: 483–490.
29. Haynes RL, Borenstein NS, Desilva TM, et al (2005) Axonal development in the cerebral white matter of the human fetus and infant. *J Comp Neurol* 484: 156–167.
30. Bruska M (2003) An ultrastructural study of the myelination of the trigeminal ganglion in human foetuses aged 10 to 23 weeks. *Folia Morphol (Warsz)* 62: 231–233.
31. Niebrój-Dobosz I, Fidzianska A, Rafallowska J, Sawicka E (1980) Correlative biochemical and morphological studies of myelination in human ontogenesis. II. Myelination of the nerve roots. *Acta Neuropathol* 49: 153–158.
32. Keene M, Hewer E (1931) Some observations on myelination in the human central nervous system. *J Anat* 66: 1–13.
33. Fidzianska A (1976) Fine structure of human fetal nerve. *Pol Med Sci Hist Bull* 15: 281–289.
34. Wozniak W, O'Rahilly R, Bruska M (1982) Myelination of the human fetal phrenic nerve. *Acta Anat (Basel)* 112: 281–296.
35. Shield LK, King RH, Thomas PK (1986) A morphometric study of human fetal sural nerve. *Acta Neuropathol (Berl)* 70: 60–70.
36. Brante G (1949) Studies on lipids in the nervous system with special reference to quantitative chemical determination and topical distribution. *Acta Physiol Scand* 18(Suppl 63): 1–189.
37. Davison A, Peters A (1970) *Myelination*. Springfield, IL: Charles C. Thomas.
38. Savolainen H, Palo J, Riekkinen P, Moronen P, Brody LE (1972) Maturation of myelin proteins in human brain. *Brain Res* 37: 253–263.
39. Savolainen H (1972) Proteins and glycoproteins of human myelin and glial cell membrane with special reference to myelin formation. *TIT J Life Sci* 2: 35–38.
40. Martinez M, Conde C, Ballabriga A (1974) Some chemical aspects of human brain development. II Phosphoglyceride fatty acids. *Pediatr Res* 8: 93–102.
41. Conde C, Martinez M, Ballabriga A (1974) Some chemical aspects of human brain development. I Neutral glycosphingolipids, sulfatides, and sphingomyelin. *Pediatr Res* 8: 89–92.
42. Fishman MA, Agrawal HC, Alexander A, Golterman J (1975) Biochemical maturation of human central nervous system myelin. *J Neurochem* 24: 689–694.
43. Ballabriga A, Martinez M (1978) A chemical study on the development of the human forebrain and cerebellum during the brain 'growth spurt' period. II Phosphoglyceride fatty acids. *Brain Res* 159: 363–370.
44. Martinez M, Ballabriga A (1978) A chemical study on the development of the human forebrain and cerebellum during the brain 'growth spurt' period. I. Gangliosides and plasmalogens. *Brain Res* 159: 351–362.
45. Poduslo SE, Jang Y (1984) Myelin development in infant brain. *Neurochem Res* 9: 1615–1626.
46. Friede RI (1961) A histochemical study of DPN-diaphorase in human white matter with some notes on myelination. *J Neurochem* 8: 17–30.
47. Matthews MA, Duncan D (1971) A quantitative study of morphological changes accompanying the initiation and progress of myelin production in the dorsal funiculus of the rat spinal cord. *J Comp Neurol* 142: 1–22.

48. Weidenheim KM, Bodhireddy SR, Rashbaum WK, Lyman WD (1996) Temporal and spatial expression of major myelin proteins in the human fetal spinal cord during the second trimester. *J Neuropathol Exp Neurol* 55: 734–745.

49. Rorke L, Riggs H (1969) *Myelination of the Brain in the Newborn*. Philadelphia: JB Lippincott.

50. Lemire RJ, Loeser JD, Leech RW, Alvord EC Jr. (1975) *Normal and Abnormal Development of the Human Nervous System*. Hagerstown, Maryland: Harper and Row.

51. Gilles FH, Shankle W, Dooling EC (1983) Myelinated tracts: growth patterns. In: Gilles FH, Leviton A, Dooling EC, editors. *The Developing Human Brain: Growth and Epidemiologic Neuropathology*. Boston: Wright-PSG, pp. 117–183.

52. Brody BA, Kinney HC, Kloman AS, Gilles FH (1987) Sequence of central nervous system myelination in human infancy, I: an autopsy study of myelination. *J Neuropathol Exp Neurol* 46: 283–301.

53. Gilles FH, Winston K, Fulchiero A, Leviton A (1977) Histologic features and observational variation in cerebellar gliomas in children. *J Natl Cancer Inst* 58: 175–181.

54. Ayer M, Brunk H, Ewing GM, Reid WT, Silverman E (1955) An empirical distribution function for sampling with incomplete information. *Ann Math Statistics* 26: 641–647.

55. Finkelstein DM (1984) A WfR methods of survival analysis. In: Cornell RG, editor. *Statistical Methods for Cancer Studies*. New York: Dekker, pp. 127–166.

56. Kinney HC, Brody BA, Kloman AS, Gilles FH (1988) Sequence of central nervous system myelination in human infancy, II: patterns of myelination of autopsied infants. *J Neuropathol Exp Neurol* 47: 217–234.

57. Hooker D (1952) *The Prenatal Origin of Behavior*. Lawrence, KS: University of Kansas Press.

58. Humphrey T (1951) The caudal extent of the descending root of the trigeminal nerve during the period of early human fetal activity (8 to 8.5 weeks of menstrual age). *Anat Rec* 109: 306–307.

59. Humphrey T (1952) The spinal tract of the trigeminal nerve in human embryos between 7.5 and 8.5 weeks of menstrual age and its relation to fetal behavior. *J Comp Neurol* 97: 143–209.

60. Humphrey T (1954) The trigeminal nerve in relation to early human fetal activity. *Res Pub Assoc Res Nerv Ment Dis* 33: 127–154.

61. Broca P (1878) Anatomie comparee circonvolutions cerebrales: le grand lobe limbique et la scissure limbique dans la serie des mammiferes. *Rev Anthropol* 1: 384–498.

62. Humphrey T (1968) The development of the human amygdala during embryonic life. *J Comp Neurol* 132: 135–165.

63. Larroche J (1966) The development of the central nervous system during intrauterine life. In: Falkner F, editor. *Human Development*. Philadelphia: WB Saunders, pp. 257–276.

64. Klosovskii B (1963) *The Development of the Brain and Its Disturbance by Harmful Factors.* Oxford: Pergamon Press.

65. Cajal R (1911) *Histologie du Systeme Nerveux*. Paris: Maloine.

66. Takashima S, Armstrong D, Becker LE, Huber J (1978) Cerebral white matter lesions in sudden infant death syndrome. *Pediatrics* 62: 155–159.

67. Kemper TL, Lecours AR, Gates MJ, Yakovlev PI (1973) Retardation of the myelo- and cytoarchitectonic maturation of the brain in the congenital rubella syndrome. *Res Publ Assoc Res Nerv Ment Dis* 51: 23–62.

68. Rorke LB, Spiro AJ (1967) Cerebral lesions in congenital rubella syndrome. *J Pediatr* 70: 243–255.

69. Alvord EC, Stevenson LD, Vogel FS, Engle RL (1950) Neuropathogical findings in phenylpyruvic oligophrenia (phenylketonuria). *J Neuropathol Exp Neurol* 9: 298.

70. Silberman J, Dancis J, Feigin I (1961) Neuropathological observations in maple syrup urine disease: branched-chain ketoaciduria. *Arch Neurol* 5: 351–363.

71. Zeman W, Demyer W, Falls HF (1964) Pelizaeus–Merzbacher disease. A study in nosology. *J Neuropathol Exp Neurol* 23: 334–354.

72. Carey EM, Foster PC (1984) The activity of 2′,3′-cyclic nucleotide 3′-phosphohydrolase in the corpus callosum, subcortical white matter, and spinal cord in infants dying from sudden infant death syndrome. *J Neurochem* 42: 924–929.

73. Foster PC, Carey EM (1983) The ontogenic development of 2′,3′-cyclic nucleotide 3′-phosphohydrolase in the corpus callosum in relation to oligodendroglial proliferation, myelination and the distribution of fat-containing glial cells. *Early Hum Dev* 9: 33–47.

74. Wiggins RC (1982) Myelin development and nutritional insufficiency. *Brain Res* 257: 151–175.

75. Davison AN, Dobbing J (1966) Myelination as a vulnerable period in brain development. *Brit Med Bull* 22: 40–44.

76. Dodge PR, Prensky AL, Feigin RD (1975) *Nutrition and the Developing Nervous System*. St. Louis: CV Mosby Co.

77. Evans D, Hansen JD, Moodie AD, van der Spuy HI (1980) Intellectual development and nutrition. *J Pediatr* 97: 358–363.

78. Morgane PJ, Austin-LaFrance R, Bronzino J, et al (1993) Prenatal malnutrition and development of the brain. *Neurosci Biobehav Rev* 17: 91–128.

79. McLennan JE, Gilles FH, Robb RM (1974) Neuropathologic correlation in Sjogren–Larsson syndrome (oligophrenia, ichthyosis and spasticity). *Brain* 97: 693–703.

80. Ostergaard JR, Christensen T (1996) The central nervous system in Tay syndrome. *Neuropediatrics* 27: 326–330.

81. Toelle SP, Valsangiacomo E, Boltshauser E (2001) Trichothiodystrophy with severe cardiac and neurological involvement in two sisters. *Eur J Pediatr* 160: 728–731.

82. Nakayama M, Tavora DG, Alvim TC, Araujo AC, Gama RL (2006) MRI and ^{1}H-MRS findings of three patients with Sjogren–Larsson syndrome. *Arq Neuropsiquiatr* 64(2B): 398–401.

83. Kinney HC, Brody BA, Finkelstein DM, Vawter GF, Mandell F, Gilles FH (1991) Delayed central nervous system myelination in the sudden infant death syndrome. *J Neuropathol Exp Neurol* 50: 29–48.

84. Barkovich AJ (1998) Neuroimaging manifestations and classification of congenital muscular dystrophies. *AJNR Am J Neuroradiol* 19: 1389–1396.

85. Ulfig N, Nickel J, Saretzki U (1998) Alterations in myelin formation in fetal brains of twins. *Pediatr Neurol* 19: 287–293.

86. Pineda M, Vilaseca MA, Artuch R, et al (2000) 3-phosphoglycerate dehydrogenase deficiency in a patient with West syndrome. *Dev Med Child Neurol* 42: 629–633.

87. Morath DJ, Mayer-Proschel M (2001) Iron modulates the differentiation of a distinct population of glial precursor cells into oligodendrocytes. *Dev Biol* 237: 232–243.

88. Morath DJ, Mayer-Proschel M (2002) Iron deficiency during embryogenesis and consequences for oligodendrocyte generation in vivo. *Dev Neurosci* 24(2–3): 197–207.

89. Ortiz E, Pasquini JM, Thompson K, et al (2004) Effect of manipulation of iron storage, transport, or availability on myelin composition and brain iron content in three different animal models. *J Neurosci Res* 77: 681–689.

90. Kanaumi T, Takashima S, Hirose S, Kodama T, Iwasaki H (2006) Neuropathology of methylmalonic acidemia in a child. *Pediatr Neurol* 34: 156–159.

91. Koch R, Verma S, Gilles FH (2008) Neuropathology of a 4-month-old infant born to a woman with phenylketonuria. *Dev Med Child Neurol* 50: 230–233.

92. Pujol J, Lopez-Sala A, Sebastian-Galles N, et al (2004) Delayed myelination in children with developmental delay detected by volumetric MRI. *Neuroimage* 22: 897–903.

93. Leviton A, Gilles FH, Dooling EC (1983) The epidemiology of delayed myelination. In: Gilles FH, Leviton A, Dooling EC, editors. *The Developing Human Brain: Growth and Epidemiologic Neuropathology*. Boston: Wright-PSG, pp. 185–192.

94. de Haas JH (1975) Parental smoking. Its effects on fetus and child health. *Eur J Obstet Gynecol Reprod Biol* 5: 283–296.

95. Romo A, Carceller R, Tobajas J (2009) Intrauterine growth retardation (IUGR): epidemiology and etiology. *Pediatr Endocrinol Rev* 6(Suppl 3): 332–336.

96. de la Monte SM, Hsu FI, Hedley-Whyte ET, Kupsky W (1990) Morphometric analysis of the human infant brain: effects of intraventricular hemorrhage and periventricular leukomalacia. *J Child Neurol* 5: 101–110.

97. Konat G, Clausen J (1976) Triethyllead-induced hypomyelination in the developing rat forebrain. *Exp Neurol* 50: 124–133.

98. Zimmerman AW, Matthieu JM, Quarles RH, Brady RO, Hsu JM (1976) Hypomyelination in copper-deficient rats. Prenatal and postnatal copper replacement. *Arch Neurol* 33: 111–119.

99. Castroviejo IP, Alonso Blanco M, Benito Casado C, Escobar H, Ciria Latre E (1977) [Menke's disease. A case report (author's transl)]. *An Esp Pediatr* 10: 205–214.

100. Dabbagh O, Swaiman KF (1988) Cockayne syndrome: MRI correlates of hypomyelination. *Pediatr Neurol* 4: 113–116.

101. Kennedy RM, Rowe VD, Kepes JJ (1980) Cockayne syndrome: an atypical case. *Neurology* 30: 1268–1272.

102. Nishio H, Kodama S, Matsuo T, Ichihashi M, Ito H, Fujiwara Y (1988) Cockayne syndrome: magnetic resonance images of the brain in a severe form with early onset. *J Inherit Metab Dis* 11: 88–102.

103. Bernal J (2002) Action of thyroid hormone in brain. *J Endocrinol Invest* 25: 268–288.

104. Hanlo PW, Gooskens RJ, van Schooneveld M, et al (1997) The effect of intracranial pressure on myelination and the relationship with neurodevelopment in infantile hydrocephalus. *Dev Med Child Neurol* 39: 286–291.

105. van der Knaap MS, Naidu S, Pouwels PJ, Bonavita S, van Coster R, Lagae L (2002) New syndrome characterized by hypomyelination with atrophy of the basal ganglia and cerebellum. *AJNR Am J Neuroradiol* 23: 1466–1474.

106. Mercimek-Mahmutoglu S, van der Knaap MS, Baric I, Prayer D, Stoeckler-Ipsiroglu S (2005) Hypomyelination with atrophy of the basal ganglia and cerebellum (H-ABC). Report of a new case. *Neuropediatrics* 36: 223–226.

107. Di Biase A, Salvati S (1997) Exogenous lipids in myelination and myelination. *Kaohsiung J Med Sci* 13: 19–29.

108. Del Bigio MR, Greenberg CR, Rorke LB, Schnur R, McDonald-McGinn DM, Zackai EH (1997) Neuropathological findings in eight children with cerebro-oculo-facio-skeletal (COFS) syndrome. *J Neuropathol Exp Neurol* 56: 1147–1157.

109. Morse RP, Kleta R, Alroy J, Gahl WA (2005) Novel form of intermediate salla disease: clinical and neuroimaging features. *J Child Neurol* 20: 814–816.

110. Pineda M, Campistol J, Vilaseca MA, et al (1995) An atypical French form of pyruvate carboxylase deficiency. *Brain Dev* 17: 276–279.

111. Kagawa T, Ikenaka K, Inoue Y, et al (1994) Glial cell degeneration and hypomyelination caused by overexpression of myelin proteolipid protein gene. *Neuron* 13: 427–442.

112. Crome L (1954) Some morbid-anatomical aspects of mental deficiency. *J Ment Sci* 100: 894–912.

113. Roessmann U, Gambetti P (1986) Pathological reaction of astrocytes in perinatal brain injury. Immunohistochemical study. *Acta Neuropathol (Berl)* 70(3–4): 302–307.

114. Saliba E, Henrot A (2001) Inflammatory mediators and neonatal brain damage. *Biol Neonate* 79(3–4): 224–227.

115. Rezaie P, Dean A (2002) Periventricular leukomalacia, inflammation and white matter lesions within the developing nervous system. *Neuropathology* 22: 106–132.

116. Inder T, Neil J, Kroenke C, Dieni S, Yoder B, Rees S (2005) Investigation of cerebral development and injury in the prematurely born primate by magnetic resonance imaging and histopathology. *Dev Neurosci* 27(2–4): 100–111.

117. Chattha AS, Richardson EP Jr. (1977) Cerebral white-matter hypoplasia. *Arch Neurol* 34: 137–141.

118. Back SA, Luo NL, Borenstein NS, Volpe JJ, Kinney HC (2002) Arrested oligodendrocyte lineage progression during human cerebral white matter development: dissociation between the timing of progenitor differentiation and myelinogenesis. *J Neuropathol Exp Neurol* 61: 197–211.

119. Schellinger D, Grant EG, Manz HJ, Lavenstein BL, Patronas NJ (1986) Ventricular shapes, distortions, and deformities: mirrors of past cerebral insults. A study based on early sonographic follow-up studies. *Pediatr Neurol* 4: 193–201.

120. Schouman-Claeys E, Picard A, Lalande G, et al (1989) Contribution of computed tomography in the aetiology and prognosis of cerebral palsy in children. *Br J Radiol* 62: 248–252.

121. Krageloh-Mann I, Hagberg B, Petersen D, Riethmuller J, Gut E, Michaelis R (1992) Bilateral spastic cerebral palsy. Pathogenetic aspects from MRI. *Neuropediatrics* 23: 46–48.

122. Truwit CL, Barkovich AJ, Koch TK, Ferriero DM (1992) Cerebral palsy: MR findings in 40 patients. *AJNR Am J Neuroradiol* 13: 67–78.

123. DeVries LS, Eken P, Groenendaal F, van-Haastert IC, Meiners LC (1993) Correlation between the degree of periventricular leukomalacia diagnosed using cranial ultrasound and MRI later in infancy in children with cerebral palsy. *Neuropediatrics* 24: 263–268.

124. Skranes JS, Vik T, Nilsen G, et al (1993) Cerebral magnetic resonance imaging (MRI) and mental and motor function of very low birth weight infants at one year of corrected age. *Neuropediatrics* 24: 256–262.

125. de Vries LS, Gunardi H, Barth PG, Bok LA, Verboon-Maciolek MA, Groenendaal F (2004) The spectrum of cranial ultrasound and magnetic resonance imaging abnormalities in congenital cytomegalovirus infection. *Neuropediatrics* 35: 113–119.

126. Magliocco AM, Demetrick DJ, Sarnat HB, Hwang WS (1992) Varicella embryopathy. *Arch Pathol Lab Med* 116: 181–186.

127. Cohen MM Jr., Kreiborg S (1990) The central nervous system in the Apert syndrome. *Am J Med Genet* 35: 36–45.

150

128. Lazzeri S, Mascalchi M, Cellerini M, Martinetti MG, Dal Pozzo G (1993) Epidermal nevus syndrome: MR of intracranial involvement. *AJNR Am J Neuroradiol* 14: 1255–1257.
129. Graf WD, Born DE, Sarnat HB (1998) The pachygyria–polymicrogyria spectrum of cortical dysplasia in X-linked hydrocephalus. *Eur J Pediatr Surg* 8(Suppl 1): 10–14.
130. Takahashi S, Makita Y, Okamoto N, Miyamoto A, Oki J (1997) L1CAM mutation in a Japanese family with X-linked hydrocephalus: a study for genetic counseling. *Brain Dev* 19: 559–562.
131. Morgagni G (1769) *The Seats and Causes of Diseases*. London: Millar A and Cadell T; and Johnson and Payne.
132. Cruveilhier J (1829–1835) *Anatomie Pathologique du Corps Humain, Part 2, XVth Liv*. Paris: JB Baillière.
133. McClelland JE (1940) The syndrome of hydromicrocephaly. *J Pediatr* 16: 36–51.
134. Benda C (1941) Microcephaly. *Am J Psychiatr* 97: 1135–1145.
135. Benda C (1945) The late effects of cerebral birth injuries. *Medicine (Baltimore)* 24: 71–110.
136. Gilles F, Murphy S (1969) Perinatal telencephalic leucoencephalopathy. *J Neurol Neurosurg Psych* 32: 404–413.
137. Huttenlocher PR (1970) Myelination and the development of function in immature pyramidal tract. *Exp Neurol* 29: 405–415.
138. Rasmussen A (1951) *Atlas of Cross Section Anatomy of the Brain: Guide to the Study of the Morphology and Fiber Tracts of the Human Brain*, 14th edn. New York: McGraw-Hill.

7
DEVELOPING BRAIN IMAGING AND MAGNETIC RESONANCE SPECTROSCOPY

MD Nelson MD, with S Bluml PhD, and A Panigrahy MD[a]

Introduction

Modern imaging technologies allow investigation of both structure and function of the brain. Ultrasonography, computed tomography (CT), and magnetic resonance imaging (MRI) are all useful methods of determining the structure and viability of brain parenchyma. MRI offers the unique ability to measure the biochemical makeup of brain parenchyma using magnetic resonance spectroscopy (MRS). In this chapter we will explore how advanced imaging technologies are used to investigate the premature and infant brain.

Prescanning evaluations

When an imaging study is ordered, every request should include an appropriate medical indication for the study. Signs and symptoms should be listed and the condition suspected by the referring physician should be stated. Most imaging examinations should be ordered as non-contrast examinations; however, if contrast is indicated (tumors, vascular malformations), the child needs to be well hydrated and renal function needs to be screened to avoid complications.

Preterm infants and neonates must be prepared for the trip to the radiology department for a CT or magnetic resonance examination. These infants are prone to hypothermia and dehydration. One way to solve these problems is to use an MRI/CT-compatible incubator[1] (Fig. 7.1a,b). The infant is placed in the incubator in the neonatal intensive care unit and is stabilized. Both temperature and humidity are controlled within the incubator. The entire unit can be transported to the radiology department and placed on the scanning table. For MRI, a special smaller-sized head coil is contained within the incubator.

Another method is to feed and bundle the infant. Most infants will sleep for 45 to 60 minutes following a bottle of formula. After feeding, the infant is wrapped in warm blankets and transported to the radiology department. Earplugs and headphones are placed to reduce magnetic resonance scanner noise.

When sedation/anesthesia is needed, chloral hydrate 50mg/kg may be administered either by mouth or intravenously. Propofol administered intravenously by anesthesiologists may be used. Heart rate, oxygen saturation, and blood pressure need to be monitored and charted during the imaging examination and during recovery.

---

[a]All at Children's Hospital Los Angeles.

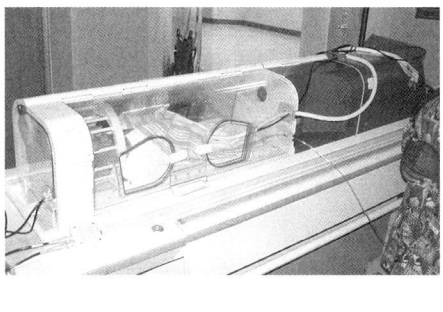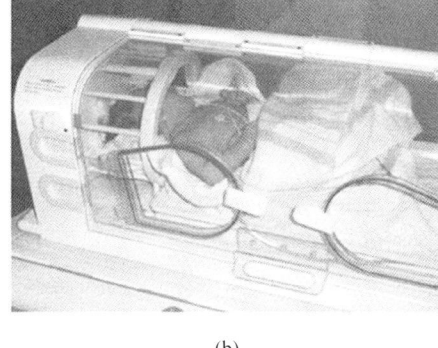

(a)　　　　　　　　　　　　　　　　　　(b)

Fig. 7.1 (a) Magnetic resonance-compatible incubator situated on magnetic resonance table. The incubator has a temperature- and humidity-controlled chamber for the infant. Either a head or body coil is also contained in the incubator. The infant is placed in the incubator in the neonatal intensive care unit and is stabilized. The entire incubator unit is transported to the magnetic resonance scanner. The unit is placed on the magnetic resonance table, the coil is plugged in, and scanning begins. Magnetic resonance-compatible ventilators and intravenous injectors are used with the unit when necessary. (b) Infant compartment of the magnetic resonance-compatible incubator.

When intravenous contrast is indicated, only nonionic agents should be used. There are many different nonionic contrasts for CT and MRI. Typical doses for CT agents are 2ml/kg. For MRI, 0.1ml/kg doses of gadolinium-based contrasts are used.

Cranial ultrasonography or neurosonography

Cranial ultrasonography (CUS) should be the first imaging study ordered after birth to evaluate the brain formation and status of brain parenchyma, and to provide evidence of intraventricular or parenchymal hemorrhage. CUS is also the imaging study of choice for assessing ventricular size as long as the anterior fontanelle is still open. CUS is inexpensive, can be performed at the bedside, and requires no sedation. However, the standard study has a limited field of view. Unless special views are done, there is limited evaluation of the vertex of the cerebral hemispheres and the posterior fossa. CUS is not the ideal study for assessing extracerebral hemorrhage or subarachnoid hemorrhage.

CRANIAL ULTRASOUND TECHNIQUE

Using a 5 to 10MHz sector transducer, a series of coronal and sagittal brain images are obtained via the anterior fontanelle. Usually six coronal and six sagittal images are obtained in a standard examination.[2]

NORMAL BRAIN SONOGRAPHIC APPEARANCE

Normal brain parenchyma has a granular baseline echogenic appearance.[3] Both the choroid plexus and cerebellar vermis are normally echogenic. On sagittal images, the para-atrial white matter appears echogenic. This is an artifact produced by the sound waves encountering the penetrating blood vessels from the cerebral surface at right angles.

There are several normal variants that must be recognized to avoid misinterpretation. Almost all preterm infants have a cavum septi pellucidi and cavum vergae. A small amount of extra-axial fluid is frequently seen.[4–6] Larger extra-axial fluid collections are seen in neonates on extracorporeal membrane oxygenation. The lateral ventricles in the neonate may be small or not seen (effaced). This should not be mistaken for a sign of cerebral edema[7] (see Chapter 3). Occasionally, there are 3- to 10-mm cysts adjacent to the superiolateral margin of the frontal horns. These may be found unilaterally or bilaterally in neonates without signs, symptoms, or laboratory evidence of infection, hemorrhage, or hypoxia. These 'cysts' are solitary and most probably represent frontal horn coarctation.[8]

CRANIAL ULTRASOUND GESTATIONAL AGE ASSESSMENT

Primary and secondary gyri and sulci form in a set sequential pattern. Using this information, gestational age may be determined by mapping the presence or absence of key gyri and sulci. The superior temporal sulcus is present at 23 weeks. The superior frontal sulcus is present at 25 weeks. The cingulate sulcus is appreciated on sagittal images at 30 weeks. The marginal branch of the cingulate gyrus is present at 32 weeks. The secondary superior temporal sulci, which give a 'sawtooth' pattern, are present at 35 weeks. The secondary long and short insular gyri are present at 40 weeks, and are the best cortical marker of a term gestation.

Both hemorrhage and infarction cause parenchyma to become echogenic.[9] Infarction typically occurs in a wedge-shaped distribution while hemorrhage tends to be more spherical in shape as if emanating from a single central source point.

Computed tomography

Computed tomography is a fast and relatively inexpensive (compared with magnetic resonance) imaging technique that is widely available. The speed of modern scanners is such that sedation is rarely needed for CT. However, CT is not the imaging modality of choice because of the radiation dose to the immature brain and the secondary scatter of radiation to the lens of the eyes. CT remains the imaging modality of choice for evaluation of acute head trauma and intracranial hemorrhage.

COMPUTED TOMOGRAPHY TECHNIQUE

Five-millimeter-thick slices are obtained in an axial plane from the foramen magnum to the vertex. The plane of the axial scans should be angled to avoid the orbit. For a term newborn, the typical parameters are a voltage of 120kV and a current of 120mA when a diagnostic scan is desired. For follow-up scans (ventricular size, etc.), a slice thickness of 10mm, voltage of 120kV, and a current of 80mA is sufficient and significantly decreases radiation dose to the patient.

NORMAL NEONATAL COMPUTED TOMOGRAPHY BRAIN APPEARANCE

For a diagnostic-quality CT scan, gray and white matter should be of different attenuation, with the cortex forming a continuous band over the lower attenuation white matter (Fig. 7.2).

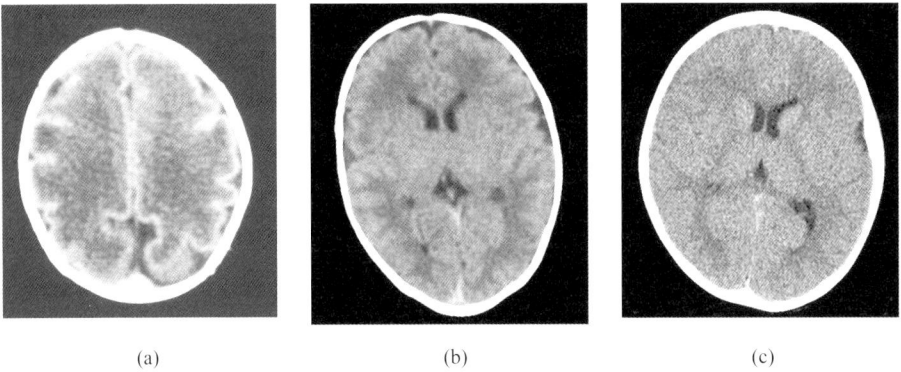

(a)   (b)   (c)

Fig. 7.2 Normal noncontrast head CT scans. (a) Typically developing 32-week preterm infant. Note the low attenuation of the unmyelinated white matter and the higher attenuation of the basal nuclei and cortex. (b) Typically developing term infant. The white matter remains of lower attenuation than the cortex. (c) Typically developing 3-year-old child. The CT now has the appearance of an adult brain CT. Normal physiologic calcifications (habenular commissure, pineal gland, choroid plexus) are unusual in the brains of children less than 5 years of age.

The basal ganglia and thalami should have the attenuation of the cortex. Low-dose techniques make the brain parenchyma appear without gray/white separation. This should not be confused with cerebral edema.

The normal neonatal brain has no CT-detectable calcifications. Physiologic choroid plexus, habenular, and pineal calcifications normally are not present before 8 years of age. If the hematocrit is high, the dural sinuses and cerebral arteries may appear hyperdense relative to the gray matter (Fig. 7.2a,b).

Magnetic resonance imaging

Overall, magnetic resonance is the imaging modality of choice for evaluating the structure and maturation of brain parenchyma at any age.[10–17] New imaging techniques allow for evaluation of both anatomic and biochemical structure of the brain as well as quantitation of basic biomolecules (magnetic resonance spectroscopy), parenchymal perfusion (arterial spin labeling, dynamic enhanced MRI), and functional activity of neurons. MRI is expensive, time-consuming, and usually requires sedation or some other intervention to keep the child motionless. The child must be transported to the scanner.

MAGNETIC RESONANCE TECHNIQUE

A complete magnetic resonance examination includes T1-weighted images in two planes (usually sagittal and axial), T2-weighted axial, axial fluid-attenuated inversion recovery (FLAIR), diffusion, and a gradient echo sequence. Intravenous contrast may be necessary when evaluating for neoplasia, infection, and vascular malformations. The smallest field of view should be used without causing a wrap-around artifact. A higher signal to noise ratio

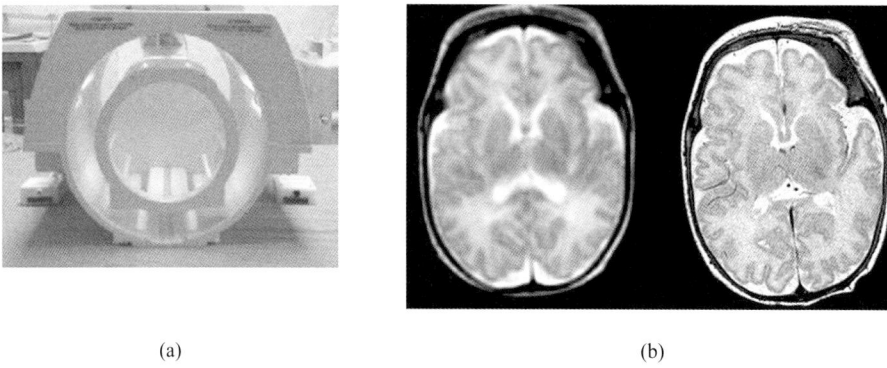

(a)   (b)

Fig. 7.3 (a) Neonatal head coil. Relative size compared with a standard adult head coil. (b) The difference in quality of an image of a newborn's brain obtained with standard adult head coil (left) and a neonatal head coil (right).

may be obtained by using head coils reduced in size to fit the neonatal head compared with the standard adult head coil (Fig. 7.3).

MAGNETIC RESONANCE SEQUENCES
Every manufacturer has a different set of labels for each sequence. We will list the generic names here for simplicity and how each sequence is useful.

T1 spin echo or T1 fluid-attenuated inversion recovery
The standard spin-echo T1 is not useful in the neonatal period as the gray–white discrimination is poor in the unmyelinated brain. The T1 FLAIR does a much better job of differentiating gray and white matter in the neonatal brain. Myelin is bright (hyperintense—short T1) and cerebrospinal fluid (CSF) is black. This sequence is excellent for studying brain structure and for assessing interval growth and myelination (Fig. 7.4a). Focal coagulation necroses in unmyelinated white matter appear as hyperintense lesions.

T2-weighted fast spin echo
This is a rapidly acquired T2-weighted sequence in which CSF is bright (hyperintense) and myelin is dark (Fig. 7.4b). This sequence is useful for identifying problems with the basic integrity of brain parenchyma. As such, hyperintensities on T2-weighted sequences are fairly nonspecific.

T2-weighted fluid-attenuated inversion recovery
This sequence combines the nonspecific sensitivity of T2 sequences for detecting parenchymal lesions with a pulse that nullifies the CSF signal, eliminating the usually bright signal of free fluid in the ventricles and around the brain (Fig. 7.4c). Any disturbance of the basic matrix of the brain parenchyma is depicted as increased signal on the T2 FLAIR sequence. As such, this sequence is very sensitive, but not very specific, for damage to brain parenchyma.

156

Gradient echo sequence

Gradient echo sequences are exquisitely sensitive for detecting by-products of hemorrhage, specifically hemosiderin. Dark areas identified on T2-weighted images may be air, calcifications, or hemosiderin (Fig. 7.4d). If the focus is hemosiderin, it will remain dark and appear to 'bloom,' that is, increase in size on the gradient echo sequence because of the magnetic influence of iron present in the hemosiderin.

Diffusion-weighted imaging

Standard diffusion-weighted imaging is based on whether brain water is free to move around or is restricted in some way. Restricted water produces a hyperintense signal whereas unbound water produces no signal. Standard diffusion imaging is done on the x-, y-, and z-axis planes (three directions). From the scan data, mathematical reconstructions of diffusion within each voxel can be made, which identify the degree of random water motion. The voxels may be grouped together within a defined region of interest (ROI). The calculated apparent diffusion coefficient (ADC) value of the tissue within the ROI may then be compared with ADCs within ROIs placed in other structures in the same brain, or with a similarly placed ROI in another brain (Fig. 7.4e).

Diffusion tensor imaging

In standard diffusion-weighted imaging (DWI), three gradient directions are applied to estimate the diffusivity of water within each voxel. These values are assigned to a grayscale and an axial image is constructed. Such images are useful in diagnosing brain infarcts, usually becoming positive within a couple of minutes of the hypoxic edema. Diffusion tensor imaging (DTI) scans are based on 6 to 30 or more gradient directions. These data are used to compute the diffusion tensor, that is the direction that the water is least restricted in moving, such as

---

Fig. 7.4 (overleaf) Normal examples of the standard magnetic resonance sequences for neonatal brain imaging. (a) Normal T1 fluid-attenuated inversion recovery (FLAIR) sequence of the brain at the ages of 25 weeks (left), 40 weeks (middle), and 3 years (right). The images have been corrected in size to match the centimeter scale to illustrate the tremendous growth changes that have occurred between the unmyelinated 25-week-old brain and the myelinated 3-year-old brain. (b) Normal T2 sequence of the brain at the ages of (left) 25 weeks, (middle) 40 weeks, and (right) 3 years. The white matter changes from high signal intensity in the 25-week-old and 40-week-old brains to low signal intensity in the 3-year-old brain. (c) Normal T2 FLAIR sequence of the brain at the ages of (left) 25 weeks, (middle) 40 weeks, and (right) 3 years. Relatively little signal change is demonstrated on this sequence in the normal brain at the various ages. Damage to the parenchyma generally causes increased signal on the gray background of the FLAIR sequence. (d) Gradient echo sequence (GRE). This sequence is useful for identifying old blood products such as hemosiderin. (i) Normal newborn brain without hemorrhage. Note the clear homogeneous background of the normal tissue. (ii) Newborn with paraventricular and intraventricular hemorrhage. Owing to the paramagnetic effect of the iron in hemosiderin, hemorrhage appears as a hypointense (dark or black) signal. (e) Diffusion-weighted imaging (DWI). Diffusion imaging evaluates the rate of the diffusion of water within each image voxel. If the water is free to randomly move about in all directions (such as the cerebrospinal fluid within the ventricles), no signal is generated and the image appears black. However, if the water is restricted in its movement, then a hyperintense, or bright, signal is produced. The standard diffusion-weighted images may be obtained in less than 1 minute and are extremely useful in identifying areas of early infarction *[continued overleaf]*

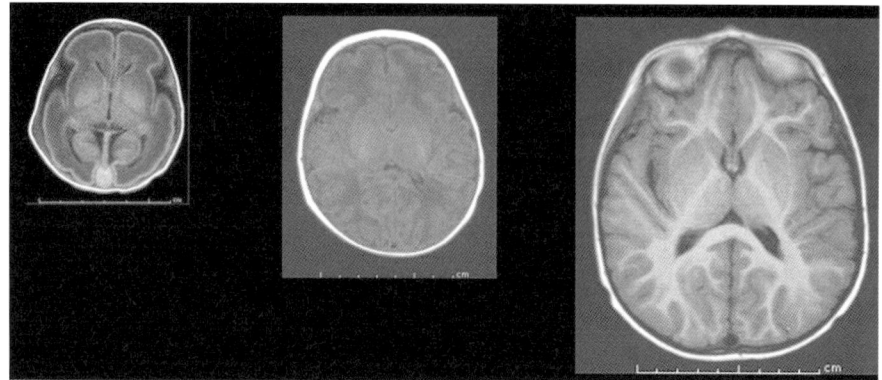

(a)

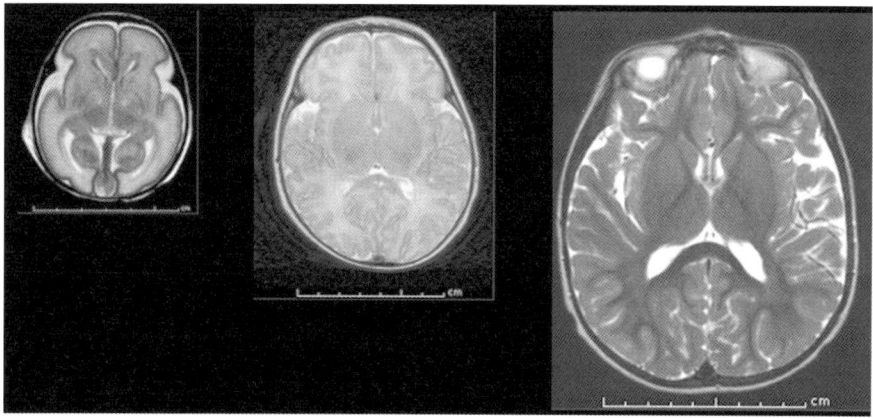

(b)

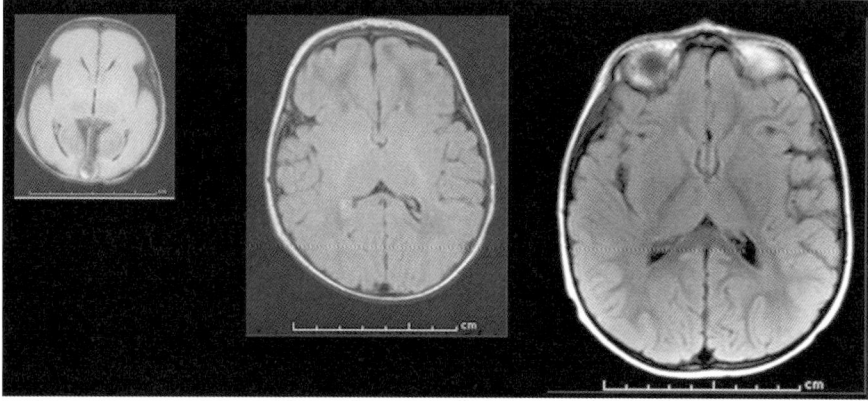

(c)

158

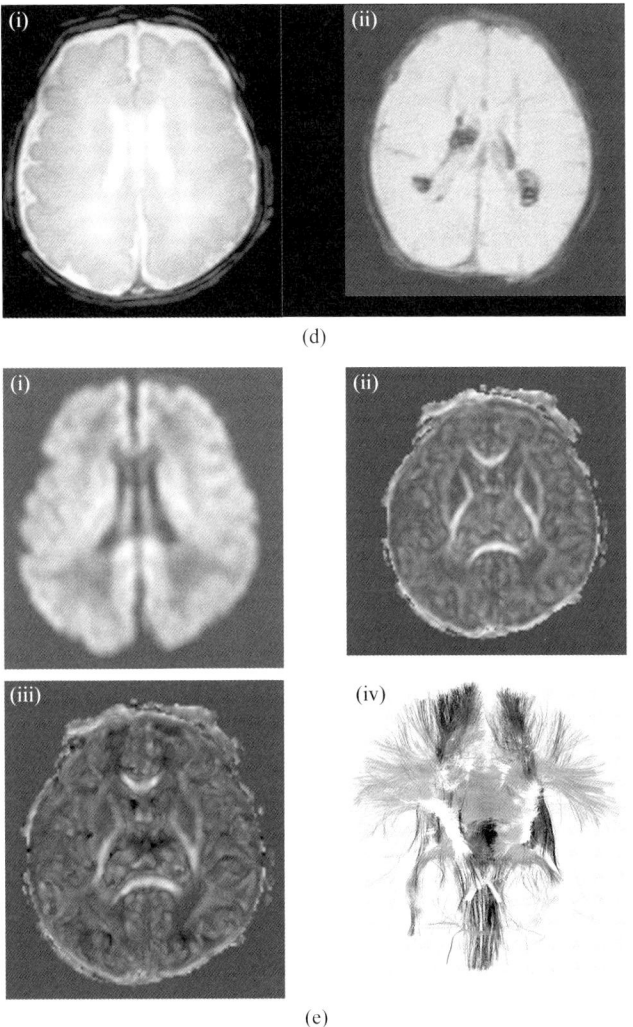

(d)

(e)

Fig. 7.4 (continued) and in identifying extra-axial epidermoids, both restricting diffusion of water molecules and causing bright signal on an otherwise gray background of normal brain parenchyma. (i) Normal diffusion-weighted image in which the brain parenchyma is gray and the cerebrospinal fluid is black. See Figure 13.24 for an example of a positive diffusion-weighted image in a child with an acute infarction. (ii) Diffusion tensor imaging (DTI). When the water molecules are restricted in some but not all directions, the bulk flow of the water can be assigned to pointing along a vector, which for DWI is termed the 'tensor.' The tensors are calculated for each voxel. The x-, y-, and z-planes are presented separately. Tensors aligned with the x-axis are bright on the x-plane, y-axis are bright on the y-plane, etc. (iii) DTI color map. In this format, the tensor information is color-coded and all three planes are presented on one image. Red is the x-axis (left/right), green is the y-axis (superior/inferior), and blue is the z-axis (anterior/posterior. A color version of this figure is available in the color plate section at the back of the book. (iv) Magnetic resonance tractography. By connecting voxels with their neighbors with a similar tensor, large groups of axons may be configured into 'tracts' and color coded by direction. A color version of this figure is available in the color plate section at the back of the book.

along an axon. By matching the tensor directions in adjacent voxels, maps of groups of white matter fibers may be 'tracked' (Fig. 7.4eii). Colors may be assigned to the primary x, y, and z directions of the fiber tracts (Fig. 7.4eiii). Groups of axons may be followed and subtracted from the basic image producing 'tractrography' (Fig. 7.4eiv).

Susceptibility-weighted imaging
Susceptibility-weighted imaging (SWI), originally termed blood oxygen level-dependent (BOLD) venographic imaging, uses a fully flow-compensated long-echo, gradient echo scan to acquire images. This method exploits the susceptibility differences between tissues and uses the phase image to detect these differences. The magnitude and phase data are combined to produce an enhanced contrast magnitude image, which is exquisitely sensitive to venous blood, hemorrhage, and iron deposition or storage. Owing to this sensitivity, SWI is commonly used in patients with traumatic brain injury.

Arterial spin labeling
Arterial spin labeling is an MRI technique capable of measuring cerebral blood flow in vivo. The water in neck blood vessels is 'tagged' by a magnetic pulse. Then, as blood flows into the brain, the tagged blood emits the 'tagged' energy, which is detected and allows the production of cerebral perfusion maps without requiring the administration of a contrast agent or the use of ionizing radiation.

Functional magnetic resonance imaging
Functional MRI measures changes in cerebral blood flow related to neuronal brain activity. A baseline resting scan is obtained, followed by a series of stimulations (paradigm) that cause increased neural activity and increased focal blood flow. By subtracting the stimulated scan from the baseline scan, the areas of 'activation' can be detected and mapped onto the structural reconstruction of the patient's brain (from T1-weighted images) (Fig. 7.5).

Voxel-based morphometry
Voxel-based morphometry is a neuroimaging analysis technique that takes advantage of the ability of MRI to obtain high-resolution three-dimensional (3D) data sets of the brain.[18] After acquiring a number of brain scans, a 'normal' template is created statistically and each study is then compared, voxel by voxel, with the template. In this way, small regional differences are detected that are not obvious to standard observation. This technique is particularly good for comparing the volume of gray matter structures between groups. When brain shape and surface anatomy are of interest, deformation-based morphometry and tensor-based morphometry are utilized. Deformation-based morphometry uses deformation-based fields to identify differences in the relative positions of brain structures, and tensor-based morphometry localizes differences in the shape of brain structures.

Magnetic resonance spectroscopy
Magnetic resonance spectroscopy is a modality that is available on most clinical magnetic resonance scanners and is readily integrated with standard MRI. For the brain in particular,

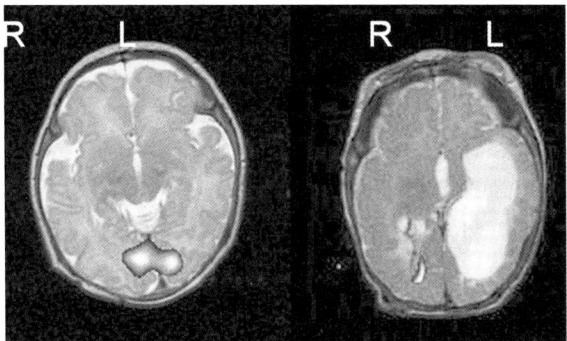

Fig. 7.5 Functional magnetic resonance imaging (MRI) study of two neonates exposed to a flashing strobe light. On the left is a normal response with activation around the primary visual cortex in the occipital lobes. On the right is a former preterm neonate with extensive parenchymal damage in which the strobe light evokes only weak activation in the right medial occipital lobe, indicating compromise of the visual pathways. A color version of this figure is available in the color plate section at the back of the book.

MRS has been a powerful research tool that has provided additional clinically relevant information for several disease families such as brain tumors, metabolic disorders, and systemic diseases.[19] The most widely available MRS method, proton (^{1}H; hydrogen) spectroscopy, has been approved by the Food and Drug Administration for general use in the USA and can be ordered by clinicians for patient studies if indicated. MRS measures small-molecular-weight amino acids, carbohydrates, fatty acids, and lipids involved in the complex network of well-regulated biosynthetic and degradative pathways. This network is particularly tightly controlled in the brain by enzymes and all but a few key molecules (magnetic resonance 'invisible' messengers and neurotransmitters) are kept at remarkably constant concentrations. For this reason, reproducible brain magnetic resonance spectra can be obtained when robust methods are applied. In sequentially studied healthy individuals, the single greatest variable may not be biologic or diet-imposed variations, but the practical, unavoidable inaccuracy of an individual's positioning, problems with the identification of a previously selected brain region, and imperfect magnetic resonance hardware stability. The biochemical fingerprint of tissue will be abnormal when there is structural damage (trauma, tumor, degenerative diseases, gliosis), altered physiologic conditions (blood flow interruption), and biochemical or genetic problems. The metabolic fingerprint also varies with the brain region studied. Because the microscopic composition (density/maturation of cells) of the brain and the activity of the enzymes that regulate its metabolism change during brain development, there will also be changes of the normal metabolic profile with brain maturation. As expected, these changes are most dramatic and interesting during early brain development. This is also the period when it is most difficult to obtain normal control data owing to the inherent difficulties of conducting research studies on small children. Although completely harmless, MRI and MRS are expensive and lengthy tests that are sensitive to an individual's motion. Unless there is a need to evaluate whether a metabolic profile is consistent with a certain disease, MRI or MRS scans are rarely performed in small children, who often require sedation to ensure studies with sufficient quality. Consequently, there are few studies published that describe normal biochemical maturation[20–26] and the numbers of children included in those studies were small and/or the study covered only a limited age range. However, over a 7-year period, hundreds of spectra from children aged 0 (term) to 18 years (young adults) that were retrospectively considered to be 'close to control' based on the MRI findings (negative) and unremarkable clinical follow-up were acquired by Panigrahy et al.[27] The goal of this chapter is to describe the metabolic changes in brain tissue as a function of age that were observed in this cohort of 'closest-to-control' individuals.

Basic principles of magnetic resonance

All atomic nuclei with an uneven number of nucleons (protons and neurons) have a *spin* and detectable *magnetic moment* when brought into a magnetic field. MRI takes advantage of the magnetic moment of the *hydrogen atom* (i.e., of water), whose nuclei comprise a single proton. In a magnetic field, the spins align themselves to form a *macroscopic magnetization*, often depicted as a vector pointing into the magnetic field direction. A *radiofrequency* pulse— basically a transient modulation of the strength and direction of the magnetic field—tips the magnetization vector out of its *equilibrium position*. After the radiofrequency pulse is switched off, the magnetization vector moves back into its equilibrium position by three basic processes:

1 Magnetization perpendicular to the magnetic field decays exponentially owing to a process often termed transversal or T2 relaxation. The decay rate depends on the environment and is different for different tissue types.

2 The magnetization parallel to the static magnetic field grows to its original length following an exponential law, a process often termed as longitudinal or T1 relaxation, again at a rate that differs with tissue type.

3 While this occurs, a radiofrequency signal (a few thousand times smaller than the radiofrequency pulse used for excitation) can be detected. This small radiofrequency signal forms the basis for all MRI and MRS. By switching additional magnetic fields (gradients) on and off before and during the readout of the radiofrequency signal, the spatial origin of the signal can be determined. Images of different contrast can be generated by using different combinations of radiofrequency pulses, by altering the time delay between the radiofrequency excitation and the signal readout [echo time (TE)], and by choosing appropriate time delays between repeated excitations [repetition time (TR)]. For example, in some tissues, the transverse magnetization may decay quicker than in others. If the readout of the signal is delayed, comparably less signal would be detected from this region and the tissue would be rendered dark. Contrast in magnetic resonance is also generated by the density of water (or protons) and to what extent water diffuses in tissue. Today, among the various imaging modalities used in clinical practice, MRI, by virtue of its availability, contrast versatility, pathophysiologic specificity, and potential for repeat studies without adverse effects on the health of the individual, is often the method of choice. MRI provides excellent soft-tissue contrast and is particularly powerful for brain imaging.

As mentioned above, the signal used by MRI to create anatomical maps is generated primarily by the hydrogen nuclei, also known as protons (^{1}H), found in water molecules (H_2O). In contrast, ^{1}H MRS analyzes signals of protons attached to other molecules. Whereas for MRI only a single peak (water) is being mapped, the output of MRS is a collection of peaks at different radiofrequencies representing proton nuclei in different chemical environments, termed the spectrum (Fig. 7.6). Because ^{1}H MRS uses the same hardware as MRI, it is by far the most widely used technique, and this chapter will focus on the application of ^{1}H MRS. Nonetheless, other methods such as phosphorus-31 (^{31}P), carbon-13 (^{13}C), or fluorine-19 (^{19}F) MRS have been successfully applied in humans. The concentration of water in the brain is high ($\approx$70–80%), and enough signal can be acquired to reconstruct magnetic resonance images covering the whole brain within a few minutes of acquisition time. MRS is more challenging and is restricted not only by the generally low concentrations of chemicals but also by the size of molecules. Only small, mobile chemicals with concentrations of $\geq$0.5µmol/g tissue can be observed. This leaves most true neurotransmitters out of reach for this method. Exceptions may be glutamate, γ-aminobutyric acid, and aspartate. Also, large immobile macromolecules and phospholipids, myelin, proteins, RNA, and DNA are rendered 'invisible' to MRS. Because of the low concentrations of magnetic resonance-detectable chemicals, MRS is also restricted to the analysis of individual ROIs much larger than the resolution of MRI (typically 1–10cm^3 for MRS vs 1–10mm^3 for MRI).

As for MRI, there are many different techniques that can be used to acquire information. It is beyond the scope of this chapter to discuss details about MRS localization methods. Today,

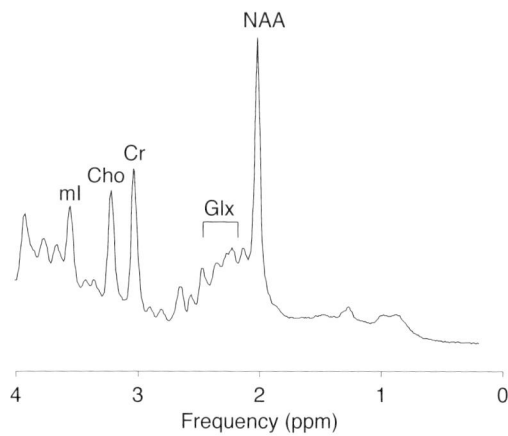

Fig. 7.6 The output of magnetic resonance spectroscopy (MRS) is a spectrum where the x-axis (chemical shift axis) is used to identify chemicals by their chemical shift, whereas the y-axis (signal amplitude) is a measure of the concentration of a chemical. Each molecule has its own typical pattern and a spectrum is a linear combination of the individual spectra. The spectrum shown is an average of many spectra acquired in older 'close-to-normal' children in parietal white matter and occipital gray matter. Spectra were acquired using a magnetic resonance scanner [echo time (TE)=35ms]. NAA, N-acetylaspartate; Cr, creatine; Cho, choline; mI, myoinositol; Glx, glutamate+glutamine; ppm, parts per million.

MRS studies of the human brain are almost exclusively conducted with either *localized single-voxel spectroscopy* or two-dimensional (2D) or 3D *chemical shift imaging* (CSI), also termed magnetic resonance spectroscopic imaging (MRSI) or spectroscopic imaging. Single-voxel MRS measures the magnetic resonance signal of a single selected ROI, and a signal outside this area is suppressed. For single-voxel MRS, the magnetic field and other parameters are optimized to obtain the best possible spectrum from a relatively small region of the brain. With CSI, many spectra from a slab (2D-CSI) or from a volume (3D-CSI) are acquired at the same time. Although CSI is more efficient than single-voxel MRS, individual spectra of a CSI acquisition sometimes do not reach the quality obtained with single-voxel MRS. CSI also requires considerable postprocessing and quality control. In magnetic resonance, the signal is derived from the ROI whereas all the tissue within the sensitive part of a radiofrequency coil contributes to the noise. Thus, the signal-to-noise ratio of magnetic resonance methods where information from a large ROI is sampled is superior to those methods where the signal from a small region is desired and the signal outside is suppressed. Single-voxel spectra can be processed and quantified using fully automated, widely available software. Single-voxel MRS (point resolved spectroscopy[28,29]) is thus more practical in clinical environments where resources are limited. Discipline and a methodologic approach are required, starting at the time of the data acquisition. With CSI, a ROI can be selected retrospectively. When single-voxel MRS is used, the appropriate ROI needs to be selected by the operator at the study time. To simplify this task, standardized regions should be examined (unless there is a focal process or a specific reason to measure in a certain anatomical region).

Material
The developmental curves for biochemical maturation of the human brain were developed from a database of 2300 children undergoing 6000 MRS studies at this institution. Of those, 320 children with a gestational age at birth of exactly 40 weeks (term) with no abnormalities on MRI (including no abnormalities on diffusion MRI), as explicitly stated on the MRI report, and unremarkable clinical follow-up (where available) were identified. These children were either enrolled in various research studies ongoing in this institution (including a small group typically of patient siblings) or had clinical indications for MRI and MRS, including suspected encephalitis, metabolic disorders, seizures (retrospectively classified as febrile seizures), hypoxic–ischemic episodes, suspected but not confirmed tumor, hypotonia, meningitis, or others. All spectra were reviewed for quality and spectra of insufficient quality (large line width or insufficient signal-to-noise ratio) were not included in the analysis. Also eliminated were studies in which patients had diseases with persistent clinical symptoms or where spectroscopic abnormalities were reported in the literature despite normal MRI, including mitochondrial myopathy, encephalopathy, lactic acidosis, stroke-like episodes, gyral atrophy, and hepatic encephalopathy.[30–32]

BRAIN REGIONS
The MRS studies routinely included the acquisition of spectra from two standardized brain regions where good quality spectra can be obtained. The first location is the occipital cortex, which contains mostly gray matter. The second region consists of mostly white matter in

the parietal/occipital region (Fig. 7.7). Typical magnetic resonance spectra from these two regions illustrating the main metabolic changes detectable by visual inspection are shown in Figure 7.8.

Data presentation

In MRS, the signal received is proportional to the number of nuclei present in the region of interest. MRS is thus inherently quantitative, albeit that obtaining the correct 'scaling' factors to translate signal amplitudes into concentrations is a significant challenge. Indeed, it has been argued that MRS cannot be used to quantify chemicals because the same chemical may be 'magnetic resonance visible,' when capable of moving freely, or 'magnetic resonance invisible,' when bound to a membrane or confined in myelin. While this is almost certainly an academic problem that can be overcome in practice by agreeing that the 'unbound magnetic resonance visible' concentrations are being measured, the complexity of magnetic resonance and the many parameters that can have an impact on the observed signal pose significant challenges. Consequently, concentrations reported by MRS of the same chemical in the same brain region have varied widely in the past. Owing to significant hardware improvements and much iteration to find the best processing and quantitation strategies, the reproducibility of MRS and the consistency of reported concentrations has greatly improved. There might still be small systematic differences, depending on how a particular sequence is implemented and which corrections are applied. All the same, observations such as choline concentrations are higher and creatine concentrations are lower in parietal white matter than in occipital gray matter are now universally true (geographically, across vendors, at different field strengths,

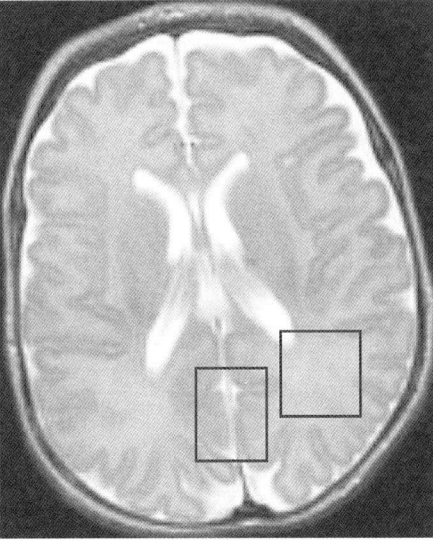

Fig. 7.7 T2-weighted magnetic resonance images and boxes that indicate the brain regions that were evaluated. WM (right-hand box), mostly white matter containing parietal/occipital tissue; GM (left-hand box), occipital gray matter.

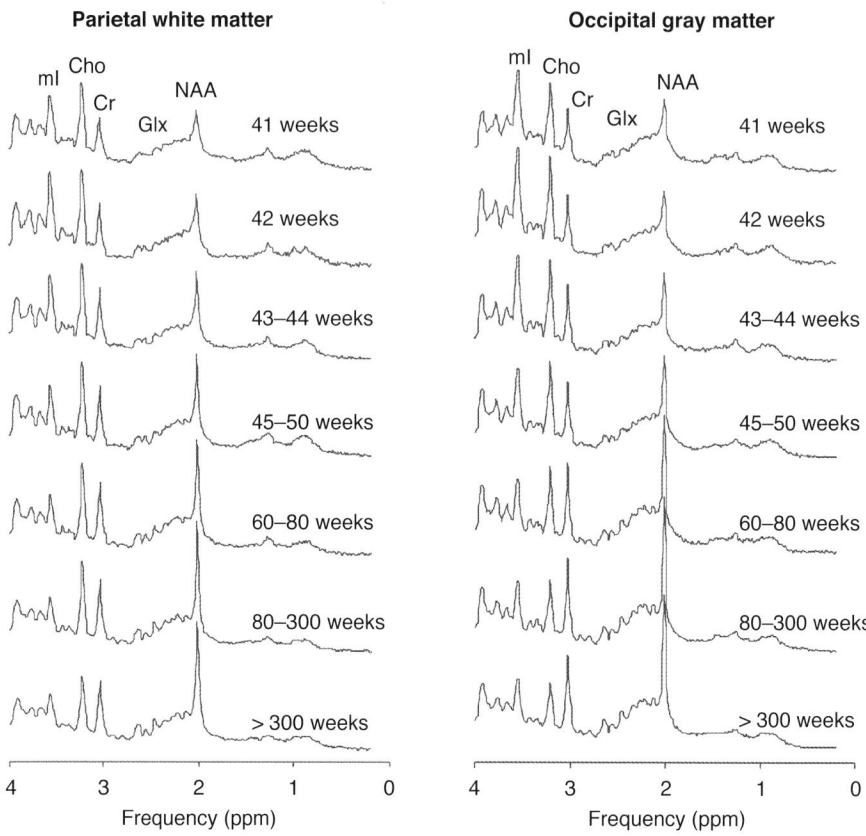

Fig. 7.8 Typical proton magnetic resonance spectra acquired from parietal white matter and occipital gray matter in children with normal magnetic resonance image at different stages of brain development. NAA, *N*-acetylaspartate; Cr, creatine; Cho, choline; mI, myoinositol; Glx, glutamate+glutamine; ppm, parts per million.

and irrespective of the acquisition method used). In this chapter, we report the concentrations as measured with our methods—which we believe are state of the art—to allow the interested reader to make comparisons with data obtained by other measurement techniques. However, we also report concentrations as a percentage of concentrations measured in the young adult brain. Reporting relative concentrations is generally more robust as correction factors have no impact on those numbers. Table 7.1 summarizes all parameters from which absolute and relative concentrations can readily be calculated for different stages of brain maturation.

MAGNETIC RESONANCE SPECTRA QUANTITATION

One commonly employed strategy for absolute quantitation is to acquire the brain water signal in the ROI and measure (or assume) the water content of tissue. This can then be used as an internal concentration reference, for instance the water signal of tissue with a water content

TABLE 7.1
Fitted parameters and fit functions for metabolites with significant changes during brain maturation

		Fit function	A_1 (mmol/kg)	A_2	A_3 (1/year)	A_4 (1/year)	A_5 (years)
NAA	WM	f_1	9.29 (0.10)	0.27 (0.02)	0.22 (0.03)	15.1 (1.2)	0.812 (0.004)
	GM		9.87 (0.05)	0.35 (0.03)	0.44 (0.06)	9.1 (0.8)	0.840 (0.005)
Cr	WM	f_2	5.13 (0.03)	–	5.83 (0.46)	3.7 (0.3)	0.848 (0.006)
	GM	f_1	7.01 (0.06)	0.13 (0.02)	0.24 (0.10)	7.2 (1.4)	0.686 (0.018)
Cho	WM	f_1	1.64 (0.01)	−0.30 (0.01)	0.41 (0.05)	10.9 (1.5)	0.544 (0.035)
	GM		1.24 (0.01)	−0.50 (0.02)	1.17 (0.09)	16.2 (1.5)	0.667 (0.013)
mI	WM	f_2	4.85 (0.02)	−0.65 (0.01)	3.00 (0.10)	46.4 (2.4)	0.737 (0.002)
	GM		5.89 (0.02)	−0.62 (0.02)	3.72 (0.12)	67.3 (8.5)	0.748 (0.004)
Glu	WM	f_2	8.08 (0.07)	–	5.70 (0.51)	3.6 (0.4)	1.005 (0.012)
	GM	f_3	11.86 (0.06)	–	9.90 (6.19)	6.4 (4.7)	0.805 (0.009)
Tau	WM	f_4	24.1 (0.9)	0.015 (0.001)	2.72 (0.04)	–	–
	GM		2.36 (0.05)	0.32 (0.04)	0.17 (0.02)	–	–

Values are mean (SD).

NAA, *N*-acetylaspartate; WM, white matter; GM, gray matter; Cr, creatine; Cho, choline; mI, myoinositol; Glu, glutamate; Tau, taurine.

$$f_1 = \frac{A_1}{A_2 e^{-A_3(PCA-A_5)} + e^{-A_4(PCA-A_5)} + 1} \qquad \text{(Equation 7.1)}$$

$$f_2 = \frac{A_1}{e^{-A_3(PCA-A_5)} - e^{-A_4(PCA-A_5)} + 1} \qquad \text{(Equation 7.2)}$$

$$f_1 = \frac{A_1}{e^{-A_3(PCA-A_5)} + e^{-A_4(PCA-A_5)} + 1} \qquad \text{(Equation 7.3)}$$

$$f_4 = A_1(A_2 + e^{-A_3 \cdot PCA}) \qquad \text{(Equation 7.4)}$$

where PCA is the postconceptional age in years.

of 80% corresponds to a concentration of 55mol/kg × 80%=44mol/kg. Use of the water signal as an absolute concentration reference eliminates several sources of error, such as differences in voxel size, total gain due to coil loading, receiver gains, and hardware changes. However, often the water content changes, as is the case in the developing brain. Data presented in the following paragraphs were thus corrected for the developing human brain varying water content by using a look-up table for water content as a function of postconceptional age.[33,34] Concentrations were also corrected for the varying fractions of CSF in the ROI, as described earlier.[35]

In a preliminary analysis, data from female and male children were analyzed separately. No significant differences were noted and data were pooled. Metabolite concentrations measured in each brain region were fitted to empirical functions using the least-squares fit routine provided by MatLab (MathWorks, Natick, MA, USA). The functions where minimum χ^2 was determined are reported. Fit functions and fitted parameters [standard deviation (SD)] are summarized in Table 7.1. The SD of the fitted parameters were determined by Monte Carlo simulation as follows. First, typical errors for the quantitation of metabolites (not accounting for systematic errors) were determined by calculating the SD of metabolite concentrations in individuals older than 10 years when metabolite concentrations were close to constant. For example, gray matter [N-acetylaspartate molecule (NAA)] in children older than 10 years was 9.89 (0.48) mmol/kg. Then random numbers within 1 SD (here 0.48mmol/kg) were generated and added to all measured data, simulating the experimental uncertainty. These synthetic data can be interpreted as a possible result if all individuals were re-examined with MRS taking into account the experimental imperfections. This new data set was then fitted to determine to what extent experimental uncertainty could alter fit parameters. This procedure was typically repeated 2000 times for each data set and the distribution of the fit parameters was analyzed. Generally, the parameters showed a close to Gaussian distribution and the reported uncertainties of the fitted parameters were the SDs of the distributions.

Normative developmental curves

N-ACETYLASPARTATE

The most prominent peak of the ^{1}H spectrum of a normal adult is the resonance at 2.0ppm (parts per million) from three equivalent protons of the acetyl group of the N-acetylaspartate molecule (NAA). NAA, because of its prominence in the spectrum, is also the chemical that can be measured most accurately. The role of NAA, and its regulation in vivo, is not well understood. In the normal brain, NAA is synthesized in neurons, diffuses along axons, and is broken down in oligodendrocytes. In the mature brain, NAA is present in high concentrations in neurons and axons,[36-38] and from an MRS perspective it is a marker for adult-type 'healthy' neurons and axons. However, it has also been reported that immature oligodendrocytes and O-2A progenitor cells may be a significant source of NAA in the developing brain.[39,40] NAA is clinically important because its reduction is an indicator for neuronal/axonal loss or damage. There is only one disease with elevated NAA, Canavan disease, in which the enzyme breaking down NAA in the oligodendrocytes (aspartoacylase) is missing.

    N-acetylaspartate in parietal white matter increased rapidly from approximately 30% to 75% of normal adult levels between 40 weeks (term) and 51 weeks postconceptional age (≈ equivalent to a 2.5-month-old infant born at term) (Fig. 7.9). Thereafter, a more gradual increase to 95% of adult levels by 7 to 8 years of age was observed. A similar time course was observed for NAA in occipital gray matter, although it appears that the white matter increase of NAA slightly precedes the increase in gray matter. NAA concentrations of the young adult brain are similar for both locations [9.3mmol/kg (white matter) vs 9.9mmol/kg (gray matter)].

CREATINE

Another prominent peak in magnetic resonance spectra of normal brains is creatine (Cr) at 3.0ppm. For normal brain tissue, the Cr peak comprises contributions from free creatine (fCr) and phosphocreatine (PCr) in approximately equal proportions. PCr is in rapid chemical exchange with fCr and is used to replenish adenosine triphosphate (ATP) levels if required.

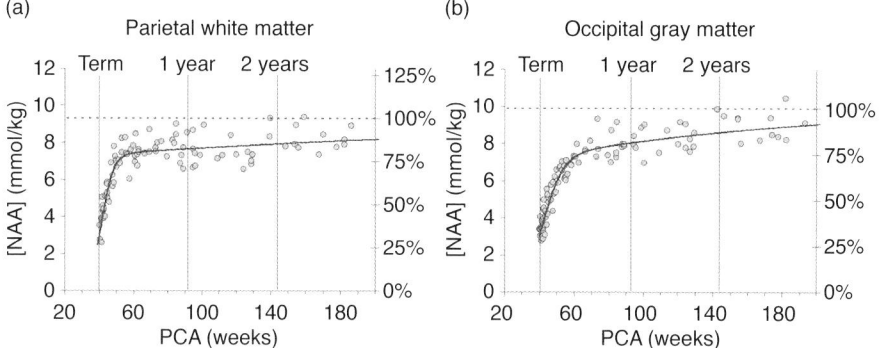

Fig. 7.9 Shown are the measured *N*-acetylaspartate (NAA) concentrations in children deemed to be 'closest-to-control' as a function of postconceptional age (PCA). Only children born exactly at term (40 weeks) with normal magnetic resonance image and unremarkable clinical follow-up are included. Superimposed are curves that were obtained by least-squares fits. Albeit, the curves for white matter and gray matter regions appear to be similar, there were significant differences in the fitted parameters. For example, the increase of NAA in white matter (left) preceded the increase in gray matter (right).

Like NAA, Cr is also low in the newborn brain. In contrast to NAA (which is believed to decline eventually in the aging brain as a result of 'normal' neuronal/axonal degradation), once Cr reaches adult levels it continues to slightly increase further in the normal brain.[25,41] As NAA is believed to be a marker for neurons/axons, this could indicate that Cr is present at higher concentrations in the glial compartment.

Parietal white matter Cr levels at term are approximately 80% of normal adult levels. Creatine rapidly increases thereafter and reaches a transient maximum (≈125% of normal) within the first 6 months of life, then declines gradually and reaches normal adult levels between 1 and 2 years of age. In a subgroup of this study, magnetic resonance spectra of right frontal white matter were obtained and a similar time course, with a transient maximum concentration within 6 months after birth, was observed. In contrast, in occipital gray matter, a transient maximum for Cr was not observed. Instead, Cr increased from ≈50% to 75% of normal adult levels within the first 2 to 3 months of life and to 95% around 4 years of age (Fig. 7.10). In young adults, the Cr concentration of gray matter was 7.0mmol/kg, whereas in white matter the Cr concentration was lower at 5.1mmol/kg.

TOTAL CHOLINE

The next prominent peak, at 3.2ppm, is commonly referred to as choline (Cho) or trimethylamine (TMA). Cho is a complex peak comprising several Cho-containing metabolites often referred to as 'total choline' or 'choline-containing metabolites.' In a previous study using ^{1}H MRS and ^{31}P MRS in vivo, it was found that the sum of phosphorylated Cho, phosphorylcholine (PCho), and glycerophosphorylcholine (GPC) accounts for most of the Cho detected with ^{1}H MRS in normal tissue.[42] Cho-containing compounds are involved in the synthesis and breakdown of phosphatidylcholine (PtdCho=lecithin). PtdCho is the major phospholipid component of eukaryotic cells, accounting for approximately 60% of total phospholipids. GPC

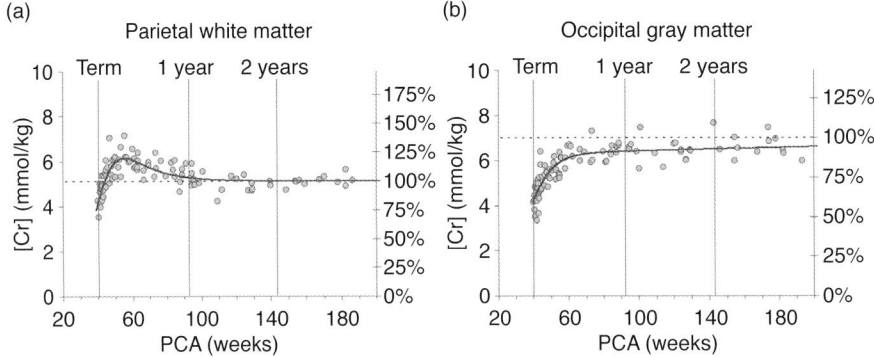

Fig. 7.10 For creatine (Cr), the developmental curves in white and gray matter-containing brain regions are remarkably different. In white matter (a), a transient maximum concentration is observed within the first 6 months of life. In contrast, in gray matter (b), a transient maximum was not observed. PCA, postconceptional age.

is also a cerebral osmolyte,[43] and a reduction (increase) of GPC in response to hypo-osmotic (hyperosmotic) conditions might be reflected by an alteration of total Cho. Cho is of particular interest in tumor spectroscopy as all forms of cancer have abnormal membrane metabolism, and thus abnormal Cho.

In young adults, Cho concentration in gray matter was 1.24mmol/kg, whereas in white matter the Cho concentration was higher, at 1.64mmol/kg. Changes of Cho during early brain development are less dramatic than those observed for NAA and Cr. Cho increased slightly in the first few weeks of life in both parietal white matter and occipital gray matter and declined gradually thereafter (Figs 7.11, 7.12). In parietal white matter, initial Cho reached approximately 130% of levels observed in young adults. In gray matter, a maximum of 150% of the Cho levels in young adults was observed. The decline of Cho was more gradual in white matter than in gray matter.

MYOINOSITOL

Myoinositol (mI) is a little-known sugar-like molecule that resonates at 3.6ppm in the proton spectrum. It has been identified as a marker for astrocytes and is elevated in glial tumors and gliosis. mI is also an osmolyte[43,44] and is altered in diseases associated with osmotic imbalance. mI is involved in the metabolism of phosphatidyl inositol, a membrane phospholipid. Similar to Cho, mI varies in response to altered membrane metabolism or damaged membrane. In contrast to NAA, Cr, and Cho, which can be observed with a wide range of MRS-acquisition methods, the mI signal decays more rapidly owing to the molecular structure. To observe mI, methods with only a short delay between initial excitation and signal readout (short TE) are required. Glycine (Gly) co-resonates with mI and cannot be distinguished from mI with the method employed in this study. However, Gly levels are low and it has previously been reported that it is unlikely that Gly varies significantly during maturation.[20]

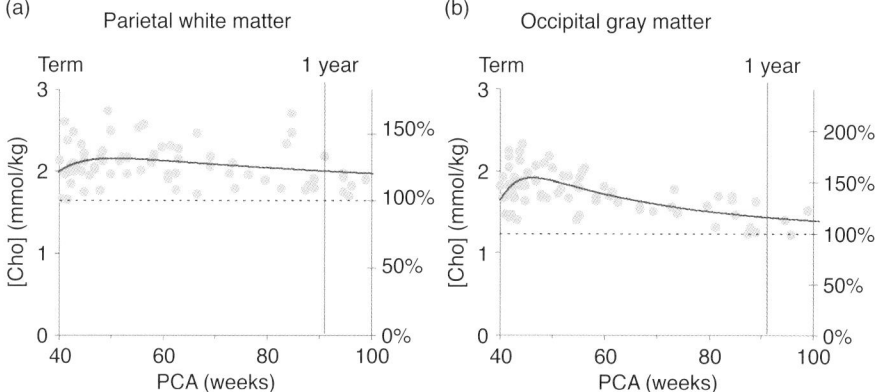

Fig. 7.11 A small increase of choline (Cho) is observed during the first few months of life. Thereafter, Cho declines in both white matter (a) and gray matter (b). PCA, postconceptional age.

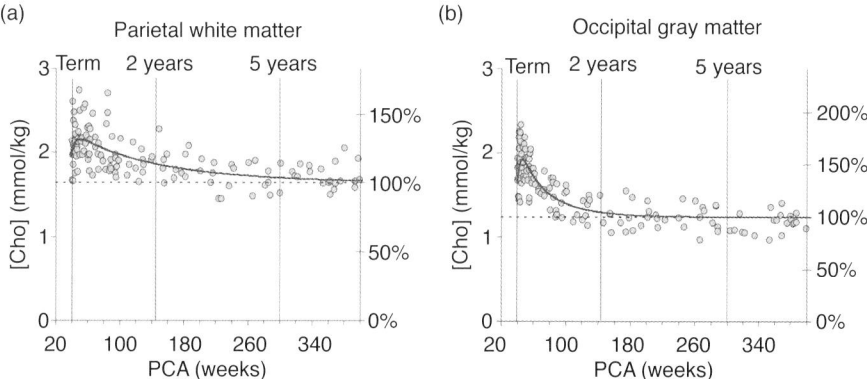

Fig. 7.12 After reaching a transient maximum within the first 6 months of life, choline (Cho) declines more gradually in white matter (a) than in occipital gray matter (b). PCA, postconceptional age.

A small increase of mI to a transient maximum at approximately 200% of normal within the first weeks after term was observed. mI concentrations then declined rapidly during further postnatal brain development (Fig. 7.13). Absolute concentrations of mI appear to be slightly higher in gray matter, particularly at birth, than in white matter.

GLUTAMATE AND GLUTAMINE
Glutamate (Glu) and glutamine (Gln) are important components of the ^{1}H spectrum. Of all metabolites, Glu is believed to have the highest concentration in normal human brain tissue. Owing to their similar chemical structures, Glu and Gln form complex and partially overlapping resonances in ^{1}H spectra. Therefore, often the more robust sum of Glu+Gln (Glx) is

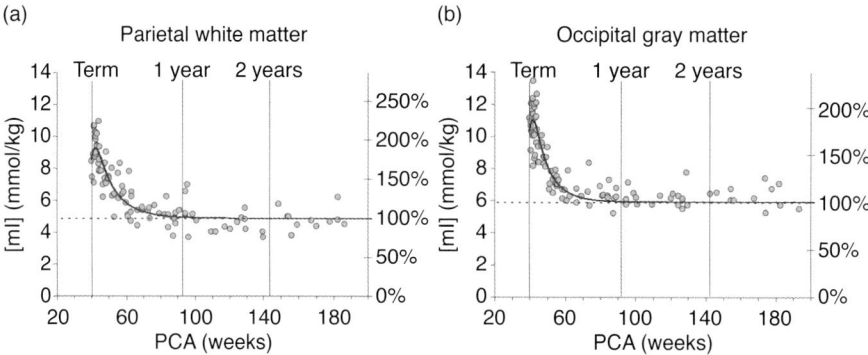

Fig. 7.13 After reaching a transient maximum within the first few months of life, myoinositol (mI) declines rapidly to levels observed in young adults in both white matter (a) and gray matter (b). PCA, postconceptional age.

determined. Both Glu and Gln have two groups of resonances: The first group (α-Glu and α-Gln) has three peaks between 3.6 and 3.9ppm, whereas the second group (β,γ-Glu and β,γ-Gln) comprises a more complex series of resonances between 2.0 and 2.6ppm. Accordingly, the quantitation of these chemicals is challenging. Magnetic resonance spectra of excellent quality and sophisticated software, such as LCModel (Stephen Provencher Inc., Oakville, ON, Canada),[45] which fit all metabolite resonances simultaneously, are essential for quantitation of these amino acids. Still, at clinical field strength (1.5-T magnets), accurate measurements in individual subjects are challenging and the scatter of the Glu (and Gln) data is significantly larger than, for example, with NAA, Cr, or Cho. At higher field strength (3T and higher), the Glu and Gln signals start to separate and independent quantitation improves considerably.

Glu and Gln constitute an important neurotransmitter cycle in the normal brain, where Glu is stored mainly in neuropil and Gln concentration is higher in astrocytes. However, the role of Glu and Gln is almost certainly much more complicated. For example, Glu can be oxidized to substitute for glucose metabolism in hypoglycemic states.[46,47] Excess synaptic Glu may cause nerve cell damage as a result of inordinate excitation. Glutamine increases under hypoxic stress and under hyperammonemic conditions.[48]

Glu concentrations increased rapidly from ≈25% at term in parietal and frontal white matter and reached a transient maximum within the first year of life. A transient maximum was not observed for occipital GM, whereas Glu increased from ≈25% to adult levels within the first year of life and remained close to constant thereafter. Glu concentration in gray matter is approximately 50% higher than in parietal white matter (Fig. 7.14). The interpretation of the transient maximum of Glu in white matter and an early plateau in gray matter is unclear. The time courses of Glu concentration suggest that maturation of glutamatergic neurons and the maximum density of their axon/dendrite network, in each location studied, is reached within the first year of life. In contrast, NAA, possibly a more general marker for adult-type neurons and axons, has a different developmental curve and does not reach a plateau before 5 years of age for both locations (see *N*-acetylaspartate above). On the other hand, developmental curves

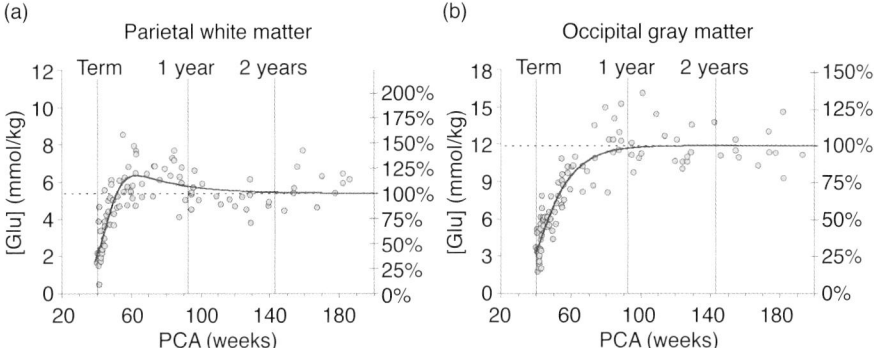

Fig. 7.14 Both in parietal white matter (a) and occipital gray matter (b) an initial rapid increase in glutamate (Glu) is observed. In white matter, a transient maximum is reached at around 6 months and thereafter Glu declines gradually to levels observed in young adults. In gray matter, a significant transient maximum was not observed. PCA, postconceptional age.

for Cr (see 'Creatinine' above) are similar to the Glu curves in both locations. A detailed analysis shows, however, that the rise of Cr slightly precedes the increase of Glu in both locations (see fit parameter A_5 in Table 7.1). No significant age-dependent changes were observed for Gln. Consequently, Glx showed a time course similar to that of Glu.

TAURINE

Taurine (Tau), an aminosulfonic acid, is abundant in developing cerebellum and isocortex[49] and its levels are generally high in less differentiated brains of preterm newborns.[20] It has been suggested that Tau has inhibitory properties and functions as an osmoregulator and neuromodulator but also has neuroprotective features in neural tissue.[50] In adults, the detection and quantitation of Tau is difficult owing to its low concentration and spectral overlap with scylloinositol. Pathologically elevated Tau has been detected in pediatric medulloblastoma.[51,52]

Tau levels decreased in both white matter and gray matter locations with age. Whereas Tau fell below the limits of detection in white matter locations within the first 2 to 4 years of life, it declined more gradually in occipital gray matter (Fig. 7.15).

LACTATE

Lactate (Lac) is an important metabolite as it signifies anaerobic metabolism. Although Lac can be detected at pathologically elevated concentrations, in healthy tissue the Lac concentration is too low for routine detection with currently available methods. Careful positioning of the region of interest is also required because the Lac concentration of CSF is approximately 1mmol/l. Consequently, a spectrum acquired from a voxel with a significant partial volume of CSF might show the typical doublet of Lac at 1.33ppm. Lac is the product of anaerobic glycolysis and increases when subsequent oxidation of Lac in the tricarboxylic acid cycle is impaired (for example, by lack of oxygen or mitochondrial disorders). Lac can also increase in necrotic tissue and cysts. Consistent with earlier reports,[20,24] we have observed Lac in typically

173

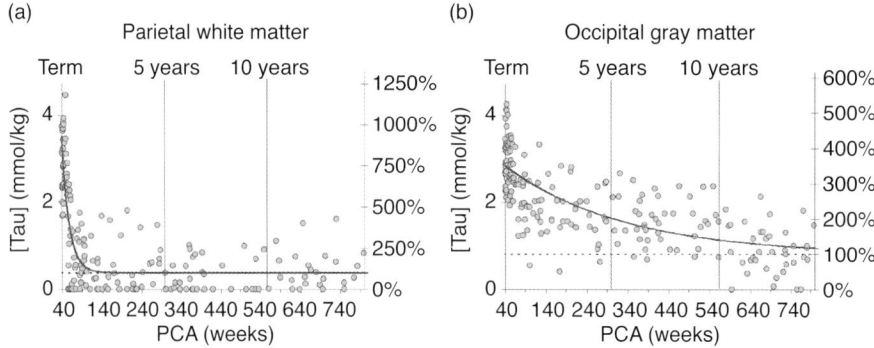

Fig. 7.15 Taurine (Tau) can be detected in white matter at the very early stages of brain development (a) but then very quickly declines to concentrations that are at or below the level of detection. In occipital gray matter (b), a more gradual decline is observed. PCA, postconceptional age.

developing preterm infants. At term or shortly thereafter, Lac is hardly detectable with the routine MRS methods that are available today (Figs. 7.7 and 7.17).

OTHER MAGNETIC RESONANCE-DETECTABLE METABOLITES

Several other metabolites are present in proton spectra. Glucose and scyllo-inositol can be routinely observed in normal brains. Also, metabolites such as NAA, Glu, γ-aminobutyrate, glutathione, glycine, aspartate, and others can be observed with optimized acquisition methods. Nevertheless, concentrations in normal brain are generally small, and thus the quantitation is unreliable. Age-dependent changes of these metabolites may become apparent as more powerful magnetic resonance scanners, providing magnetic resonance spectra with improved resolution and signal-to-noise ratios, and more robust acquisition methods, become available for future clinical research.

LIPIDS AND MACROMOLECULES

The protons of the methyl groups ($-CH_3$) of lipid molecules resonate at 0.9ppm (LipMM09), whereas protons of the methylene groups ($-CH_2^-$) resonate at 1.3ppm (LipMM13) in the ^{1}H spectrum. Both resonances are broad and may also include contributions from other macromolecules. Because the number of equivalent protons per lipid molecule or macromolecule is unknown, these entities cannot be quantified in absolute concentrations and arbitrary absolute intensities are often reported. In normal tissue, the concentration of free lipids is small and there should be very little signal in this part of the spectrum. The lipids signal increases when there is a breakdown/injury of cell membrane and release of fatty acids. Visual inspection of spectra in Fig. 7.3 shows that there are no dramatic changes of the magnetic resonance-detectable lipid content during brain maturation. When all individual data were plotted against age, the signal intensity of LipMM09 declined slightly in both white matter and gray matter (Fig. 7.17). However, owing to the unspecific nature of this signal, it is not clear whether this

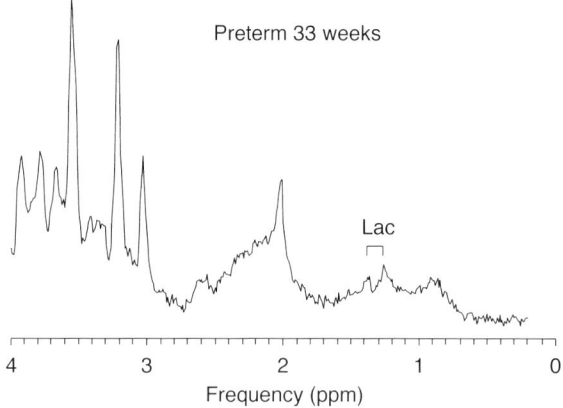

Preterm 33 weeks

Lac

Frequency (ppm)

Fig. 7.16 Lactate (Lac) forms a typical doublet at 1.3ppm and is readily detected (unless obscured by a huge lipid peak from necrosis) if present, as shown in this spectrum acquired from a preterm infant with normal MRI. However, it is not reliably detectable in term or older children (Fig. 7.9). ppm, parts per million.

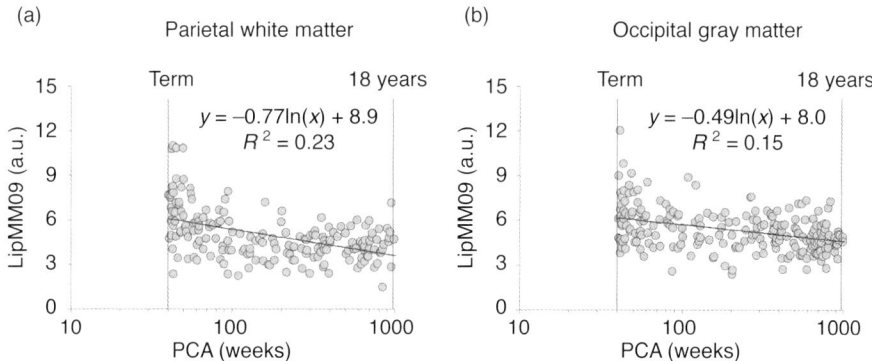

Fig. 7.17 Lipids (and possibly macromolecules) (LipMM09) are generally low in the structurally intact brain. A mild decline of the resonance at 0.9ppm is observed for both white matter (a) and gray matter (b). No trend was observed for lipid signal at 1.3ppm (not shown). a.u., arbitrary units; ppm, parts per million; PCA, postconceptional age.

represents declining levels of free lipids or whether the macromolecule content decreases with age. No trend was observed for LipMM13.

Regional variations

Significant differences in age-dependent changes in white matter and gray matter were observed for several metabolites. Most striking was Tau, which is detectable in white matter reliably around term but thereafter quickly decreases to levels virtually undetectable. In contrast, in gray matter, Tau remains detectable in children aged 5 years and older. Both Glu and Cr reach a transient maximum in white matter within the first year of life, not observed in gray matter. Other metabolites exhibit less apparent regional variation. NAA increases in both gray matter and white matter locations without reaching a plateau. However, a detailed analysis shows that the increase of white matter NAA precedes the increase of gray matter NAA slightly. Similarly, small differences in the developmental curves were also observed for Cho and mI. Apart from different time courses, metabolite levels in the two brain regions showed differences with respect to initial (at term) and final (young adults) concentrations. Consistent with what has been published by other groups independently, in young adults, Cho is higher in white matter than in gray matter whereas Glu and Cr concentrations are lower; at term, mI was lower in white matter than in gray matter, whereas the levels of other metabolites were in the same range.

Conclusions

In this chapter, we provided information about age-dependent changes of the metabolites that can be observed on most state-of-the-art magnetic resonance scanners. There are several mechanisms that underlie metabolism changes in the developing brain. The metabolism of different cell types varies and a relative increase of one cell population over another due to migration, formation/loss of neurons, axonal sprouting, synaptic pruning, and myelination will result in altered metabolic profiles. There are also metabolic changes associated with cell maturation and brain function. Examples are the switch to aerobic energy metabolism and increased pyruvate dehydrogenase activity or increased energy demand owing to increased neuronal activity. In addition, the role, regulation, and location of some of the metabolites and their 'magnetic resonance visibility' are often not well known and may vary with age. That provides many expanded parameters, and the interpretation of observed time courses and their correlation with specific neurodevelopmental events is currently very daunting. Still, there is a 'normal' spectrum for each anatomical brain region at each step of the developing brain. It is expected that future studies, beyond the two regions evaluated for this chapter, and careful comparison with events in brain development obtained by other means, may result in the elimination of some (or all) uncertainties and thereby complement our understanding of normal brain maturation. The fact that MRS is completely harmless, noninvasive, and nondestructive, that it does not require preparation, it shows the 'real thing' (repeatedly if desired), and it can readily be combined with MRI to provide insights at a microscopic/cellular level makes it a powerful tool for neuroscience.

REFERENCES

1. Bluml S, Friedlich P, Erberich S, Wood JC Seri I, Nelson MD Jr. (2004) MR imaging of newborns by using an MR-compatible incubator with integrated radiofrequency coils: initial experience. *Radiology* 231: 594–601.
2. Ment LR, Bada HS, Barnes P, et al (2002) Practice parameter: neuroimaging of the neonate: report of the Quality Standards Subcommittee of the American Academy of Neurology and the Practice Committee of the Child Neurology Society. *Neurology* 59: 1663.

3. Ramji FG, Slovis TL (1998) Normal neonatal head ultrasound. In: Haller JO, editor. *Textbook of Neonatal Ultrasound*. New York: Parthenon Publishing, pp. 1–30.
4. Babcock DS, Han BK, Dine MS (1988) Sonographic findings in infants with macrocrania. *AJR Am J Roentgenol* 150: 1359–1365.
5. Fessell DP, Frankel DA, Wolfson WP (2000) Sonography of extraaxial fluid in neurologically normal infants with head circumference greater than or equal to the 95th percentile for age. *J Ultrasound Med* 19: 443–447.
6. Slovis TL, Kelly JK, Eisenbrey AB, et al (1982) Detection of extracerebral fluid collections by real-time sector scanning through the anterior fontanelle. *J Ultrasound Med* 1: 41–44.
7. Nelson MD Jr., Tavare CJ, Petrus L, Kim P, Gilles FH (2003) Changes in the size of the lateral ventricles in the normal-term newborn following vaginal delivery. *Pediatr Radiol* 33: 831–835.
8. Osenfeld DL, Schonfeld SM, Underberg-Davis S (1997) Coarctation of the lateral ventricles: an alternative explanation for subependymal pseudocysts. *Pediatr Radiol* 27: 895–897.
9. Babcock DS (1995) Sonography of the brain in infants: role in evaluating neurologic abnormalities. *AJR Am J Roentgenol* 165: 417–423.
10. Schaefer PW, Grant PE, Gonzalez RG (2000) Diffusion-weighted MR imaging of the brain. *Radiology* 217: 331–345.
11. Triulzi F, Baldoli C, Parazzini C (2001) Neonatal MR imaging. *Magn Reson Imaging Clin N Am* 9: 57–82
12. Arthur R (2006) Magnetic resonance imaging in preterm infants. *Pediatr Radiol* 36: 593–607.
13. Bydder GM, Rutherford MA (2001) Diffusion-weighted imaging of the brain in neonates and infants. *Magn Reson Imaging Clin N Am* 9: 83–98.
14. Hüppi PS, Barnes PD (1997) Magnetic resonance techniques in the evaluation of the newborn brain. *Clin Perinatol* 24: 693–723.
15. Jones RA, Palasis S, Grattan-Smith JD (2004) MRI of the neonatal brain: optimization of spin-echo parameters. *AJR Am J Roentgenol* 182: 367–372.
16. Rutherford M, Malamateniou C, Zeka J, Counsell S (2004) MR imaging of the neonatal brain at 3 Tesla. *Eur J Paediatr Neurol* 8: 281–289.
17. Williams L-A, Gelman N, Picot PA, et al (2005) Neonatal brain: Regional variability of in vivo MRI imaging relaxation rates at 3.0T—initial experience. *Radiology* 235: 595–603.
18. Ashburner J, Friston KJ (2000) Voxel-based morphometry—the methods. *Neuroimage* 11: 805–821.
19. Ross BD and Bluml S (1999) Neurospectroscopy. In: Greenberg JO, editor. *Neuroimaging Second Edition; A Companion to Adams and Victor's Principles of Neurology*. New York: McGraw Hill, pp. 727–773.
20. Kreis R, Hofmann L, Kuhlmann B, Boesch C, Bossi E, Huppi PS (2002) Brain metabolite composition during early human brain development as measured by quantitative in vivo ^{1}H magnetic resonance spectroscopy. *Magn Reson Med* 48: 949–958.
21. van der Knaap M, van der Grond J, van Rijen P, Faber J, Valk J, Willemse K (1990) Age-dependent changes in localized proton and phosphorus MR spectroscopy of the brain. *Radiology* 176: 509–515.
22. Huppi PS, Posse S, Lazeyras F, Burri R, Bossi E, Herschkowitz N (1991) Magnetic resonance in preterm and term newborns: [1]H-spectroscopy in developing human brain. *Pediatr Res* 30: 574–578.
23. Toft PB, Leth H, Lou HC, Pryds O, Henriksen O (1994) Metabolite concentrations in the developing brain estimated with proton MR spectroscopy. *J Magn Reson Imaging* 4: 674–680.
24. Cady EB, Penrice J, Amess PN, et al (1996) Lactate, *N*-acetylaspartate, choline and creatine concentrations, and spin–spin relaxation in thalamic and occipito-parietal regions of developing human brain. *Magn Reson Med* 36: 878–886.
25. Kreis R, Ernst T, Ross BD (1993) Development of the human brain: in vivo quantification of metabolite and water content with proton magnetic resonance spectroscopy. *Magn Reson Med* 30: 424–437.
26. Pouwels PJ, Brockmann K, Kruse B, et al (1999) Regional age dependence of human brain metabolites from infancy to adulthood as detected by quantitative localized proton MRS. *Pediatr Res* 46: 474–485.
27. Panigrahy A, Tavare J, Nelson MD, Gilles FH, Seri I, Bluml S (2008) *Age and Regional Dependent Changes of Glutamate in Human Brain: In vivo Quantitation with MR Spectroscopy*. Toronto, Canada: International Society of Magnetic Resonance in Medicine (ISMRM).
28. Bottomley PA (1984) Selective volume method for performing localized NMR spectroscopy. US patent 4 480 228. USA, 1984.
29. Bottomley PA (1987) Spatial localization in NMR spectroscopy in vivo. *Ann N Y Acad Sci* 508: 333–348.

30. Castillo M, Kwock L, Green C (1995) MELAS syndrome: imaging and proton MR spectroscopic findings. *AJNR Am J Neuroradiol* 16: 233–239.
31. Nanto-Salonen K, Komu M, Lundbom N, et al (1999) Reduced brain creatine in gyrate atrophy of the choroid and retina with hyperornithinemia. *Neurology* 53: 303–307.
32. Ross BD, Danielsen ER, Bluml S (1996) Proton magnetic resonance spectroscopy: the new gold standard for diagnosis of clinical and subclinical hepatic encephalopathy? *Dig Dis* 14(Suppl 1): 30–39.
33. Dobbing J, Sands J (1973) Quantitative growth and development of human brain. *Arch Dis Child* 48: 757–767.
34. Lentner C (1981) *Geigy Scientific Tables*. *Units of Measurement Body Fluids Nutrition, Vol. 1*. Basel, Switzerland: Ciba-Geigy, pp. 220, 222, 223.
35. Ernst T, Kreis R, Ross BD (1993) Absolute quantitation of water and metabolites in the human brain. I Compartments and water. *J Magn Reson B* 102: 1–8.
36. Tallan HH (1957) Studies on the distribution of *N*-acetyl-L-aspartic acid in brain. *J Biol Chem* 224: 41–45.
37. Baslow MH (2000) Functions of *N*-acetyl-L-aspartate and *N*-acetyl-L-aspartylglutamate in the vertebrate brain: role in glial cell-specific signaling. *J Neurochem* 75: 453–459.
38. Bjartmar C, Battistuta J, Terada N, Dupree E, Trapp BD (2002) *N*-acetylaspartate is an axon-specific marker of mature white matter in vivo: a biochemical and immunohistochemical study on the rat optic nerve. *Ann Neurol* 51: 51–58.
39. Urenjak J, Williams SR, Gadian, DG, Noble M (1992) Specific expression of *N*-acetylaspartate in neurons, oligodendrocyte-type-2 astrocyte progenitors, and immature oligodendrocytes in vitro. *J Neurochem* 59: 55–61.
40. Urenjak J, Williams SR, Gadian DG, Noble M (1993) Proton nuclear magnetic resonance spectroscopy unambiguously identifies different neural cell types. *J Neurosci* 13: 981–989.
41. Pfefferbaum A, Adalsteinsson E, Spielman D, Sullivan EV, Lim KO (1999) In vivo spectroscopic quantification of the *N*-acetyl moiety, creatine, and choline from large volumes of brain gray and white matter: effects of normal aging. *Magn Reson Med* 41: 276–284.
42. Bluml S, Seymour, KJ, Ross BD (1999) Developmental changes in choline- and ethanolamine-containing compounds measured with proton-decoupled^{31}P MRS in in vivo human brain. *Magn Reson Med* 42: 643–654.
43. Lien YH, Shapiro JI, Chan L (1990) Effects of hypernatremia on organic brain osmoles. *J Clin Invest* 85: 1427–1435.
44. Videen JS, Michaelis T, Pinto P, Ross BD (1995) Human cerebral osmolytes during chronic hyponatremia. A proton magnetic resonance spectroscopy study. *J Clin Invest* 95: 788–793.
45. Provencher SW (1993) Estimation of metabolite concentrations from localized in vivo proton NMR spectra. *Magn Reson Med* 30: 672–679.
46. Daikhin Y, Yudkoff M (2000) Compartmentation of brain glutamate metabolism in neurons and glia. *J Nutr* 130: 1026S–1031S.
47. Erecinska M, Silver IA (1990) Metabolism and role of glutamate in mammalian brain. *Prog Neurobiol* 35: 245–296.
48. Kreis R, Ross BD, Farrow NA, Ackerman Z (1992) Metabolic disorders of the brain in chronic hepatic encephalopathy detected with H-1 MR spectroscopy. *Radiology* 182: 19–27.
49. Flint AC, Liu X, Kriegstein AR (1998) Nonsynaptic glycine receptor activation during early neocortical development. *Neuron* 20: 43–53.
50. Saransaari P, Oja SS (2000) Taurine and neural cell damage. *Amino Acids* 19: 509–526.
51. Kovanlikaya A, Panigrahy A, Krieger MD, et al (2005) Untreated pediatric primitive neuroectodermal tumor in vivo: quantitation of taurine with MR spectroscopy. *Radiology* 236: 1020–1025.
52. Moreno-Torres A, Martinez-Perez I, Baquero M, et al (2004) Taurine detection by proton magnetic resonance spectroscopy in medulloblastoma: contribution to noninvasive differential diagnosis with cerebellar astrocytoma. *Neurosurgery* 55: 824–829; discussion 829.

8
ANGIOGENESIS

Introduction

Angiogenesis is a key prerequisite for all vertebrate embryos. Streeter (1918)[1] generalized from his studies of human cerebral vascular development that vascular growth occurs *pari passu* with brain development; the number and distribution of vessels is continuously adequate for brain portions existing at any particular stage; the developing vascular system continuously adapts to the growing and changing brain; and, finally, no anticipatory vessels precede structures that have not yet appeared. This chapter will display the interplay of these guidelines in human embryonic forebrain microvascular development, particularly during the growth spurt during the last half of gestation (see Chapter 2).

FORMATION OF CRANIAL BLOOD SUPPLY AND LEPTOMENINGEAL PLEXUSES

Neural tissue grows as a defined organ to a certain stage (Carnegie stage 11 or 12; approximately 4mm crown–rump length; 24–26 days) before leptomeningeal vascular bed development. The proximal internal carotid artery arises from the third aortic arch, while the first and second arches contribute to the distal carotid. Later, at the 12–14mm stage (~41 days), the dorsal aortae, between the third and fourth arches, regress, leaving the internal carotid continuous with the third arch. At completion, the internal carotid artery consists of three portions:[2] a root portion, partially or wholly developed from the third aortic arch; an intermediate portion, from the dorsal aorta, between the third and original first arch site; and a cranial portion, a dorsal aortae continuation, probably representing the first pharyngeal arch branch. A rudimentary carotid siphon, first seen at 3 months, is fully formed by the fifth month. The basilar artery is formed from two longitudinal neural arteries (first apparent at about 26 days), which lie dorsal and parallel to the internal carotid arteries. According to Padget, large leptomeningeal channels foreshadow prospective carotid, basilar, and trigeminal arteries by stage 14 (~32 days) and their positions are set by 40 days, predating sprouting of endoneural endothelial sinusoidal channels.[3] The circle of Willis is not completed until stage 20 (~50 days) (Table 8.1). Other estimates place internal carotid artery appearance at about 20 days; distinct basilar and vertebral arteries at about 31 days; the posterior cerebral, middle cerebral, and anterior cerebral arteries at about 41 days; and anterior communicating artery at about 45 days.

179

TABLE 8.1

First endothelial sprouts

	Carotid	Trigeminal	Basilar	Circle of Willis
Stage 9 (20 days)	Begins	0	0	0
Stage 14 (32 days)	+	0	+[a]	0
Stage 20 (50 days)	+	+	+	+

'Begins'=carotid endothelial sprouts arise from the first aortic arch (the arch is also a simple endothelium at this stage). Note: The major cerebral arteries do not attain an adult configuration until about 40mm (about 2.5 months).

[a]The endothelial precursors to bilateral longitudinal arteries that antedate the basilar artery. Initially, the basilar bilateral longitudinal arteries are supplied by the trigeminals; later the first cervical segment will reinforce it caudally. Later in this stage the basilar artery proper starts to form followed by endothelial precursors to the vertebral arteries. Throughout these stages there are many interruptions of basilar precursors by angioblastic islands. 0, not present; +, present.

Following primary cerebral artery formation, an extensive leptomeningeal arterial and arteriolar bed is established after closure of rostral neuropore (stage 11) and caudal neuropore (stage 12) (24–26 days).[4] The epineural leptomeningeal plexus of endothelium-lined sinusoidal channels, derived from primordial angioblastic islands at the brain base,[5] arises at 3mm (~24 days); a few days later arteries, veins, and capillaries have differentiated (~28 days or 4mm). These vessels spread in the primitive leptomeninges from base to convexity[3,5] (rabbit[6] and rat),[7,8] gradually differentiating into veins or arteries also in the same direction.[1,4] Leptomeningeal epineural vascular beds give rise to all endoneural vessels.[3,5,6,9–12] Extensive anastomoses characterize fetal and neonatal leptomeningeal vascular beds,[13,14] continually increasing throughout gestation and the first two[15] or three postnatal months,[16] and are essentially completed by the end of the third postnatal month. These findings stand in distinct contrast to *Gray's Anatomy*, which states that leptomeningeal vessel branching is complete by 28 weeks.[17] The postnatal increase parallels the burst in neuronal cell body and dendritic growth rate occurring during the first 2 months.[18]

In summary, central nervous system blood supply develops in several steps in the same sequence, no matter the nervous system location, but its timing varies for each location. With advancing developmental time, leptomeningeal vascularization proceeds from anterior, basal, or ventral to dorsal or posterior, complicated by variation in timing of telencephalic convexity vascularization in different lobes and timing of subventricular neuroblast proliferation and migration (see Chapters 4 and 5).[19] The individual steps at any specific location follow a distinctive sequence: formation of a leptomeningeal plexus, transpial endothelial penetration, and growth of endothelial penetrators through the neural wall, without branching, until nearby subventricular matrix is entered and penetrated.

ENDOPARENCHYMAL MICROVASCULATURE

Capillaries first penetrate the basal or ventral neural wall surface at stages 12 (~26 days) (hindbrain), 13 (~30 days) (midbrain), and 16 (~37 days) (cerebral hemispheres),[20] spreading laterally and dorsally. Before this time, neural nourishment is entirely dependent upon amniotic fluid. Thereafter, the brain becomes increasingly dependent upon its blood supply. Endothelial channels enter the brain at roughly right angles to the surface[6,12,21,22] and grow toward the nearest lateral ventricular surface, where they branch and anastomose to form a plexus within the germinal matrix lining the ventricular system. Subsequently, endoparenchymal endothelial channels branch and establish a continuous capillary network throughout the telencephalon. Subsequent crops of penetrators branch in marginal and, finally, mantle layers; cerebral cortex is the last to receive branches of penetrators.

CURRENT MODELS

Many years ago, the speculation took hold that a vascular borderzone existed in deep cerebral white matter, between ventriculofugal and ventriculopetal arteries.[23–25] These earlier studies of human fetal telencephalic microvasculature, done with radiographs of vessels filled with radio-opaque intravascular contrast material, referred to the arterial nature of some deep extrastriatal vessels without any histologic verification and were repeatedly quoted (Fig. 8.1).[17,26–30] Furthermore, these two-dimensional radiographs of injected specimens precluded inspection of very small channels or delineation of separate superimposed vessels. De Reuck[25] described ventriculopetal and ventriculofugal arteries, the latter supposedly arising from striate arteries and from choroid plexus tela choroidea, supplying deep white matter near the ventricles. According to their accounts, ventriculopetal and ventriculofugal arteries made no anastomotic connections and formed a deep white matter borderzone.

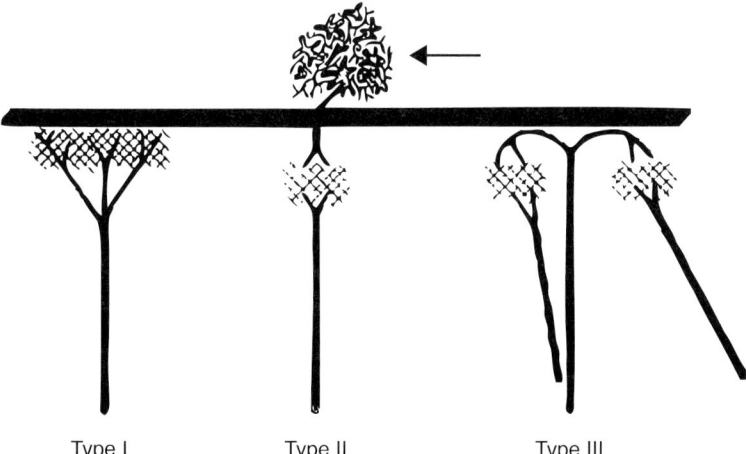

| Type I | Type II | Type III |

Fig. 8.1 Model of de Reuck (1971) illustrates the three types of claimed paraventricular arterial borderzones. Type I, terminal arterial bed formed by a ventriculopetal perforating or medullary branch ending adjacent to ventricular wall. Type II, borderzone formed by ventriculopetal perforating or medullary branch and ventriculofugal branch from choroidal arteries of choroid plexus (arrow) traversing lateral ventricle and ependyma to reenter parenchyma. Type III, borderzone formed by ventriculopetal perforating or medullary branches between one another. Heavy black line represents ventricular wall. Reproduced with permission of S. Karger AG from de Reuck.[25]

181

Nonetheless, three-dimensional studies of thick brain slabs with Microfil®-filled vascular trees (Microfil, Flow Tech, Carver, MA, USA) found no ventriculofugal arteries arising from lateral striate arteries or from the choroid plexus as claimed,[25] the ventriculofugal arteries traversing the lateral ventricular spinal fluid, and penetrating the ependymal layer to supply deep white matter.[21,22,31] Subsequent studies using thick sections of celloidin-embedded fetal brains, stained with alkaline phosphatase, claimed separation of veins and arteries in the fetal brain,[32–34] even though these channels contained only endothelium without muscularis or adventitia. In adult neural vessels, alkaline phosphatase-stained endothelial cells appear to distinguish differentiated arteries and veins. All the same, in undifferentiated fetal endoneural capillaries, while alkaline phosphatase is present in endothelial cells, it is not necessarily limited to future arteries,[35–37] it varies by species (for example, in developing mouse brain the arteries, veins, and capillaries are stained),[38] and sometimes is found in other cell types.

Endoparenchymal Capillary Remodeling

Brain capillary beds change extensively during the fetal period and first postnatal year; there is constant vascular remodeling as the cerebrum enlarges and grows away from the ventricular walls. Within the cerebral and cerebellar cortex, relative capillary volume is said to increase linearly from the third gestational month until the fourth postnatal year; in contrast, others claim there is no change in capillary density in telencephalic white matter over the same period.[39,40] Nevertheless, adult levels of cortical capillary density are not reached at 4 years. Others place the burst in deep telencephalic vasculogenesis later in gestation, possibly not until the middle.[39,41] During fetal telencephalic vasculogenesis, white matter capillary density is always greater than that of cortex and decreases (relative to cortex) after major myelination is completed.

Embryonic, fetal, and early childhood angiogenesis

Specimens

The data reported here are based on 108 human embryos, ranging from stage 11 (~24 days) to stage 23 (~8 weeks), particularly in telencephalon. These specimens are in the Carnegie Collection of serially sectioned human embryos presently located at the Armed Forces Institute of Pathology in Washington; previous studies depicted many of these embryos.[1,3,5,42] In addition, 60 human fetal and childhood autopsied brains, ranging from 16 weeks' gestation to 15 years' postconceptional age, constituted our material. The fetal group had respiratory distress syndrome, congenital heart disease, asphyxia, white matter necrosis, sepsis, and germinal matrix and intraventricular hemorrhage. The older children died as a result of trauma, sepsis, leukemia, or neoplasia not involving the brain. Forty-three brains were from specimens 44 weeks old or less.[21] Fetal gestational age was estimated by Dubowitz criteria when available and/or by congruency of body weight, crown–rump length, head circumference, and brain weight with the approximate fetal postconceptional age.[43,44]

METHODS

The Carnegie embryos had been serially sectioned in various planes (horizontal, sagittal, coronal) and stained with hematoxylin and eosin, Mallory-azan, or alum cochineal. The vascular systems of seven embryos, at several different stages, had been injected with India ink before specimen fixation. Complete photographic sets of each serial section were made of 22 representative specimens.

In fetal material, one or both internal carotid arteries or the sagittal sinus were cannulated before scalp incision. The cranial vascular bed was flushed with saline and infused, under near-physiologic injection pressures, with a liquid silicone rubber compound (Microfil®) designed to fill and opacify microvascular beds of nonsurviving animals and postmortem tissues. For details, see the original papers.[21,22] One half of each brain slab was used for routine processing; the other half was carried through graded alcohols and cleared in methyl salicylate. The slabs were examined under a stereomicroscope equipped with a drawing tube. Microvasculature was either drawn or photographed with a combination of direct and indirect lighting, in single field or stereoscopic pairs, while in methyl salicylate. Microscopic sections of blocks of photographed, cleared slabs were used for histologic determination of arteries, arterioles, sinusoids, capillaries, venules, or veins. We measured the least vessel lumen diameters using a calibrated reticle and stage micrometer. Densities of microvessels were estimated by counting the number of vascular lumina of specified diameters within a calibrated grid at a magnification of ×200. The superior frontal gyrus cortex and subjacent corona radiata white matter to the ventricular wall, just anterior to the foramen of Monro, were sampled.

In four fetal specimens, the entire parasylvian and lateral convexity leptomeninges, including borderzone regions between the anterior, middle, and posterior cerebral arteries, with their Microfil®-filled vascular beds, were lifted off the cerebral hemispheres and examined stereoscopically and photographed while submerged in methyl salicylate. Removal of leptomeninges was not difficult because they floated free after the slightest nick and manipulation. The lateral surface of one 26-week-old hemisphere was removed in an oblique sagittal plane down to the lateral ventricle in order to expose germinal matrix vascular supply.

For operational purposes, we designated vessels of less than two red cell diameters as 'capillaries' and endothelial sinusoids of greater diameter 'channels.' One or more of three criteria distinguished arteries and veins: (1) *connections*—vessels arising from identified surface arteries and veins were considered the same as the parent vessel until the main trunk divided; (2) *location*—large arteries or veins, in known locations, were assumed to be the designated vessel, for example a large single midline vessel anterior to pons was the basilar artery; and (3) *histology*—channels with at least one layer of smooth muscle cells were designated 'arteries'; channels with only a collagenous adventitial sheath, 'veins.' We defined 'striatal vessels' as those supplying the corpus striatum (caudate and putamen, namely lateral or medial striate vessels) and 'extrastriatal vessels' as those supplying the remaining telencephalon (except for amygdala), including both the cortex and white matter.

Embryonic and fetal head vascularization

Stages 6 to 9 (until 20 days), dorsal aortae formation
Some leptomeningeal endothelial channels eventually develop into the great vessels supply-ing the cerebrum.[42] The chorionic mesoblast is the site of first angiogenesis at stage 6 (~13 days); blood vessel formation precedes blood cell formation. At stage 8 (~18 days), the neural groove is evident before the heart and other organs. The neural plate and groove are open to the amniotic cavity. By stage 9 (~20 days), concomitant with the rise of rostral neural groove sides, a series of endothelial sprouts develops from the first pair of aortic arches, forming the dorsal aortae. These consist of only simple endothelial sinusoids and begin growth toward the developing nervous system while the neural groove remains open. Caudal endothelial sprouts eventually supply the spinal cord; more rostral sprouts supply the rhombencephalon and mesencephalon; and the most rostral sprouts coalesce into large endothelial channels, destined to become the internal carotid arteries (Table 8.1).

Stages 11 to 15 (~24 to 33 days), primitive plexus brain base
The rostral neuropore closes during these stages, and once this is accomplished amniotic fluid no longer supplies the nervous system's nutritional needs.[42] The heart begins beating, causing a simple to and fro blood movement. Before this stage, no central nervous system vascularization exists. As the simple dorsal aortae endothelial channels approach the rostral nervous system, primitive mesenchyme surrounding the nervous system gives rise to lepto-meningeal angioblastic islands, endothelial sprouts, and endothelial channels, which anasto-mose. Dorsal aortae endothelial sprouts form a primitive basal brain plexus (Tables 8.1 and 8.2), although most telencephalic perineural primitive mesenchyme is still free of endothelial channels. These endothelial channels, at first, are filled with an acellular fluid, followed by a few erythroblasts. The superior cardinal vein cephalad extension (called the primitive head vein), located lateral to the rhombencephalon, becomes prominent, suggesting establishment of a caudal basal plexus circulation.

The endothelial channels join, proliferate, and form a basal plexus, which spreads rapidly, and begins differentiating arterial and venous circulations at about stage 12 (about 3–5mm; ~26 days). However, in one case we reviewed at this stage (Carnegie Accession #9154), a basal plexus had not yet formed. A rudimentary leptomeningeal circulation is established at stage 13 (~30 days, about the time of the initial telencephalic outpouching). By stage 14 the endothelial channels rapidly form a dense plexus growing over the base by stage 15 (~33 days), and eventually spreading over the convexity to become a perineural plexus.

Throughout stages 15–20, the telencephalic perineural leptomeningeal capillary plexus was very dense, with most superficial forebrain regions lying within 15μm of a leptomenin-geal capillary. After stage 20 (about 21–23mm; ~50–51 days), leptomeningeal plexus density gradually decreased with cerebral growth, and most superficial forebrain regions were at a greater distance from leptomeningeal capillaries (Table 8.2).

TABLE 8.2
Perineural plexus and endothelial penetrators

	Perineural capillary plexus	Endothelial penetrators matrix striatum	Endothelial penetrators matrix extrastriatal	Subependymal veins	Choroid plexus
Stage 11 (24 days)	±	NA	NA	0	NA
Stage 14 (32 days)	+	0	0	0	NA
Stage 15 (33 days)	+ +	0	0	0	NA
Stage 16 (37 days)	+ +	+ +	0	0	0
Stage 20 (50 days)	+ +	+	+	0	+ +
40mm (2.5 months)	+	+	+	0	+

The transneural penetrating capillaries to the matrix reach the medial hemisphere during stage 23. Subependymal veins are present after 16 weeks, but we do not have the appropriately aged specimens to determine their time of appearance. The superior choroidal vein is the sole supply to the internal cerebral vein until between the third gestational month and term. The basal vein appears between 60 and 80mm. 0, absent; ±, present in only a few brains; +, present; ++, prominent. NA, not available.

Stages 14–20 (~32–50 days), first formation of endothelial penetrators

The first endothelial central nervous system penetrators are occasionally mesencephalic at stage 14 (about 5–7mm; ~32 days);[20,42] in some cases, we found them only in rhombencephalon, but, in larger specimens at the same stage, they were present also in the mesencephalon. The brainstem penetrators enter the basal plate ventricular layer germinal matrix only. At stage 15 (about 7–9mm; ~33 days), internal carotid artery precursors lie lateral to the adenohypophyseal pouch, penetrating capillaries are found in mesencephalon, rhombencephalon, cervical, and thoracic spinal cord, and, for the first time, a few in the diencephalon. As cerebral evagination occurs, diencephalic penetrators become more extensive than rhombencephalic penetrators, with one tier of ventricular matrix branching. The first transcerebral channels penetrate to the lateral and medial eminence subventricular germinal matrix, that is the matrix overlying the future caudate nucleus head and the matrix overlying the prospective olfactory ventricular outpouching root (stage 17: about 11–14mm; ~41 days). They penetrate the pia; traverse the entire cerebral wall; bifurcate in the subventricular germinal matrix of these two regions; and form a latticework, which persists throughout the second trimester, shrinking in extent with matrix depletion at the end of the second trimester. As in other nervous system regions, at this embryonic stage there are no separate subventricular venous channels. By stage 17, mesencephalic alar penetrators are present; by stage 19 (about 17–20mm; ~47–48 days), a second set of penetrators branch deep in the prospective corpus striatum, just before the matrix layer.

Penetrating vessels are always similar histologically, consisting of simple endothelium without recognizable arterial or venous features. Later in gestation, there is no histologic differentiation between extrastriatal channels connected to leptomeningeal arteries or leptomeningeal veins. Arteries and veins both branch at acute and right angles. Separation of arterial from venous endoneural channels is partially possible only by identification of parent surface vessels.

Stage 16 (about 11–14mm; ~37 days), extrastriatal telencephalic endothelial sprouts
Penetrators traversing the remaining telencephalic regions first develop near the base, in extrastriatal locations lateral to striatal penetrators, and gradually spread laterally and dorsally to reach the hemispheral dorsolateral surface, where they meet penetrators spreading from the medial hemispheral surface at stage 20 (~50 days) (Table 8.2). These early extrastriatal penetrators proceed directly through the hemispheral wall, reaching the subventricular matrix before branching to form a germinal matrix latticework (Fig. 8.2). With time, additional endothelial penetrators develop and create endothelial plexuses more peripherally in telencephalic wall mantle and marginal zones (Fig. 8.3), particularly in regions undergoing migration or maturation, where they form more or less concentric plexuses. While the process is similar in all cerebral locations, the timing differs depending on age and location in the brain, whether basal or convexity, and position in differing lobes.

Leptomeningeal vascular beds from midgestation
By midgestation, many leptomeningeal vessel walls have developed sufficient muscularis or collagenous adventitia to be recognizable as arteries or veins. In general, fetal muscularization is far more robust in basal than convexity vessels. All vascular channels lie external to the pia within the future arachnoid except for penetrating branches as they enter the cerebrum. At all ages, basal leptomeningeal arteries have larger diameters and more smooth muscle layers than convexity arteries. Leptomeningeal veins contain a single endothelial layer, with surrounding collagen layers constituting an adventitia; larger diameter leptomeningeal veins have more collagenous layers than smaller veins. Arteriolar smooth muscle coat extends only as far as the

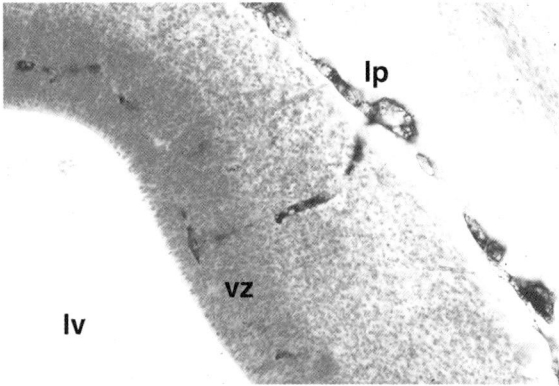

Fig. 8.2 Photomicrograph of hemispheral penetrating capillary at about stage 20 (50 days). The leptomeningeal plexus (lp) has been filled with India ink and the penetrating capillary extends through the pia directly to the ventricular zone (vz) where it first divides. The lateral ventricle is indicated by lv.

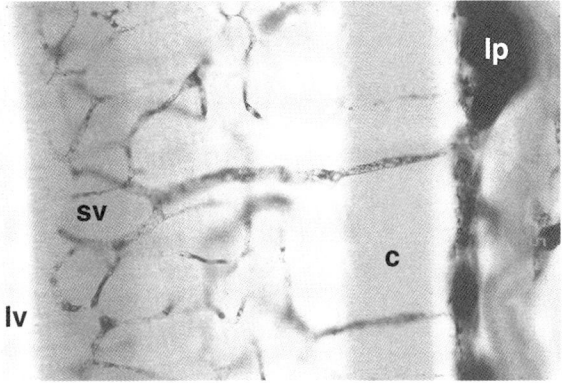

Fig. 8.3 Photomicrograph of hemispheral penetrating capillaries at a slightly older age at approximately the same site. Subsequent crops of penetrators derived from the India ink-filled leptomeningeal plexus (lp) branch in intermediate zones of the cerebral wall. The penetrating capillaries pass directly through the prospective cortex (c), and contribute several branches to the subventricular zone (sv) after providing branches to intermediate cerebral layers. lv, lateral ventricle.

pia. In all 60 fetal specimens, smaller vessels branch from leptomeningeal arteries, arterioles, veins, and venules toward the cerebral surface, immediately perforate the pia and penetrate the cerebrum. These branches usually cross the pia at right or oblique angles and rarely contain a muscularis below the pia, except for large basal striatal branches, with increasing numbers in infants, children, and adolescents. Following leptomeningeal vessel differentiation into arteries and veins, no leptomeningeal capillary beds remain. Leptomeningeal veins larger than 1mm tend to lie superficial to remaining leptomeningeal plexus, but smaller arterial and venous branches interweave; hence, no general statement concerning the relative arterial and venous positions can be made (for instance, veins were not always superficial to arteries).[45] Larger leptomeningeal arteries divide into smaller branches that are frequently interconnected (Table 8.3 and Fig. 8.4); leptomeningeal veins also are interconnected, but less frequently than arteries or arterioles. In all specimens, both arterial and venous networks are continuous over the borderzones between the anterior, middle, and posterior cerebral arteries.

Leptomeningeal arteries vary from 15 to 75µm in luminal diameter at 16 weeks; the largest diameters (excluding the first two segments of anterior, middle, and posterior cerebral arteries) increase to 200µm at birth and to 260 to 280µm at 15 years of age. Leptomeningeal vein diameters (excluding the vein of Galen and large superficial collecting veins draining into the dural sinuses) vary from 50 to 100µm at 16 weeks; the maximal venous luminal diameter increases to 225 to 250µm at birth and to 280 to 300µm at 15 years of age.

There were no leptomeningeal 'terminal' arteries in any specimen, despite reports of others,[46] even after specific searches of major borderzones between the anterior, middle, and posterior cerebral arteries, but rather the same anastomosing vessels continued throughout the remaining leptomeningeal plexus (Fig. 8.4). Similarly, the cerebellar borderzone between the superior and inferior cerebellar arteries is a continuous capillary bed (Fig. 8.5).

TABLE 8.3

Muscularization of human telencephalic arteries

	Perineural plexus	Striatum	Extrastriatal
Stage 20 (50 days)	+[a]	0	0
78.5mm (4 months)	+	+	0
Term	+	+	±
First postnatal year	+	+	+

[a]A muscularis consisting of a single cell layer is found on only a few major trunks in the perineural plexus at the brain base. 0, absent; ±, present in some brains; +, present.

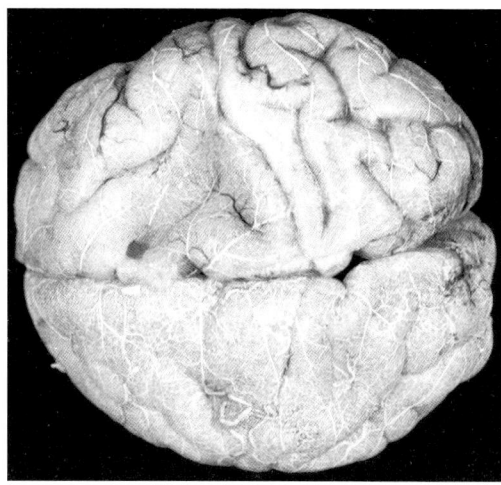

Fig. 8.4 The white leptomeningeal plexus has been filled with Microfil®. Veins have not been filled and are black. There is a dense arteriolar and capillary bed that is continuous across the borderzone between the anterior and middle cerebral arteries.

Striatal vascular bed from midgestation

Striatal channels support the growth of caudate, putamen, and medial and lateral eminences by branching, enlarging in diameter, and increasing in length with brain expansion. In specimens of 16 to 20 weeks, striatal vessels branch from the first middle cerebral artery segment and penetrate the basilar pia; these channels pass through the putamen and caudate, distally entering either the medial or lateral eminence (Fig. 8.6). In general, basal striatal vessels are larger, progressively branching into smaller channels as they course toward the lateral ventricles. The longest striatal channel measures 60μm in diameter at its base and 15mm in length; side branches diverge at acute angles. Smaller channels, both in length and diameter, branch in the middle and inferior putamen. No striatal vessels in this age group had a muscularis or adventitia.

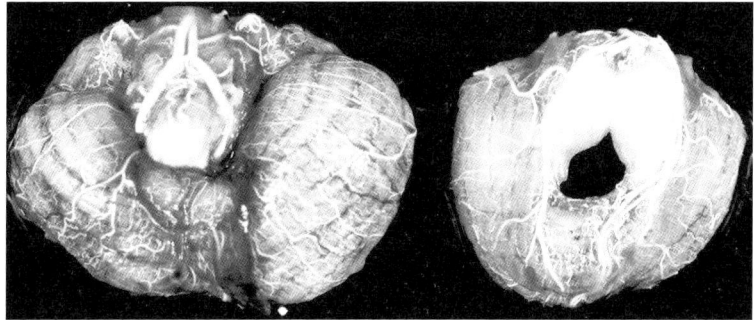

Fig. 8.5 The white leptomeningeal plexus has been filled with Microfil®. The inferior cerebellar (left) surface also demonstrates the medulla and pons with vertebral and paired basilar and anterior spinal arteries. The dense plexus is usually supplied by the posterior inferior cerebellar arteries. On the right, the pons has been cut through its upper portions and demonstrates the superior cerebellar arteries encircling the pons and supplying the leptomeningeal plexus. The superior and inferior leptomeningeal plexuses are continuous across the borderzone at the cerebellar periphery.

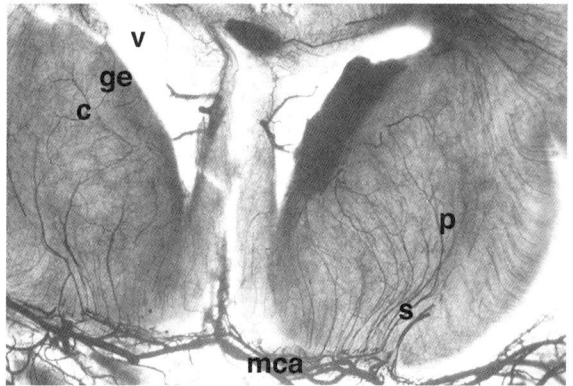

Fig. 8.6 Photograph of cleared thick coronal section of striatum anterior to foramen of Monro at 28 weeks. Striatal channels (s) branch from the middle cerebral artery (mca) and course through the putamen (p) and caudate (c) to end in the subventricular ganglionic eminence (ge). There is a small hemorrhage in the right ganglionic eminence. v, lateral ventricle.

Specimens of 22 to 26 weeks have approximately the same number of long striatal channels reaching the medial or lateral eminence germinal matrix as the 16 to 20 week group; however, these channels are larger and longer (longest, 18mm). Basal striatal channels may be up to 75μm in diameter and taper to 10 to 20μm distally before entering the germinal matrix eminence (Fig. 8.6). Long striatal channels, persisting beyond 16 weeks, are lateral striate arterial precursors. In all specimens with an identifiable blood supply source to the lateral, eminence was present, coming from the middle cerebral arterial striate branches. We could

189

TABLE 8.4

Muscularization of telencephalic arteries as identified on photomicrographs

Arterial area	First identification of smooth muscle layer
Leptomeningeal	Present at 16 weeks' gestation
Striatal	20 to 22 weeks' gestation
Extrastriatal	
Medullary	Term to 1 month after birth
Cortical	6–9 months after birth

not find a large source of blood from Heubner's recurrent artery and in none of our specimens was there a germinal tissue blood supply from choroidal arteries.[29]

Differentiation of striatal endothelial channels into histologically identifiable arteries or veins occurred; by the end of the second trimester, muscularization of some caudate lateral striate arteries, within 60 or 100μm of ganglionic eminence, appeared in all specimens at 24 to 26 weeks[21] (Table 8.4), as the ganglionic eminence reaches its maximum absolute volume[47] (see Chapter 4). In specimens of 28 to 30 weeks' gestation, several large channels (50–100μm in diameter), situated between germinal tissue and the caudate nucleus head, developed adventitial layers characteristic of veins and could be followed in injected specimens as they anastomosed with collecting veins from the internal cerebral venous system. Muscularis was not present in any germinal matrix vessel at any age. A true ependymal layer does not develop until ventricular matrix regression; hence, submatrix veins do not become subependymal veins until after this happens. Submatrix veins first were evident after 2.5 months; subependymal veins were absent at 8 weeks (the embryonic period end) and in one specimen at 12 weeks, but were present at 16 weeks. At the end of the second trimester, as the germinal matrix regresses, matrix endothelial plexuses also regress, leaving subependymal veins in place. The subependymal veins reach diameters of 200μm at birth and 300μm at 15 years. Others have found these human fetal submatrix veins.[29,48]

The longest striatal arteries increased in length from 20mm at birth to 45mm at 15 years, and increased in maximal diameter from 250μm at birth to 500μm at 15 years of age. Striatal vessels and their major branches never coursed superior or lateral to the lateral ventricular outer corner to end in the corona radiata in any of our 60 specimens. The capillary bed itself was continuous between striatal and extrastriatal circulations in all specimens of all ages; precapillary anastomotic channels were located between extrastriatal insular and most lateral striatal channels.

A distinct media develops much earlier in striatal than in extrastriatal endoneural vessels. It begins first in basal striatal vessels, in continuity with the muscularized leptomeningeal middle cerebral artery branches, and extends upward across the putamen with advancing gestational age. A media is discernible in basal putamenal vessels at 24 weeks, and in intervening internal capsule anterior limb and caudate a few weeks later. Capillaries are encountered throughout the caudate and putamen at all fetal ages.

Extrastriatal telencephalic endothelial sprouts, penetrators,
and channels from midgestation

Penetrating channels, 15 to 50μm in diameter, branch at right or acute angles from lepto-meningeal vessels at approximately 100-μm intervals in all 16- to 20-week specimens. These channels cross the pia and cerebral surface to extend variable lengths toward the nearest lateral ventricle before their subventricular matrix branching (Figs. 8.7 and 8.8). Larger channels,

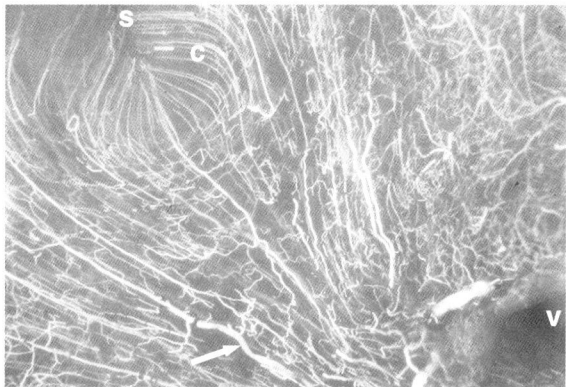

Fig. 8.7 Photomicrograph of a cleared thick coronal section of cerebrum anterior to foramen of Monro. The lateral ventricle (v) is at the lower right. The cortex around the depths of a sulcus (s) is seen at the upper left. Large numbers of transcerebral channels extend from the sulcus toward the ventricular wall. Many channels end in collecting veins in the ventricular wall when focusing through this thick section. Some channels enlarge in their course through the cerebrum (arrow). The lack of cortical channel branching is seen particularly well (c). Note the rich vascularity in subsulcal and deep white matter.

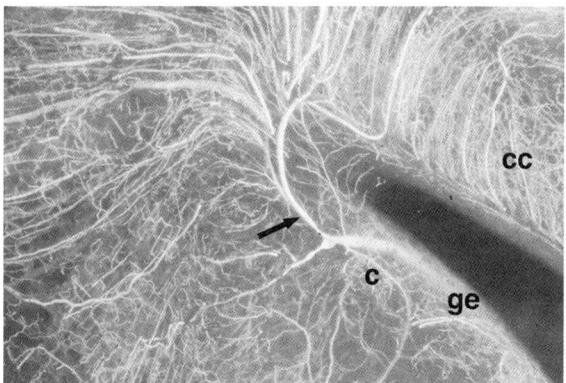

Fig. 8.8 Photomicrograph of a cleared thick section of cerebrum anterior to foramen of Monro (end of the second trimester). Multiple capillaries and channels pass through the corpus callosum (cc) and collect on its undersurface in the lateral ventricle roof. The caudate (c) lies under the densely vascularized residual ganglionic eminence (ge). Transcerebral channels in their courses through telencephalic wall have given off many branches in prospective white matter and collect in large or small venous structures in the ventricular wall (arrow).

50μm in diameter, nearly spanning the entire cerebral wall thickness, branch into smaller vessels that anastomose with other vessel branches in the subependymal germinal matrix, lateral to the ganglionic eminence. Transcerebral channels are either larger or narrower at their ventricular ends; but some remain approximately the same diameter throughout their transcerebral course. In specimens of 22 to 26 weeks, transcerebral channels are longer (9–14mm in length) and larger in diameter than at 16 to 20 weeks. Transcerebral channels persist throughout gestation, gradually enlarging and lengthening with brain growth. In all nervous system locations, the first endothelial penetrators are simple endothelial structures, either capillaries (early) or sinusoids (later). Penetrators and plexuses, whether in the matrix or in regions undergoing migration or differentiation, have the same gamut of capillaries or sinusoids. Specifically, plexus channels in embryonic telencephalon tend to remain small in caliber, namely capillary size throughout the embryonic period; only later do transcerebral channels enlarge to become sinusoids. Endothelial channels eventually form more endothelial channels, arteries, or veins, but the fetal ages when this occurs vary with site, whether striatal or extrastriatal, and, among the extrastriatal vessels, whether of basolateral, convexity, or hemispheral location; and whether in white matter or the cortex. The growing forebrain surface area increases concomitantly with cerebral bulk[47] and development of additional extrastriatal channels seem governed by this large increase in cortical surface area, maintaining penetrating channels at approximately 80 to 100μm intervals, throughout the second gestational half. Endothelial channels are constantly remodeled, with new connections and new channels forming, as the supplied tissue bulk increases; some channels were removed if hemodynamically unnecessary.[6] Penetrators supplying the cortical plate capillary plexus are the last to form; some appearing toward term, but the bulk after birth.

Transcerebral channels form a basic scaffold for telencephalic microvasculature, which branch with subsequent crops of intermediate and short penetrators, vascularizing portions of deep and more superficial intermediate and subplate regions with telencephalic growth. The extrastriatal plexus supplies all ventricular layer germinal matrixes except for the medial and lateral eminences (supplied largely by striatal channels). Subsequent crops of small channels, 4 to 15μm in diameter, divide short of the germinal matrix in the intermediate layer to branch out and anastomose with side branches from other larger channels and/or equal, or smaller, diameter vessels at various distances from the cortical surface. All channels pass through the cortex or cortical plate in younger specimens without branching and then provide right angle, acute, or oblique branches to connect with other channels (Fig. 8.7). Histologically, all extrastriatal endoneural channels consist initially of a single layer of endothelium. These subsequent crops of intermediate and shorter penetrating channels are similar to those in rabbits and rodents.[6,8] In contrast to the transcerebral striatal penetrators, muscularizing late in the second trimester, most extrastriatal channels remain, to a large extent, sinusoidal with a single layer of endothelial cells and no apparent muscularis until the final weeks of gestation and into the postnatal period (Table 8.3). At midgestation, many become quite large with transpial diameters of 10 to 20μm and twice that at the ventricular end; by term, peripheral ends enlarge and central ends measure 50 to 120μm. Thus, many transcerebral trunks are larger in diameter at their ventricular ends. We did not find that branching angle gave any clue as to their arterial or venous nature.[45]

A new series of short, penetrating channels branch from the leptomeningeal plexus and anastomose within the cortex without entering white matter between 22 and 24 weeks, as previously noted;[29] the longest channels are the largest, measuring up to 75μm in diameter. Larger transcerebral channels occasionally provide a few side branches to this new cortical network before entering the white matter. Isocortical regions that differentiate early in the third trimester, such as calcarine and motor cortices, do not vascularize ahead of other regions. Cortical channels that branch and anastomose solely within the cortex measured up to 25μm in diameter at birth and up to 40μm at 15 years of age; the longest channels increased in length from 3mm at birth to 3.5mm at 15 years of age. Intracortical channels develop a muscularis between 6 and 9 postnatal months (Table 8.1). Similarly, some cortical channels, connected to leptomeningeal veins, develop an adventitia between 6 and 9 postnatal months, whereas others remain simple endothelial sinusoids.

Gyri develop with advancing age after midgestation (see Chapter 5). Throughout gyral formation, penetrating endoneural channels remain perpendicular to the pia and cortical plate, requiring pre-existing channels to bend considerably before reaching deep white matter (Fig. 8.7). Thus, channels that pass through the cortex into deep white matter turn another 90° below the corticomedullary junction before proceeding toward the nearest corner or other lateral ventricular surface.

Least and maximal distances from the cerebral surface to the nearest lateral ventricle vary with age (Table 8.5). At 16 weeks' gestation, only primary fissures are present and the maximal transcerebral width is 10mm; increasing to 21mm at birth and 40mm at 15 years of age. Interestingly, the distance from the bottoms of primary sulci to the nearest lateral ventricle is never more than 10 to 15mm; moreover, no regions of consistently hypovascularized white matter are present either near the ventricular corner[25] or in subsulcine white matter.[27] The density of microvessels, 5 to 100μm in diameter, is greater in white matter than in cortical gray matter throughout the last half of gestation (Table 8.6); in contrast, toward the end of the first postnatal year the opposite pattern develops: density of cortical vessels becomes much greater than white matter (Table 8.3).

Muscularized extrastriatal endoneural vessels are first identified in 38- to 40-week specimens when the largest transcerebral channels are approximately 200μm in diameter (Table 8.4). They develop layers of smooth muscle from the channel's leptomeningeal end, as the layers of smooth muscle are thickest at leptomeningeal ends. Long transcerebral channels, connected to leptomeningeal veins, develop an adventitia between 40 and 48 weeks (Fig. 8.5).

Blood–brain barrier development

Endothelial cells, astrocytic end-feet, and pericytes are the blood–brain barrier cellular components. Its formation starts shortly after intraneural vascularization in rodents. Endothelial fenestrations are initially frequent, but decrease rapidly. Tight junctions between cerebral endothelial and choroid plexus epithelial cells form the morphologic barrier to large molecules. Astrocytic end-feet form tight sheaths around the vessel and appear essential for tight junction induction and maintenance;[49] but tight junctions sometimes precede development of astrocytic end-feet. As soon as cerebral capillaries and choroid plexus differentiate, they have tight junctions; in the germinal matrix, 'strap' junctions are also present.[50] Gröntoft[51]

TABLE 8.5

Critical dimensions in fetal telencephalic vascular development

Dimension	Measurement (mm)		
	16 weeks	40 weeks	15 years
Cortical plate/cortex	0.8	2	3.5
Surface to lateral ventricle	10	21	40
Bottom (fundus) of sulcus to lateral ventricle	—[a]	10	10–15
Base of brain to top of caudate	15	20	42

Note: Measurements were subject to distortions caused by specimen fixation and dehydration.
[a]No sulci were present at this age.

TABLE 8.6

Density of microvessels 5–100μm in diameter per 500μm² area

Area	Number of microvessels per 500μm²		
	19 weeks' gestation	40 weeks' gestation	2 years old
Cortex	6 (2)	9 (2)	29 (5)
White matter	11 (3)	13 (2)	17 (3)

Values are mean (SD).

showed that when trypan blue solution was perfused through human fetal cerebral vessels of 10 weeks' and 16 to 27 weeks' gestation, within 10 minutes of placental separation, no dye penetrated into the brain. Much prior confusion about fetal blood–brain barrier 'immaturity' existed owing to investigators using either toxic dye concentrations or experiments of long duration (summarized in reference 50).

Claudin-5, occludin, and junctional adhesion molecule (JAM-1) (protein markers of tight junctions) are expressed in the fetal brain at 16 weeks in germinal matrix, cortex, and white matter; their concentration in these locations does not differ throughout the remaining gestational weeks.[52] Other tight junction protein markers were not expressed. Tight junction molecules are fundamental to the control of paracellular permeability.

Conclusion

CURRENT MODELS

Models dominating current thought about telencephalic microvasculature are not consistent with the literature or the studies reported in this chapter, which directly contradict their concepts.[17,25,28,30] Our findings indicate that there are no ventriculofugal arteries, no periventricular arterial rings, and no transventricular arterial supplies. Furthermore, muscularization of extrastriatal transcerebral trunks and shorter channels does not begin until term; thus, there are no extrastriatal arteries to form deep hemispheral borderzones at any time during gestation. Concepts of shifts in blood supply from basal ganglia to cortex between 24 and 34 weeks (see, for example, reference 29) found no support in our material. Various aspects of telencephalic angiogenesis have been described,[3,5,6,8–13,21,24,46,53–59] but we have provided new observations and interpretations on leptomeningeal vascular development, sequence of endoneural vessel wall maturation, and differences between telencephalic striatal and extrastriatal vascularization (Table 8.4).

BÄR'S MODEL

Bär, building on the rabbit model of Strong,[6] demonstrated that the developing rat telencephalic vasculature is initially composed of transcerebral trunks and, subsequently, of shorter intertruncal vessels, similar to microvascular development in other organs.[7,8,60] He proposed that transcerebral trunks, and shorter vascular beds, constitute a system of hexagonally packed vascular supply units, of differing length, developing in response to brain growth: as cerebral depth and surface area increase, addition of regularly spaced shorter vessels between larger transcerebral trunks maintains perfusion to newer and more superficial cerebral regions. The regularity of intertrunk distance and, later, shorter penetrating vessels in our human embryonic and fetal specimens are consistent with Bär's model (Fig. 8.9). The shorter vessels appear to compensate for the disproportionate tissue increase in more superficial brain regions during fetal growth.

We were unable to find isolated capillary loops, without anastomotic connections, extending from primitive meninges deep into embryonic brain and returning back to the meninges, as reported in lizard, newt, necturus, lamprey, or human.[45,61–64] At early stages, all vessels were simple endothelium-lined capillaries; sinusoids (endothelium-lined channels more than two erythrocytes in diameter) were not usually present.

MAJOR POINTS

1   Large perineural plexus arteries (such as carotid) acquire a muscular coat partway through the embryonic period, and leptomeningeal muscularized arterioles are widespread by midgestation.

2   The first vascular penetration from leptomeningeal plexus takes place in the basal forebrain, below the striatum, followed by subsequent pial penetration progressively more laterally, extending to convexity.

3   Primary endothelial penetrators first branch to supply germinal matrix lining ventricles, no matter where in the nervous system, whether the spinal cord, brainstem, or telencephalon (previously observed),[65] and do not branch to form a capillary plexus in their course from the pia through the cortex and white matter until they reach the germinal tissue. They create a basic pattern of transcerebral telencephalic endothelial channels (trunks) that persist and enlarge as gestation progresses. In all nervous system locations, the first endothelial penetrators were simple endothelial channels, either capillaries (early) or sinusoids (later). Penetrators and plexuses, whether in the matrix or in regions undergoing

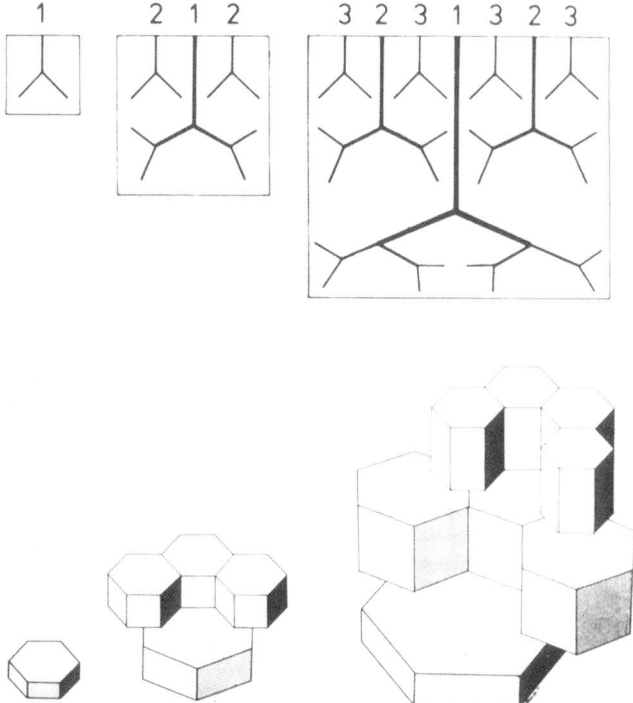

Fig. 8.9 Model proposed by Bär (1980) of telencephalic angiogenesis for the rat. Top: On the left, transcerebral channels [1] first ramify in the subventricular zone. As the fetal brain grows (middle), branching of transcerebral channels in the subventricular zone continues [1] and additional large channels are added, which branch deep in the telencephalon [2]. With continued growth in width and surface (right), subventricular branches of transcerebral channels become more extensive [1], deep telencephalic branches are added [2], and additional penetrating channels [3] branch more superficially. Bottom: Hexagonally packed regions of supply for each of these crops of branching vessels are indicated. Reproduced with permission of Springer Science+Business Media from Bär.[8]

migration or differentiation, all had the same range of capillaries or sinusoids. Endothelial channels eventually produced more endothelial channels, or arteries or veins, but the fetal ages when this occurred varied with site: striatal or extrastriatal, basolateral or convexity. Subventricular-zone endothelial channels formed a latticework of interconnecting channels, which persisted, shrinking only in extent with matrix depletion at the end of the second trimester.

4 Subsequent crops of shorter extrastriatal penetrators grew into and branched in prospective white matter, just short of germinal tissue, with brain growth.

5 Long extrastriatal transcerebral channels were found throughout gestation, forming a basic network of endothelial cells from which deep capillary plexuses sprouted, and also

contributing to more superficial capillary plexuses, which had arisen from successive crops of intermediate length and superficial penetrators, supplying superficial white matter and, finally, isocortex. These interconnected plexuses eventually formed a continuous capillary network throughout the central nervous system.[45]

6   As vascular channels branch from muscularized leptomeningeal arterioles, they lose their muscularis when penetrating the pia.[5,21,22,31,54,66]

7   Channels supplying the striatum (caudate and putamen) are the first to muscularize, from the base toward the caudate. Muscularization of lateral striate branches begins by midgestation and, close to the end of the second trimester, extends almost to the germinal matrix overlying the caudate.

8   In contrast, muscularization of long transcerebral trunks and shorter intertruncal vessels occurs in late gestation or postnatally.

9   During the first trimester, there are no subependymal veins; they form from 12 to 16 weeks between the layer of germinal tissue and the underlying neural tissue. Thus, some transcerebral channels must be afferent and some efferent, even though the lack of muscularis or angle of branching failed to distinguish these two varieties of vessels. The undifferentiated networks of anastomosing endothelial channels have the capacity to become arteries or veins, or to regress if hemodynamically superfluous.[6] The extrastriatal transcerebral channels ultimately develop into medullary arteries and veins. Their transcerebral nature and multiple interconnections persist into adolescence and are the basis for both arterial and venous collateral flow. At midgestation, the telencephalic endoneural microvascular bed consisted of vascular channels and capillaries differing markedly in size, distribution, degree of muscularization, and patterns of branching. In striatal and extrastriatal microvascular beds, simple endothelium-lined sinusoidal channels antedated arteries or veins, and their patterns of branching and distribution were distinctly different. Penetrators supplying the cortical plate capillary plexus were the last to form: some toward term, but the majority after birth.

REFERENCES

1. Streeter G (1918) The developmental alterations in the vascular system of the brain of the human embryo. *Contr Embryology (Carnegie Institution of Washington)* 8: 5–38.
2. Lie T (1968) *Congenital Anomalies of the Carotid Arteries, Including the Carotid-Basilar and Carotid-Vertebral Anastomoses; An Angiographic Study and Review of the Literature.* Amsterdam: Excerpta Medica Foundation.
3. Padget D (1948) The development of the cranial arteries in the human embryo. *Contr Embryology (Carnegie Institution of Washington)* 32: 205–261.
4. Klosovskii B (1963) *The Development of the Brain and Its Disturbance by Harmful Factors.* Oxford, New York: Pergamon Press.
5. Mall F (1904) On the development of the blood vessels of the brain in the human embryo. *Am J Anat* 4: 1–18.
6. Strong LH (1964) The early embryonic pattern of internal vascularization of the mammalian cerebral cortex. *J Comp Neurol* 123: 121–138.
7. Wolff JR, Goerz C, Bar T, Guldner FH (1975) Common morphogenetic aspects of various organotypic microvascular patterns. *Microvasc Res* 10: 373.
8. Bär T (1980) The vascular system of the cerebral cortex (Review). *Adv Anat Embryol Cell Biol* 59: 1–62.

9. Cohnheim J (1882) *Vorlesungen über allgemeine Pathologie. Pathologie: Ein Handbuch für ärtze und Studierende.* Berlin: A Hischwald.
10. Craigie E (1955) *Vascular patterns of the developing nervous system.* New York: Academic Press.
11. Duckett S (1971) The establishment of internal vascularization in the human telencephalon. *Acta Anat (Basel)* 80: 107–113.
12. Marin-Padilla M (1985) Early vascularization of the embryonic cerebral cortex; Golgi and electron microscopic studies. *J Comp Neurol* 241: 237–249.
13. Pfeifer R (1931) Anastomosen der hirngefässe dargestellt am asphyktisch hyperämischen kindergehirn. *J Psychol Neurol* 42: 1–173.
14. Ruckes J (1967) Die arterielle Vascularisation der Pia mater des Nerugeborenen. *Frankfurt Z Path* 76: 227–234.
15. Rhodes AJ, Hyde JB (1965) Postnatal growth of arterioles in the human cerebral cortex. *Growth* 29: 173–182.
16. Harnarine-Singh D, Hyde JB (1970) Post-natal growth of the arterial net in the human cerebral pia mater. *Nature* 225: 86–87.
17. Standing S (2005) *Gray's Anatomy,* 39th edition. Edinburgh: Elsevier, Churchill Livingstone.
18. Schade J, van Groenigen W (1961) Structural organization of the human cerebral cortex. 1. Maturation of the middle frontal gyrus. *Acta Anat (Basel)* 47: 74–111.
19. His W (1880–1885) *Anatomie Menschlichen Embryonen.* Leipzig: F. C. W. Vogel.
20. O'Rahilly R, Müller F (1994) *The Embryonic Human Brain: An Atlas of Developmental Stages.* New York: Wiley-Liss.
21. Kuban KCK, Gilles FH (1985) Human telencephalic angiogenesis. *Ann Neurol* 17: 539–548.
22. Nelson MD, Gonzalez-Gomez I, Gilles FH (1991) The search for human telencephalic ventriculofugal arteries. *Am J Neuroradiol* 12: 215–222.
23. Van Den Bergh R (1969) The periventricular intracerebral blood supply. In: Meyer JS, Lechner H, Eichhorn O, editors. *Research on the Cerebral Circulation Third International Salzburg Conference.* Springfield, IL: Charles C. Thomas, pp. 52–65.
24. Van der Eecken H (1969) Arterial topography and architecture of the intracerebral arterial demarcation zones of the human adult and fetus. In: Meyer JS, Lechner H, Eichhorn O, editors. *Research on the Cerebral Circulation.* Springfield, IL: Charles C. Thomas, pp. 42–51.
25. de Reuck J (1971) The human periventricular arterial blood supply and the anatomy of cerebral infarctions. *Eur Neurol* 5: 321–334.
26. Larroche JC (1977) *Developmental Pathology of the Neonate.* Amsterdam: Excerpta Medica.
27. Takashima S, Tanaka K (1978) Development of cerebrovascular architecture and its relationship to periventricular leukomalacia. *Arch Neurol* 35: 11.
28. Wigglesworth JS, Pape KE (1978) An integrated model for haemorrhagic and ischaemic lesions in the newborn brain. *Early Hum Dev* 2: 179–199.
29. Pape KE, Wigglesworth JS (1979) *Haemorrhage, Ischemia and the Perinatal Brain.* London: Heinemann.
30. Volpe JJ (1994) *Neurology of the Newborn.* Philadelphia: WB Saunders.
31. Gilles FH, Nelson MDJ, Gonzalez-Gomez I (1992) Human telencephalic angiogenesis: an update. In: Fujisawa K, Morimatsu Y, editors. *Development and Involution of Neurons.* Tokyo: Japan Scientific Societies Press, pp. 31–41.
32. Ghazi-Birry HS, Brown WR, Moody DM, Challa VR, Block SM, Reboussin DM (1997) Human germinal matrix: venous origin of hemorrhage and vascular characteristics. *AJNR Am J Neuroradiol* 18: 219–229.
33. Anstrom JA, Brown WR, Moody DM, Thore CR, Challa VR, Block SM (2002) Anatomical analysis of the developing cerebral vasculature in premature neonates: absence of precapillary arteriole-to-venous shunts. *Pediatr Res* 52: 554–560.
34. Anstrom JA, Brown WR, Moody DM, Thore CR, Challa VR, Block SM (2004) Subependymal veins in premature neonates: implications for hemorrhage. *Pediatr Neurol* 30: 46–53.
35. Betz AL, Firth JA, Goldstein GW (1980) Polarity of the blood–brain barrier: distribution of enzymes between the luminal and antiluminal membranes of brain capillary endothelial cells. *Brain Res* 192: 17–28.
36. Bell MA, Weddell AG (1984) A morphometric study of intrafascicular vessels of mammalian sciatic nerve. *Muscle Nerve* 7: 524–534.
37. Mori S, Nagano M (1985) Electron-microscopic cytochemistry of alkaline-phosphatase activity in endothelium, pericytes and oligodendrocytes in the rat brain. *Histochemistry* 82: 225–231.

38. Lierse W (1963) [Alkaline phosphatase in the cerebral blood vessels of mice (*Mus muris*) during postnatal development.]. *Z Mikrosk Anat Forsch* 70: 48–61.
39. Diemer K, Henn R (1964) The capillary density in the frontal lobe of mature and premature infants. *Biol Neonat* 7: 270–279.
40. Otto K, Leirse W (1970) Die Kappillarisierung verschiedener Teile des menschlichen Gehirns in der Fetal periode und in den ersten Lebensjahren. *Acta Anat Basel* 77: 25–36.
41. Pessacq T, Reissenweber N (1972) Structural aspects of vasculogenesis in the central nervous system. II Histogenesis of blood vessels in periventricular regions of the brain. *Acta Anat (Basel)* 81: 439–447.
42. O'Rahilly R, Müller F (1987) *Developmental Stages in Human Embryos*. Washington: Carnegie Institution of Washington.
43. Lubchenco LO (1970) Assessment of gestational age and development of birth. *Pediatr Clin North Am* 17: 125–145.
44. Dubowitz LM, Dubowitz V, Goldberg C (1970) Clinical assessment of gestational age in the newborn infant. *J Pediatr* 77: 1–10.
45. Pfeifer RA (1940) *Die angioarchitektonische areale Gliederung der Grosshirnrinde*. Leipzig: Georg Thieme.
46. Vander Eecken HM, Adams RD (1953) The anatomy and functional significance of the meningeal arterial anastomoses of the human brain. *J Neuropathol Exp Neurol* 12: 132–157.
47. Jammes JL, Gilles FH (1983) Telencephalic development: matrix volume and isocortex and allocortex surface areas. In: Gilles FH, Leviton A, Dooling EC, editors. *The Developing Human Brain Growth and Epidemiologic Neuropathology*. Littleton, CO: Wright-PSG, Inc, pp. 87–93.
48. Kedzia A (1995) Characteristics of periventricular matrix vascularization in image computer transformation system. *Folia Neuropathol* 33: 267–270.
49. Ballabh P, Braun A, Nedergaard M (2004) The blood–brain barrier: an overview: structure, regulation, and clinical implications. *Neurobiol Dis* 16: 1–13.
50. Møllgård K, Saunders NR (1986) The development of the human blood–brain and blood–CSF barriers. *Neuropathol Appl Neurobiol* 12: 337–358.
51. Gröntoft O (1954) Intracranial haemorrhage and blood–brain barrier problems in the new-born; a pathologico-anatomical and experimental investigation. *Acta Path Microbiol Scand Suppl C* 100: 8–109.
52. Ballabh P, Hu F, Kumarasiri M, Braun A, Nedergaard M (2005) Development of tight junction molecules in blood vessels of germinal matrix, cerebral cortex, and white matter. *Pediatr Res* 58: 791–798.
53. Pfeifer RA (1928) *Die Angioarchitektonik der Groshirnrinde*. Berlin: Verlag Julius Springer.
54. Rhodes A, Hyde J (1965) Postnatal growth of arterioles in the human cerebral cortex. *Growth* 29: 173–182.
55. Kennedy JC, Taplin G (1967) Shunting in cerebral microcirculation. *Am J Surg* 33: 763–771.
56. Hasegawa T, Ravens JR, Toole JF (1967) Pre-capillary arteriovenous anastomoses. *Arch Neurol* 16: 217–224.
57. Anderson B, Anderson W (1978) Shunting in intracranial microvasculature demonstrated by SEM of corrosion-casts. *Am J Anat* 153: 617–624.
58. Duvernoy HM, Delon S, Vannson JL (1981) Cortical blood vessels of the human brain. *Brain Res Bull* 7: 519–579.
59. Moody DM, Bell MA, Challa VR (1990) Features of the cerebral vascular pattern that predict vulnerability to perfusion or oxygenation deficiency: an anatomic study. *AJNR Am J Neuroradiol* 11: 431–439.
60. Bar T (1983) Patterns of vascularization in the developing cerebral cortex. *Ciba Found Symp* 100: 20–36.
61. Lazzari M, Franceschini V (2000) Structural and spatial organisation of brain parenchymal vessels in the lizard, *Podarcis sicula*: a light, transmission and scanning electron microscopy study. *J Anat* 197(Pt 2): 167–175.
62. Ciani F, Franceschini V (1984) Ultrastructural study and cholinesterase activity of paired capillaries in the newt brain. *J Hirnforsch* 25: 11–20.
63. Craigie E (1940) Vascularity in the brains of tailed amphibians. II Necturus Maculosus Rafinesque. *Proc Am Phil Soc* 82: 395–410.
64. Bundgaard M (1982) Brain barrier systems in the lamprey. I Ultrastructure and permeability of cerebral blood vessels. *Brain Res* 240: 55–64.
65. Allsopp G, Gamble HJ (1979) Light and electron microscopic observations on the development of the blood vascular system of the human brain. *J Anat* 128: 461–477.
66. Haruda F, Blanc WA (1981) The structure of intracerebral arteries in premature infants and the autoregulation of cerebral blood flow. *Ann Neurol* 10: 103.

Section 2

9
DEVELOPMENTAL HUMAN FETAL REACTIONS: AVOID, SQUINT, SCOWL, SNEER, AND PUCKER

Introduction

The earliest human embryonic and fetal behavior is purely reflex in nature. Intricate neural connections, underlying embryonic and fetal reflexes, grow and lay the functional foundation for future postnatal voluntary acts. Receptors, internuncial neurons, and neuromuscular connections, used in early fetal reflex behavior, are the structural basis of later motor action patterns, and reflex arcs continue to serve the organism throughout its life. Muscles contract from electrical or mechanical stimuli before motor innervation exists. Synapses become functional well after histologic connections are in place. The motor system develops before the sensory system and reflex activity starts much later. Subsequently, behavior develops first as a total pattern, with partial patterns later individuated. Function, then, is an expression of structure as well as of other changes under normal circumstances. The developmental rate of various organs and structures, including the nervous system, varies considerably in different individuals of the same biologic age.[1] Very early human fetal activity reports were of individual cases observed fortuitously (for instance, movements in a 4-month-old fetus).[2] The early portion of this chapter depends on Davenport Hooker's[3] work at the University of Pittsburgh for direct observations of embryonic and fetal behavior using graded standardized stimuli (1932–1956), expanding Minkowski's extensive observations from the 1920s.[4] Both investigators relied on a huge amount of earlier work in nonhuman vertebrates. The second portion of this chapter uses ultrasonographic and other fetal imaging observations available since 1976.

To set the stage, human embryonic somites first arise at approximately 20 days of postovulatory age. Neural folds begin to fuse at 22 days, when there are 4 to 12 lowermost rhombencephalic and adjacent upper cervical region somites. The rostral neuropore closes at 24 days and the caudal neuropore at 26 days. Hypoglossal roots first become evident at 26 days. Dorsal and ventral roots of first and second cervical nerves contain nerve fibers at day 33. The trigeminal spinal tract appears at about 32 days, before the main trigeminal sensory nucleus at about 44 days. The embryonic central nervous system grows and matures in two directions: upper cervicocaudal and upper cervicorostral. Cervical axial musculature maturation, development of functionally active cervical spinal cord synaptic connections, cervical responsiveness, and cervical reflexes follow the same pattern. The embryonic period ends at stage 23, usually at about 8 weeks.[5]

Reflexes evoked by trigeminal skin stimulation and early extremity reflexes mediated through spinal nerves are stereotyped. Each response secured from a given area is, in amplitude, character, and duration, almost exactly like every other elicited by similar site stimulation in any fetus at the same response age. As long as a response can be secured after delivery, it follows the same stereotyped pattern. The early stereotypic reflex character does not disappear until the fetus reaches 13 or 14 weeks of age. Furthermore, all reflexes that are evident later in fetal life are also stereotyped when first elicited, and remain so for a period thereafter before losing this quality.

Much early work and many ultrasound studies are based on small numbers of cases at any given conceptional age. Nevertheless, there is much variation in development from fetus to fetus, and one needs to think about the 'critical' fetal age, the age at which half of fetuses exhibit a particular function.[6]

Background

Minkowski's early studies[7] included 75 individuals, and the later Pittsburgh group studies[1,3,8–12] included 149 individuals. All studies reported were done on embryos or fetuses that were either exposed because of a compelling maternal operation or had recently been delivered. All fetal responses were stereotyped and persistent until they gradually faded out within 7 to 20 minutes after placental separation, forming a continuous series consistent with the stage of morphologic development.[13,14] The Pittsburgh group, using motion pictures, continuously recorded the embryo or fetus from the time of exposure or delivery until demise. Carefully calibrated human and horse hairs ensured that the maximum pressure exerted did not exceed 10, 25, 50, or 100mg or 2, 5, or 10g. Most responses reported were from hairs with pressure values of 10 to 50mg. The Pittsburgh studies were reported in weeks (menstrual age).

Results

Earliest Responses

Trunk
Mouth and nasal alae stimulation (a limited region of upper lip and nasal wing innervated by trigeminal nerve maxillary and mandibular branches) during the seventh week (menstrual age) resulted in contralateral neck flexion in some fetuses (avoiding response).[3] Ipsilateral responses rarely occurred at 8 weeks (Table 9.1). At 8 weeks, the sensory receptive area had enlarged and the response spread caudally to include the uppermost trunk; by 8.5 to 9.5 weeks, the entire trunk was involved in a contralateral flexion response. During this same period, the sensitive skin gradually increased in area, attaining trigeminal maxillary and mandibular division distribution at 11 to 11.5 weeks. Pelvic rotatory responses developed by 8.5 to 9.5 weeks. Most trunk flexions were contralateral, but occasional ipsilateral flexions occurred. As the trunk response extended below the shoulders, the arms extended usually backward at the shoulder. There was no elbow, wrist, or hand movement. The arms moved only with the trunk, without capacity for independent movements, before 10.5 weeks.

TABLE 9.1

Human embryonic and early fetal fifth cranial nerve reflexes: somatic reflexes

Menstrual age in weeks	Region of stimulation	Divisions of fifth cranial nerve involved	Nature of response
7.5	Perioral	V_2 and V_3 (limited)	Contralateral flexion of neck (avoiding)
7.5–8	Perioral	V_2 and V_3 (limited)	Contralateral flexion of neck and uppermost trunk, with, at most, slight quivering of upper extremities
7.5–8.5	Perioral	V_2 and V_3 (expanding)	Chiefly contralateral flexion of neck and upper trunk, with extension of both brachia at shoulder and slight rotation of pelvis toward contralateral side. All movements becoming more pronounced and trunk flexion extending further caudad as age of 7.5 weeks is approached
10.5	Perioral	V_2 and V_3	Contralateral trunk flexion, with occasional trunk extension
11–12	Perioral	V_2 and V_3	Trunk extension, with medial rotation of both arms and head away from stimulus, sometimes returning to contralateral flexion

Underlying anatomy

The sensory limb of this reaction involves maxillary or mandibular trigeminal fibers in the descending spinal tract (Fig. 9.1). These axons presumably form synapses on ipsilateral internuncial neurons in the upper cervical lamina VIII, whose axons, in turn, innervate contralateral ventral horn motor neurons after crossing midline anterior or ventral commissure. Cervical motor neuron axons extend well into the mesenchyme and some motor neuron cell bodies begin to develop dendrites in human embryos at 3 weeks (menstrual age).[15] The cervical ventral commissure is well formed at 3 weeks and by the fifth week is particularly well represented rostrally. At 3 weeks, descending trigeminal fibers are still in the medulla, barely below incoming vestibular fibers.[16] Certain trigeminal fibers constitute the earliest receptor pathway to develop in man.[15–17] In 1954, Humphrey[14] showed that at around 6.5 weeks, maxillary and mandibular fibers reach the fourth cervical cord segment, and ophthalmic fibers extend as far caudally as do those from the other two divisions by 7.5 weeks (Fig. 9.2). All three divisions of the trigeminal reach the first cervical segment by 4.5 weeks, and 1 week later the fibers had grown through the first and into the second cervical segments. Initially, the maxillary and mandibular fibers outdistance ophthalmic fibers in caudal growth, but at around 7.5 weeks the ophthalmic fibers reach the same caudal levels. All elements needed for a functional spinal reflex system are laid down by the sixth menstrual week.[15] At 5.5 weeks, the fibers connect the trigeminal spinal tract termination with contralateral ventral horn motor neurons,[17] and Humphrey suggested that this pathway constituted the reflex arc whereby contralateral neck flexion occurred in response to perioral stimulation. Similar commissural connections with

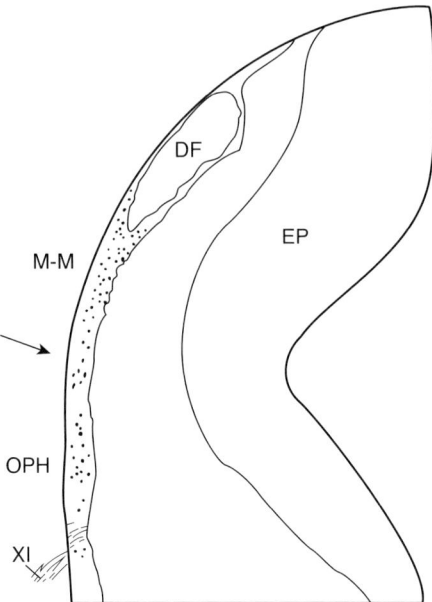

Fig. 9.1 14mm (6.5 weeks) embryo. A transverse spinal cord section at C1. Cervical subventricular matrix (EP) is prominent adjacent to future central canal. Dots at the periphery represent descending fibers of trigeminal spinal tract. The arrow points to the junction between ophthalmic (OPH) and maxillomandibular (M-M) trigeminal divisions. DF, dorsal funiculus (the division between fasciculus gracilis and fasciculus cuneatus has not yet occurred); XI, a rootlet of cranial nerve 11. Reproduced with permission of Elsevier from Humphrey.[16]

the contralateral spinal accessory nucleus enable the sternomastoid and trapezius muscles to participate in this reflex. These trigeminal connections and early functional reflexes occur long before trigeminal nerve myelination, which takes place at about 20 weeks.[18]

In human embryonic skin there are no structures comparable to adult sensory endings at the time the lip first responds to stimulation, resulting in orbicularis oris contraction. Most nerve fibers terminate 40–50μm below the epithelium.[13] Hair follicles are innervated and responsive at about the twelfth week.

Local facial responses
The first local facial response is active, but incomplete, mouth opening by mandible lowering at about 9.5 weeks (menstrual age) following lower lip stimulation. It occurs only with lower lip mandibular division sensory fiber stimulation (Table 9.2).[3] The involved sensory fibers pass through the trigeminal spinal tract to the spinal trigeminal nucleus, then by internuncials to the ipsilateral seventh nucleus to innervate the suprahyoid and the other first three cervical internuncials, which innervate the infrahyoid muscles participating in mouth opening.[16] There is no other indication of facial nerve activity until 10 to 10.5 weeks, when there is eyelid

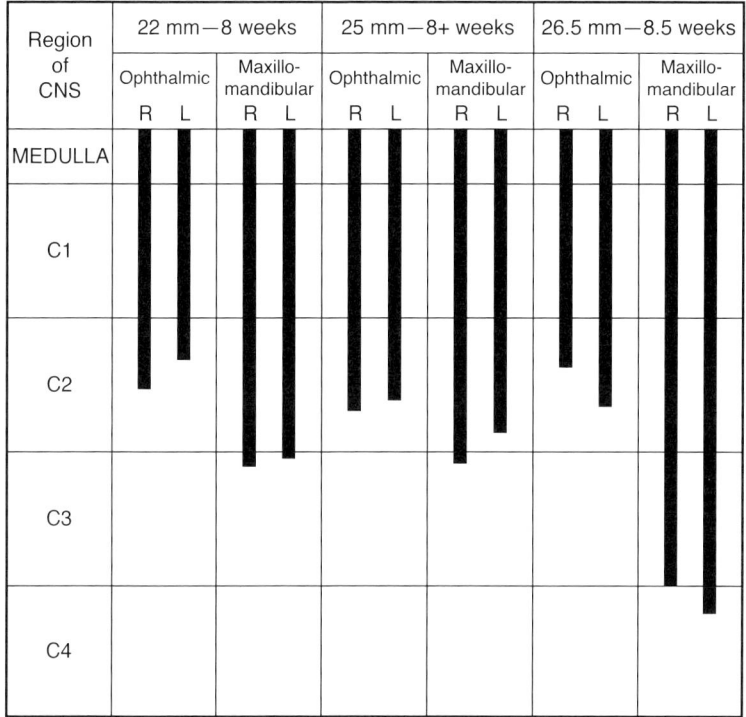

Region of CNS	22 mm—8 weeks				25 mm—8+ weeks				26.5 mm—8.5 weeks			
	Ophthalmic		Maxillo-mandibular		Ophthalmic		Maxillo-mandibular		Ophthalmic		Maxillo-mandibular	
	R	L	R	L	R	L	R	L	R	L	R	L
MEDULLA												
C1												
C2												
C3												
C4												

Fig. 9.2 A graphic representation of trigeminal ophthalmic and maxillomandibular divisions of right and left sides of the spinal cord of five human embryos from 22mm to 26.5mm in crown–rump length (~8 weeks to 8.5 weeks), showing the descent of trigeminal spinal sensory fibers. Reproduced with permission of Elsevier from Humphrey.[16]

squinting, and no indication of action of trigeminal mandibular division motor fibers before 12.5 weeks, when mouth closure happens.

The skin over the upper eyelids (trigeminal ophthalmic division) becomes sensitive to tactile stimulation causing upper eyelid squinting at 10 to 10.5 weeks, a contraction of most of the orbicularis oculi fibers, a response that becomes fixed by 11 to 12 weeks. A squint follows upper lip (trigeminal maxillary division) or lower lip (trigeminal mandibular division) stimulation at 12.5 to 13 weeks, through the descending spinal trigeminal tract to internuncials passing the stimulation to the facial nucleus.

Repeated stimulation of both lips sometimes causes swallowing movements at 10.5 weeks, but full deglutition is not regularly observed until near midgestation. Receptivity spreads onto the forehead by 11 weeks, and stimulation sometimes causes scowling. These reflexes become constant a week later, thus indicating the beginning of functioning of intermediate neurons between descending trigeminal and facial nuclei at these ages.[16]

The mouth at these ages is rarely open enough for tongue stimulation without touching the lips. The earliest that tongue stimulation occurs is at 14 weeks, resulting in its withdrawal.

TABLE 9.2

Human fetal fifth cranial nerve reflexes: local facial reflexes

Menstrual age in weeks	Region of stimulation	Divisions of fifth cranial nerve involved	Nature of response
9.5	Edge of lower lip	V_3	Active mouth opening by lowering of mandible
10–10.5	Upper eyelid	V_1	Occasional contraction of orbicularis oculi muscle
10.5	Rima oris	V_2 and V_3	Deglutition
11	Upper eyelid	V_1	Occasional contraction of corrugator supercilii muscle
12.5	Tongue and/or rima oris	V_2 and V_3	Momentary lip closure and, if repeated, deglutition
12.5–13	Upper lip or, rarely, lower lip	V_2 and V_3	Contraction of orbicularis oculi muscle
13	Rima oris	V_2 and V_3	Maintained lip closure
13–14	Upper lip and nose ala	V_2	Contraction of quadratus labii superioris muscle and rotation of head away from stimulus
17	Upper lip at rima oris	V_2	Protrusion of upper lip
20	Lower lip at rima oris	V_3	Protrusion of lower lip
22	Rima oris	V_2 and V_3	Simultaneous protrusion and pursing of both lips
29 or before	Rima oris	V_2 and V_3	Audible sucking

Sensory fibers from the tongue (anterior two-thirds) pass along the lingual nerve (mandibular division of trigeminal). All the tongue muscles concerned with its retraction receive hypoglossal innervation. Evidence exists for a functional reflex arc, consisting of descending trigeminal spinal tract mandibular fibers to medullary tegmental internuncial neurons to the hypoglossal nucleus, by 14 weeks, if not before.

Upper or lower lip stimulation more regularly elicits swallowing at 12.5 weeks, giving evidence of functional connections to the facial nucleus for lip closure and to the glossopharyngeal and vagal nuclei for swallowing. Lip stimulation sometimes causes maintained lip closure by 13 weeks and mandibular movement follows trigeminal mandibular stimulation, giving additional evidence of sensory mandibular trigeminal connections to trigeminal motor neurons via internuncial neurons. The motor root itself accompanies mandibular division fibers to the masticatory muscles.

General trunk responses to maxillary and mandibular division stimulation tend to cease between 13 and 14 weeks, and stimulation of skin supplied by the trigeminal causes chiefly local reflexes. Upper lip and nose ala (wing) stimulation elicits quadratus labii superioris contraction, which elevates the upper lip and the nose wing, producing a sneer accompanied

TABLE 9.3
TABLE 9.3
Human fetal spinal nerve reflexes: local upper extremity reflexes

Menstrual age in weeks	Region of stimulation	Nature of response
10.5	Shoulder	Rare independent extension of brachium
10.5	Palm	Occasional partial finger closure, rarely with pollex flexion
11	Palm	Constant partial finger closure, usually with wrist flexion, sometimes with elbow flexion, medial rotation of brachium, or forearm pronation
11.5	Shoulder	Occasional abduction of brachium
13	Palm	Occasional nearly complete finger closure, rarely with pollex opposition
13.5–14	Palm	Occasional complete finger closure
15–15.5	Palm	Maintained finger closure
18.5	Palm	Weak, true grasp
27	Palm	Sufficient grasp almost to support body weight momentarily

by head rotation, carrying the face away from the stimulus. Both this response as well as the earliest head movement, contralateral flexion at 7.5 weeks and older, are avoiding reactions, each response separating the sensitive area of facial skin from the stimulus. At 13 to 14 weeks, the same avoiding reaction is not part of a general trunk response but a local response. This is a much more complicated response in that both cranial nerve nuclei and the contralateral cervical neurons are stimulated through internuncials, but now without the remaining truncal responses. The various branches of cranial nerve VII do not become functional at the same time. During the eleventh to twelfth week, the reflexogenous area gradually extends to include almost the whole body.[13]

Upper extremity local reflexes
Shoulder stimulation occasionally produces arm extension (cervical 5, 6) at 10.5 weeks (Table 9.3). Light palmar stimulation (cervical 6–8 spinal segments) sometimes causes a quick partial finger closure without the thumb (cervical 8; thoracic 1). Thumb flexion is rare at any fetal age. At 11 weeks, nearly every fetus exhibits partial finger closure (cervical 8; thoracic 1 spinal segments) on palmar stimulation. Usually, the wrist also flexes (cervical 6–8). At times, elbow flexion (cervical 5, 6), medial arm rotation, forearm pronation (cervical 6, 7), or all three movements accompany finger flexion. Arm abduction (cervical 5, 6) followed by adduction (cervical 6–8) occurs as the local reflex at 11.5 weeks. Neither movement occurs independently before 27 weeks. These movements are mediated by spinal cord reflex arcs, consisting of spinal ganglion cells, internuncial neurons, and motor neurons. More importantly, the reflexes from a limited point of stimulation spread to multiple cervical anterior horn cells.

Prehension in children involves two elements, finger closure and grasp, developing in that order.[19] The appearance of partial finger closure at about 10.5 weeks and its development into a constant response at 11 weeks are mentioned above. Finger closure remains only partial until 14 weeks, when a few fetuses exhibit almost complete finger flexion. The finger closure is still quick, with almost immediate hand opening. The rapid opening ceases in a few fetuses at 15 or 15.5 weeks. A true grasp occurs by 18.5 weeks, when a glass rod or a stimulating hair is retained inside the closed fist. The grasp remains weak until 27 weeks, when it supports body weight momentarily. No instance of bimanual grasp was observed as grasp was immediately released when a similar object was placed in the other palm, and it proved impossible to secure grasp when both hands were simultaneously presented with any object.

Stretch reflex

The Pittsburgh studies demonstrated stretch reflexes at 9.5 weeks. Stretch reflexes at this age were highly localized and affected only the part stimulated. Fetal behavior was influenced only to a minor extent as these reflexes remained localized in nature even in the adult.[20]

Lower extremity local reflexes

The first reflex elicited by sole stimulation (lumbar 5; sacral 1) occurs at 10 to 10.5 weeks, somewhat later than the finger closure reflex (Table 9.4). The earliest mixed responses [toe flexion (sacral 1, 2) and great toe extension (sacral 1)] are not found until 11.5 weeks. Whichever type of response was exhibited, it was often accompanied by knee flexion (lumbar 4, 5; sacral 1, 2), then quick leg extension (lumbar 2–4) in a kick. The thigh sometimes flexed, rotated in either direction, or abducted, with subsequent return to resting position.

From about 12.5 weeks until birth, the plantar reflex takes the form of great toe dorsiflexion and other toe fanning. Toe plantar flexion occurs at any age, but it is an isolated response after 12.5 weeks. Toe dorsiflexion occasionally occurs after plantar stimulation at 12.5 weeks; still, this was rarely observed.

Local trunk reflexes

The beginning of trunk reflexes is marked at 7.5 weeks in response to exteroceptive stimulation around the mouth. The amount of trunk musculature participating in the response spreads caudally into the pelvic region, along with cervicocaudal neuromuscular differentiation; the

TABLE 9.4
Human fetus spinal reflexes: local lower extremity reflexes

Menstrual age in weeks	Region of stimulation	Nature of response
10–10.5	Sole of foot	Plantar flexion of all toes
11.5	Sole of foot	Either plantar flexion of all toes or dorsiflexion of hallux and fanning of other toes, sometimes with knee flexion, then extension (as a kick) and with hip flexion, rotation, or abduction
12.5	Sole of foot	Principally dorsiflexion of hallux and toe fanning, dorsiflexion of foot at ankle, flexion at knee and hip
13.5	Sole of foot	Occasional dorsiflexion of all toes
32 or before	Inside thigh	Cremasteric reflex

TABLE 9.5

Human fetal spinal reflexes: local trunk reflexes

Menstrual age in weeks	Region of stimulation	Nature of response
13	Chest	Isolated respiratory chest contractions
15	Abdomen	Abdominal muscle contractions
22	Chest	Temporary diaphragmatic contractions
23.5	Chest	Temporary, effective respiratory chest contractions and phonation
27	On delivery	Permanent respiration established

arms and lower extremities move with the trunk. As the nervous system continues its differentiation and new neuromuscular connections are established, specific local reflexes arise; first facial, and then upper and, finally, lower extremities and trunk.

Chest skin stimulation results in isolated respiratory chest contractions at 13 weeks (Table 9.5). Two weeks later, abdomen stimulation results in abdominal muscle contractions. At 22 weeks, chest stimulation results in temporary diaphragmatic contractions, and at 23.5 weeks chest stimulation gives effective respiratory chest contractions and phonation. At 27 weeks, if delivered, permanent respiration is established.

Feeding responses
At 17 weeks, upper lip mucous membrane stimulation causes that lip to protrude; the lower lip merely closes from 12.5 and 20 weeks. At 20 weeks, both lips protrude on stimulation and, at 22 weeks, pucker as well. The earliest sucking movements occur at 29 weeks. In general, preterm infants born before 28 to 29 weeks are not capable of nursing effectively.

Neuroimaging
Many investigators of fetal behavior began using neuroimaging in the early 1970s (initially ultrasonography, later fetal magnetic resonance).[21,22] Fetal heart rates were detected at 7 weeks, fetal trunk movement at 8 weeks, and individual fetal limb movements at 9 weeks.[23] During the first gestational half, a developmental trend was usually found: either a gradual increase in incidence as the fetus grew older (breathing movement, head rotation, jaw opening, sucking, and swallowing); or an increase in incidence until a plateau was reached (general movement, isolated arm movement); or an increase in incidence followed by a decrease (startle, hiccup, hand-to-face contacts, head retroflexion). In a few infrequently occurring movements, no developmental trends could be observed (isolated leg movement, head anteflexion, yawn, stretch). A few movement patterns were generated at a more or less regular interval (implying the development of a central pattern generator); hiccups occurred every 1 to 3 seconds and isolated arm movements about every second. Breathing movements showed a clear developmental shift in interval: between 10 and 19 weeks, changing from 2 to 3 seconds to less than 1 second. Total absence of movements never lasted longer than 13 minutes between 8 and 19 weeks.[24]

211

We organize these studies into general movements: motor bursts, fetal limb movement, thumb sucking and handedness, fetal breathing, swallowing, hiccup, gastric emptying, bladder emptying, auditory responses, light responses, sleep–wakefulness cycle, sexual dimorphism, and maternal stress effects.

GENERAL MOVEMENTS

General movements are complex movements involving all body parts.[25] A healthy fetus aged between 16 and 20 weeks reveals pronounced rhythms of activity.[26] Several movement patterns occur, including sideways bending, hiccup, breathing, mouth opening, and facial changes.[27] There is a general decrease in gross body movement frequency, a significant

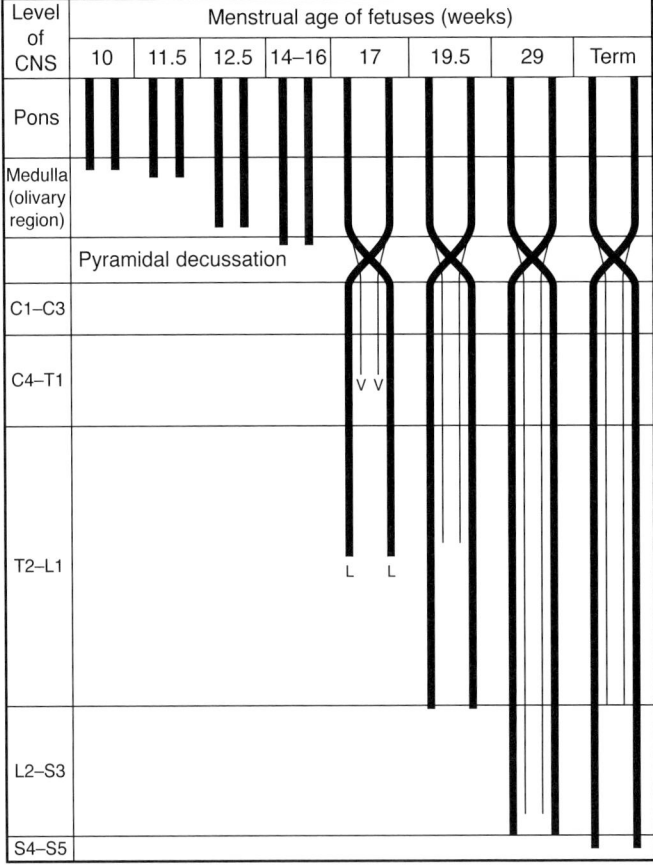

Fig. 9.3 A graphic representation of corticospinal tract (L) development in human fetuses from 10 weeks (menstrual age) to term. Note that it lags spinal trigeminal development by many weeks. The fine lines (V) originating at the pyramidal decussation represent the direct corticospinal tract. Reproduced with permission of Elsevier from Humphrey.[16]

increase in mouthing movements between 28 and 38 weeks, and a short association between body and eye movements after 28 weeks.[28] Linkage occurred among general movements, eye movements, and fetal heart rate pattern between 32 and 34 weeks.[29]

From 20 to 41 weeks, whole trunk movements are grouped into six fundamental movements: flexion, stretch, rolling, startle, stepping, and writhing. In 1988, Kuhlman et al[30] showed startle responses to noise external to the mother between 26 and 41 weeks. Startle is always observed as a single movement, but other movements are more frequently observed as a part or combination rather than as a single movement. The incidence of flexion and stretch movements peaks at 28 to 31 weeks, whereas startle and stepping decrease during this period. The incidence of rolling and upper half trunk movements increases at 40 to 41 weeks.[31]

Underlying anatomy

Functional corticospinal connections are established late in gestation. Eyre demonstrated from morphologic studies that corticospinal axons reach the lower cervical cord by 24 weeks. The axons progressively innervate spinal neurons before birth (Fig. 9.3). Functional monosynaptic corticomotoneuronal projections are present neurophysiologically from term, but are also likely to be present from as early as 26 weeks. At term, direct corticospinal projections to group Ia inhibitory interneurons occur. Corticospinal axons retain a high degree of plasticity during axon growth and synaptic development.[32]

Motor bursts

Fetal motor bursts occur from 11 weeks of pregnancy.[33] Fetal movement incidence and number does not change appreciably during the third trimester, they are sometimes cyclic and sometimes have a circadian rhythm.[34–36] Spontaneous movements appear randomly distributed during the early second trimester, later in that trimester the intervals of quiescence increase in duration and result in activity that appears cyclically distributed, with the duration of quiet cycles progressively increasing to term.

Fetal limb movements

Isolated arm movements and movements placing the hand near the head, mouth, face, eye, or ear are seen from 13 weeks. Two varieties of facial activities are easily differentiated: smiling and scowling. Simultaneous eyelid and mouthing movements dominated between 30 and 33 weeks. Pure mouth movements such as mouth opening, tongue expulsion, yawning, and pouting are sometimes present.[37] Decreasing numbers of leg movements per minute are displayed (30–37 weeks), followed by increasing numbers from birth to 6 weeks of age.[38]

Thumb sucking and handedness

Lateralized behavior is first seen at 10 weeks. Behavioral asymmetries, in particular handedness, occur from 15 weeks to term with a marked bias for sucking the right thumb. This preference, maintained throughout pregnancy, is unrelated to fetal position in utero.[39] Significantly more right arm movements than left arm movements occur at every gestational age. The number of arm movements observed peaks at 15 to 18 weeks and declines rapidly during midgestation.[40] Fetal and neonatal movements are not random, and seem to be directed or aimed at specific targets.[41] The number of movements exhibited with the preferred arm does not differ, whether right or left. Independent finger movements develop much later, between 6 and 12 months postnatally.

Fetal breathing movements
Changes in patterns of fetal breathing occur from 30 to 38 weeks. The duration of a complete respiratory cycle, the inspiratory phase, and the expiratory phase is shorter at 33 to 36 weeks than in younger and older fetuses. Fetuses of 30 to 32 weeks have slower breathing rates than older fetuses.[42] Fetal mouthing and breathing are linked with cyclic behavior from the time they start. Fetal heart rate patterns are recognized from around 30 weeks.[43] The incidence of trunk movements is high in rapid eye movement periods.[44]

Swallowing
In fetuses of 15 to 39 weeks, mandibular and/or labial movements and their rhythmic activity are seen in an increasing percentage of fetuses as gestational age increases. Doppler findings show an increase of nose–mouth flow signals, larynx–esophagus flow signals, and effective swallowing as gestational age increased.[45] The mean percentage of time spent in fetal swallowing increases from 16.1% before to 44.3% after maternal acoustic stimulation.[46] In term fetuses, two to six sucking movements and the introduction of an amniotic fluid bolus into the oral cavity characterize an initial stage of fetal swallowing. The soft palate, superiorly, and the tongue, posteriorly and inferiorly, further obstruct flow, and low-frequency tongue movements characterize the final stage of swallowing with upward laryngeal and epiglottic movements and pharyngeal lumen narrowing, directing the fluid bolus caudally.[47]

Hiccups
Throughout the second and third trimesters, hiccups are the predominant diaphragmatic movement and there is a significant negative correlation with age. There is a pronounced reduction between 24 and 26 weeks, a result of a decrease in the number of episodes of hiccups rather than a change in duration of episodes. In contrast, fetal breathing is positively correlated with gestational age, the greatest increase in breathing occurring between 26 and 32 weeks. This results from an increase in both number and duration of breathing episodes. Both breathing and hiccups are dependent on behavioral state or cycle, occurring predominantly during active episodes. This association between quiet and active behavior and breathing does not alter with increasing gestational age.[48]

Sleep–wakefulness cycle in the fetus
The frequency of rapid eye movements significantly increases between 20 and 40 weeks.[44,49] Rapid eye movement and nonrapid eye movement periods become distinguishable between 28 and 31 weeks, and subsequently increase with fetal age. The correlation between rapid eye movements and breathing movements is high after 27 weeks and increases with gestational age. Trunk movements have no correlation to rapid eye movements, but the incidence of trunk movements is high in rapid eye movement periods.[44]

Gastric emptying

Fetal swallowing contributes greatly to amniotic fluid homeostasis and fetal somatic development. The highest peak gastric emptying cycles before 24 weeks can be of any length between 30 and 100 minutes. At 32 to 35 weeks, cycles are focused at approximately 40 minutes. At term, the cycles increase to more than 80 minutes. Thus, fetal gastric emptying cycles normalize during the early third trimester.[50] Fetal swallowed volume linearly increases until 28 to 30 weeks. Daily swallowed volume exponentially increases to a maximum of 1006ml/day at term. This model indicates that the normal reduction in amniotic fluid volume beginning at 34 weeks results from a marked increase in swallowed volume during the third trimester.[51]

Bladder emptying

In a normal pregnancy, the fetal bladder volume increases linearly with time and then decreases rapidly with micturition. The mean cycle length does not change significantly with gestation, but both the mean bladder volume and the hourly fetal urine production rate increase.[52]

Auditory responses

Application of a vibratory acoustic stimulation to the maternal abdomen has shown that fetal hearing is present at 27 weeks. Acoustic stimulation later evoked a standard fetal heart rate and motor response, fetal voiding, and a startle reflex.[53-56] In addition, an auditory stimulus applied to the maternal abdomen sometimes results in significant activation in one or both temporal lobes between 37 and 41 weeks.[57]

It has been reported that applying music to the maternal abdomen over several days at the end of gestation causes more alterations in fetal heart rate than detected in fetuses not exposed to music. These effects are carried over into the neonatal period, with prenatally exposed newborns manifesting more state transitions from sleep to awake and spending a higher proportion of time in awake states when exposed to the same music stimulus.[58]

Fetal responses to light on maternal abdomen

There was significant fetal brain activation on functional magnetic resonance imaging (localized in fetal frontal, but not occipital, cortex) in most women who had light shone on their abdomen.[59]

Fetal sexual dimorphism

In 3889 fetuses of both sexes, aged 20 to 42 weeks, the total body weight and the weight of internal organs, except adrenals, were more advanced in female fetuses at any specific gestational age.[60] Males displayed greater numbers of leg movements per minute than females during both antenatal and postnatal development and females displayed a stronger and different movement continuity pattern than males, suggesting disparate time courses for neurobehavioral development of male and female fetuses and neonates.[38]

Furthermore, there are cerebral structural differences. The corpus callosum thickness, measured in the midcoronal plane, was significantly larger in female than male fetuses between 16 and 36 weeks, while length and width did not differ significantly between the sexes during gestation.[61]

215

Embryo and behavior states

The four fetal behavioral states are comparable to neonatal states: quiet sleep, active state, quiet awake, and active awake. Crying was not considered to have a fetal correlate, but in a study assessing the effects of exposure to tobacco and cocaine during pregnancy on fetal response and habituation to vibroacoustic stimulation, a fetal homolog of crying was observed on ultrasound and captured on video recordings. It included an initial exhalation movement associated with mouth opening and tongue depression, followed by a series of three augmented breaths, the last breath ending in an inspiratory pause followed by an expiration and settling.[62]

Most movements during gestation emerge before 16 weeks, and the presence of diurnal variation in human fetal behavior was demonstrated from as early as 20 weeks. Up to 26 weeks, quiet intervals rarely exceed 5 minutes. After this age, quiet intervals progressively increased in duration so that behavior appeared cyclic rather than randomly distributed.[63]

Maternal stress effects

Adverse early experience, including prenatal maternal psychosocial stress, has the potential to negatively influence developmental processes through both physiologic and behavioral mechanisms. The maternal environment exerts a significant influence on fetal autonomic nervous system and on central nervous system processes related to recognition, memory, and habituation, and sometimes persists after birth.[64] DiPietro et al[65] used a benign cognitive stressor to study fetal responses to maternal sympathetic activation, and found that maternal environmental intrusions routinely disrupted fetal neurobehavioral regulation. There was no evidence of a protective effect of diminished maternal sensitivity on fetal stress.

Conclusion

We have shown the details of human embryonic and fetal responsiveness as well as the underlying neuroanatomic substrates (in so far as known). One remarkable aspect is that these early brainstem and upper cervical responses occur at a time when many central nervous system regions are still forming, and while cerebral hemispheral neuroblasts are still forming or are migrating to future cerebral cortex. The first reactions were related to early lip sensitivity and the embryonic responses summarized in the chapter title: avoid, squint, scowl, sneer, and pucker.

REFERENCES

1. Hooker D (1938) The origin of the grasping movement in man. *Proc Am Phil Soc* 79: 597–606.
2. Erbkam WH (1837) Lebhafte Bewegungen eines vier monatliche Foetus. *Neue Zeitschr f Geburisk* 5: 324–326.
3. Hooker D (1957, 1958) *Evidence of Prenatal Function of the Central Nervous System in Man*. James Arthur Lecture on the Evolution of the Human Brain. New York: The American Museum of Natural History.
4. Minkowski M (1928) Neurobiologische studien am menschlichen foetus. In: Aberhalden E, editor. *Handbuch der biologischen Arbeitsmethoden*. Berlin: Urban & Schwarzenberg, pp. 511–618.
5. O'Rahilly R, Muller F (1994) Neurulation in the normal human embryo. *Ciba Found Symp* 181: 70–82; discussion 82–89.
6. Gesell A, Thompson H (1934) *Infant Behavior; Its Genesis and Growth*. New York: McGraw-Hill.

7. Minkowski M (1923) Zur Entwicklungsgeschichte, Lokalization und Klinik des Fussohlen-reflexes. *Schweizer Arch f Neurol u Psychiat* 13: 475–514.
8. Hooker D (1939) Fetal behavior. *Res Pub Assoc Res Nerv Ment Dis* 19: 237–243.
9. Hooker D (1942) Fetal reflexes and instinctual processes. *Psychosom Med* 4: 199–205.
10. Hooker D (1944) *The Origin of Overt Behavior*. Ann Arbor: University of Michigan.
11. Hooker D (1952) *The Prenatal Origin of Behavior*. Lawrence, KS: University of Kansas Press.
12. Hooker D (1954) Early human fetal behavior, with a preliminary note on double simultaneous fetal stimulation. *Res Pub Assoc Res Nerv Ment Dis* 33: 98–113.
13. Hogg ID (1941) Sensory nerves and associated structures in the skin of human fetuses of eight to fourteen weeks of menstrual age, correlated with functional capability. *J Comp Neurol* 75: 371–410.
14. Humphrey T (1955) Pattern formed at upper cervical spinal cord levels by sensory fibers of spinal and cranial nerves. *Arch Neurol Psychiat* 73: 36–46.
15. Windle WF, Fitzgerald JE (1937) Development of the spinal reflex mechanism in human embryos. *J Comp Neurol* 67: 493–509.
16. Humphrey T (1954) The trigeminal nerve in relation to early human fetal activity. *Res Pub Assoc Res Nerv Ment Dis* 33: 127–154.
17. Humphrey T (1952) The spinal tract of the trigeminal nerve in human embryos between 7.5 and 8.5 weeks of menstrual age and its relation to fetal behavior. *J Comp Neurol* 97: 143–209.
18. Williams P, Warwick R, editors (1980) *Gray's Anatomy*. Philadelphia: WB Saunders Co.
19. Halverson HM (1937) Studies on the grasping responses of early infancy. *J Genet Psychol* 51: 371–449.
20. Humphrey T (1953) The relation of oxygen deprivation to fetal reflex arcs and the development of fetal behavior. *J Psychol* 35: 3–43.
21. Schillinger H (1976) [Characterization of active fetal movements in early pregnancy using ultrasound (time-motion technic)]. *Fortschr Med* 94: 1439–1442.
22. Higgenbottom J, Bagnall KM, Harris PF, et al (1976) Ultrasound monitoring of fetal movements. A method for assessing fetal development? *Lancet* 1(7962): 719–721.
23. Shawker TH, Schuette WH, Whitehouse W, et al (1980) Early fetal movement: a real-time ultrasound study. *Obstet Gynecol* 55: 194–198.
24. de Vries JI, Visser GH, Prechtl HF (1985) The emergence of fetal behaviour. II Quantitative aspects. *Early Hum Dev* 12: 99–120.
25. Hadders-Algra M (1996) The assessment of general movements is a valuable technique for the detection of brain dysfunction in young infants. A review. *Acta Paediatr Suppl* 416: 39–43.
26. Kintraia PI, Zarnadze MG, Kintraia NP, et al (2005) Development of daily rhythmicity in heart rate and locomotor activity in the human fetus. *J Circadian Rhythms* 3: 5.
27. Andonotopo W, Medic M, Salihagic-Kadic A, Milenkovic D, Maiz N, Scazzocchio E (2005) The assessment of fetal behavior in early pregnancy: comparison between 2D and 4D sonographic scanning. *J Perinat Med* 33: 406–414.
28. D'Elia A, Pighetti M, Moccia G, et al (2001) Spontaneous motor activity in normal fetuses. *Early Hum Dev* 65: 139–147.
29. Nijhuis IJM, ten Hof J, Nijhuis JG, et al (1999) Temporal organization of fetal behavior from 24-weeks gestation onwards in normal and complicated pregnancies. *Dev Psychobiol* 34: 257–268.
30. Kuhlman KA, Burns KA, Depp R, et al (1988) Ultrasonic imaging of normal fetal response to external vibratory acoustic stimulation. *Am J Obstet Gynecol* 158: 47–51.
31. Kozuma S, Okai T, Nemoto A, et al (1997) Developmental sequence of human fetal body movements in the second half of pregnancy. *Am J Perinatol* 14: 165–169.
32. Eyre JA, Miller S, Clowry GJ, et al (2000) Functional corticospinal projections are established prenatally in the human foetus permitting involvement in the development of spinal motor centres. *Brain* 123(Pt 1): 51–64.
33. Bursian AV, Konstantinova NN, Natsvlishvli VV, et al (1992) [The temporal organization of human fetal motor function]. *Zh Evol Biokhim Fiziol* 28: 591–595.
34. Robertson SS (1985) Cyclic motor activity in the human fetus after midgestation. *Dev Psychobiol* 18: 411–419.
35. Valentin L, Marsal K (1986) Fetal movement in the third trimester of normal pregnancy. *Early Hum Dev* 14(3–4): 295–306.
36. Liedtke B (1982) [Intrauterine fetal movements and their significance for the condition of the fetus]. *Z Geburtshilfe Perinatol* 186: 219–229.

37. Kurjak A, Azumendi G, Vecek N, et al (2003) Fetal hand movements and facial expression in normal pregnancy studied by four-dimensional sonography. *J Perinat Med* 31: 496–508.
38. Almli CR, Ball RH, Wheeler ME (2001) Human fetal and neonatal movement patterns: Gender differences and fetal-to-neonatal continuity. *Dev Psychobiol* 38: 252–273.
39. Hepper PG, Shahidullah S, White R (1991) Handedness in the human fetus. *Neuropsychologia* 29: 1107–1111.
40. McCartney G, Hepper P (1999) Development of lateralized behaviour in the human fetus from 12 to 27 weeks' gestation. *Dev Med Child Neurol* 41: 83–86.
41. Sparling JW, Van Tol J, Chescheir NC (1999) Fetal and neonatal hand movement. *Phys Ther* 79: 24–39.
42. Florido J, Cortes E, Gutierrez M, Soto VM, Miranda MT, Navarrete L (2005) Analysis of fetal breathing movements at 30–38 weeks of gestation. *J Perinat Med* 33: 38–41.
43. Pillai M, James DK, Parker M (1992) The development of ultradian rhythms in the human fetus. *Am J Obstet Gynecol* 167: 172–177.
44. Shinozuka N, Okai T, Kuwabara Y, et al (1989) The development of sleep–wakefulness cycle and its correlation to other behavior in the human fetus. *Asia Oceania J Obstet Gynaecol* 15: 395–402.
45. Grassi R, Farina R, Floriani I, et al (2005) Assessment of fetal swallowing with gray-scale and color Doppler sonography. *AJR Am J Roentgenol* 185: 1322–1327.
46. Petrikovsky BM, Schifrin B, Diana L (1993) The effect of fetal acoustic stimulation on fetal swallowing and amniotic fluid index. *Obstet Gynecol* 81: 548–550.
47. Petrikovsky BM, Kaplan GP, Pestrak H (1995) The application of color Doppler technology to the study of fetal swallowing. *Obstet Gynecol* 86(4 Pt 1): 605–608.
48. Pillai M, James D (1990) Hiccups and breathing in human fetuses. *Arch Dis Child* 65(10 Spec No): 1072–1075.
49. Okai T, Kozuma S, Shinozuka N, et al (1992) A study on the development of sleep–wakefulness cycle in the human fetus. *Early Hum Dev* 29(1–3): 391–396.
50. Sase M, Miwa I, Sumie M, et al (2005) Gastric emptying cycles in the human fetus. *Am J Obstet Gynecol* 193(3 Pt 2): 1000–1004.
51. Mann SE, Nijland MJ, Ross MG (1996) Mathematic modeling of human amniotic fluid dynamics. *Am J Obstet Gynecol* 175(4 Pt 1): 937–944.
52. Nicolaides KH, Rosen D, Rabinowitz R, et al (1988) Urine production and bladder function in fetuses with open spina bifida. *Fetal Ther* 3: 135–140.
53. Ke X, Gu Z, Wu R (1995) [Vibratory acoustic stimulation test in fetal hearing monitor]. *Zhonghua Er Bi Yan Hou Ke Za Zhi* 30: 264–266.
54. Pereira LN, Pereira LC, Germany PL, et al (1980) Auditory evoked response: a new approach for the evaluation of the unborn fetus. *Reproduction* 4: 255–263.
55. Zimmer EZ, Chao CR, Guy GP, et al (1993) Vibroacoustic stimulation evokes human fetal micturition. *Obstet Gynecol* 81: 178–180.
56. Divon MY, Platt LD, Cantrell CJ, et al (1985) Evoked fetal startle response: a possible intrauterine neurological examination. *Am J Obstet Gynecol* 153: 454–456.
57. Moore RJ, Vadeyar S, Fulford J, et al (2001) Antenatal determination of fetal brain activity in response to an acoustic stimulus using functional magnetic resonance imaging. *Hum Brain Map* 12: 94–99.
58. James DK, Spencer CJ, Stepsis BW (2002) Fetal learning: a prospective randomized controlled study. *Ultrasound Obstet Gynecol* 20: 431–438.
59. Fulford J, Vadeyar SH, Dodampahala SH, et al (2003) Fetal brain activity in response to a visual stimulus. *Hum Brain Map* 20: 239–245.
60. Waszak M, Cieslik K (2003) Sex dimorphism in development dynamics and in development progression of morphological features in human foetuses. *Folia Morphol (Warsaw)* 62: 33–39.
61. Achiron R, Lipitz S, Achiron A (2001) Sex-related differences in the development of the human fetal corpus callosum: in utero ultrasonographic study. *Prenat Diagn* 21: 116–120.
62. Gingras JL, Mitchell EA, Grattan KE (2005) Fetal homologue of infant crying. *Arch Dis Child Fetal Neonatal Ed* 90: F415–418.
63. Pillai M, James D (1990) Development of human fetal behavior: a review. *Fetal Diagn Ther* 5: 15–32.
64. Wadhwa PD, Sandman CA, Garite TJ (2001) The neurobiology of stress in human pregnancy: implications for prematurity and development of the fetal central nervous system. *Prog Brain Res* 133: 131–142.
65. DiPietro JA, Costigan KA, Gurewitsch ED (2003) Fetal response to induced maternal stress. *Early Hum Dev* 74: 125–138.

10
BLAKE'S POUCH AND RETROCEREBELLAR CYSTS: POSTERIOR FOSSA CYSTS

Normal posterior fossa development and anatomy

Early cerebral development has been reviewed in Chapters 2, 3, and 4. During stage 14, cerebellar development commences as two symmetric dorsal rhombencephalic alar plate thickenings lateral to the isthmus (the short narrow neural tube region between the midbrain and hindbrain) and first rhombomere. A few days later, as the pontine flexure develops (fourth ventricular floor bend) and the hindbrain enlargement (basis pontis) develops (ventral to the bend), dorsolateral cerebellar bulges protrude externally and inwardly into the fourth ventricle as rhombic lips, one on each side. Isthmus-derived cells (caudal mesencephalon), contributing to midline vermal fusion, are essential for additional signals responsible for further cerebellar fusion.[1] Absence of one fibroblast growth factor receptor gene results in inferior collicular and cerebellar vermal deletion.[2] At around 51 days, the cerebellar hemispheres unite in midline only in the rostral medullary vellum. By the end of the embryonic period (~57 days), cerebellar hemispheres and lateral recess roofs are very wide, without much dorsal growth; a few days later (~60 days) the early vermis forms from anterior to posterior.[3] The pontine flexure deeply indents the fourth ventricular floor. Sonographically, and with magnetic resonance imaging (MRI), the rostral vermis is seen, but the caudal vermis is undeveloped. The vermis finally closes the furrow between cerebellar hemispheres between 14 and 17 weeks, leaving only a shallow groove, the vallecula.[4,5] Thereafter, the vermis grows either linearly throughout gestation[6] or with an accelerated growth spurt between 34 and 41 weeks.[7] The vermis is believed by some to be derived entirely from mesencephalon.[8] The normal adult vermis has nine lobules, identified by the central white matter spikes of each lobule, starting with the lingula, lying upon the superior medullary velum, and counting in a clockwise manner the central, culmen, declive, folium, tuber, pyramis, uvula, and nodulus. The individual lobules appear around 14 weeks,[8,9] with middle vermian lobules taking longer to reach full size. The number of folia in each lobule continues increasing until birth, except in the lingula.

The brainstem and cerebellum fill the normal posterior fossa, leaving only small cerebrospinal fluid spaces between the cerebellar hemispheres, just inferior and posterior to the vermis, known as the vallecula, and below the cerebellum (Fig. 10.1). The supraoccipital bone caps the cerebellar hemispheres, leaving only a small cerebrospinal fluid space between the inner table, dura, arachnoid, and pial cerebellar surface. The straight sinus, within the inferior falcine edge at the tentorial leaf union, courses superior to the vermal culmen on the way to the torcular Herophili (dural sinus confluence). The fourth ventricular choroid plexus exists as a midline paired structure from the fastigium through the midline aperture (foramen Magendie) to end at the lowest tonsillar point (Fig. 10.2). The fastigial end of each choroid plexus half extends from the fastigium through the lateral apertures (foramina of Luschka) to end just anterior to the flocculi (Fig. 10.3). The choroid plexus normally

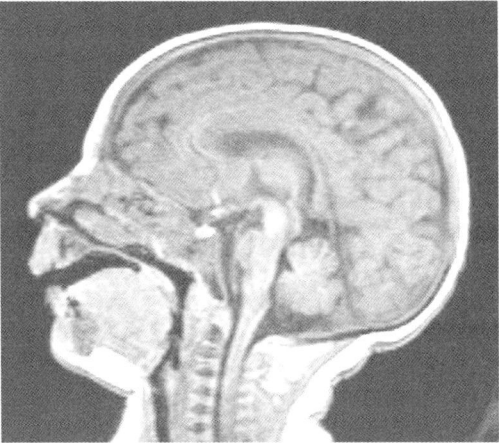

Fig. 10.1 Newborn. Normal posterior fossa. Sagittal T1-weighted magnetic resonance image. The occipital bone is normally adjacent to the cerebellar hemispheres. The cerebellum extends almost as far caudally and posteriorly as does the occipital pole. Note the small dark cerebrospinal fluid space behind the medulla and below the cerebellum, the normal cisterna magna. Reproduced with permission of Springer Verlag from Nelson et al.[68]

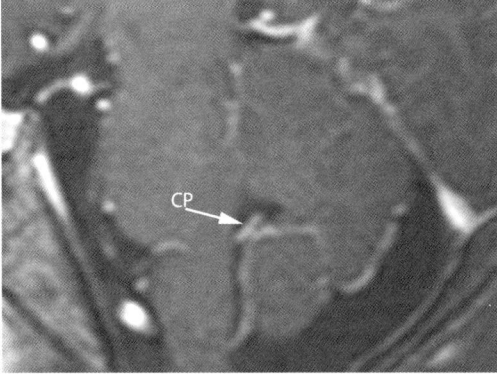

Fig. 10.2 Normal postcontrast sagittal T1-weighted magnetic resonance image showing the normal choroid plexus (CP) enhancement in the fourth ventricular roof along the inferior medullary velum. Reproduced with permission of Springer Verlag from Nelson et al.[68]

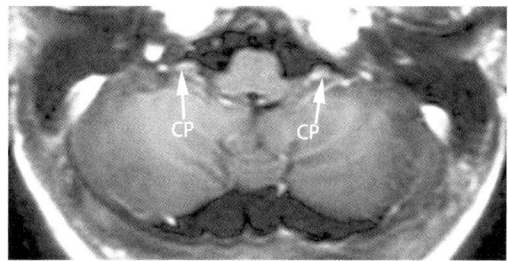

Fig. 10.3 Postcontrast axial T1-weighted magnetic resonance image showing the normal choroid plexus (CP) enhancement in the lateral recess just anterior to the flocculli. Reproduced with permission of Springer Verlag from Nelson et al.[68]

enhances with intravenous contrast and is usually identified on every postcontrast sagittal T1-weighted MRI series. When a posterior fossa fluid collection is present and the inferior vermis is missing, the question arises as to whether the inferior vermis ever formed (suggesting absence) or was present and compressed by the fluid collection. Sometimes the central white matter branch to each lobule is identified, implying inferior vermal compression; otherwise, if its inferior lobules and central white matter branches cannot be identified, the question cannot be answered.

Leptomeningeal development

Mesenchyme, derived from various sources, surrounds the brain and spinal cord as a delicate meshwork (primitive meninx) and contains a rudimentary vasculature at about 25 days. Pia develops on the brain surface subjacent to the vessels.[10–12] Small arteries lie external to the pia and small veins usually lie more peripherally, closer to the future dense skeletogenous layer. Cartilage and intramembranous bone form within the skeletogenous layer. A cellular dural limiting layer develops between the pia and the skeletogenous layer at about 41 days and becomes arachnoid.[12] The dural limiting layer appearance between the pia mater and skeletogenous sheath initiates subarachnoid space formation at around 47 to 48 days,[13] before development of the fourth ventricular roof choroid plexus; however, there is ventricular fluid (presumably derived from ependyma) as soon as the anterior neuropore is closed. Separately, the loose primitive meninx also seems to exude fluid (presumably derived from the leptomeningeal plexus) while forming the subarachnoid space,[13] but these two fluids are not commingled as the fourth ventricular roof separates them. The falx and tentorium are present by the end of the embryonic period. The torcular Herophili is in its normal position at about 12 weeks.

The arachnoid is normally attached to the cerebellum along the horizontal fissure, forming a membrane, which, during the years of pneumoencephalography, was known as the posterior fossa diaphragm;[14] before that, Key and Retzius[15] had demonstrated several different attachments, but always to the inferior cerebellar surface. The arachnoid over the inferior cerebellum is loose with few septations; in contrast, the arachnoid over the superior cerebellum is normally very dense with numerous septations.

Fourth ventricular roof development

At around 4 to 5 weeks, with both neuropores closed and the future ventricular system no longer communicating with amniotic fluid, the choroid plexus appears in the fourth ventricular roof (stage 19, approximately 44 days). Sonographically demonstrable around the eighth week, the choroid plexus divides the thin, flattened ependymal fourth ventricular roof into a rostral and caudal portion relative to the plexus.[9,16] At about 48 days, the fourth ventricle possesses lateral recesses (but no aperture), each with its own choroid plexus; by the end of the embryonic period, the lateral recesses contain a laterally oriented choroid plexus without caudal fourth ventricular roof extensions. Lateral and midline ventricular apertures are not yet present. Occasionally, the tubular lateral recesses wind around the medulla on either side, past the inferior cerebellar peduncle, on its rostral and inferior aspect. The future lateral aperture (foramen of Luschka), in the distal lateral recess, is identified by a tuft of choroid plexus, continuous with the fourth ventricular roof plexus.[15,17] While the exact timing of lateral aperture opening is unknown, it probably occurs between 14 and 17 weeks.[18,19] The lateral apertures remain closed in about 20% of humans.[20]

The adult midline fourth ventricular roof aperture (foramen of Magendie) is 4 to 6mm in diameter (Fig. 10.4).[21] Magendie's peer, Cruveilhier,[22] thought the fourth ventricular roof remained closed throughout life. A tuft of the choroid plexus marks the median aperture rostral lip continuous with the fourth ventricular roof plexus and is a useful imaging landmark (Fig. 10.2).[23,24] In most humans, the choroid plexus extends only into the midline aperture rostral lip and not into the cisterna magna. In 56% (of 118 human brains), the foramen is a wide opening; in 23%, the pial–ependymal membrane does not extend posteriorly along the vermal inferior surface; in 10%, the choroid plexus is prolonged along the inferior vermis reaching considerably beyond paramedian lobule posterior limits (and even up and over the inferior vermal surface); and in 7%, the membranous roof covers the calamus anterior to the obex, in some cases extending horizontally and attaching to cisterna magna posterior wall arachnoid. In 3%, there is only a minute midline aperture, and in 1% to 4% it is absent.[25,26] In some adults, the midline aperture rostral edge is carried over the inferior vermis along with its choroid plexus, reflecting an incomplete persistence of Blake's outpouching. The foramen opens at approximately 7 to 8 weeks, with the cisterna magna developing a few days later. Luschka recognized that in some vertebrates (horses) the midline foramen remains closed.

Cisterna magna

'At certain parts of the base of the brain, the arachnoid is separated from the pia mater by wide intervals, which communicate freely with each other and are named subarachnoid cisterns; in these the subarachnoid tissue is scanty and may be absent'.[27] The term cisterna magna refers to the wide subarachnoid space below the inferior cerebellar surface, behind the medulla, and inside the dura and external arachnoidal membrane over the lower and medial supraoccipital bone (Fig. 10.1).[28] The midline aperture (foramen of Magendie) lies at the anterior apex, rostral and tucked under the lower vermal surface. There is considerable variation in cisterna magna size behind the cerebellum. It usually extends 2.5cm up from the foramen magnum along the occipital bone inner table to a point midway between the foramen magnum posterior lip and the internal occipital protuberance. The depth is usually 5mm; the width is variable but about

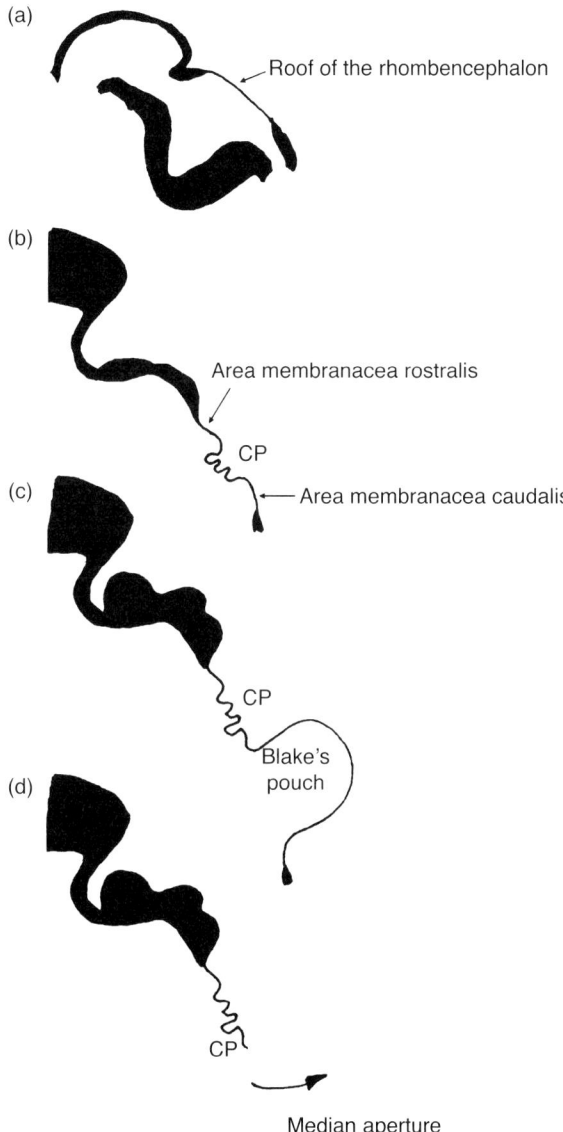

(a)

Roof of the rhombencephalon

(b)

Area membranacea rostralis

CP

(c)

Area membranacea caudalis

CP

Blake's pouch

(d)

CP

Median aperture

Fig. 10.4 Normal formation of fourth ventricle median aperture. Median sections: (a) stage 17 (41 days), (b) stage 19 (46 days), (c) stage 23 (56 days), (d) 9 to 10 weeks. In (a), the rhombencephalic roof is thin and only one or two cells thick. In (b), the choroid plexus (CP) is forming, separating the roof into area membranacea rostralis above, and area membranacea caudalis below. In (c), the area membranacea caudalis evaginates creating Blake's pouch. The apex of this outpouching normally thins and disappears, creating the fourth ventricular median aperture (foramen Magendie) as in (d). Reproduced with permission of Springer Verlag from Nelson et al.[68]

TABLE 10.1

Type	Connective tissue	Blood vessels	Arachnoid	Ependyma	Choroid plexus	Glia	Neurons
Dandy–Walker	+	+	+	+	–	+	+
Blake's pouch	+	+	+	+	+	+	–
Arachnoid	+	+	+	–	–	–	–
Ependymal	+	+	±	+	–	–	–
Choroid plexus	+	+	±	±	+	–	–

+, present; –, absent; ±, may be present or absent.

2cm; occasionally, it rises to the internal occipital protuberance. The cisterna magna is visible sonographically at around 16 weeks.[29]

Posterior fossa cysts: general

The identification of any body cyst depends on its wall histology, location, or associated structures. Its designation generally reflects the inner cyst wall cell lining; as, for instance, bronchogenic cyst, where lining cells are respiratory epithelium. Posterior fossa cyst walls obtained surgically contain various combinations of thin fibrous tissue, thin delicate arachnoid, complex membranes composed of glia, arachnoid and choroid plexus, and, sometimes, neurons (Table 10.1). Posterior fossa cysts are easily missed at autopsy unless the fixed whole brain is examined under water.[28,30] This maneuver allows the delicate cyst wall to float away from the cerebellum, demonstrating bridging veins stretched around the cyst in their course from inferior and caudal cerebellar surfaces to lateral, or straight sinus or tentorial terminations. The normal midline and lateral fourth ventricle apertures are marked with robust choroid plexus buttons that protrude slightly through the foramina into the subarachnoid space. The normal midline plexus button is caudal to nodulus and uvula and defines the rostral midline aperture limit.

Fibrous arachnoidal cysts

The first kind of cyst, and most understandable, is a cyst wall composed solely of fibrous tissue, or dense fibrous tissue and arachnoid. This is an arachnoidal fibrosis, such as the fibrosis following leptomeningeal inflammation from subarachnoid hemorrhage, bacterial or fungal leptomeningitis,[31] or mucopolysaccharidosis arachnoidal thickening.[32]

Arachnoidal duplications: Arachnoidal cysts proper

The second kind of cyst contains a thin, delicate arachnoidal wall (Figs. 10.5 and 10.6), namely the outer wall of a true intra-arachnoidal cyst or, more explicitly, an arachnoidal duplication with subarachnoid space vessels still within the inner layer of arachnoid.[28,33–35] Arachnoidal cysts are sometimes huge,[36] familial,[37] located above, below, or behind the cerebellum,[38,39] or

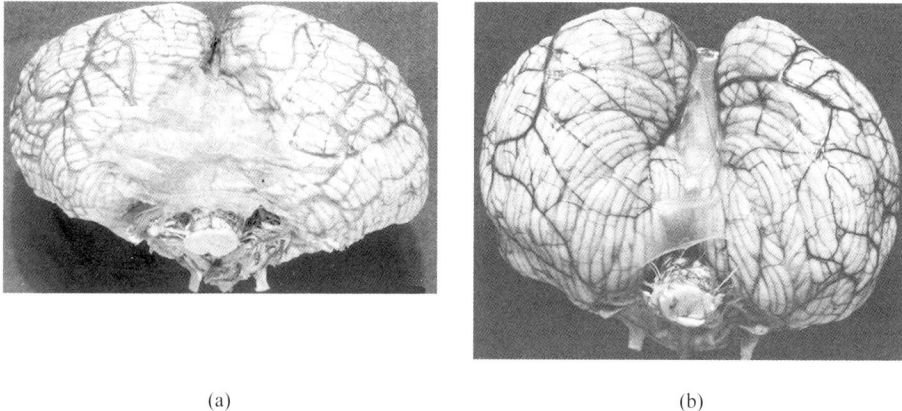

(a)   (b)

Fig. 10.5 Arachnoid cyst. (a) The outer arachnoidal membrane of this large cisterna magna has floated away from the cerebellum while under water. Horizontal arrows indicate its lateral attachments to the lower cerebellar surface. (b) Removal of the outer membrane reveals the inner membrane, which is the normal arachnoid covering the cisterna magna. The normal cerebellar arteries and veins lie within the arachnoid external to the pia. The inferior cerebellar surface has been slightly indented by this arachnoid cyst. Reproduced with permission of Springer Verlag from Nelson et al.[68]

bulge down through the foramen magnum and compress the upper cervical cord.[40] They rarely occur within the fourth ventricle; moreover, they are not part of Dandy–Walker malforma-tion.[33] Unfortunately, several articles claim to discuss posterior fossa arachnoidal cysts without pathologic study.[41,42]

Arachnoidal duplications are very common, producing fluid-filled cysts that occupy space between the cerebellum and occipital bone, or if supratentorial between cerebrum and bone. The cyst walls are too thin to visualize with neuroimaging. These cysts sometimes enlarge and produce mass effect on the cerebellum or cause secondary ventricular system obstruction, producing hydrocephalus and/or pressure-inducing occipital bone erosion or remodeling. These retrocerebellar cysts do not communicate with the fourth ventricle, when the fourth ventricular choroid plexus is in the normal position. On cross-sectional imaging studies, these cysts appear as cerebrospinal fluid spaces between the cerebellum and occipital bone. The tor-cular Herophili is usually normal in position, but with early fetal formation it may sometimes be elevated. The falx cerebelli is normally present. Occasionally, there is the appearance of compression or absence of the inferior vermis. Other central nervous system malformations are rarely associated with arachnoid duplication cysts.

Blake's pouch and the opening of foramen of magendie

The third kind of cyst is a persistent Blake's pouch with ependyma, glia, and choroid plexus in the wall. Blake[43] and Wilson[44–46] independently identified a human midline fourth ventricle roof evagination lined by ependyma as a step in normal midline aperture development. This diverticulum extended posterior and upward into the primitive meninx caudal to the cerebel-lum and was subsequently identified in dogs, cats, goats, pigs, sheeps, chicks, horses, and

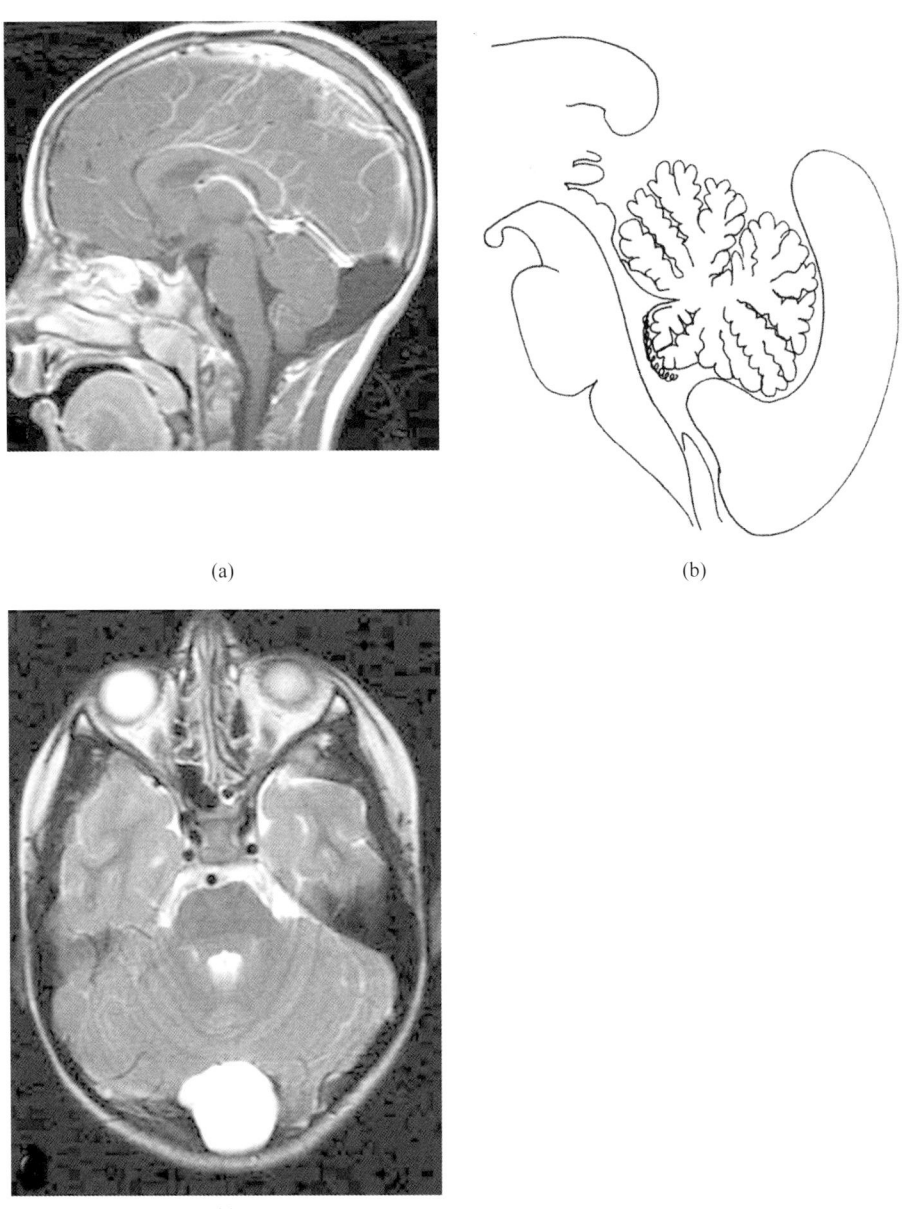

(a)

(b)

(c)

Fig. 10.6 Posterior fossa arachnoid cyst. (a) Sagittal postcontrast T1-weighted magnetic resonance image. The retrocerebellar fluid collection bulges above the torcula and causes remodeling of the occipital bone inner table. Note the normal choroid plexus position. (b) Midline posterior fossa drawing illustrating how an arachnoid duplication does not communicate with the fourth ventricle and how the choroid plexus is in normal position. (c) Axial T2-weighted magnetic resonance image showing the large retrocerebellar fluid collection behind the cerebellar hemispheres and vermis. Reproduced with permission of Springer Verlag from Nelson et al.[68]

marsupials, but not in rodents.[43,47] This evagination has in its wall the same histologic elements as the fourth ventricular wall and roof: ependyma, glia, and choroid plexus. The ependyma thins, becoming indistinguishable from the arachnoid at its apex. In humans, the evagination, plastered to vermal inferior surface, eventually ruptures and forms a midline aperture opening into the subarachnoid space between 7 and 8 weeks.[48] If this opening does not form, or is late in forming, the fourth ventricular cerebrospinal fluid causes the evagination to expand, eventually forming a retrocerebellar cyst, with the same histologic composition as mentioned above. This type of retrocerebellar cyst was named 'Blake's pouch' after the man who initially identified the outpouching (Fig. 10.7).[30,44]

Choroid plexus, displaced from the midline aperture anterior lip into the cyst lying under the posterior vermal borders, is continuous with the lower fourth ventricular roof, and as the cyst extends upward between the cerebellar hemispheres, the plexus follows the vermis posteriorly and upward.[25,26] The cyst, containing choroid plexus, sometimes spreads the cerebellar hemispheres apart and continues all the way over the vermis to the collicular plate. Some cysts communicate with subarachnoid space, but many are closed; if closed, there is no midline aperture. When completely separated from the fourth ventricle, the Blake's pouch cyst still becomes quite large because of its functional choroid plexus (Fig. 10.8). These cyst walls contain glia and ependyma (Fig. 10.9) and choroid plexus (Fig. 10.10). The large cysts stretch bridging veins and modify the cranium, and displace supraoccipital bone posteriorly along with the bridging vein attachments to the lateral and straight sinuses. Figure 10.11 shows an underwater view of a Blake's pouch behind the cerebellum with fourth ventricular roof

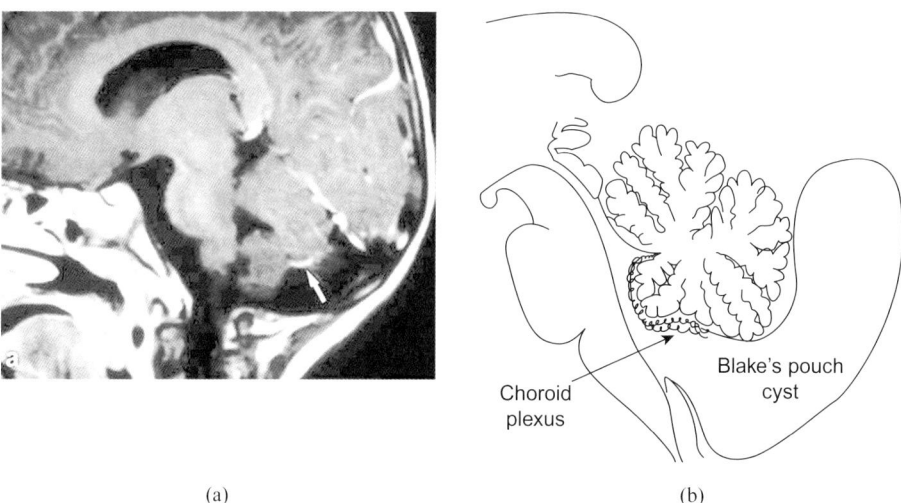

(a)   (b)

Fig. 10.7 Blake's pouch cyst. (a) Sagittal T1-weighted postcontrast magnetic resonance image. Note the enhancing choroid plexus under the vermis (arrow) running in the superior wall of the Blake's pouch cyst. (b) Midline posterior fossa drawing illustrating the abnormal choroid plexus position along the superior cyst wall and that the cysts usually communicate with the fourth ventricle. Reproduced with permission of Springer Verlag from Nelson et al.[68]

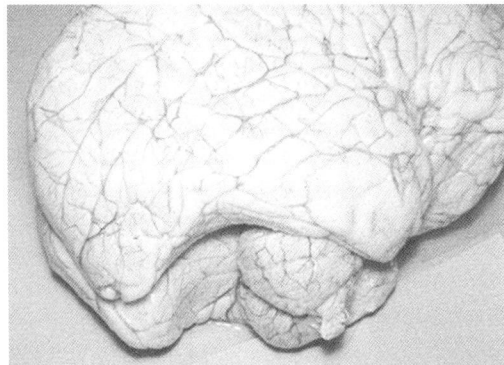

Fig. 10.8 This large hydrocephalic brain resulted from a massive Blake's pouch cyst occupying the space posterior and inferior to the cerebellum. The cyst fully occupied the space between the cerebellum and the occipital poles. In this child, the aqueduct was fully patent, the leptomeninges were delicate and transparent, and the arachnoid villi were adequate in number and size along the sagittal sinus.

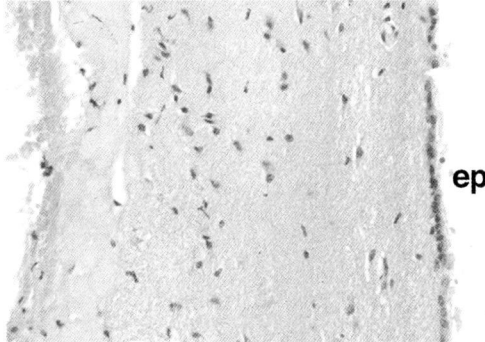

Fig. 10.9 This photomicrograph of a Blake's pouch cyst wall demonstrates the ependymal cells (ep) lying on a layer of glia. Reproduced with permission of Springer Verlag from Nelson et al.[68]

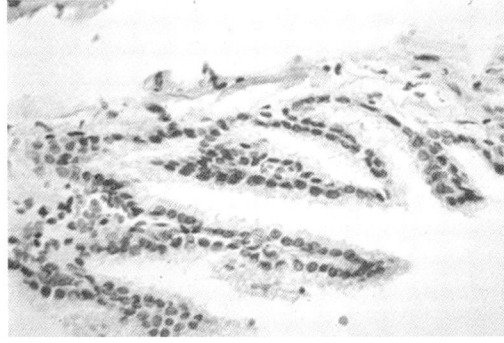

Fig. 10.10 This photomicrograph of a Blake's pouch cyst wall demonstrates the choroid plexus. Reproduced with permission of Springer Verlag from Nelson et al.[68]

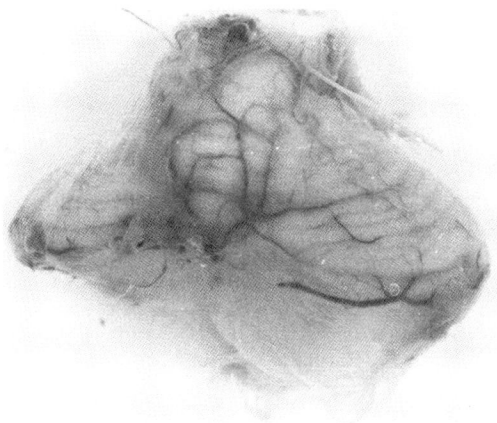

Fig. 10.11 This large persistent Blake's pouch cyst did not obstruct the outflow of cerebrospinal fluid from the fourth ventricle but demonstrates the marked stretching of the bridging veins. It also displaced the supraoccipital bone posteriorly.

posterior extensions and secondarily elongated cerebellar bridging veins, and Figures 10.12 and 10.13 show the cyst wall continuity with fourth ventricular roof. Thus, in the absence of vermal hypoplasia, there is only rostral or dorsal cerebellar displacement.[30,49] The cyst sometimes communicates with the fourth ventricle and is a persistent Blake's pouch.[43] Often, Blake's pouches form retrocerebellar cysts that do not obstruct the fourth ventricle (Fig. 10.13). Extracerebellar cyst walls sometimes consist predominantly of ependymal or glial cells and have been given these names; nevertheless, we think that these are merely variations of Blake's pouches (Table 10.1).

Blake's pouches have the same radiographic appearance as arachnoidal cysts, except that in some cases the choroid plexus is identified as it extends through the midline aperture along the superior cyst wall (Fig. 10.7a), carrying the anterior median aperture lip far up the vallecula. Care should be taken to distinguish the enhanced choroid plexus from a prominent inferior vermian vein, which continues to the straight sinus. Blake's pouches usually communicate with the fourth ventricle and sometimes produce mass effect on the cerebellum. The falx cerebelli is usually present. The torcular is usually in the normal position or elevated with occipital bone pressure erosion. Occasionally, there is the appearance of inferior vermal compression or absence. Other central nervous system malformations are rarely associated with Blake's pouches.

Lateral recess cysts
The lateral recess cyst is a subset of Blake's pouch cyst. The normal cerebellopontine angle contains the lateral recess with its choroid plexus tuft (Fig. 10.3). Cysts histologically similar to persistent Blake's pouches arise in relation to Luschka's foramen when the latter does not open into the subarachnoid space[50] (Fig. 10.14). The figure, from Virchow's original description, shows the cyst closed peripherally. These cerebellopontine angle cysts contain ependyma,

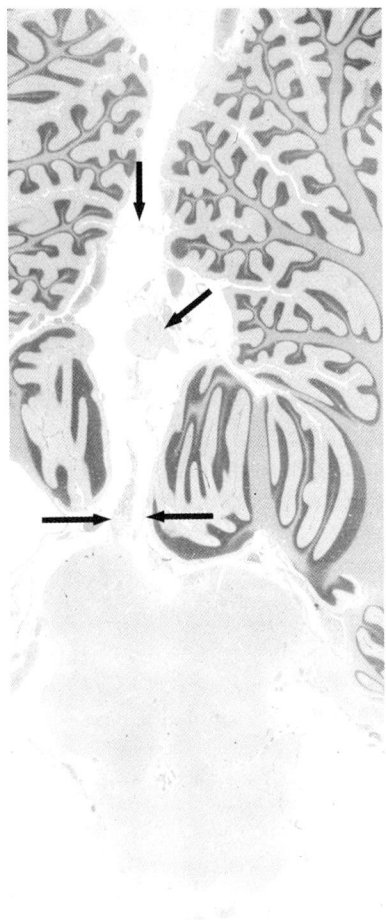

Fig. 10.12 In this axial section at the medullary–pontine junction from a child with a persistent, ruptured, Blake's pouch, the fourth ventricular roof has been carried posteriorly and upward between the biventral lobules just below and behind the vermis (not shown). The vertical arrow demonstrates the cyst roof; the single oblique arrow shows a fragment of glia in cyst wall and the opposing horizontal arrows show the cyst walls carrying choroid plexus out of the fourth ventricle up between the cerebellar hemispheres. Reproduced with permission of Springer Verlag from Nelson et al.[68]

glia, choroid plexus, and arachnoid;[51–54] for these reasons they are not simple arachnoid cysts.[51] Cerebellopontine angle cysts are sometimes symptomatic;[50,55–57] rarely are they associated with other malformations.[58] Cerebellopontine angle cysts are fluid collections with or without mass effect on the cerebellum and/or brainstem (Fig. 10.15). As previously discussed, these cysts are usually either Blake's pouch-like (containing plexus, ependyma, or glia), arachnoid duplication, or acquired, and are generally indistinguishable by imaging.

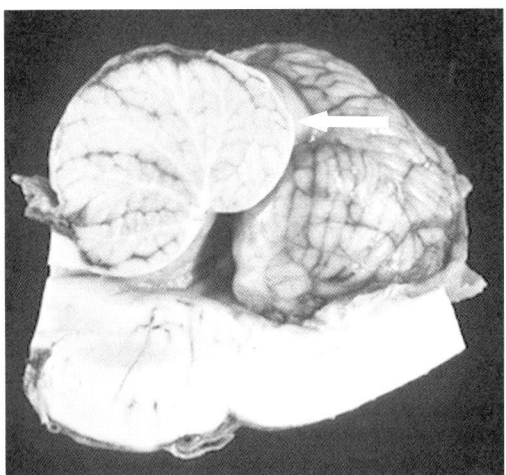

Fig. 10.13 Midline section of cerebellum, pons, and medulla showing how the Blake's pouch wall is continuous with the fourth ventricular roof. Here the white roof is plastered to the distorted caudal vermis (arrow) and continues around the under vermal surface. The vermal distortion has reduced the apparent number of vermal lobules.

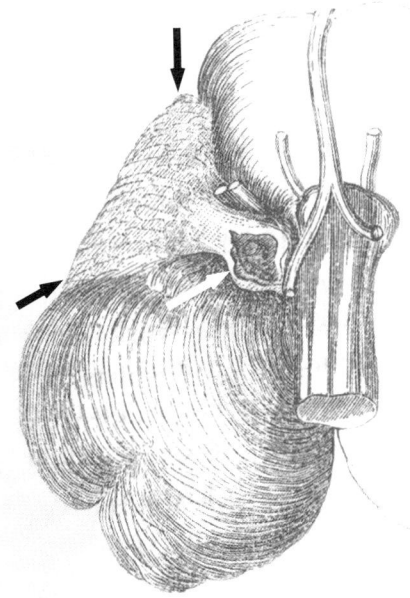

Fig. 10.14 The lateral recess cyst, from Virchow's original description, shows that the cyst is distally closed (black arrows). The artificial cyst opening (white arrow) shows choroid plexus within the cyst. Cerebellopontine angle cysts contain ependyma, glia, choroid plexus, and arachnoid. Reproduced with permission of Springer Verlag from Nelson et al.[68]

231

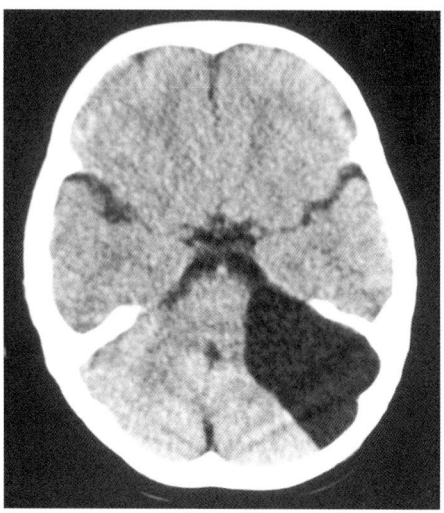

Fig. 10.15 Cerebellopontine angle cyst. Noncontrast CT of cerebellopontine angle cyst not obstructing cerebrospinal flow from the ventricular system. The left cerebellopontine angle fluid collection caused a cerebellar mass effect.

Dandy–Walker cysts

The fourth variety of posterior fossa cyst wall contains neurons in addition to arachnoid, glia, and ependyma, but not choroid plexus, and occurs in patients with a very large fourth ventricle, and complete or partial vermal agenesis (Fig. 10.16).[59] In the Dandy–Walker malformation, there are usually other central nervous system malformations, such as corpus callosum agenesis or heterotopic gray matter. This type of malformation, first described by Dandy and Blackfan[60] and later by Taggert and Walker,[61] results from dysgenetic rhomben-cephalic roof development and not from a failure of fourth ventricular outlet formation, as previously thought.

Dandy–Walker cysts have a spectrum of radiographic appearances (Fig. 10.17). Barkovich suggested using the term 'Dandy–Walker complex' to account for the various imaging mani-festations of this malformation.[62] The classic malformation consists of a huge posterior cyst, which is the fourth ventricle, with absent, or markedly hypoplastic, vermis and cerebellar hemispheres and elevated lateral and straight sinuses and torcular Herophili. No choroid plexus is identifiable. Milder forms have only a mildly hypoplastic vermis with a large fourth ventricle filling a normal-sized posterior fossa with a torcular Herophili in the normal position (Fig. 10.18). The falx cerebelli is usually absent. The normal-sized posterior fossa Dandy–Walker cyst sometimes simulates an arachnoid cyst or a persistent Blake's pouch with imag-ing. In contrast, a normal fourth ventricular choroid plexus in the inferior medullary velum rules out a Dandy–Walker malformation. If the choroid plexus is elongated or displaced under the inferior vermal surface, a Blake's pouch should be considered (Table 10.2).

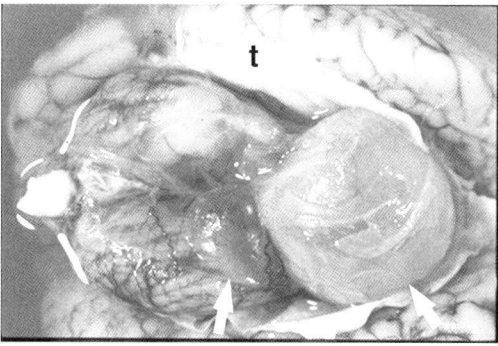

Fig. 10.16 Dandy–Walker cyst; underwater view. The medulla is to the left. There is no vermis in the midline and the fourth ventricle opens into two large multiloculated cysts filled with air (arrows). The cysts press against the undersurface of the dural tentorium (t).

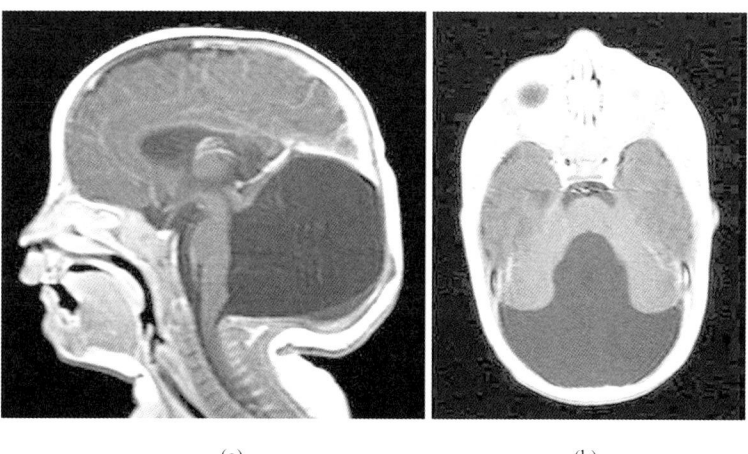

(a)   (b)

Fig. 10.17 Classic Dandy–Walker cyst. (a) Sagittal T1-weighted magnetic resonance image demonstrating a small brainstem, hypoplastic vermis, torcula high position, and large posterior fossa fluid collection. (b) Axial T1-weighted magnetic resonance image demonstrating the hypoplastic cerebellar vermis and hemispheres and large posterior fossa. Reproduced with permission of Springer Verlag from Nelson et al.[68]

The term 'Dandy–Walker variant' was introduced to describe an 'outpouching of an ependymal lined cyst from the fourth ventricle' associated with vermal dysplasia.[63] This was probably a Blake's pouch. Some define a Dandy–Walker variant as a hypoplastic cerebellar vermis, cystic fourth ventricular dilatation with a normal-sized posterior fossa,[62] while others use the term for individuals with a large fourth ventricle with at least one patent foramina.[64] Because there is no standard definition of a 'Dandy–Walker variant,' this term should be avoided completely.

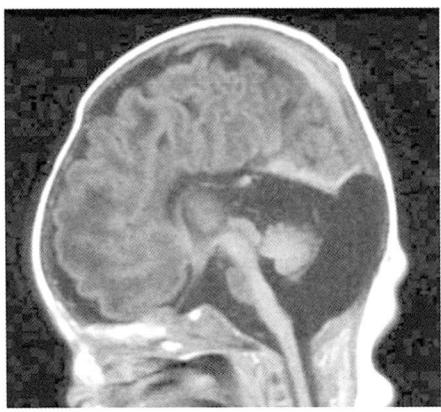

Fig. 10.18 Dandy–Walker cyst. Sagittal T1-weighted magnetic resonance image. There is a normal downward straight sinus slant, normal torcular position, small posterior fossa, slightly hypoplastic vermis, and corpus callosum agenesis. Reproduced with permission of Springer Verlag from Nelson et al.[68]

The Dandy–Walker malformation is associated with other central nervous system malformations in up to 70% of cases [usually corpus callosum agenesis (Fig. 10.19) and heterotopias] and carries genetic risks not associated with the other histologic types of posterior fossa cysts.[65] These genetic risks become important when counseling patients and their parents.

'Mega' cisterna magna

The term 'mega cisterna magna' was first used to describe a series of adult patients with grossly enlarged posterior fossa cisterns ascribed to cerebellar atrophy.[66] More recently, the term has been loosely applied to a large retrocerebellar space with a normal vermis and cerebellar hemispheres. We agree with Gonsette et al[66] that the cisterna magna should enlarge only in response to the removal of damaged cerebellum. If there exists a cerebrospinal fluid space between the normal cerebellum and occipital bone, there must be something occupying that space for it to exist; otherwise, the occipital bone would form snugly against the cerebellar hemispheres. To use this term to describe an enlarged subarachnoid cistern that causes cerebellar mass effect, enlarges the posterior fossa, and/or splits the falx and extends supratentorially defies all logic.[67] In our experience, when such spaces are carefully examined at autopsy (the fixed brain submerged under water), the delicate retrocerebellar cyst membranes become apparent and histologically are usually arachnoidal cysts or Blake's pouches.

Conclusion

In conclusion, posterior fossa fluid collections are common findings on MRI. These fluid collections often are asymptomatic but have secondary effects on the surrounding structures (cerebellum, torcula, occipital bone) that identify their presence. Imaging studies demonstrate that all cysts have similar imaging appearances but can only be differentiated pathologically. The presence (or absence) and position of the fourth ventricular choroid plexus helps to distinguish some cysts. As the cyst wall histology is not known radiologically, the radiologist should

TABLE 10.2

TABLE 10.2

Imaging characteristics of posterior fossa cysts

Cyst type	Posterior fossa	Fourth ventricular choroid plexus	Torcula	Occipital bone	Falx cerebelli	Other nervous system malformations
Dandy–Walker	Normal to very large	Absent	Normal to elevated	Normal to thinned	Usually absent	Frequent
Blake's pouch	Usually normal to large	Normal to displaced	Usually normal to elevated	Normal to thinned	Usually present	Rare
Arachnoid	Usually normal to large	Normal	Usually normal to elevated	Normal to thinned	Usually present	Rare

describe the cyst by its location (retrocerebellar, supracerebellar, or cerebellopontine angle) and secondary effects. For example, 'retrocerebellar cyst, not obstructing the cerebrospinal flow' is the preferred alternative to speculation ('arachnoid cyst'). Such terms as 'Dandy–Walker variant' and 'mega cisterna magna' should be avoided because these terms only confuse, add nothing to patient management, and, with the Dandy–Walker variant, imply genetic implications (by association with true Dandy–Walker malformation) that are not warranted.

REFERENCES

1. Louvi A, Alexandre P, Metin C, Wurst W, Wassef M (2003) The isthmic neuroepithelium is essential for cerebellar midline fusion. *Development* 130: 5319–5330.
2. Trokovic R, Trokovic N, Hernesniemi S, et al (2003) FGFR1 is independently required in both developing mid- and hindbrain for sustained response to isthmic signals. *EMBO J* 22: 1811–1823.
3. Loeser JD, Lemire RJ, Alvord EC Jr. (1972) The development of the folia in the human cerebellar vermis. *Anat Rec* 173: 109–113.
4. Bromley B, Nadel AS, Pauker S, Estroff JA, Benacerraf BR (1994) Closure of the cerebellar vermis: evaluation with second trimester US. *Radiology* 193: 761–763.
5. Babcook CJ, Chong BW, Salamat MS, Ellis WG, Goldstein RB (1996) Sonographic anatomy of the developing cerebellum: normal embryology can resemble pathology. *AJR Am J Roentgenol* 166: 427–433.
6. Malinger G, Ginath S, Lerman-Sagie T, Watemberg N, Lev D, Glezerman M (2001) The fetal cerebellar vermis: normal development as shown by transvaginal ultrasound. *Prenat Diagn* 21: 687–692.
7. Huang CC, Liu CC (1993) The differences in growth of cerebellar vermis between appropriate-for-gestational-age and small-for-gestational-age newborns. *Early Hum Dev* 33: 9–19.
8. Yachnis AT, Rorke LB (1999) Cerebellar and brainstem development: an overview in relation to Joubert syndrome. *J Child Neurol* 14: 570–573.
9. Müller F, O'Rahilly R (1990) The human brain at stages 21–23, with particular reference to the cerebral cortical plate and to the development of the cerebellum. *Anat Embryol (Berl)* 182: 375–400.
10. Harvey SC, Burr HS (1926) The development of the meninges. *Arch Neurol Psychiat Chicago* 15: 545–567.
11. Gil DR, Ratto GD (1973) Contribution to the study of the origin of leptomeninges in the human embryo. *Acta Anat (Basel)* 85: 620–623.
12. O'Rahilly R, Müller F, Bossy J (1986) [Atlas of the stages of development of the external forms of the brain in the human embryo]. *Arch Anat Histol Embryol* 69: 3–39.

13. O'Rahilly R, Müller F (1994) *The Embryonic Human Brain: An Atlas of Developmental Stages*. New York: Wiley-Liss.
14. Taveras JM, Wood EH (1976) *Diagnostic Neuroradiology*. Baltimore, MD: Williams and Wilkins.
15. Key A, Retzius G (1875) *Studien in der Anatomie des Nerversystems und des Bindegewebes*. Stockholm: Norstedt & Söner.
16. Blaas HG, Eik-Nes SH, Kiserud T, Hellevik LR (1995) Early development of the hindbrain: a longitudinal ultrasound study from 7 to 12 weeks of gestation. *Ultrasound Obstet Gynecol* 5: 151–160.
17. von Luschka H (1855) *Die Adergeflechte der menschlichen Gehirnes. Eine Mongraphie*. Berlin: Reimer.
18. Rasmussen A (1926) Additional evidence favoring the normal existence of the lateral apertures of the fourth ventricle in man. *Anat Rec* 33: 179–182.
19. Lemire RJ, Loeser JD, Leech RW, Alvord EC Jr. (1975) *Normal and Abnormal Development of the Human Nervous System*. Hagerstown, Maryland: Harper and Row.
20. Alexander L (1931) Die Anatomie der Seitentaschen der vierten Hirnkammer. *Z Anat* 95: 531–707.
21. Magendie F (1827) Troisième et dernière partie du second mémoire sur le liquide qui se trouve dans le crâne et l'épine de l'homme et des animaux vértebrés. *J Physiol Exp Path Paris* 7: 66–82.
22. Cruveilhier J (1829–1835) *Anatomie Pathologique du Corps Humain*, Part 2, XVth Liv. Paris: JB Baillière.
23. Rogers L, West CM (1931) The foramen of Magendie. *J Anat* 65: 457–467.
24. Hayman LA, Evans RA, Hinck VC (1979) Choroid plexus of the fourth ventricle: a useful CT landmark. *AJR Am J Roentgenol* 133: 285–288.
25. Hess C (1885) Das Foramen Magendie und die Oeffnungen an den Recessus des 4. Ventricle. *Morph Jahrb* 10: 578–602.
26. Barr ML (1948) Observations on the foramen of Magendie in a series of human brains. *Brain* 71: 281–289.
27. Williams P, Warwick R (1980) *Gray's Anatomy*. Philadelphia: WB Saunders Co.
28. Robertson EG (1949) Developmental defects of the cisterna magna and dura mater. *J Neurol Neurosurg Psych* 12: 39–51.
29. Serhatlioglu S, Kocakoc E, Kiris A, Sapmaz E, Boztosun Y, Bozgeyik Z (2003) Sonographic measurement of the fetal cerebellum, cisterna magna, and cavum septum pellucidum in normal fetuses in the second and third trimesters of pregnancy. *J Clin Ultrasound* 31: 194–200.
30. Gilles FH, Rockett FX (1971) Infantile hydrocephalus: Retrocerebellar 'arachnoidal' cyst. *J Pediatr* 79: 436–443.
31. Horrax G (1924) Generalized cisternal arachnoiditis simulating cerebellar tumor: Its surgical treatment and end-results. *Arch Surg* 9: 95–112.
32. Neuhauser EBD, Griscom T, Gilles FH, Crocker AC (1968) Arachnoid cyst in the Hurler–Hunter syndrome. *Annales de Radiologie* 11: 453–470.
33. Kaplan A (1948) Pia-arachnoid cysts of the posterior fossa. *Am J Surg* 76: 102–106.
34. Starkman SP, Brown TC, Linell EA (1958) Cerebral arachnoid cysts. *J Neuropath Exp Neurol* 17: 484–500.
35. Rengachary SS, Watanabe I, Brackett CE (1978) Pathogenesis of intracranial arachnoid cysts. *Surg Neurol* 9: 139–144.
36. Sugata S, Niiro M, Tanioka K, Yano T, Kuratsu J (2003) Huge arachnoid cyst of the posterior fossa with cerebellar tentorium dysplasia associated with juvenile polyposis. *Pediatr Neurosurg* 38: 253–257.
37. Suzuki H, Takanashi J, Sugita K, Barkovich AJ, Kohno Y (2002) Retrocerebellar arachnoid cysts in siblings with mental retardation and undescended testis. *Brain Dev* 24: 310–313.
38. Ucar T, Akyuz M, Kazan S, Tuncer R (2000) Bilateral cerebellopontine angle arachnoid cysts: case report. *Neurosurgery* 47: 966–968.
39. Krisht AF, O'Brien MS (1992) Acquired mirror-image cerebellopontine angle arachnoid cysts: case report. *Neurosurgery* 30: 798–800.
40. Shukla R, Sharma A, Vatsal DK (1998) Posterior fossa arachnoid cyst presenting as high cervical cord compression. *Br J Neurosurg* 12: 271–273.
41. Erdincler P, Kaynar MY, Bozkus H, Ciplak N (1999) Posterior fossa arachnoid cysts. *Br J Neurosurg* 13: 10–17.
42. Jallo GI, Woo HH, Meshki C, Epstein FJ, Wisoff JH (1997) Arachnoid cysts of the cerebellopontine angle: diagnosis and surgery. *Neurosurgery* 40: 31–7; discussion 7–8.
43. Blake JA (1900) The roof and lateral recesses of the fourth ventricle, considered morphologically and embryologically. *J Comp Neurol* 10: 79–108.

44. Wilson JT (1936–1937) On the nature and mode of origin of the foramen of Magendie. *J Anat* 71: 423–428.
45. Wilson JT (1906) Part II: On the anatomy of the calamus region in the human bulb; with an account of a hitherto undescribed 'nucleus postremus.' *J Anat Physiol* 40 (Pt. 4): 357–386.
46. Wilson JT (1906) Part I: On the anatomy of the calamus region in the human bulb; with an account of a hitherto undescribed 'nucleus postremus.' *J Anat Physiol* 40 (Pt. 3): 210–241.
47. Coben LA (1967) Absence of a foramen of Magendie in the dog, cat, rabbit, and goat. *Arch Neurol* 16: 524–528.
48. Brocklehurst G (1969) The development of the human cerebrospinal fluid pathway with particular reference to the roof of the fourth ventricle. *J Anat* 105: 467–475.
49. Sharpe JA, Deck JH (1977) Neuroepithelial cyst of the fourth ventricle. Case report. *J Neurosurg* 46: 820–824.
50. Virchow R (1864–1865) Die Krankhaften Geschulste. Berlin: August Hirschwald.
51. Schuhmann MU, Tatagiba M, Hader C, Brandis A, Samii M (2000) Ectopic choroid plexus within a juvenile arachnoid cyst of the cerebellopontine angle: cause of cyst formation or reason of cyst growth. *Pediatr Neurosurg* 32: 73–76.
52. Ho KL, Chason JL (1987) A glioependymal cyst of the cerebellopontine angle. Immunohistochemical and ultrastructural studies. *Acta Neuropathol (Berl)* 74: 382–388.
53. Monaco P, Filippi S, Tognetti F, Calbucci F (1995) Glioependymal cyst of the cerebellopontine angle. *J Neurol Neurosurg Psychiatry* 58: 109–110.
54. Nakase H, Ohnishi H, Touho H, Karasawa J (1994) Large ependymal cyst of the cerebello-pontine angle in a child. *Brain Dev* 16: 260–263.
55. Takano S, Maruno T, Shirai S, Nose T (1998) Facial spasm and paroxysmal tinnitus associated with an arachnoid cyst of the cerebellopontine angle—case report. *Neurol Med Chir (Tokyo)* 38: 100–103.
56. Heier LA, Comunale JP Jr., Lavyne MH (1997) Sensorineural hearing loss and cerebellopontine angle lesions. Not always an acoustic neuroma—a pictorial essay. *Clin Imaging* 21: 213–223.
57. Babu R, Murali R (1991) Arachnoid cyst of the cerebellopontine angle manifesting as contralateral trigeminal neuralgia: case report. *Neurosurgery* 28: 886–887.
58. Hassan J, Sepulveda W, Teixeira J, Cox PM (1996) Glioependymal and arachnoid cysts: unusual causes of early ventriculomegaly in utero. *Prenat Diagn* 16: 729–733.
59. Walsh J, Gilles FH, Welch K (1978) Infantile retrocerebellar cyst with immature neural tissue. Case report. *J Neurosurg* 48: 628–631.
60. Dandy WE, Blackfan KD (1914) Internal hydrocephalus: an experimental, clinical, and pathological study. *Am J Dis Child* 8: 406–482.
61. Taggert JK Jr., Walker AE (1942) Congenital atresia of the foramens of Luschka and Magendie. *Arch Neurol Psychiatry* 48: 583–612.
62. Barkovich AJ, Kjos BO, Norman D, Edwards MS (1989) Revised classification of posterior fossa cysts and cystlike malformations based on the results of multiplanar MR imaging. *AJNR Am J Neuroradiol* 10: 977–988.
63. Harwood-Nash DC, Fitz CR (1976) *Neuroradiology in Infants and Children*. Saint Louis: C.V. Mosby Company.
64. Raybaud C, Girard N, Sevely A, Leboucq N (1996) *Neuroradiologie Pediatrique (I)*. Paris: Elsevier.
65. Volpe JJ (1994) *Neurology of the Newborn*. Philadelphia: WB Saunders.
66. Gonsette R, Potvliege R, Andre-Balisaux G, Stenuit J (1968) Mega-cisterna magna: clinical, radiologic and anatomopathologic study. *Acta Neurol Psychiatr Belg* 68: 559–570.
67. Kollias SS, Ball WS Jr., Prenger EC (1993) Cystic malformations of the posterior fossa: differential diagnosis clarified through embryologic analysis. *Radiographics* 13: 1211–1231.
68. Nelson MD Jr., Maher K, Gilles FH (2004) A different approach to cysts of the posterior fossa. *Pediatr Radiol* 34: 72-–732.

11
DEVELOPMENTAL CENTRAL NERVOUS SYSTEM ABERRATION

Introduction

Severe embryonic and early fetal life insults are generally thought to result in death or malformations. Later fetal insults result in damage to more organized brain previously acquired, and are the focus of this and succeeding chapters. Developmental anomalies related to genetic metabolic antecedents will not be considered in this book.

NEURAL DAMAGE: VARIATION DURING GESTATION

Background

The anatomic and histologic evidence of neuronal, glial, and white matter damage changes dramatically during fetal development and advancing age.[1-7] In part, this is because the fetal brain manifests shifting gross and microscopic features that vary from week to week during its development, and understanding abnormalities at any fetal age requires familiarity with normal morphology at each stage. As very immature neural tissue does not 'react' like its adult counterpart, the pathologist's criteria for assessing brain damage during gestation must differ at various developmental stages and recognize confounding artifacts. Furthermore, some immature brain insults are the same in the mature brain (for instance, infarct in a specific arterial distribution, borderzone necrosis, or focal necrosis) and some are merely quantitatively different, such as the immature brain apparently having more reserve to low arterial oxygen than the adult,[8] as seen after umbilical cord occlusion of up to 20 minutes.[9] Other insults appear unique to the developing brain (for instance, subpial or matrix hemorrhages, status marmoratus, hydrencephaly, or multicystic encephalopathy). To complicate the situation further, fetal brain vulnerability to some agents is limited to very specific developmental times.

The first section of this chapter addresses the ways in which fetal and neonatal brains react to insult, the second deals with specific events, the third reviews other abnormal histologic changes in the brain, and the fourth summarizes brain damage locations in National Collaborative Perinatal Project (NCPP) brains.

Complicating variables

Two complicating variables create difficulties in fetal brain lesion interpretation. The first variable is that the noxious influence itself modifies the timing of cellular and tissue response during fetal brain development. For instance, standard neuropathology texts assume that the incubation period for hypertrophic astrocytes following damage is the same for all insults; this is unsupportable in the immature brain based upon information about insults in neonatal feline telencephalon.[10,11] Simply changing the nature of the insult modifies the hypertrophic astrocyte incubation period several-fold.

The second complicating variable is fetal brain plasticity and repair capability. Whether this 'repair' completely reconstitutes a damaged region is unknown. This capability appears in some experimental situations, but not in others.[3,12] For instance, rat fetal brain does not regenerate if damaged late in gestation.[13] Evidence for plasticity also exists in human material; some growing axons arriving at a normal destination will grow abnormally if the local target cells are missing, or be widely diverted to abnormal targets.

Misleading notions

Unfortunately, attention is often focused only upon neuronal loss. Neuronal loss evaluation as loss/unit area on a microscopic slide is difficult and overlooks maintenance of apparent packing density from tissue shrinkage when neurons are lost. Neuronal and dendritic field growth additionally modifies neuronal packing density at different fetal ages.

Three notions, widely held among pathologists, potentially confuse interpretations about pathogenetic mechanisms. The first notion is that acute neonatal brain morphologic abnormalities arise from the same antecedents as neuronal depletion and glial scars in children surviving a fetal or neonatal insult; the acute morphologic changes are likely to have occurred during brain death. The question, then, is which of the many acute morphologic changes reflect only the sequential cascading of systemic abnormalities leading to the child's death? Such changes cannot be argued a priori to arise from the same constellation of antecedents as those found in children who survived superficially similar insults. Arbitrarily grouping many kinds of brain necrosis (acute and chronic changes, for instance) mitigates a work's potential importance.[14]

The second notion is that brain abnormalities in neonates with a common systemic illness (for instance, hyaline membrane disease) reflect damage wrought by that illness. Although this may be the case, the argument does not rest on firm ground until it is shown that the brain changes are quantitatively or qualitatively different from morphologic abnormalities found in dead neonates comparable in every way except for the systemic disease in question.

The third notion is that multiple different pathologic conditions, such as hemorrhage in various locations, gray matter necrosis, and white matter necrosis, can all be accounted for by a single etiologic entity, say hypoxic–ischemic encephalopathy.[15,16]

Changes in brain components

DELAY OR FAILURE TO ACQUIRE A COMPONENT

Failure to acquire an entire component or an adequate component amount at an appropriate developmental time constitutes a large group of fetal brain abnormalities that can be either subtle (such as white matter hypoplasia) or blatantly obvious (such as missing olfactory tract and bulb). The component whose acquisition is delayed may be estimated using bulk (brain weight or head size),[17,18] degree of gyral development,[19] myelin tract development,[20–22] or proportionate lobar or brain component growth (for instance, overall hemispheral white matter paucity).[23–25] A group subset is total acquisition failure of some component (olfactory tracts and bulbs aplasia, for example, or genetic dysmyelinogenic syndromes)[26] or pyramidal absence in genetic syndromes.[27]

COMPONENT LOSS

Programmed cell death in human telencephalic development exists in two distinct types: *embryonic*, synchronous with neuronal cell proliferation and migration, and *fetal* apoptosis, coinciding with differentiation and synaptogenesis.[28] Apoptosis is normal in the frontal lobe intermediate zone, but not in the cortex.[29] Glial cells probably start dying around the middle of gestation.

Some components are normally lost during central nervous system development.[30] For instance, portions of tuberculum olfactorium,[31] trochlear nucleus,[32] dorsal root ganglia, and anterior neuronal cell column[33,34] are lost in part after being laid down in excess; the germinal cell mass lining the lateral ventricle and its blood vessels is lost entirely. There is an approximately 35% decline in human spinal cord motoneuron numbers from 11 to 25 weeks, but none thereafter,[35] occurring more or less simultaneously with connections between the spinal trigeminal root and upper cervical anterior horn cells and fetal head movement onset (see Chapter 9). In human isocortex, neuronal number reaches a maximum at 28 weeks and declines by approximately 70% by term.[36]

Changes in response to insults during specific developmental periods

NECROSIS

Early signs of cellular necrosis include karyorrhexis, eosinophilia, nuclear membrane loss, and nuclear or cytoplasmic stain failure. Other cellular changes rest on less certain grounds as reliable signs of necrosis. One change commonly encountered in fetal, perinatal, or neonatal material is nuclear, cytoplasmic, or pericellular vacuolization, possibly reflecting the brain death mode,[37] and therefore contributing little to our evaluation of antenatal events. A similar problem arises with the dark or pyknotic neuron. Although sometimes alluded to as 'ischemic' or 'anoxic' neurons, there is no histologic way to differentiate this from the dark neuron artifact.[38]

Other abnormalities, short of focal necroses, found in neonatal telencephalic white matter include hypertrophic astrocytes, acutely damaged glial cells, and amphophilic globules.[39] They will be discussed later in this and the next chapter.

Necrosis evolution in the fetus, neonate, and infant

For nongenetically determined cerebral abnormalities, few guidelines detail when in gestation specific responses or repair capabilities develop, how they change during development, what the incubation periods are for each specific cellular change, how the insult itself influences the reacting cellular systems, or how these capabilities evolve over development.

Necrosis of mature neurons is similar to that in the adult with the exception that necrotic neurons rapidly disintegrate and one rarely sees cytoplasmic eosinophilia except when these neurons are located in the thalami, basal ganglia, or brainstem. Thus, regional variation in neuronal necrosis sometimes makes acute neuronal lesion evaluation in the immature brain difficult to assess. Midgestational fetal necrosis proceeds directly to dissolution with few hypertrophic astrocytes and little or no fibrillary gliosis. Lesions later in gestation result in small neurons with narrow eosinophilic cytoplasm and less vesicular nuclei than the adult. In fetal brains, mature (glial fibrillary acidic protein immunohistochemical staining) astrocytes are found throughout the central nervous system at around 15 gestational weeks, varying in density in different parts,[40] but their ability to react with hypertrophy appears later. Repair and reconstitution attempts within late embryonic or fetal human neural tissue are largely unrecognized. For instance, during the first 2 gestational months, one does not expect macrophages to participate in necrosis, and hypertrophic astrocytes and glial fibrils do not appear in lesion evolution. Furthermore, at this age, no usual inflammation is expected when the brain is faced with a predatory organism. Whether the tissue is merely resorbed following insult or whether some other heretofore unrecognized reaction takes place is unknown.[41]

The developing central nervous system literature is silent about the changing histologic responses to insult at 3 (possibly 2) to 6 gestational months. Prospective cavum septi pellucidi contains histiocytes during early corpus callosum formation at about 12 weeks,[42] and leptomeningeal histiocytes appear at approximately 20 weeks.[2] The literature is also unclear as to when histiocytes first appear in parenchymal lesions. Repair capabilities during the last half of gestation are known, such as malformations described (for instance, micropolygyria in a vascular bed distribution)[43] as possibly reflecting abortive repair after a vascular insult. Surprisingly, two recent pediatric neuropathology texts do not address the gestational ages at which histologic repair features first appear or the incubation periods for specific features following insult. Spatz[44] recognized that very damaged immature neural tissue liquefies and dissolves much faster than adult tissue. In rabbit neonatal spinal cord, necrotic neural tissue organization is almost complete at around 8 days and phagocytes disappear around the twelfth day without fibrillary gliosis.

In general, the more regional the maturation that produces neuronal and glial cells comparable to adult (sixth fetal month to term), the more similar the brain response to destructive events. These basic morphologic observations reflect (1) specific regional characteristics in the developing nervous system, (2) fetal organ and tissue maturation elsewhere, and (3) changes in insult damage capability with advancing developmental time. When these three processes interact, they give rise to tissue reactions varying with developmental age and brain location.

Some events leave permanent markers. Markers, although fading with time, may indicate the adverse process anatomic location, but not, usually, its nature or antecedent events. Permanent markers retained far into childhood, if not throughout life, include (1) lost neural tissue component previously attained (neuronal depletion, cystic defect, sclerotic microgyria), (2) mineralized debris, (3) abnormal arrangement, (4) acquisition failure (absent normal structural component such as neuron, brain volume, myelin, or a structure such as medullary pyramid), or (5) focal or diffuse glial scarring. These structural deficits are not usually replaced, although there is experimental evidence that some white matter cystic defects are replaced if occurring early enough.[11] Some permanent markers give a clue to the developmental time when the insult occurred. Thus, sclerotic microgyria in parietal and occipital lobe gyri imply that the insulting process occurred after 28 weeks, when these gyri are first delineated, as one would not expect gyri to appear in an already scarred region. Abnormal neuronal arrangement (for example, heterotopias) implies insult during migration very early in gestation, and a fibrillary gliosis in telencephalic white matter implies that an adverse event occurred after forebrain astrocytes at that site acquired the ability to generate glial fibrils.

Hemorrhage

Fetal hemorrhage occurs in several well-defined locations. In order of prevalence: (1) arachnoid;[45,46] (2) dural, falx, and tentorium;[46] (3) subdural;[47–51] (4) ganglionic eminence (many authors); (5) choroid plexus;[52,53] (6) intraventricular (from either ganglionic eminence and/ or choroid plexus); and (7) parenchymal rarely resulting in superficial hemosiderosis.[54] 'Periventricular' or 'peri-intraventricular' are not anatomically specific and encompass hemorrhages occurring in several locations; thus, we do not use these terms. Hemorrhage is described in detail in Chapter 14.

Fetal and Neonatal Edema

Acutely necrotic tissue swells, as does brain with a parenchymal hematoma.[55–58] Others, nevertheless, consider that fetal and neonatal brain swells without accompanying necrosis. Clinically important cerebral swelling, without concomitant necrosis or hematoma, is thought to contribute to necrosis. The few pathologic studies of fetal, term, or neonatal brain edema are in conflict, and whether edema occurs without necrosis remains in dispute. This confusion resulted from supposed analogies to adult swelling, poorly defined criteria, and high fetal brain water content relative to myelinated adult brain. Furthermore, the fetal and neonatal brain adds weight during fixation, often attaining a postfixation weight that is 30% greater than fresh weight (see Chapter 2). What some call edema in fixed fetal or neonatal brain (cerebral hemisphere enlargement, sulcal and ventricular narrowing) is likely to reflect initial high brain water content plus fluid accumulated during fixation. As immature brain differs from mature brain so markedly in its structure and composition as well as in its responses to insult, one cannot directly extrapolate information from the adult to neonatal brain.

Many neonatal brain edema experimental studies used lethal asphyxia or anoxia (for example, references 59–61). Whether or not this adequately measures uncomplicated water accumulation in cerebral tissue is a moot point; it certainly measures tissue swelling associated with functional endothelial and other cellular loss. Following asphyxia in an airtight jar until death, a 5-day-old rat pup brain exhibits only a 0.3% to 0.4% increase in water content, but no change in brain weight. Similar results were obtained with nitrogen anoxia and asphyxia with carbon dioxide. As expected with cellular death, shifts in sodium and potassium occur concomitantly with water shift. Whether the fluid and electrolyte changes concomitant with complete cellular function loss is tantamount to uncomplicated edema, as the term is used for the mature brain, is not clear. Other experiments support the conclusion that 'neonatal brain does not have a tendency to edema'.[62–64] In contrast, Anderson and Belton[65] studied brain swelling ('… increased tension of dura, pallor, and flattening of gyri') in 16 'freshly stillborn' or dead neonates considered asphyxiated, less than 1 week old, autopsied 14 to 78 hours after death (mean 40–41h), and felt that brain swelling did occur. Brain swelling was found in only four, a grossly obvious infarction in one, and small cortical hemorrhages in two. Thus, 12 had no brain swelling using these criteria. Of interest, eight had multiple visceral infarcts, suggesting a widely spread necrotizing process. Finally, two of their criteria (increased dural tension and brain pallor) are too nonspecific to provide any value in brain swelling diagnoses.

A prospective study of all neonatal autopsies in a maternity hospital, defining brain swelling as cerebral hemisphere enlargement, gyral flattening, and sulcal narrowing, observed that, without intraventricular hemorrhage, swelling was not found under 33 weeks.[66,67] Yet, at about term, 89% of brains were 'pathologically swollen.' They did not attribute the swollen brain proportion to prolonged postmortem interval, but found that flattened gyri were more likely in stillbirths than early neonatal deaths. The most swollen brains contained the least water.

In the NCPP material, all external and cut surface photographs were inspected specifically for signs of swelling. No cases were encountered with sufficient gyral crown flattening to approximate adjacent sulcal lips without underlying gross necrosis or hemorrhage. We excluded cases where edema was attributed to encephalitis, meningitis, metabolic abnormality, or congenital nephrotic syndrome.

HERNIATION

Neonatal brain herniation is even more vexing. Mechanical transtentorial parahippocampal gyral herniation was demonstrated experimentally in fetal cadavers.[68] Even so, neonatal transtentorial parahippocampal gyrus herniation with necrosis must be rare without hemispheral necrosis. Cases of neonatal transmagnal or upward transtentorial cerebellar herniation with necrosis along the impaction point at the foramen magnum or tentorial edge are even more difficult to find.[69] Herniation was not found in 29 dead meningitic neonates,[70] nor was fontanelle bulging.[65,71] Parahippocampal gyral cortical grooves without necrosis were so common they did not assist decisions about herniation.

In the NCPP sample, necrosis was not found along the parahippocampal gyral edge or lower cerebellar edges without widespread cerebral or cerebellar necrosis. Furthermore, neither hippocampal sector CA_1 nor subicular necrosis was found. Adult sector CA_1 necrosis is sometimes associated with parahippocampal gyral herniation and is thought to be a secondary lesion.

For these reasons, we are forced to conclude that (1) swelling accompanies neonatal brain necrosis and not uncomplicated fluid accumulation alone; (2) the evidence, both experimental and human, that excessive water accumulation occurs without necrosis in the immature brain is poor; and (3) although mechanical brain herniation during birth possibly occurs, parahippocampal cortical necrosis along the free tentorial edge secondary to herniation, or in hippocampal sector CA_1, must be very uncommon, as is lower cerebellar surface (biventral lobule) necrosis where it impacts the foramen magnum free edge.

GANGLIONIC EMINENCE CYSTS

Ganglionic eminence cysts overlying the caudate head were recognized in the first congenital rubella syndrome descriptions[72–76] (Fig. 11.1), but had been mentioned earlier and were thought to be posthemorrhagic cavities.[77] These lesions are usually bilateral and apparently occur at a time when the ganglionic eminence germinal cell mass is maximal (around 24–25

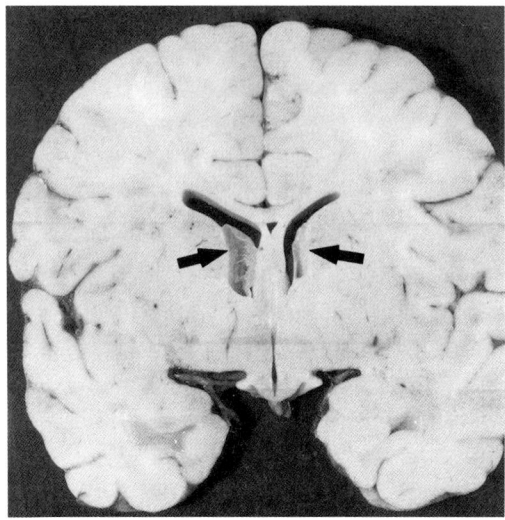

Fig. 11.1 Coronal section through frontal lobes at level of caudate head anterior to the anterior commissure and the interventricular foramen. This is the region of the main ganglionic eminence mass in the fetus at the end of the second trimester. On each side, large cysts lying ventromedial in the frontal horn have replaced the mass (arrows). Many small trabeculae lie in the left cyst.

weeks). Shaw and Alvord[75] proposed the term 'germinolysis'; it is ideal in its emphasis on loss secondary to a process different to that usually encountered in older brains. It also implies that the insult occurred at a gestational time when the germinal mass was voluminous. Thus, these lesions are likely to have occurred before the third trimester even though the cysts persist well after birth. The cysts, small or large, often contain glial trabeculae or germinal cell nodules. Most are located over the caudate head anterior to the anterior commissure and the interventricular foramen, and some continue as small cysts along the caudate body in the striothalamic groove to the atrium (Fig. 11.2). They are usually not seen along the temporal horn caudate tail. It seems likely that a large proportion reflect an encounter between the fetus and a virus;[75] the proportion remaining as posthemorrhagic cavities must be very small, as hemosiderin-filled macrophages are uncommon in their walls. In the NCPP material, 26 brains had cysts in this location, but little new information about their morphology or etiology was elucidated except to support previous observations of rare hemosiderin-filled macrophages.

Sudanophilic Lipids and Wallerian Degeneration
The late gestational fetus or infant brain contains sudanophilic lipid deposits in white matter glial cells at specific sites prior to myelination (see Chapter 6). Depending on age and site, the amount varies considerably. The fetus, similar to the adult, also accumulates sudanophilic lipid in macrophages at necrotic sites. Glial lipid deposition 'normality' or 'abnormality' has been debated for over a century; there is no argument about lipid-filled macrophages. We conclude (see Chapter 6) that glial lipid deposits antedate myelination, appearing just before

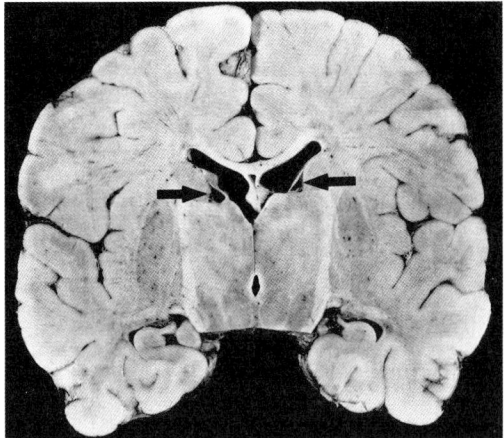

Fig. 11.2 Coronal section through frontal lobes behind the interventricular foramen through midthalamus and the caudate body. Small cysts lie on either side ventromedial to the caudate body (arrows). These small cysts are continuous with those over the caudate head and extend occipitally as far as the atrium. They usually do not extend into the temporal horn over the caudate tail.

myelin sheath deposition and disappearing just after myelination at any specific site.[78-83] Unfortunately, for the pathologist who must make decisions as to 'normality,' the criteria separating these two conditions, premyelin glial lipid deposit and glial fatty metamorphosis, are still confusing and the subject remains unsettled. The NCPP material was not usable for a study of this material, as it requires frozen sections.

In the corticospinal tract, fetal Wallerian degeneration was defined as sudanophilic lipid within the tract following cerebral lesions,[84] but these brief reports did not mention the gliosis and macrophage deposition that accompany adult Wallerian degeneration. There were no NCPP cases with tract gliosis and macrophage deposition, the adult Wallerian degeneration hallmarks.

Other histologic changes in fetal brain

MICROGLIA

Microglial colonization of fetal brain is well recognized.[85,86] Thus, diffuse microglia with pleomorphic, elongated, and frequently hyperchromatic nuclei are not diagnostic in fetal brain unless concentrated in microglial nodules. Their presence was coded in one site, the striatum, even though they were widely present in gray and white matter above and below the tentorium. They gradually disappear over the first year. Striatal microglia cell distribution in the NCPP material is displayed in Table 11.1.

Microglia are located in various sites in the human fetal brain.[86-89] They first appear in the fetal brain at about 8 weeks,[90,91] 10 weeks,[92] or 13 weeks.[93] They are probably antigen-presenting cells;[89] lipopolysaccharide is a potent stimulus for microglia but not for astrocytes. Microglia may be key astrocyte response regulators.[94]

245

TABLE 11.1

The proportion of cases containing microglia in the forebrain

Gestational weeks	Cases in each gestational period (%)
11–19	21
20–23	32
24–27	43
28–31	64
32–35	58
36–39	77
>40	73

MACROPHAGES

Inflammatory responses change with age in human fetuses and differ from the adult responses.[95,96] Macrophages are present immunohistochemically from 10 to 12 weeks.[84,92,97] Macrophage participation in response to late fetal brain necrosis is similar to that in the adult, insofar as is known. Some think macrophages contribute to white matter damage.[98] Its vacuolar or granular cytoplasm distinguishes it from hypertrophic astrocytes, acutely damaged glial cells, and premyelin glial cells (see Chapter 6). Frequently encountered in fetal leptomeninges, the macrophage in this location carries little significance and is likely to represent primitive meninx remodeling as the leptomeninges are formed, a process continuing throughout late gestation. Parenchymal macrophages, nonetheless, are distinctly abnormal and seem to be largely a third trimester telencephalic phenomenon. Parenchymal macrophages were more prevalent than cavitary necroses in the NCPP material. They appear at some sites much earlier in gestation, such as an early cavum septi pellucidi at the end of the first trimester.[84] Thus, macrophages respond much earlier in gestation than astrocytes.

INFLAMMATION

Inflammatory response markers, either acute or subacute, were rarely encountered in the NCPP population. Although polymorphonuclear leukocytes, lymphocytes or plasma cells, perivascular inflammatory cell cuffs, and microglial nodules were separately coded, they were usually encountered with neonatal leptomeningitis.

MINERALIZATION

Basophilic neuronal, axonal, or parenchymal debris encrustation was included in this category. Amphophilic globules were not included. Cases of adventitial or medial vascular mineralization were not encountered in the NCPP population.

VASCULAR OCCLUSION

Venous or arterial occlusions were extremely rare, even in serially sectioned cases with germinal matrix, choroid plexus, or ventricular hemorrhage. There were no internal cerebral or terminal vein thromboses in the NCPP material, making it unlikely that they cause germinal matrix hemorrhage.[99] Vascular occlusions will be further discussed in Chapter 13.

Pathologic process locations

There were marked differences in lesions tending to occur at the various sites screened in the NCPP study. Hemorrhage was the most likely lesion encountered, located either in leptomeninges, transient subventricular germinal tissue, or in deep hemispheral white matter. For the most part, necrotizing processes were microscopic rather than macroscopic and had a striking predilection for cerebral white matter when compared with gray matter.

GRAY MATTER

Only 2% of NCPP cases had small focal necroses in the cerebral cortex and only a few of these contained macrophages, hypertrophic astrocytes, or mineralization; no cavitary lesions were encountered. Similarly, only a few focal necroses were found in the thalamus or striatum. In 3% of cases, amphophilic globules were present in gray structures (see Chapter 12). In the cerebellar cortex or deep cerebellar nuclei, hemorrhage was present in 3% and focal necroses in 1%, similar to cerebral cortex figures.

The midbrain, pons, and medulla were striking for their lack of focal necrosis or hemorrhage. No brainstem midline necroses or hemorrhagic necroses were recognized analogous to the secondary midline lesions regularly following supratentorial parahippocampal gyral herniations. There were no lesions analogous to the cerebral peduncle necrosis contralateral to a large supratentorial lesion. These negative findings stand in mute testimony to the lack of transtentorial herniation from any supratentorial mass in neonatal brain (discussed above).

WHITE MATTER

Necrosis and hemorrhage were frequent in cerebral white matter. To gain perspective, white matter hemorrhages were found in about the same case proportion as germinal tissue hemorrhage. The white matter hemorrhages were separate and distinct from those in germinal tissue and generally seemed far smaller, sometimes consisting of only a few erythrocytes. Differences in deep white matter hemorrhage size compared with those in germinal tissue were striking; they were almost always much larger at the latter site, but there was no clear evidence of germinal matrix hematoma dissecting into the adjacent white or gray matter. Regularly, the germinal matrix hemorrhages, found adjacent to white matter or caudate, did not extend into either site.

Far more frequent than hemorrhage, though, were hypertrophic astrocytes in telencephalic white matter (38%). In addition, 15% of NCPP cases contained acutely damaged glia, 25% amphophilic globules, and 8% focal necroses. Macrophages, mineralized debris, and inflammatory responses occurred only in a very small number of cases. The paraventricular white matter, within 0.5cm of the ventricular wall, contained the same lesions, but in a far smaller case proportion.

The posterior limb, brainstem, and cerebellar white matter were infrequently necrotic, in distinct contrast to cerebral white matter.

GERMINAL MATRIX

The transient germinal matrix contained hemorrhage, as noted above, in a very large case proportion. A much smaller case proportion had hemosiderin, attesting to a rebleed or persistence of an initial oozing site. Focal areas of karyorrhexis were found in 2% and cavitary lesions were found in 27 cases (2%).

HIPPOCAMPUS

The hippocampus must be mentioned in passing. No frank necrosis was encountered. Perineuronal vacuolization, pyknosis, and hyperchromasia we ascribed to agonal changes and felt that they offered little to our long-term understanding of lesions. There were no cases with Sommer's sector sclerosis, necrosis, or gliosis; again, an observation denying hippocampus sclerosis of neonatal origin based on significant lesions in this population (see section on herniation).

One source of possible hippocampal lesion misunderstanding might be neonatal neuronal immaturity in hippocampal sector CA_1 compared with sector CA_2.[100] CA_2 neurons were larger than CA_1 neurons in 65% of cases and equal in size in 29%. In the remaining 6%, there was no clear distinction.

Summary and conclusions

This chapter shows that shifting developmental neuroanatomy potentially makes lesion interpretation difficult. Further, the inciting agent can, in and of itself, change the incubation period for the reacting cellular population. In summary, there is marked variation in gestational ages when specific lesions occur, as well as marked differences in the sites where they are likely to occur in late fetal or neonatal life, if the NCPP population is representative. In this large group, there was no hippocampal or mesial temporal sclerosis or necrosis.

REFERENCES

1. Spatz H (1920) A special reaction of the immature central nervous system. *Z Neur* 53: 363–394.
2. Dąmbska M (1968) Encephalic necrosis and inflammatory reaction in fetuses and newborns. *Pol Med J* 7: 404–434.
3. Demeyer WE (1973) Development of axonal pathways after neurosurgical lesions in the septum of the fetal rat: fornix ventralis, commissure of the fornix ventralis, corpus callosum and anterior commissure. *Res Publ Assoc Res Nerv Ment Dis* 51: 269–282.
4. Myers RE (1969) Brain pathology following fetal vascular occlusion: an experimental study. *Invest Ophthalmol* 8: 41–50.
5. Dąmbska M, Dydyk L, Szretter T, Wozniewicz J, Myers RE (1976) Topography of lesions in newborn and infant brains following cardiac arrest and resuscitation. Damage to brain and hemispheres. *Biol Neonate* 29(3–4): 194–206.
6. Gilles FH (1983) Neural damage: Inconstancy during gestation. In: Gilles F, Leviton A, Dooling E, editors. *The Developing Human Brain: Growth and Epidemiologic Neuropathology*. Boston: Wright-PSG, pp. 227–243.
7. Myers RE (1989) Cerebral ischemia in the developing primate fetus. *Biomed Biochim Acta* 48(2–3): S137–142.
8. Boyle R (1670) New pneumatical experiments about respiration. *Phil Trans R Soc Lond (Biol)* 5: 2011–2031.

9. Keunen H, Blanco CE, van Reempts JL, Hasaart TH (1997) Absence of neuronal damage after umbilical cord occlusion of 10, 15, and 20 minutes in midgestation fetal sheep. *Am J Obstet Gynecol* 176: 515–520.

10. Gilles FH, Averill Jr. DR, Kerr CS (1977) Neonatal endotoxin encephalopathy. *Ann Neurol* 2: 49–56.

11. Gilles FH, Averill Jr. DR, Kerr CS (1977) Changes in neonatally induced cerebral lesions with advancing age. *J Neuropathol Exp Neurol* 36: 666–679.

12. Schneider GE (1979) Is it really better to have your brain lesion early? A revision of the 'Kennard principle.' *Neuropsychologia* 17: 557–583.

13. Banister CM, Chapman SA (1986) Response of the fetal rat brain to trauma during the 17th to 21st days of gestation. *Dev Med Child Neurol* 28: 600–609.

14. Grunnet ML (1979) Periventricular leukomalacia complex. *Arch Pathol Lab Med* 103: 6–10.

15. Rorke LB (1992) Anatomical features of the developing brain implicated in pathogenesis of hypoxic–ischemic injury. *Brain Pathol* 2: 211–221.

16. Sladky JT, Rorke LB(1986) Perinatal hypoxic/ischemic spinal cord injury. *Pediatr Pathol* 6: 87–101.

17. Kozlowski PB, Sher JH, Nicastri AD, Rudelli RD (1989) Brain morphology in the Galloway syndrome. *Clin Neuropathol* 8: 85–91.

18. Mercuri E, Ricci D, Cowan FM, et al (2000) Head growth in infants with hypoxic–ischemic encephalopathy: correlation with neonatal magnetic resonance imaging. *Pediatrics* 106(2 Pt 1): 235–243.

19. Chi JG, Dooling EC, Gilles FH (1977) Gyral development of the human brain. *Ann Neurol* 1: 86–93.

20. Leviton A, Gilles FH, Dooling EC (1983) The epidemiology of delayed myelination. In: Gilles FH, Leviton A, Dooling EC, editors. *The Developing Human Brain: Growth and Epidemiologic Neuropathology*. Boston: Wright-PSG, pp. 185–192.

21. de Koning TJ, Jaeken J, Pineda M, Van Maldergem L, Poll-The BT, van der Knaap MS (2000) Hypomyelination and reversible white matter attenuation in 3-phosphoglycerate dehydrogenase deficiency. *Neuropediatrics* 31: 287–292.

22. Rousset CI, Chalon S, Cantagrel S, et al (2006) Maternal exposure to LPS induces hypomyelination in the internal capsule and programmed cell death in the deep gray matter in newborn rats. *Pediatr Res* 59: 428–433.

23. Chattha AS, Richardson EP Jr. (1977) Cerebral white-matter hypoplasia. *Arch Neurol* 34: 137–141.

24. Huppi PS, Schuknecht B, Boesch C, et al (1996) Structural and neurobehavioral delay in postnatal brain development of preterm infants. *Pediatr Res* 39: 895–901.

25. Pujol J, Lopez-Sala A, Sebastian-Galles N, et al (2004) Delayed myelination in children with developmental delay detected by volumetric MRI. *Neuroimage* 22: 897–903.

26. Benda C (1941) Microcephaly. *Am J Psychiatr* 97: 1135–1145.

27. Chow CW, Halliday JL, Anderson RM, Danks DM, Fortune DW (1985) Congenital absence of pyramids and its significance in genetic diseases. *Acta Neuropathol (Berl)* 65(3–4): 313–317.

28. Rakic S, Zecevic N (2000) Programmed cell death in the developing human telencephalon. *Eur J Neurosci* 12: 2721–2734.

29. Anlar B, Atilla P, Cakar N, Tombakoglu M, Bulun A (2003) Apoptosis in the developing human brain: a preliminary study of the frontal region. *Early Hum Dev* 71: 53–60.

30. Saunders JW Jr. (1966) Death in embryonic systems. *Science* 154: 604–612.

31. Humphrey T (1967) The development of the human tuberculum olfactorium during the first three months of embryonic life. *J Hirnforsch* 9: 437.

32. Cowan W, Wenger E (1967) Cell loss in the trochlear nucleus of the chick during normal development and after radical extirpation of the optic vesicle. *J Exp Zool* 164: 264.

33. Romanes GH (1946) Motor localization and effects of nerve injury on ventral horn cells of spinal cord. *J Anat* 80: 117.

34. Levi-Montalcini R (1950) The origin and development of the visceral system in the spinal cord of the chick embryo. *J Morphol* 86: 253–283.

35. Forger NG, Breedlove SM (1987) Motoneuronal death during human fetal development. *J Comp Neurol* 264: 118–122.

36. Rabinowicz T, de Courten-Myers GM, Petetot JM, Xi G, de los Reyes E (1996) Human cortex development: estimates of neuronal numbers indicate major loss late during gestation. *J Neuropathol Exp Neurol* 55: 320–328.

37. Lindenberg R (1956) Morphotropic and morphostatic necrobiosis: investigations on nerve cells of the brain. *Am J Pathol* 32: 1147.

38. Cammermeyer J (1962) An evaluation of the significance of the 'dark' neuron. *Ergeb Anat Entwicklungsgesch* 36: 1.
39. Gilles F, Murphy S (1969) Perinatal telencephalic leucoencephalopathy. *J Neurol Neurosurg Psych* 32: 404–413.
40. Roessmann U, Gambetti P (1986) Astrocytes in the developing human brain. An immunohistochemical study. *Acta Neuropathol (Berl)* 70(3–4): 308–313.
41. Becker H (1949) Uber Hirngefassausschatungen; intrakranielle Gefassverschlusse; uber experimentell Hydranencephalie (Blasenhirn). *Dsch Ztschr Nervenh* 161: 446–505.
42. Rakic P, Yakovlev PI (1968) Development of the corpus callosum and cavum septi in man. *J Comp Neurol* 132: 45–72.
43. Richman DP, Stewart RM, Caviness VS Jr. (1974) Cerebral microgyria in a 27-week fetus: an architectonic and topographic analysis. *J Neuropathol Exp Neurol* 33: 374–384.
44. Spatz H (1921) Über die Vorgänge nach experimenteller Rückenmarksdurchtrennung mit besonderer Berücksichtigung der Unterschiede der Reaktionsweise des reifen und des unreifen Gewebes nebst Beziehungen zur menschlicheden Pathologie (Porenzephalie und Syrinomyelie). In: Nissl F, Alzheimer A, editors. *Histologische und Histopathologische Arbeiten, Ergänzungsband*. Jena: Fischer, pp. 49–367.
45. Vlasiuk VV, Keshelava SD (1986) [Pathomorphology and pathogenesis of leptomeningeal hemorrhages in fetuses and newborn infants]. *Arkh Patol* 48: 36–42.
46. Gilles FH (1991) Perinatal neuropathology. In: Davis R, Robertson D, editors. *Textbook of Neuropathology*. Baltimore: Williams & Wilkins, pp. 281–330.
47. Gilles FH, Shillito JS (1970) Infantile hydrocephalus: retrocerebellar subdural hematoma. *J Pediatr* 76: 529–532.
48. Blank NK, Strand R, Gilles FH, Palakshappa A (1978) Posterior fossa subdural hematomas in neonates. *Arch Neurol* 35: 108–111.
49. Gunn TR, Becroft DM (1984) Unexplained intracranial haemorrhage in utero: the battered fetus? *Aust N Z J Obstet Gynaecol* 24: 17–22.
50. Green PM, Wilson H, Romaniuk C, May P, Welch CR (1999) Idiopathic intracranial haemorrhage in the fetus. *Fetal Diagn Ther* 14: 275–278.
51. Folkerth RD, McLaughlin ME, Levine D (2001) Organizing posterior fossa hematomas simulating developmental cysts on prenatal imaging: report of 3 cases. *J Ultrasound Med* 20: 1233–1240.
52. Larroche JC (1972) Post-haemorrhagic hydrocephalus in infancy. Anatomical study. *Biol Neonate* 20: 287–299.
53. Donat JF, Okazaki H, Kleinberg F, Reagan TJ (1978) Intraventricular hemorrhages in full-term and premature infants. *Mayo Clin Proc* 53: 437–441.
54. Kidron D, Tepper R, Beyth Y, Bernheim J (1995) Superficial hemosiderosis in a second trimester fetus: pathological and clinical manifestations. *Hum Pathol* 26: 1038–1040.
55. Lindenberg R (1955) Compression of brain arteries as pathogenetic factor for tissue necroses and their areas of predilection. *J Neuropathol Exp Neurol* 14: 223–243.
56. Richardson JC, Chambers RA, Heywood PM (1959) Encephalopathies of anoxia and hypoglycemia. *Arch Neurol* 1: 178–190.
57. Levine S, Klein M (1960) Ischemic infarction and swelling in the rat brain. *AMA Arch Path* 69: 544–553.
58. Lupton BA, Hill A, Roland EH, Whitfield MF, Flodmark O (1988) Brain swelling in the asphyxiated term newborn: pathogenesis and outcome. *Pediatrics* 82: 139–146.
59. Myers RE, Beard R, Adamsons K (1969) Brain swelling in the newborn rhesus monkey following prolonged partial asphyxia. *Neurology* 19: 1012–108.
60. De Souza SW, Dobbing J (1973) Cerebral edema in developing brain. II Asphyxia in the five-day-old rat. *Exp Neurol* 39: 414–423.
61. De Souza SW, Dobbing J (1973) Cerebral oedema in developing brain. 3. Brain water and electrolytes in immature asphyxiated rats treated with dexamethasone. *Biol Neonate* 22: 388–397.
62. Spector RG (1962) Water content of the immature rat brain following cerebral anoxia and ischemia. *Br J Exp Pathol* 43: 472–479.
63. Streicher E, Wisniewski H, Klatzo I (1965) Resistance of immature brain to experimental cerebral edema. *Neurol* 15: 833.
64. Tweed WA, Pash M, Doig G (1981) Cerebrovascular mechanisms in perinatal asphyxia: the role of vasogenic brain edema. *Pediatr Res* 15: 44–46.

65. Anderson JM, Belton NR (1974) Water and electrolyte abnormalities in the human brain after severe intrapartum asphyxia. *J Neurol Neurosurg Psychiatry* 37: 514–520.

66. Pryse-Davies J (1973) Brain swelling in the newborn: artifact, development, or pathology. *Arch Dis Child* 48: 161–162.

67. Pryse-Davies J, Beard RW (1973) A necropsy study of brain swelling in the newborn with special reference to cerebellar herniation. *J Pathol* 109: 51–73.

68. Earle KM, Baldwin M, Penfield W (1953) Incisural sclerosis and temporal lobe seizures produced by hippocampal herniation at birth. *AMA Arch Neurol Psychiatr* 69: 27–42.

69. Fischer EG, Strand RD, Gilles FH (1972) Cerebellar necrosis simulating tumor in infancy. *J Pediatr* 81: 98–100.

70. Berman PH, Banker BQ (1966) Neonatal meningitis. A clinical and pathological study of 29 cases. *Pediatrics* 38: 6–24.

71. Gibson N, Ball M, Kelsey D (1975) Anterior fontanelle herniation. *Pediatrics* 56: 466–469.

72. Rorke LB, Spiro AJ (1967) Cerebral lesions in congenital rubella syndrome. *J Pediatr* 70: 243–255.

73. Larroche JC (1972) Sub-ependymal pseudo-cysts in the newborn. *Biol Neonate* 21: 170–183.

74. Shaw CM (1973) Subependymal germinolysis. *J Neuropathol Exp Neurol* 32: 153.

75. Shaw CM, Alvord EC Jr. (1974) Subependymal germinolysis. *Arch Neurol* 31: 374–381.

76. De León GA, Girling DJ (1975) Cystic degeneration of the telencephalic subependymal germinal layer in newborn infants. *J Neurol Neurosurg Psychiatry* 38: 265–271.

77. Schwartz P (1961) *Birth Injuries of the Newborn, Morphology, Pathogenesis, Clinical Pathology and Prevention*. New York: Hafner Publishing.

78. Mickel HS, Gilles FH (1970) Changes in glial cells during human telencephalic myelinogenesis. *Brain* 93: 337–346.

79. Virchow R (1867) Zur pathologischen anatomie des gehirns: I Congenitale encephalitis und myelitis. *Virch Arch* 38: 129–138.

80. Jellinger K, Seitelberger F, Kozik M (1971) Perivascular accumulation of lipids in the infant human brain. *Acta Neuropathol* 19: 331–342.

81. Sumi SM, Leech RW, Alvord EC Jr., Eng M, Ueland K (1973) Sudanophilic lipids in the unmyelinated primate cerebral white matter after intrauterine hypoxia and acidosis. *Res Publ Assoc Res Nerv Ment Dis* 51: 176–197.

82. Larroche JC, Amakawa H (1973) Glia of myelination and fat deposit during early myelogenesis. *Biol Neonate* 22: 421–435.

83. Leech RW, Alvord EC (1974) Glial fatty metamorphosis: an abnormal response of premyelin glia frequently accompanying periventricular leukomalacia. *Am J Pathol* 74: 603–612.

84. Lemire RJ, Loeser JD, Leech RW, Alvord EC Jr. (1975) *Normal and Abnormal Development of the Human Nervous System*. Hagerstown, MD: Harper and Row.

85. del Rio-Hortega P (1932) Microglia. In: Penfield W, editor. *Cytology and Cellular Pathology of the Nervous System*. New York: Hoeber, pp. 483–534.

86. Kershman J (1939) Genesis of microglia in the human brain. *Arch Neurol Psychiatry* 41: 24–50.

87. Del Rio-Hortega P (1921) Estudios sobre la neuroglia. La glia de escasas radiciones (oligodendroglia). *Mem Real Soc Esp d Hist Nat* 11: 213.

88. Graeber MB, Streit WJ (1990) Microglia: immune network in the CNS. *Brain Pathol* 1: 2–5.

89. Streit WJ, Graeber MB, Kreutzberg GW (1988) Functional plasticity of microglia: a review. *Glia* 1: 301–307.

90. Wierzba-Bobrowicz T, Gwiazda E, Poszwinska Z (1995) Morphological study of microglia in human mesencephalon during the development and aging. *Folia Neuropathol* 33: 77–83.

91. Wierzba-Bobrowicz T, Kosno-Kruszewska E, Gwiazda E, Lechowicz W (1998) The comparison of microglia maturation in different structures of the human nervous system. *Folia Neuropathol* 36: 152–160.

92. Choi BH (1981) Hematogenous cells in the central nervous system of developing human embryos and fetuses. *J Comp Neurol* 196: 683–694.

93. Hutchins KD, Dickson DW, Rashbaum WK, Lyman WD (1990) Localization of morphologically distinct microglial populations in the developing human fetal brain: implications for ontogeny. *Brain Res Dev Brain Res* 55: 95–102.

94. Lee SC, Liu W, Dickson DW, Brosnan CF, Berman JW (1993) Cytokine production by human fetal microglia and astrocytes. Differential induction by lipopolysaccharide and IL-1 beta. *J Immunol* 150: 2659–2667.

95. Dąmbska M, Laure-Kamionowska M (1998) The morphological picture of developing meningo-enceph-alitis in central nervous system. *Folia Neuropathol* 36: 205–210.

96. Darrow VC, Alvord EC Jr., Mack LA, Hodson WA (1988) Histologic evolution of the reactions to hemor-rhage in the premature human infant's brain. A combined ultrasound and autopsy study and a comparison with the reaction in adults. *Am J Pathol* 130: 44–58.

97. Esiri MM, al Izzi MS, Reading MC (1991) Macrophages, microglial cells, and HLA-DR antigens in fetal and infant brain. *J Clin Pathol* 44: 102–106.

98. Dammann O, Durum S, Leviton A (2001) Do white cells matter in white matter damage? *Trends Neurosci* 24: 320–324.

99. Manterola A, Towbin A, Yakovlev PI (1966) Cerebral infarction in the human fetus near term. *J Neuropathol Exp Neurol* 25: 479–488.

100. Friede RL (1972) Ponto-subicular lesions in perinatal anoxia. *Arch Pathol* 94: 343–354.

12
CEREBRAL WHITE MATTER ABNORMALITIES

Introduction

By the early nineteenth century, the concept of cortical and white matter damage from infarct was well established.[1–3] Clinicians ignored abnormalities largely limited to cerebral white matter in preterm and term newborns even though white matter abnormalities were well known to pathologists from the mid-nineteenth century.[4–6] Schmorl[7] summarized the large numbers of cases in previous descriptions (those of Moebius, Vivius, Herschfeld, and Hlava) when he documented his own 280 cases of neonates with white matter focal necroses in 1904. Nevertheless, these early investigators overlooked white matter abnormalities other than focal necroses, although adequate microscopes had been available from the late nineteenth century.[8] Careful investigators of the twentieth century, additionally, noted mild loss of cortical and thalamic neurons in cases with white matter focal necroses.[9] More recent investigators have often conflated other white matter abnormalities into single entities under new names, such as periventricular leukomalacia, a commonly used term combining focal necroses and diffuse white matter hypertrophic astrocytes.

PREVALENCE OF WHITE MATTER ABNORMALITIES

There are four distinct white matter abnormalities: diffuse hypertrophic astrocytes; acutely damaged glial cells; amphophilic globules; and focal necroses; as well as their combinations. Diffuse white matter hypertrophic astrocytes were the most prevalent abnormality in the National Collaborative Perinatal Project (NCPP) material (Table 12.1), fourfold that of focal necrosis and much greater than the number of cases with neuronal necrosis. Amphophilic globules and acutely damaged glial cells were intermediate in prevalence. Are these histologic abnormalities markers of a single entity or several different entities? Are the glial cell abnormalities part of normal white matter development? This chapter will (1) briefly discuss each entity with its history, (2) describe a clustering strategy to help decide whether the four abnormalities constitute single or multiple entities, (3) show the risk factor similarities and differences of each histologic entity, and (4) demonstrate how risk factors and histologic entities are related.

TABLE 12.1

Prevalence of white matter abnormalities

	Percentage of cases in 20–40 weeks
Hypertrophic astrocytes	38
Amphophilic globules	26
Acutely damaged glial cells	15
Focal necrosis	8
Neuronal necrosis	2

Diffuse white matter hypertrophic astrocytes

The most prevalent abnormality in fetal forebrain white matter, astrocytic cytoplasmic hypertrophy, occurred in about one-third of NCPP brains.[10–13] The diminutive, yet distinct, cloud of eosinophilic cytoplasm that distinguishes this cell from other telencephalic glial cells antedating myelination is readily recognized and is not 'myelination gliosis'[14] (Fig. 12.1a,b). Cells contain star-shaped eosinophilic cytoplasm and have medium-to-large vesicular nuclei with a fine chromatin stippling, distinguishing them from the many other glial cell types in immature white matter. The cytoplasm tends to extend from the nucleus in rays or narrow bands and accompanies glial fibril production.[8] In kittens, this persists into adulthood following neonatal white matter lesions.[11] In focally damaged neonatal, child, and adult brains, hypertrophic astrocytes increase in number adjacent to the lesion. Nonetheless, in late fetal and neonatal white matter with diffuse hypertrophic astrocytes, there is little increase in the total number of astrocytes. Hence, there are two varieties of hypertrophic astrocytes in fetal white matter: the first is a widespread diffuse change in white matter glial cells converting some into hypertrophic astrocytes without much increase in total number; the second is a focal increase in hypertrophic astrocytes around necrotic lesions.

These statements about the human infant's forebrain white matter are in distinct contrast to Spatz's assertions that glial scar does not develop after neonatal insult, there is no fibrillary gliosis, and the development of astrocytic hypertrophy is rare.[15] The difference between these two sets of observations is likely to reflect the different species used in each set of experiments (rabbit,[15] human,[8] and kitten);[16] regional differences in responsiveness between the forebrain and spinal cord;[17,18] or differences in histologic techniques. Late fetal hypertrophic astrocyte production includes an increase in cytoplasmic glycogen,[19] and is probably derived from a separate class of astrocytes.[20] The incubation period for astroglial cell hypertrophy to develop is very short at 2 to 3 days (kitten), varies with different insults, and is delayed after some insults.[16,21] The fetal human brain hypertrophic astrocytic incubation period is unknown, as is its life cycle; nevertheless, cytoplasmic hypertrophy diminishes with time.

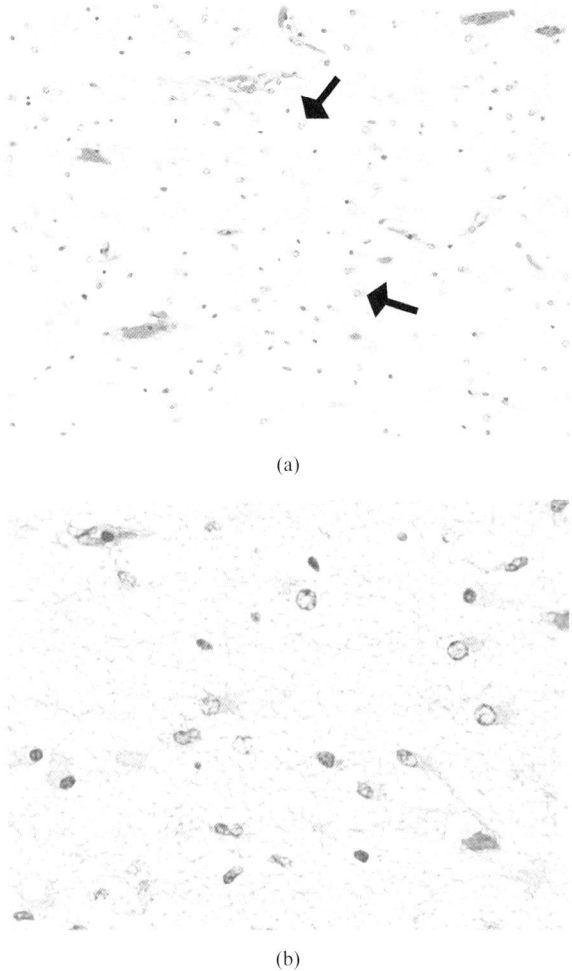

(a)

(b)

Fig. 12.1 Diffuse white matter hypertrophic astrocytes. (a) This low-power view contains multiple glial cells, each with a splash of eosinophilic cytoplasm (arrows). Note that the total glial cell population is not particularly increased. The capillaries in this field are unremarkable. (b) At higher power, the diffuse hypertrophic astrocytes usually contain fairly large nuclei with a distinct nucleolus, although some in this field have smaller darker nuclei. Several have a process that extends toward a neighboring capillary.

The ability of a subset of glial cells to alter and become hypertrophic astrocytes originates after midgestation in humans[22,23] (Table 12.2), whereas in the rat, cortical astrocytic capacity to hypertrophy develops around the second postnatal week.[24] Either the capability or insults capable of inducing these astrocytic changes appear during the third trimester. The diffuse hypertrophic astrocyte proportion of NCPP cases by gestational age is displayed in Table 12.2, confirming their appearance in the second half of gestation.

255

TABLE 12.2

Hypertrophic astrocytes

Gestational weeks	Percentage of cases in each gestational period
20–23	9
24–27	14
28–31	34
32–35	46
36–39	59
>40	63

In human fetal forebrain after midgestation, the location of diffuse hypertrophic astrocytes is remarkable in its bilateral lobar symmetry. When present, the small hypertrophic astrocytes are usually located in the frontal, parietal, and occipital white matter, and unusually in the temporal lobe. These astrocytes are limited to white matter and are not found in the nearby caudate, putamen, thalamus, or cortex, unlike focal lesions, which may damage both gray and white matter.

This diffuse astrocytic hypertrophy is easily separable from those mature human central nervous system regions normally containing glial fibrils, including the ventricular wall, subpial layer, brainstem, spinal cord, and dentate nuclear hilus. Brainstem and spinal cord glial fibril deposition is a late gestational phenomenon[25] and is variable within any section (that is, there is a different density subpially, subependymally, and within neuronal aggregates). The developmental timing for the lateral and third ventricular subependymal glial fibril is unknown.

Amphophilic globules

Amphophilic globules consist of small amphophilic or basophilic deposits, sometimes laminated, in telencephalic white matter, usually in proximity to sinusoids or capillaries, suggesting that their presence reflects local vascular integrity loss (Fig. 12.2a–c). They contain carbohydrate residues, calcium, and protein, but no iron.[8] In any given affected fetal forebrain section, globules may be few or frequent and do not elicit a focal glial response. Found preferentially in white matter, they occasionally occur in striatum. Although of doubtful usefulness as an index of perinatal 'anoxia' (because this vague term lacks specificity),[26] they are well recognized.[8,10,16,17,27–34] Amphophilic globules were frequently encountered in the NCPP material and the case proportion gradually increased with advancing gestational age (Table 12.3), indicating that they develop well after the development of the blood–brain barrier. Insults specific to late gestation must be related to this timing, but their nature is unknown.

Acutely damaged glial cells

Normal glial cells in unmyelinated white matter have an almost unstainable cytoplasm (in conventional stains) and either a large pale vesicular nucleus or a small dark hyperchromatic nucleus. Another glial cell abnormality, beyond astrocytic cytoplasmic hypertrophy of

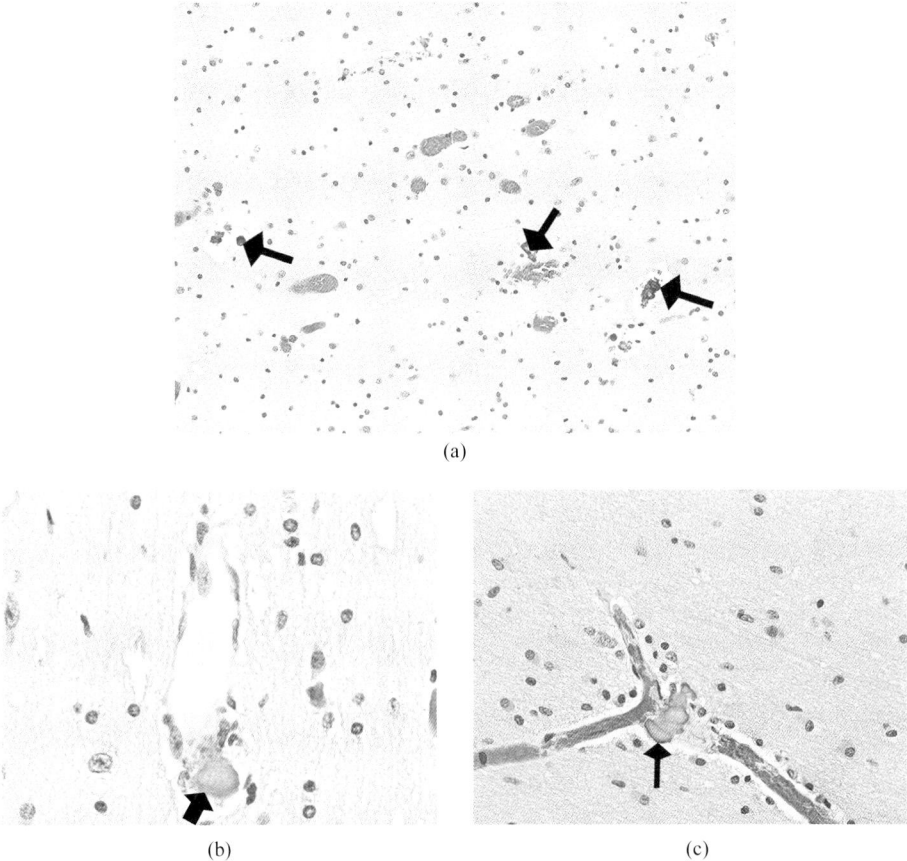

(a)

(b)   (c)

Fig. 12.2 (a) This low-power view of white matter containing amphophilic globules (arrows) demonstrates the relatively large numbers sometimes encountered. Several lie adjacent to a nearby capillary or sinusoid. There are no hypertrophic astrocytes in this field. This field also demonstrates the relatively normal glial cell density expected in frontal white matter at this age. (b) A higher-power view of a small sinusoid demonstrates an amphophilic globule occupying the sinusoidal wall (arrow). (c) This amphophilic globule (arrow) crosses a large capillary adjacent to a branching point. There are no hypertrophic astrocytes.

astrocytes, occurs when their nuclei are pyknotic, irregular, or hyperchromatic and their cytoplasm becomes globular, amphophilic, or darkly eosinophilic without apparent cellular processes. The nucleus remains small, round, or oval and does not undergo karyorrhexis; whereas nuclear chromatin is clumped, the nuclear membrane remains intact. The hyaline or faintly granular eosinophilic or amphophilic cytoplasm of these cells bears little or no resemblance to the vesiculate cytoplasm of macrophages, to pleomorphic, hyperchromatic microglial nuclei, or even to hypertrophic astrocytes, even though intermediate stages may be encountered. Acutely damaged glial cells are distinct from the diffuse white matter hypertrophic astrocytes mentioned above, necrotic glial cells undergoing karyorrhexis or apoptosis, and premyelin

257

TABLE 12.3

Amphophilic globules

Gestational weeks	Percentage of cases in each gestational period
20–23	8
24–27	14
28–31	31
32–35	30
36–39	32
>40	35

oligodendroglial cell precursors. We specifically designated these cells as acutely damaged glial cells.[8] Like diffuse white matter hypertrophic astrocytes, there is little, if any, increase in total white matter glial cell numbers when these glial changes are present. They are either partially damaged glial cells or altered by an unknown tissue insult. Neither their incubation period nor their evolution is known. These cellular changes are largely found in late gestation and were approximately one-third as prevalent as hypertrophic astrocytes (Table 12.4).

Focal necroses

Encompassed within this category is white matter focal necrosis in any stage; ranging from simple coagulative necrosis to organized small or large cystic lesions, frequently located adjacent to linear or globular, eosinophilic or mineralized, axonal retraction balls and other debris. Some focal necroses are small or microscopic simple coagulative necroses (Fig. 12.3). When coagulative necroses are located subcortically below sulci, they are sometimes called 'subcortical leukomalacia,' suggesting a separate entity. Slightly older focal necroses appear grossly as chalky white small lesions (containing fat-filled macrophages, microscopically) (Figs. 12.4, 12.5, and 12.6), and are scattered from ventricular wall to subcortical U-fibers. They strongly resemble their magnetic resonance images (Fig. 12.7). Some appear linear,[30,31] seemingly following the transmural radial vascular channels extending from gyral white matter core to the ventricular wall (see Chapter 8). This linearity of some small focal necroses has been noted by others.[35,36] While focal necroses occur in both hemispheres, they are rarely exactly symmetric in location. Many are located in parietal or occipital white matter, often interrupting the external sagittal stratum (optic radiation), internal sagittal stratum (corpus callosum forceps major, tapetum), or both. One expects residual homonymous defects in the lower visual fields from the prevalence and location of the latter focal necroses.

Larger lesions also sometimes appear linear, oriented roughly perpendicular to the ventricular wall. Still larger lesions are cavitary, of many sizes, located anywhere from the ventricular wall to the overlying cortex[37] (Fig. 12.8), or may include all of the white matter from the ventricular wall to the cortex (Fig. 12.9). The large focal necroses usually have chalky edges and shaggy walls with trabeculi composed of a few retained vessels. These large lesions are much less common than the small focal necroses. Sonographs and magnetic resonance scans show

TABLE 12.4

Acutely damaged glial cells

Gestational weeks	Percentage of cases in each gestational period
20–23	2
24–27	5
28–31	10
32–35	20
36–39	30+13
>40	25

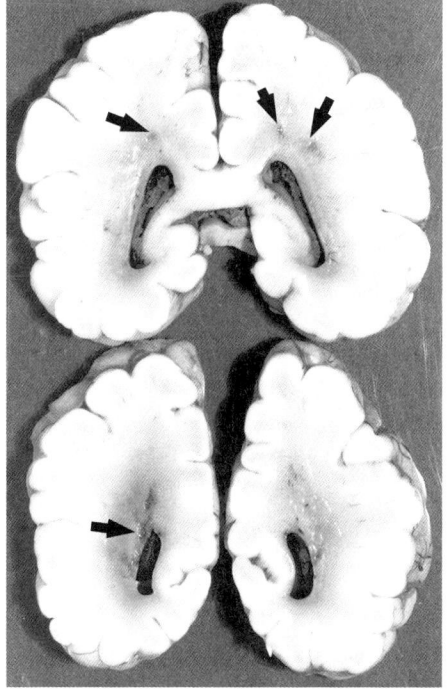

Fig. 12.3 Coronal slices of late fetal brain through the splenium, atrium, and occipital horns. Many scattered coagulative necroses (arrows) lie external to the external sagittal stratum (upper slice) or in both sagittal strata closer to the ventricle (lower slice). These necroses have not yet begun to organize.

persistent large cavitary lesions for some months after birth (Figs. 12.10 and 12.11). Older lesions remain as large or small cysts surrounded by dense astrocytosis (Fig. 12.12), or cysts sometimes shrink or collapse, leaving a residual glial vestige. Focal necroses sometimes exist with local narrow dense zones of hypertrophic astrocytes, but without the diffuse hypertrophic

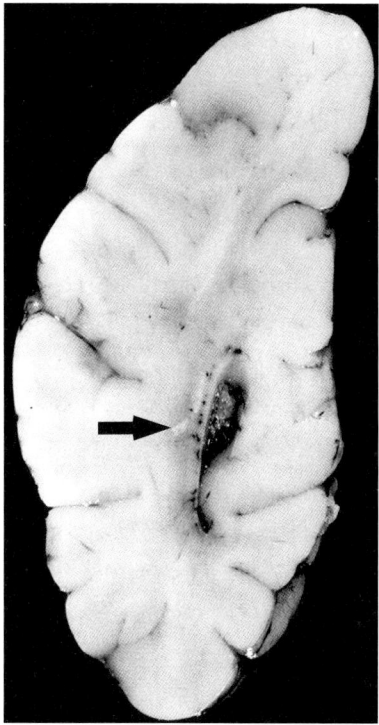

Fig. 12.4 Coronal slice of left parieto-occipital lobe just behind atrium. There is a chalky white focal necrosis (arrow) in the external sagittal stratum. Early necrosis organization with large numbers of macrophages underlies the chalky white color.

astrocytes mentioned previously. Focal white matter lesions are sometimes hemorrhagic, as expected when capillary or sinusoidal endothelium is damaged and erythrocytes leak into necrotic regions (Figs. 12.13 and 12.14).

Necrosis, used in this context, signifies the death of all white matter components in a specific, limited region, including vessels, all varieties of immature glia, and axons. This is the entity described throughout the last half of the nineteenth and first half of the twentieth centuries as focal necrosis, until eventually renamed 'periventricular leukomalacia' in 1962.[9] Necrosis has many antecedents; many factors, endogenous and exogenous, increase its risk. Several authors have shown that focal necroses seem largely a late gestational phenomenon (Table 12.5).

Thus, histologically, focal necroses are widely spread throughout telencephalic white matter from the frontal to occipital pole and from the ventricular wall to the cortex.[7,35,36] Their distribution is far too variable in deep paraventricular and superficial white matter or in gyral white matter cores to implicate any specific arterial bed or arterial borderzone.[9] They are usually located dorsal and lateral to the hemispheral ventricular wall, rarely inferiorly or medially. Focal necroses involve almost all telencephalic white matter regions except for the

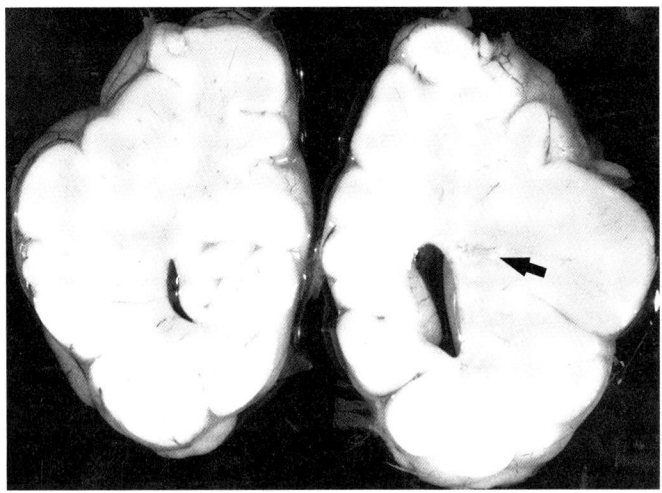

Fig. 12.5 Coronal slice of late fetal brain through the posterior thalamus. There are two small chalky lesions in the deep right parietal white matter and two larger chalky lesions more inferiorly in the external sagittal stratum (arrow).

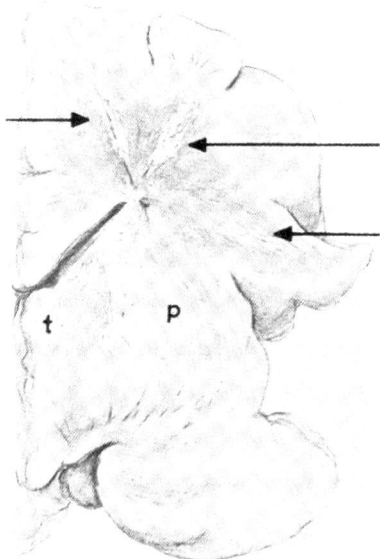

Fig. 12.6 The previous two images are similar to this image by Schwartz. In this picture, note the chalky necroses (arrows) and the linear nature of their deposition. Reproduced with permission of S. Karger AG from Schwartz.[120]

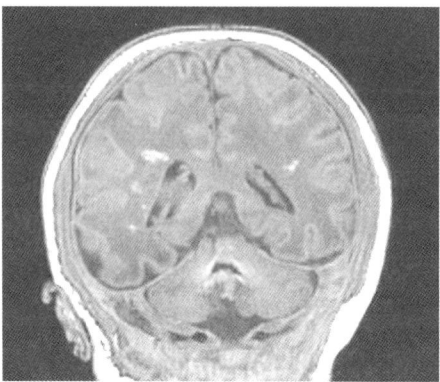

Fig. 12.7 Coronal T1-weighted magnetic resonance scan through the splenium and lateral ventricle atria. The four focal hyperintense lesions (white spots) in the left (image side) lie in the internal and external sagittal strata. The lesions are similar in location, except for the sides. Both the top lesion (left) and the single lesion (right) are linear. All of these focal necroses seem of the same age and probably reflect coagulative necrosis or early macrophage organization of the focal necroses. These lesions are not hemorrhagic, because there was not evidence of hemosiderin on T2 or susceptibility-weighted images.

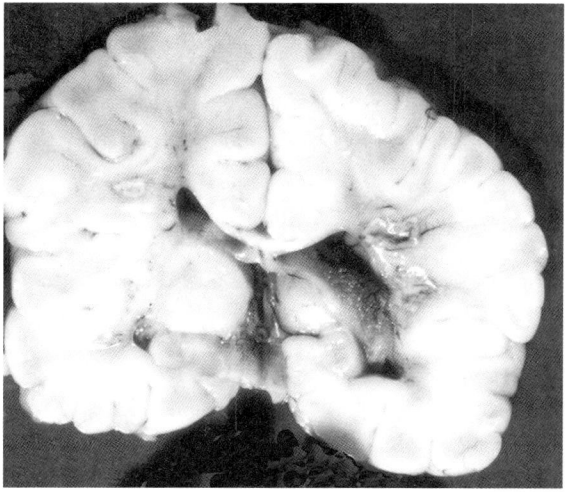

Fig. 12.8 Coronal late fetal brain slice through the posterior thalamus. There are three large focal necroses with early central cavitation. The two on the right extend from the ventricular wall far out into the white matter; in the left hemisphere, a single large lesion lies in the white matter just below the cortex. Note the absence of lesions in the temporal white matter.

anterior temporal lobe, and occur in a wide variety of perinatal conditions: preterm birth, difficult labor, neonatal meningitis, rubella, posterior fossa subdural hematoma, herpes simplex, kernicterus, phenylketonuria, cystic fibrosis, hyaline membrane disease, congenital heart disease, intraventricular hemorrhage, ganglionic eminence hemorrhage, erythroblastosis fetalis

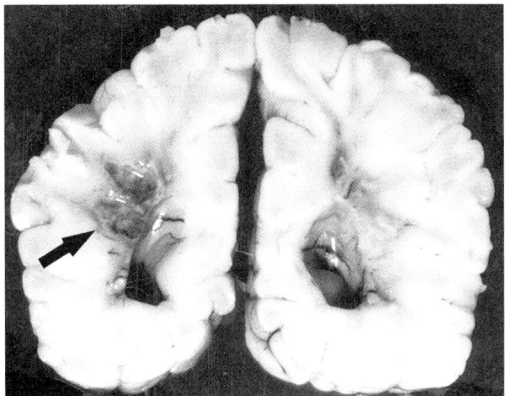

Fig. 12.9 Anterior surface of a coronal slice of fetal brain through the occipital horn. In both hemispheres, focal necroses range in size from small chalky white lesions to larger lesions lying intermediate between the ventricular wall and the cortex (right). On the left, two larger cavitary lesions extend from the ventricular wall (intact) to the white matter just below the cortex (arrow). Both large cavitary lesions interrupt both the internal and external sagittal strata as well as the more superficial white matter. Note that all lesions, large or small, are dorsal or lateral, but not medial, to the ventricle.

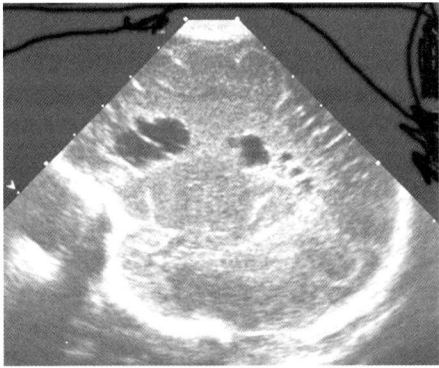

Fig. 12.10 Oblique sagittal sonographic image of large cavitary necroses in a neonate. The nose is to the left. The striatum and temporal lobe lie below.

without kernicterus, agranulocytosis, and sagittal sinus thrombosis. Of interest, although most of the hemispheral white matter may contain large numbers of focal necrosis, the isocortex, hippocampus, striatum, globus pallidus, amygdala, and thalamus are spared.

FOCAL NECROSES HISTORY
Necrotic lesions in neonatal telencephalic white matter attracted pathologists' attention for a century before popularization with a different nonspecific name in 1962.[4–7,9,38–41] Virchow[5] found multiple white matter focal necroses with smallpox or syphilis during pregnancy,

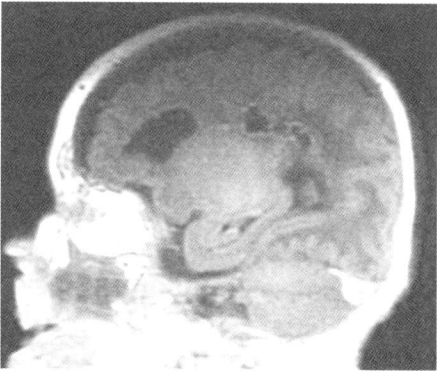

Fig. 12.11 Sagittal T1-weighted image of the same patient as in Fig. 12.10 at a later date showing the cavitary lesions. Remarkably, cavitary lesions even of this size sometimes collapse.

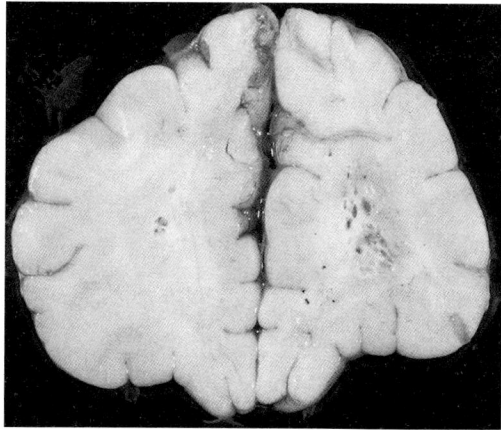

Fig. 12.12 Coronal slice of late fetal brain through the frontal poles anterior to the corpus callosum rostrum. Note many small cysts surrounded by a dense white band of glial fibrils. There are considerably more on the right than the left. During organization, after macrophages remove necrotic debris a small cyst remains surrounded by a narrow dense astrocytic glial layer. The latter are quite distinct from the diffuse widespread hypertrophic astrocytes demonstrated in Fig. 12.1, in which there is little overall glial cell increase in density.

calling the condition congenital interstitial encephalitis. Parrot[38] pointed out that neonates with these lesions were often preterm and that there were no associated inflammatory cells, and attributed them to nutritional and circulatory disturbances. Other nineteenth-century investigators felt that thrombosis, icterus, omphalitis, or emboli caused them. In the early twentieth century, Schwartz[39,40] initially felt that they were ischemic, resulting from venous stasis (a position Larroche refuted),[42,43] but later changed his opinion to birth trauma. Single large regional necroses involving gray and white matter were not included in this entity. The

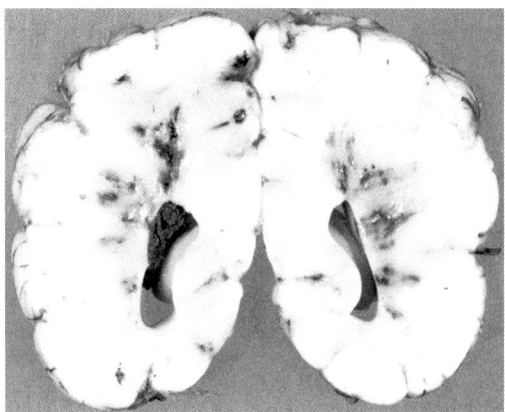

Fig. 12.13 Coronal slice of late fetal brain through the atrium. Multiple linear or globular hemorrhagic focal necroses are present in both cerebral hemispheres. At some locations, they are confluent.

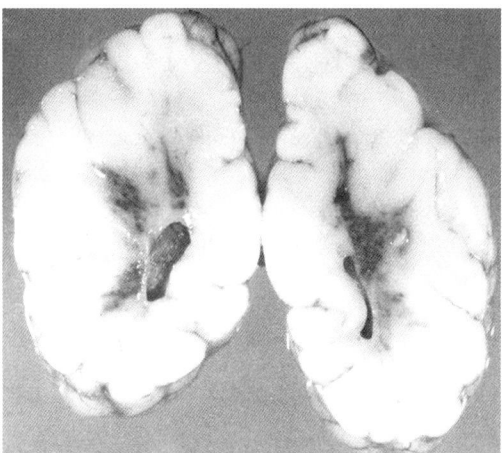

Fig. 12.14 Coronal slice of late fetal brain through the occipital horns. Multiple linear, globular, or confluent hemorrhagic focal necroses are present in the white matter.

early descriptions were also consistent in emphasizing that these necroses occurred at multiple sites (both deep and superficial) including gyral cores, and later descriptions concurred.[35] Focal necrotic lesions with macrophages must be distinguished from diffuse fatty changes in cerebral white matter related to the normal accumulation of sterol esters in premyelin glial cells (see Chapter 6).[5]

In 1962, a subset of focal white matter necrosis was termed 'periventricular leukomalacia'.[9] Before 1962, original definitions of focal necroses were consistent among multiple authors emphasizing their minute size, ranging from a few millimeters in diameter, and often below ultrasound resolution, to much larger lesions. Early investigators overlooked the wide

265

TABLE 12.5

Focal necroses

Gestational weeks	Percentage of cases in each gestational period
11–19	0
20–23	1
24–27	8
28–31	6
32–35	8
36–39	6
>40	2

variability in size of some lesions. Although common in frontal white matter, anterolateral to the anterior frontal horn and in parietal and occipital lobes, lateral to and in the optic radiation, they are less common in posterior frontal and rostral parietal white matter underlying motor and sensory cortices of pre- and postcentral gyri.[36,41,44] Therefore, the smaller necrotic foci are not likely to constitute the anatomic basis for most diplegia,[45] despite claims to the contrary.[9,46] In the 1962 paper, the term 'periventricular leukomalacia' was used only to refer to focal necroses, not to any or all of the other neonatal white matter histologic abnormalities. We prefer the historically accurate definition even though some researchers extend the definition of periventricular leukomalacia to almost any white matter abnormality (for instance, ventriculomegaly, extensive cystic leukoencephalopathy,[47] or lesions of white or gray matter).[48]

Recent investigators have often conflated focal necroses and diffuse white matter astrocytosis. The commonly used name, 'periventricular leukomalacia,' is anatomically and pathologically inappropriate as the term 'leukomalacia' means widespread white matter softening instead of focal necroses.[26] Topologically, these small focal necroses do not surround (are not 'peri' strictly speaking) the lateral ventricle but lie at multiple sites, in several patterns, within the deep to superficial white matter, with deep necroses sometimes larger than superficial necroses.[49]

Despite the fact that these small focal necrotic lesions are just that, *focal* necroses, with loss of all tissue components, they have been thought to derive from systemic 'anoxia',[9] or as a result of ischemic lesions from hypotension,[36,50] or from 'hypoxischemia'[51] in hypothetical white matter arterial borderzones (see Chapter 8). Each model implies that small focal necroses arise in systemic conditions of hypoxia or hypotension, conditions which also are expected to produce widespread necrosis or bilateral lesions in borderzone territories of arterial supply (see Chapter 13). Friede's recognition (1975)[26] that these lesions are small focal necroses is important, as the usual size and distribution of these lesions speak eloquently for local ischemic changes and not for systemically lowered blood flow. The focality of white matter necroses suggests, if anything, local microvessel damage, and not systemic problems. Typical large systemic borderzone lesions, involving gray and white matter, do occur in neonatal brains; they appear unrelated to the hypothetic deep white matter borderzones, postulated, yet never proven.[36,52,53]

Thus, we describe four frequently found white matter histologic abnormalities. The following exercises will try to assist in understanding whether any are normal white matter developmental phenomena or whether they are different manifestations of a single or multiple entities.

Role of clustering in understanding relationships of various white matter histologic features

Fetal and neonatal white matter glial cells respond in a very limited set of ways to a variety of insults. Thus, each is expected to have multiple risk factors, which may overlap. The four abnormalities are either independent or represent differing manifestations of a single entity. Histologic feature clustering, temporal patterns of occurrence of each feature, or histologic feature associations with risk factors or with clinical features assist decisions.[27] While histologic feature clusters are more likely to be etiologically homogeneous than entities defined by a single histologic characteristic, neither the four histologic entities nor their clusters are likely to have single etiologies. That is, each is likely to be multifactorial in origin, an additive model in which disease risk increases as the weight of all contributions to the occurrence of that disease increases.[54,55] Thus, every child with a perinatal leukoencephalopathy cannot be expected to have exactly the same risk factor set as another child with the same disorder.

The four histologic features occurred in several clusters. In the original review, three clusters emerged: diffuse hypertrophic astrocytes with amphophilic globules without necrotic foci; diffuse hypertrophic astrocytes and amphophilic globules with necrotic foci; and acutely damaged glial cells with amphophilic globules.[27] In the larger NCPP population, clustering of diffuse hypertrophic astrocytes and necrotic foci was relatively weak,[56] and risk factor identification was sought for only the two remaining clusters as well as the individual four histologic features. For this chapter, we review only one cluster (diffuse hypertrophic astrocytes and amphophilic globules) because of the uncertain meaning of acutely damaged glial cells.

Perinatal telencephalic leukoencephalopathies and their risk factors

We are reviewing these old studies because they are derived from the only carefully collected database of fetal brain pathology. Two observers collected the NCPP histologic data, reading the slides simultaneously (a tactic to reduce observer variability)[57] without knowledge of clinical data. The NCPP clinical variable file initially included more than 1200 clinical variables, all collected prospectively during the mother's pregnancy, labor, and delivery. First, a single parameter univariate analysis identified clinical variables of interest for each leukoencephalopathy. Second, a multivariate analysis was performed on the clinical variables associated with each histologic subset. For the latter, relative risk point estimates had to fall between the 95% confidence limits (further limiting the data mass), and, as there were several variables that could be subsumed under simpler overarching terms, these latter are presented here. For the full analyses, please refer to references 12, 56, and 58–61. 'Total age' as used here refers to gestational plus survival age, sometimes called conceptual age.

The risk factors were assembled into five groups for all leukoencephalopathies in order to facilitate understanding of their relationships: total age, endotoxemia, congenital anomaly, uterine environment, and socioeconomic status.

Total age

The risk of diffuse hypertrophic astrocytes in telencephalic white matter increased with advancing gestational age after 28 weeks, with maximal risk occurring at gestational end, confirming the increased risk associated with older gestational age.[58,62] This risk factor may represent an increasing ability of white matter to respond to insult with diffuse hypertrophic astrocytes or changing risk factor exposure with advancing age.[28,63] Others feel that the appearance of glial cell changes represents damage to oligodendroglial progenitors.[64–66]

Risk factors associated with older maternal age that also increased the risk of diffuse hypertrophic astrocytes included previous child with retarded development (28-fold), non-perineal laceration during delivery (13-fold), maternal hematocrit <24.9 (12-fold), Protestant religion (~fourfold), and maternal pregnancy weight gain of more than 30 pounds or a final maternal weight of more than 150 pounds (~threefold each). How nonperineal lacerations or religion increase risk is open to speculation. Even so, low maternal hematocrit and excessive weight gain are also related to uterine environment.

Endotoxemia

Neonatal sepsis increased the risk of diffuse white matter hypertrophic astrocytes almost fivefold. In more recent studies, motor deficits occurring among very low birthweight children at 6 years, without focal white matter necroses, were significantly associated with neonatal septicemia.[67] Older infants tended to develop endotoxemia from their own septicemia, whereas younger infants were potentially exposed in utero when their mothers had (transient) endotoxemia with a urinary tract infection. In both human and experimental animals, white matter hypertrophic astrocytes were associated with endotoxemia.[17,30,68–70]

Congenital anomaly effect

Cyanotic congenital heart disease, older sibling with retarded development, and alimentary tract malformation all increased the risk of developing diffuse white matter hypertrophic astrocytes. The association between diffuse white matter hypertrophic astrocytes and cyanotic congenital heart disease is an old observation.[31] It seems that increased risk occurs in families and with other associated malformations. Although infants with life-threatening congenital anomalies are at increased risk of nosocomial infections via catheterization, prolonged intravenous hydration, and surgery, other mechanisms by which cyanotic heart disease leads to astrocytosis deserve consideration. These include persistent viral infection, undernutrition, hypoglycemia, hypoxia, and oxygen toxicity.[31,71]

TABLE 12.6

**Grouped variables that increase the risk of white
matter hypertrophic astrocytes**

Umbrella term	Variables
Older total age	Final weight of gravida ≥150lb
	Pregnancy weight gain=30lb
	Nonperineal laceration
	Protestant religion
	Alimentary tract condition
Endotoxemia	Septicemia
	Puerto Rican heritage
	Edema of hands and face
Congenital anomaly effect	Alimentary tract conditions
	Retarded development of sibling
Unfavorable uterine environment (includes toxemia and maternal age effect)	Edema of hands and face
	Retarded development of sibling
	Protestant religion
Low socioeconomic state	Puerto Rican heritage
	Protestant religion

The original study also described clinical variables associated with decreased risk of white matter hypertrophic astrocytes.
From Leviton and Gilles.[61]

Unfavorable uterine environment

Toxemia, birth order, and maternal age all increased the risk of diffuse white matter hypertrophic astrocytes. Edema of hands and face and body weight variables are potential manifestations of toxemia. Whether maternal behaviors as such are related to delayed weight gain and add to white matter damage is unknown.[72]

Socioeconomic effect

The manner in which low socioeconomic factors contribute to the increased risk of diffuse hypertrophic astrocytes is unclear, but it is likely to be related to low birthweight antecedents, which include socioeconomic status[73] (see Table 12.6).

LEUKOENCEPHALOPATHY CHARACTERIZED BY AMPHOPHILIC GLOBULES

Risk factors

Total age
Birthweight of greater than 1kg, among the clinical variables identified in multivariate analysis, increased the risk of white matter amphophilic globules; this is consistent with the idea

269

that preterm infants need a certain amount of brain before these deposits can occur.[28,59,63] Maternal syphilis and higher education of gravida also increased the risk of white matter amphophilic globules.

Endotoxemia

Maternal endotoxemia from a urinary tract infection and maternal insulin or oral hypoglycemics increased the risk of white matter amphophilic globules, suggesting that fetuses and infants acquired endotoxins either from their mothers or from a fetal inflammatory response induced by maternal endotoxemia. Transplacental effects of transient maternal endotoxemia from urinary tract infection or periodontal disease have been demonstrated for many years,[74,75] and were proposed long ago.[76,77] Finally, the high prevalence of elevated fetal immunoglobulin M to *Campylobacter rectus* among preterm infants raises the possibility that this specific oral pathogen serves as a primary fetal infectious agent stimulating preterm birth.[78]

Congenital anomaly effect

There was a single associated risk factor in this category, namely 'eye condition,' but unfortunately it was ambiguously defined in the NCPP clinical variable file. In any case, it correlated with cardiac enlargement and alimentary tract malformation.

Unfavorable uterine environment

This term includes a heterogeneous group of clinical variables consistent with a suboptimal intrauterine setting including insulin or oral hypoglycemics (or maternal diabetes), gynecologic tumor, seizures in an older sibling, and low birthweight of the last previous pregnancy. The last two variables are markers of sibling morbidity. Again, there is no way to precisely define those uterine characteristics common to these disorders; they all contribute to the risk of amphophilic globules.

Socioeconomic

Although there is an association between higher socioeconomic status and maternal diabetes, there is no way to postulate the ways in which socioeconomic correlates contribute to amphophilic globule production (see Table 12.7).

THE LEUKOENCEPHALOPATHY CHARACTERIZED BY ACUTELY DAMAGED GLIA

Acutely damaged glial cells tended to occur with one or more of the other white matter abnormalities, and their risk factors are similar to those of white matter hypertrophic astrocytes.[60]

Risk factors

Age

The newborn brain's ability to produce acutely damaged glia is age dependent. Ten risk factors provided information about infant maturation. The most prominent examples were birthweight greater than 1kg and dysmaturity. Nevertheless, septicemia, neonatal antibiotic receipt, and

TABLE 12.7

**Grouped variables that increase the risk of
white matter amphophilic globules**

Umbrella term	Variables
Older total age	Maternal syphilis
	Birthweight greater than 1kg
	Higher education of gravida
Congenital anomaly effect	Eye condition
Unfavorable uterine environment	Insulin or oral hypoglycemics
	Gynecologic tumor
	Seizures in previous offspring
	Low birthweight of last previous child
Endotoxemia	Insulin or oral hypoglycemics
	Urinary tract infection
Socioeconomic effect	Higher education
	Insulin or oral hypoglycemics

From Leviton and Gilles.[61]

gynecologic surgery before pregnancy correlated with higher birthweight or higher gestational age indicators. In addition, gestational age of last previous child, chromosome studies, omphalocele, and afebrile seizure in a sibling correlated with indicators of maturation.

Endotoxemia

There is overwhelming evidence that endotoxin exposure is indeed a major mechanism by which other risk factors contribute to acutely damaged glia occurrence. Not only was septicemia a risk factor in its own right, but also multivariate analysis identified three other risk factors correlated with septicemia (for instance, neonatal antibiotic receipt). This latter risk factor is a marker of identified septicemia, but also a marker of other infections. Maternal rhesus antigen and first-trimester uterine bleeding also correlated with newborn septicemia. In addition, omphalocele correlated with central nervous system infection, chromosome studies correlated with lumbar puncture (a correlate of septicemia), and low gestational age of the last prior outcome correlated with maternal costovertebral angle tenderness.

Congenital anomaly effect

The two risk factors with the highest relative risk estimates, chromosome studies and omphalocele, are indicators of congenital anomalies. In addition, other congenital anomalies are identified risk factors of other manifestations of telencephalic white matter damage. Therefore, it seems that congenital anomalies or correlates of such anomalies increase the risk of acutely damaged glia and other neonatal white matter aberrations.

Unfavorable uterine environment

The fourth postulated umbrella term, unfavorable uterine environment, included a placental insufficiency effect (first-trimester uterine bleeding), a maternal age effect (gynecologic surgery), a presumed toxemic effect (rhesus antigen in gravida), and unidentified mechanisms associated with a familial tendency to neurologic disorders (seizure in a sibling).

Socioeconomic effect

The fifth heading, which represents a heterogeneous group of mechanisms, was given the name socioeconomic effect. Both low socioeconomic index and high housing density were identified as risk factors for acutely damaged glia (see Table 12.8).

LEUKOENCEPHALOPATHY CHARACTERIZED BY WHITE MATTER FOCAL NECROSES

Risk factors

Gestational age

At one institution, necrotic foci were seen in older infants with the perinatal telencephalic leukoencephalopathy characterized by white matter focal necroses, but not in younger newborns with this entity.[28,61] In the NCPP material, the risk of white matter focal necroses increased with advancing gestational age beyond 26 weeks, confirming the previous observation, with increasing postnatal age and with increasing maternal age.[61]

Endotoxemia

Infants with either septicemia or infection were at a 40-fold increased risk of white matter focal necroses. Most newborns with documented bacteremia have organisms that produce endotoxins, and this hypothesis has laboratory support.[17]

Congenital anomaly effect

The two risk factors with the highest relative risk were both congenital anomalies, namely omphalocele and abnormalities of external genitalia. Other abnormalities also contributed to the congenital anomaly effect, one umbilical artery rather than two, renal cysts, and any other definite alimentary tract condition. It is unlikely that congenital anomalies themselves cause necrotic foci, but that factors contributing to congenital anomalies also contribute to focal necroses.

Unfavorable uterine environment

Women who had gynecologic surgery during pregnancy and a maternal age greater than 20 years were at increased risk of delivering a child with white matter necrotic foci. The specific mechanisms by which these risk factors contribute to the risk of necrotic foci are unknown.

Socioeconomic effect

High housing density (six or more persons supported and eight or more siblings) increased the risk of white matter focal necroses (see Table 12.9).

272

TABLE 12.8

**Grouped variables that increase the risk of
white matter acutely damaged glia**

Umbrella term	Variables
Congenital anomaly effect	Chromosome studies
	Omphalocele
	First trimester uterine bleeding
Endotoxemia	Chromosome studies
	Omphalocele
	Septicemia in neonate
	Gestational age of last prior outcome
	Rhesus antigen in gravida
	First trimester uterine bleeding
	Antibiotics given to neonate
Age-related phenomena	Chromosome studies
	Omphalocele
	Afebrile seizures in sibling
	Septicemia
	Birthweight >1kg
	Postnatal age <48h
	Gestational age of last prior outcome
	Antibiotics given to neonate
Unfavorable uterine environment	Chromosome studies
	Gestational age of last prior outcome
	Low socioeconomic index
	Rhesus antigen in gravida
	First-trimester uterine bleeding
Socioeconomic effect	Low socioeconomic index
	High housing density[a]

From Leviton and Gilles.[61]

[a]Six or more persons supported and eight or more siblings.

LEUKOENCEPHALOPATHY CHARACTERIZED BY DIFFUSE HYPERTROPHIC
ASTROCYTES AND AMPHOPHILIC GLOBULES

Diffuse white matter hypertrophic astrocytes and amphophilic globules are not independent of each other,[27,58] suggesting phenomena of biologic importance sharing etiologies.

Risk factors

The early evidence that endotoxin exposure increased the risk of this leukoencephalopathy included (1) infants with documented bacteremia or at risk of bacteremia; (2) infants who received antibiotics; and (3) the similar secular trends of bacteremia and this

TABLE 12.9

Grouped variables that increase the risk of focal white matter necrosis

Umbrella term	Variables
Congenital anomaly effect	Omphalocele
	Abnormality of external genitalia
	Abnormality of alimentary tract
	Septicemia
Endotoxemia	Alimentary tract malformation
Unfavorable intrauterine environment (includes toxemia and maternal age/birth order effect)	Gynecologic surgery
	Registration during first trimester
	Age of gravida ≥20 years
	Septicemia
	No prior pregnancy
Socioeconomic effect	High housing density[a]

From Leviton and Gilles.[61]

[a]Six or more persons supported and eight or more siblings.

leukoencephalopathy at one institution.[30,33] Infants with this entity tended to have smaller thymuses and spleens than infants without,[34] and intraperitoneal administration of endotoxin to newborn kittens produced white matter necroses, hypertrophic astrocytes, and amphophilic globules.[17]

Age

The risk of this entity tended to decrease with decreasing gestational age and birthweight and increase with postnatal age greater than 6 days, maternal weight gain of more than 30 pounds, and an alimentary tract condition. Six of the nine risk factors correlated with gestational age greater than 27 weeks, leading to the thought that this disorder parallels the onset of early telencephalic myelination and is more likely to be an aberration of preoligodendroglia.[30,64,79]

Infection: remote

Two risk factors, impressive for the magnitude of their relative risk estimates, were maternal fever with urinary tract infection (420-fold increase in risk) and cervical lacerations (325-fold increase in risk). The first risk factor correlated strongly with costovertebral angle tenderness, positive urine culture, and pyuria, and could be included under several of our blanket terms. The second risk factor correlated with a large number of conditions, and thus conveyed information about multiple factors.

Congenital anomaly effect

Alimentary tract abnormality increased the risk of this entity in multivariate analysis.

Unfavorable uterine environment

Eight of the nine variables identified by multivariate analysis could be subsumed under this blanket term. One adversity was toxemia. While maternal weight gain of greater than 30 pounds in this sample was not associated with measures of hypertension, it nevertheless was associated with albuminuria. Pre-eclampsia without hypertension would, in part, explain how fever with urinary tract infection, maternal weight gain greater than 30 pounds, postnatal age greater than 6 days, and non-infectious alimentary tract condition contribute to the occurrence of hypertrophic astrocytes and amphophilic globules. Infants with cardiac, gastrointestinal, and urologic anomalies are also at a considerably increased risk of endotoxin exposure due to bacteremia acquired during prolonged intravenous administration of fluids, diagnostic procedures, and surgery. We cannot account for the elevated risk if their mothers had had a previous pregnancy.

Socioeconomic effect

This blanket term has a weak effect for this white matter entity, yet was important in other perinatal telencephalic leukoencephalopathies (see Table 12.10).

Etiologic relationships among the five perinatal telencephalic leukoencephalopathies

From this review of some risk factors of the five histologic entities, the overlapping risk factors indicate that they are not likely to be five completely separate entities. Nonetheless, their interrelationships are sufficiently complex that some explication is in order. There are five groups of risk factors.

AGE

Four of the five entities have age-related risk factors; gestational age factors are more important than postnatal age, consistent with changing white matter vulnerability with fetal development, or increasing capacity of developing white matter to respond to insult. Changes in telencephalic white matter glial cell populations supporting developing axons, developing vascular beds, and the glial cell transformation from nonspecific glial cells to oligodendroglial or astrocytic precursors, and eventually to astrocytes or oligodendroglia, reflect glial cell capacity to respond to insult. Alternatively, age-related white matter abnormalities represent risk factors that increase with age.

Interestingly, in children with necrotic foci, age-related phenomena were not prominent, suggesting that they differ from the other leukoencephalopathies in that congenital anomalies are their most prominent risk factors. Congenital anomalies are unlikely to directly contribute to necrotic foci and are likely to indicate other risk factors.

ENDOTOXIN

The second most prominent and consistent risk factor is exposure to endotoxin, an hypothesis originally proposed by Perrin and Landing in 1962.[80] The evidence consists of three sets. First, neonatal bacteremia was a risk factor for most telencephalic leukoencephalopathies. Second, a number of risk factors correlated with bacteremia, including alimentary tract malformation,

TABLE 12.10

Grouped variables that increase the risk of white matter
hypertrophic astrocytes and amphophilic globules

Umbrella term	Variables
Endotoxin	Fever with urinary tract infection
	Maternal weight gain >30lb
	Postnatal age >6 days
	Puerto Rican ancestry
	Alimentary tract condition
Age-related phenomena (older gestational and postnatal age)	Postnatal age >6 days
	Puerto Rican ancestry
	Alimentary tract condition
	Nonperineal lacerations
Unfavorable uterine environment (includes toxemia and birth order effects)	Fever with urinary tract infection
	Maternal weight gain >30lb
	Postnatal age >6 days
	Alimentary tract condition
	Nonperineal lacerations
	Duration of labor <8h
	Marked head molding
	One living full sibling aged <5y
	Puerto Rican ancestry
Congenital anomaly effect (includes hydramnios)	Maternal weight gain >30lb
	Alimentary tract condition
	Fever with urinary tract infection
Socioeconomic effect	Fever with urinary tract infection
	Duration of labor <8h

From Leviton and Gilles.[61]

postnatal age between 13 and 48 hours, and birthweight greater than 1kg. Third, the association of urinary tract infection with three leukoencephalopathies: hypertrophic astrocytes, amphophilic globules, and their combination. The markers of urinary tract infection included pyuria, positive urine culture, costovertebral angle tenderness, and urinary tract infection with fever. Febrile urinary tract infection is the most prominent risk factor of hypertrophic astrocytes and amphophilic globules, but multivariate analysis identified four other risk factors associated with urinary tract infection indicators. 'Fever associated with a urinary tract infection' discriminated best between infants with and without hypertrophic astrocytes and amphophilic globules in their telencephalic white matter. The finding here that urinary tract infection is a very prominent risk factor suggests that maternal endotoxin crosses the placenta and prenatal exposure (presumably during the last trimester) contributes to hypertrophic astrocytes and amphophilic globules.[69] That endotoxin is capable of transplacental effects is known,[81,82] and newborns are deficient in their ability to inactivate endotoxin.[83] Another finding compatible with the endotoxin hypothesis is that 'postnatal age greater than 6 days' correlates with neonatal sepsis.

The relationship strength between endotoxemia and the perinatal telencephalic leuko-encephalopathies is the relative risk point estimate magnitude. For neonatal bacteremia, the relative risk of necrotic foci is increased 41.5-fold; of acutely damaged glia, 16.7-fold; and of hypertrophic astrocytes, 4.8-fold. For maternal febrile urinary tract infection, the relative risk of hypertrophic astrocytes and amphophilic globules is increased 420-fold. Neonates were at increased risk of white matter hypertrophic astrocytes and amphophilic globules if they had bacteria cultured from blood at autopsy;[30] all other risk factors were either bacteremia risk factors or bacteremia markers.[33] Neonates with the same leukoencephalopathy also had thymus atrophy.[34]

Dammann and Leviton[84–86] produced epidemiologic evidence that proinflammatory cyto-kines are induced in the preterm brain, simultaneous with the demonstration that presence of amniotic fluid inflammatory cytokines increase the risk of white matter lesions in the neonate and that focal necroses are associated with high levels of tumor necrosis factor alpha (TNF-α) and interleukin 6 (IL-6).[87–91] Cytokines are important signaling proteins involved in neuron–glia interactions and in microglial–astroglial cross-talk, modulating the glial response to brain injury, and are increased as part of the inflammatory response to both infection and ischemia. TNF-α is present in glial cells near focal necroses.[37,92–94] Preterm infants with mag-netic resonance imaging (MRI)-defined cerebral white matter injury had higher cerebrospinal fluid levels of IL-6, IL-10, and TNF-α than those without.[95] Intraperitoneal lipopolysaccharide in newborn kittens produces focal necroses in telencephalon.[17] Lipopolysaccharide injected directly into neonatal rat brain or *Escherichia coli* injected into guinea-pig cervix increased TNF-α and IL-1β and induced white matter rarefaction, ventricular dilatation, damage to oligodendroglial precursors, hypomyelination, and white matter astrocytosis without gray matter lesion.[96–99]

CONGENITAL ANOMALY EFFECT

All perinatal telencephalic leukoencephalopathies have risk factor relationships to congenital anomalies or correlates of congenital anomalies. How congenital anomalies increase the risk of white matter disturbances is open to speculation. One possibility is that infants with life-endangering anomalies are at increased risk of bacteremia and endotoxemia.

UNFAVORABLE UTERINE ENVIRONMENT

All perinatal telencephalic leukoencephalopathies have risk factors fitting under this heading, including correlates of toxemia, birth order, maternal age, and familial neurologic disorders.

SOCIOECONOMIC EFFECT

Measures of lower socioeconomic status were risk factors of some perinatal telencephalic leukoencephalopathies and correlates of risk factors of others. Clinic rather than private status of mother, low socioeconomic index, and high housing density all increased the risk of white matter acutely damaged glial cells and necrotic foci.

Ultrasonographic white matter abnormalities and clinical associations

If ultrasonography reliably reflects what is present histologically in developing white matter, then carefully performed clinical studies of antecedents and predictions using ultrasound can further our understanding of white matter lesions in the prematurely born infant. For instance, focal white matter echolucent lesions and ventriculomegaly predict an increased risk of subsequent microcephaly[100] or cerebral palsy.[101]

Elevated concentrations of vascular endothelial growth factor receptor 1, serum amyloid A, and macrophage inflammatory protein 1-β on day 1 and IL-8 on day 7 are associated with increased risk of ventriculomegaly. Elevated concentrations of macrophage inflammatory protein 1-β and intercellular adhesion molecule on day 7 are associated with increased risk of an echolucent lesion. Infants with elevated concentration of inflammation-related proteins on two separate days were at increased risk for ventriculomegaly but at less risk for echolucent lesion.[102] Further, brain damage in very preterm infants is associated with microorganisms in placental parenchyma.[103]

If present at birth, microcephaly, placental α-hemolytic streptococci, male sex, and a single mother each increased the risk of microcephaly at the age of 2 years.[104] Elevated concentrations of circulating inflammation-related proteins shortly after preterm birth are associated with increased risk of microcephaly at the age of 2 years,[105] and about half of second-trimester placentas harbor organisms within the chorionic plate.[106] Even though there is considerable evidence accumulating that neonatal inflammation-related proteins are associated with white matter damage, fetal postnatal hypotension is not associated with developmental delay at the age of 2 years.[107]

The curious change in glial cells in unmyelinated, but myelinating, white matter needs emphasis. Normal glial cells in unmyelinated or in myelinating white matter have no appreciable cytoplasm, a point long recognized.[14] Usually in an astrocytosis, one expects a locally increased density of hypertrophic astrocytes, even though transient. In fetal white matter with what we are calling hypertrophic astrocytes, the overall cell density is not increased. One could speculate that a subset of glial cells was changed from its expected differentiation into astrocytes and oligodendroglia into hypertrophic astrocytes. Interestingly, it has been recently shown that oligodendrocyte-type 2 astrocyte progenitor cells (that normally generate oligodendrocytes and astrocytes) can give rise to astrocytes in response to interferon-gamma (IFN-γ) in vitro,[108] suggesting that neuroinflammation involving increased IFN-γ can reduce progenitor numbers and contribute to astrocyte generation. Others have invoked cytokine injury or nitrosative and oxidative stress to oligodendroglial precursors in the causation of diffuse white matter injury.[109]

What about the antecedents of preterm delivery? There seem to be two patterns of disorders leading to preterm delivery: those associated with intrauterine inflammation and those associated with aberrations of placentation.[109,110]

Summary

Different prevalence rates, secular trends, histologic feature clustering, and risk factor profiles are all consistent with the notion that these individual histologic features and one of their clusters represent distinct but related entities. For these reasons, diffuse white matter hypertrophic astrocytes are not a normal developmental phenomenon.

Those who lump all of these entities together under a single appellation of 'periventricular leukomalacia' or 'encephalopathy of preterm birth' fail to realize the difficulty in which they place themselves if trying to understand etiology, as many of these entities have differing risk factor profiles. Further, they ignore the microvascular abnormality, and, finally, in the large NCPP database, the clustering between diffuse telencephalic white matter astrocytosis and focal necroses was weak, reflecting a weak association.

While the white matter distribution and orientation of focal white matter necroses suggests an abnormality of radial transcerebral microvessel channels, diffuse hypertrophic astrocytes reflect a widely spread abnormality of immature glia,[64] including astrocytic and oligodendroglial precursors,[109] and the vulnerability of oligodendroglia to oxidative damage.[65,111,112]

There is a huge, old literature on anterograde, retrograde, and trans-synaptic neuronal atrophy (for early references see 113–115). Nevertheless, some investigators seem surprised that axonal interruptions in telencephalic white matter are associated with both anterograde and retrograde atrophy of cortical or thalamic neurons,[116–118] as noted in the 1962 Banker and Larroche paper.[9] Loss of cortical or thalamic volume is expected with white matter damage. Confirmation that thalamocortical fibers were interrupted in prematurely born infants was recently documented.[119]

Conclusion

The perinatal telencephalic leukoencephalopathies represent responses to disturbances of maturational processes (such as glial cell differentiation or myelinogenesis) unique to fetal or infant white matter. Notably absent in the NCPP epidemiologic results were specific markers of asphyxia, such as newborn hypotension or cardiorespiratory support. In fact, impaired Apgar scores were weakly associated with a decrease in white matter hypertrophic astrocytes and amphophilic globules. We have summarized the NCPP epidemiologic studies and some of the extensive literature detailing this subject. The risk of white matter astrocytosis increases with gestational age and, separately, with the presence of sepsis. One major point was that white matter focal necroses of all tissue elements are quite different from white matter diffuse astrocytosis, a difference often conflated when the appellation 'periventricular leukomalacia' is used clinically.

REFERENCES

1. Morgagni G (1769) *The Seats and Causes of Diseases*. London: A. Millar, T. Cadell and Johnson and Payne.
2. Cruveilhier J (1829–1835) *Anatomie Pathologique du Corps Humain, Part 2*, XVth Liv. Paris: JB Baillière.
3. Abercrombie J (1828) *Pathological and Practical Researches on Diseases of the Brain and the Spinal Cord*. Edinburgh: Waugh and Innes.
4. Bednar A (1850) *Die Krankheiten der Neugeborenen und Säuglinge*. Wien: C. Gerold.
5. Virchow R (1867) Zur pathologischen anatomie des gehirns: I Congenitale encephalitis und myelitis. *Virch Arch* 38: 129–138.

6. Parrot MJ (1868) Etude sur la stèatose interstitielle diffuse de l'encèphale chez le nouveau-nè. *Arch Physiol Norm Patholol (Paris)* 1: 530–550, 622–642, 706–715.
7. Schmorl CG (1904) Zur kenntniss des ikterus neonatorum, inbesondere der dabei auftretenden gehirn-veranderungen. *Verhandl deutsch Path Gesellsch* 6: 109–115.
8. Gilles F, Murphy S (1969) Perinatal telencephalic leukoencephalopathy. *J Neurol Neurosurg Psych* 32: 404–413.
9. Banker BQ, Larroche JC (1962) Periventricular leukomalacia of infancy. A form of neonatal anoxic encephalopathy. *Arch Neurol* 7: 386–410.
10. Leviton A, Gilles FH (1973) Are hypertrophic astrocytes a sufficient criterion of perinatal telencephalic leukoencephalopathy? *J Neurol Neurosurg Psychiatry* 36: 383–388.
11. Gilles FH, Averill DR Jr., Kerr CS (1977) Changes in neonatally induced cerebral lesions with advancing age. *J Neuropathol Exp Neurol* 36: 666–679.
12. Dooling EC, Chi J, Gilles FH (1983) Telencephalic development: changing gyral patterns. In: Gilles FH, Leviton A, Dooling EC, editors. *The Developing Human Brain: Growth and Epidemiologic Neuropathology*. Boston: Wright-PSG, pp. 94–104.
13. Dạmbska M, Maslinska D, Kuchna I (1992) Astrogliosis in the temporal lobe of newborn infants who died in the perinatal period. *Neuropatol Pol* 30(3–4): 245–253.
14. Roback HN, Scherer HJ (1935) Über die feinere Morphologie des frünkindlichen Gehirns unter besonderer Berücksichtigung der Gliaentwicklung. *Virchows Arch Path Anat* 294: 365–413.
15. Spatz H (1920) A special reaction of the immature central nervous system. *Z Neur* 53: 363–394.
16. Gilles FH, Averill DR Jr., Kerr CS (1977) Neonatal endotoxin encephalopathy. *Ann Neurol* 2: 49–56.
17. Gilles FH, Leviton A, Kerr CS (1976) Endotoxin leukoencephalopathy in the telencephalon of the newborn kitten. *J Neurol Sci* 27: 183–191.
18. Spatz H (1921) Über die Vorgänge nach experimenteller Rückenmarksdurchtrennung mit besonderer Berücksichtigung der Unterschiede der Reaktionsweise des reifen und des unreifen Gewebes nebst Beziehungen zur menschlicheden Pathologie (Porenzephalie und Syrinomyelie). In: Nissl F, Alzheimer A, editors. *Histologische und Histopathologische Arbeiten über d Großhirnrinde mit bes Berücksichtigung d pathol Anat d Geisteskrankheiten*. Jena: Fischer, pp. 49–367.
19. Friede RI, Knoller M (1965) A quantitative mapping of acid phosphatase in the brain of the rhesus monkey. *J Neurochem* 12: 441–450.
20. Miller RH, Abney ER, David S, et al (1986) Is reactive gliosis a property of a distinct subpopulation of astrocytes? *J Neurosci* 6: 22–29.
21. Cajal R (1902) *Degeneration and Regeneration of the Nervous System* (reprint of English translation, 1959). New York: Hafner.
22. Dạmbska M (1968) Encephalic necrosis and inflammatory reaction in fetuses and newborns. *Pol Med J* 7: 404–434.
23. Gilles FH, Leviton A, Dooling EC (1983) *Developing Human Brain: Growth and Epidemiologic Neuropathology*. Boston: Wright-PSG.
24. Sumi S, Hager H (1968) Electron microscopic study of the reaction of the newborn rat brain to injury. *Acta Neuropath* 10: 324–335.
25. Martin JJ, Guazzi GC, Th dB (1969) Sur l'incidence et la signification de certaines glioses fibrillaires du tronc cerebral chez les tres jeunes enfants. *J Hirnforsch* 11: 7–12.
26. Friede RL (1975) *Developmental Neuropathology*. Vienna: Springer.
27. Leviton A, Gilles FH (1971) Clustering of the morphological components of perinatal telencephalic leukoencephalopathy. *J Neurol Neurosurg Psych* 34: 642–645.
28. Leviton A, Gilles FH (1971) Morphologic correlates of age at death of infants with perinatal telencephalic leukoencephalopathy. *Am J Pathol* 65: 303–309.
29. Brack M (1973) Perinatal telencephalic leukoencephalopathy in chimpanzees (Pan troglodytes). *Acta Neuropathol (Berl)* 25: 307–312.
30. Leviton A, Gilles FH (1973) An epidemiologic study of perinatal telencephalic leukoencephalopathy in an autopsy population. *J Neurol Sci* 18: 53–66.
31. Leviton A, Gilles FH (1974) Morphologic abnormalities in human infant cerebral white matter related to gestational and postnatal age. *Pediatr Res* 8: 718–720.
32. Murofushi K (1974) [Symmetrical pseudocalcium deposits in the basal ganglia and white matter of the brain with moderate leukoencephalopathy in Down's syndrome]. *Neuropadiatrie* 5: 103–108.

280

33. Leviton A, Gilles F, Neff R, Yaney P (1976) Multivariate analysis of risk of perinatal telencephalic leuko-encephalopathy. *Am J Epidemiol* 104: 621–626.
34. Leviton A, Gilles FH, Vawter GF (1978) The thymus in infants with perinatal telencephalic leukoencephalopathy. *Arch Neurol* 35: 377–381.
35. Leech RW, Alvord EC Jr. (1974) Morphologic variations in periventricular leukomalacia. *Am J Pathol* 74: 591–602.
36. Shuman RM, Selednik LJ (1980) Periventricular leukomalacia. A one-year autopsy study. *Arch Neurol* 37: 231–235.
37. Deguchi K, Oguchi K, Takashima S (1997) Characteristic neuropathology of leukomalacia in extremely low birth weight infants. *Pediatr Neurol* 16: 296–300.
38. Parrot MJ (1873) Etude sur le ramollissement de lencephale chez le nouveau-ne. *Arch Physiol Norm Patholol (Paris)* 5: 59–73, 176–195, 283–303.
39. Schwartz P (1927) Die traumatischen schadigungen des zentralnerversystems durch die geburt. *Anat Untersuchungen Ergebn Inn Med u Kinderh* 31: 165–372.
40. Schwartz P, Fink L (1926) Morphologie und Entstehung der geburtstraumatischen Blutungen in Gehirn und Schädel des Neugeborenen. *Z Kinderheilkd* 40: 427–474.
41. Clark DB, Anderson GW (1961) Correlation of complications of labor with lesions in the brains of infants. *J Neuropathol Exp Neurol* 20: 275–278.
42. Larroche JC (1964) Developpement du système nerveux central pendant la vie intrauterine. Etude regionale et pathologie specifique. *Acta Paediatr Latina* 17 (Suppl 6): 676–696.
43. Larroche JC, Amiel CI, Relier JP, Korn G (1975) Leucomalacie et avenir cérébral en relation avec les soins intensifs néonataux. *J Anest Fr* 16: 171–175.
44. DeReuck J, Vander Eecken H (1983) Brain maturation and types or perinatal hypoxic–ischemic encephalopathy. *Eur Neurol* 22: 261–264.
45. Crawford CL, Hobbs MJ (1994) Anatomy of diplegia: an hypothesis. *Dev Med Child Neurol* 36: 513–517.
46. Levene MI, Wigglesworth JS, Dubowitz V (1983) Hemorrhagic periventricular leukomalacia in the neonate: a real-time ultrasound study. *Pediatrics* 69: 794–797.
47. Bernert G, Gottling A, Rosenkranz A, Zoder G (1988) Hemorrhagic and hypoxic–ischemic intracranial lesions in neonates diagnosed by realtime sonography: incidence and short-term outcome. *Padiatr Padol* 23: 25–37.
48. Grunnet ML (1979) Periventricular leukomalacia complex. *Arch Pathol Lab Med* 103: 6–10.
49. Leech RW, Alvord EC (1974) Glial fatty metamorphosis: an abnormal response of premyelin glia frequently accompanying periventricular leukomalacia. *Am J Pathol* 74: 603–612.
50. DeReuck J, Chattha AS, Richardson EPJ (1972) Pathogenesis and evolution of periventricular leukomalacia in infancy. *Arch Neurol* 27: 229–236.
51. Takashima S, Tanaka K (1978) Development of cerebrovascular architecture and its relationship to periventricular leukomalacia. *Arch Neurol* 35: 11.
52. DeReuck J (1971) The human periventricular arterial blood supply and the anatomy of cerebral infarctions. *Eur Neurol* 5: 321–334.
53. Takashima S, Armstrong DL, Becker LE (1978) Subcortical leukomalacia. Relationship to development of the cerebral sulcus and its vascular supply. *Arch Neurol* 35: 470–472.
54. Vitaliano PP, Urbach F (1980) The relative importance of risk factors in nonmelanoma carcinoma. *Arch Dermatol* 116: 454–456.
55. Vitaliano PP (1978) The use of logistic regression for modeling risk factors: with application to nonmelanoma skin cancer. *Am J Epidemiol* 108: 402–414.
56. Leviton A, Gilles FH (1983) Classification of the perinatal telencephalic leukoencephalopathies. In: Gilles FH, Leviton A, Dooling EC, editors. *The Developing Human Brain: Growth and Epidemiologic Neuropathology*. Boston: Wright-PSG, pp. 244–250.
57. Cochran AL, Davis I, Flecter CM (1951) 'Entente Radioloque.' A step towards international agreement on the classification of radiographs in pneumoconiosis. *Br J Ind Med* 8: 244–255.
58. Leviton A, Gilles FH (1983) The epidemiology of the perinatal telencephalic leukoencephalopathy characterized by hypertrophic astrocytes and amphophilic globules. In: Gilles FH, Leviton A, Dooling EC, editors. *The Developing Human Brain: Growth and Epidemiologic Neuropathology*. Boston: Wright-PSG, pp. 287–295.

59. Leviton A, Gilles FH (1983) The epidemiology of the perinatal telencephalic leukoencephalopathy characterized by amphophilic globules. In: Gilles FH, Leviton A, Dooling EC, editors. *The Developing Human Brain: Growth and Epidemiologic Neuropathology*. Boston: Wright-PSG, pp. 262–269.
60. Leviton A, Gilles FH (1983) The epidemiology of the perinatal telencephalic leukoencephalopathy characterized by acutely damaged glial cells. In: Gilles FH, Leviton A, Dooling EC, editors. *The Developing Human Brain: Growth and Epidemiologic Neuropathology*. Boston: Wright-PSG, pp. 278–286.
61. Leviton A, Gilles FH (1983) The epidemiology of the perinatal telencephalic leukoencephalopathy characterized by focal necroses. In: Gilles FH, Leviton A, Dooling EC, editors. *The Developing Human Brain: Growth and Epidemiologic Neuropathology*. Boston: Wright-PSG, pp. 270–277.
62. Roessmann U, Gambetti P (1986) Pathological reaction of astrocytes in perinatal brain injury. Immunohistochemical study. *Acta Neuropathol (Berl)* 70(3–4): 302–307.
63. Leviton A, Gilles FH (1974) Astrocytosis without globules in infant cerebral white matter. An epidemiologic study. *J Neurol Sci* 22: 329–340.
64. Back SA, Luo NL, Borenstein NS, Volpe JJ, Kinney HC (2002) Arrested oligodendrocyte lineage progression during human cerebral white matter development: dissociation between the timing of progenitor differentiation and myelinogenesis. *J Neuropathol Exp Neurol* 61: 197–211.
65. Haynes RL, Folkerth RD, Keefe RJ, et al (2003) Nitrosative and oxidative injury to premyelinating oligodendrocytes in periventricular leukomalacia. *J Neuropathol Exp Neurol* 62: 441–450.
66. Volpe JJ (2003) Cerebral white matter injury of the premature infant—more common than you think. *Pediatrics* 112: 176–180.
67. Marlow N, Roberts BL, Cooke RW (1989) Motor skills in extremely low birthweight children at the age of 6 years. *Arch Dis Child* 64: 839–847.
68. Fan LW, Pang Y, Lin S, Rhodes PG, Cai Z (2005) Minocycline attenuates lipopolysaccharide-induced white matter injury in the neonatal rat brain. *Neuroscience* 133: 159–168.
69. Duncan JR, Cock ML, Suzuki K, Scheerlinck JP, Harding R, Rees SM (2006) Chronic endotoxin exposure causes brain injury in the ovine fetus in the absence of hypoxemia. *J Soc Gynecol Investig* 13: 87–96.
70. Pang Y, Cai Z, Rhodes PG (2000) Effects of lipopolysaccharide on oligodendrocyte progenitor cells are mediated by astrocytes and microglia. *J Neurosci Res* 62: 510–520.
71. Creasy RK, Resnik R (1981) Intrauterine fetal growth retardation. In: Milunsky A, Friedman EA, Gluck L, editors. *Advances in Perinatal Medicine*. New York: Plenum Medical Book Co, pp. 117–164.
72. DeWitt SJ, Sparks JW, Swank PB, Smith K, Denson SE, Landry SH (1997) Physical growth of low birthweight infants in the first year of life: impact of maternal behaviors. *Early Hum Dev* 47: 19–34.
73. Fawer CL, Besnier S, Forcada M, Buclin T, Calame A (1995) Influence of perinatal, developmental and environmental factors on cognitive abilities of preterm children without major impairments at 5 years. *Early Hum Dev* 43: 151–164.
74. Ornoy A, Altshuler G (1976) Maternal endotoxemia, fetal anomalies, and central nervous system damage: a rat model of a human problem. *Am J Obstet Gynecol* 124: 196–204.
75. Offenbacher S, Katz V, Fertik G, et al (1996) Periodontal infection as a possible risk factor for preterm low birth weight. *J Periodontol* 67 (10 Suppl): 1103–1113.
76. Miller WD (1891) The human mouth as a focus of infection. *Dental Cosmos* 33: 689–713.
77. Mayo OH (1922) Focal infection of dental origin. *Dental Cosmos* 64: 1206–1208.
78. Madianos PN, Lieff S, Murtha AP, et al (2001) Maternal periodontitis and prematurity. Part II: Maternal infection and fetal exposure. *Ann Periodontol* 6: 175–182.
79. Panigrahy A, Barnes PD, Robertson RL, et al (2001) Volumetric brain differences in children with periventricular T2-signal hyperintensities: a grouping by gestational age at birth. *AJR Am J Roentgenol* 177: 695–702.
80. Perrin EV, Landing BH (1962) 'The Schmorl lesion' in jaundiced infected infants. *Am J Dis Child* 104: 551.
81. Campbell LV Jr., Gilbert EF (1967) Experimental giant-cell transformation in the liver induced by *E. coli* endotoxin. *Am J Pathol* 51: 855–868.
82. Haesaert B, Ornoy A (1986) Transplacental effects of endotoxemia on fetal mouse brain, bone, and placental tissue. *Pediatr Pathol* 5: 167–181.
83. Scheifele DW, Melton P, Whitchelo V (1981) Evaluation of the Limulus test for endotoxemia in neonates with suspected sepsis. *J Pediatr* 98:899–903.
84. Dammann O, Leviton A (1997) Maternal intrauterine infection, cytokines, and brain damage in the preterm newborn. *Pediatr Res* 42: 1–8.

85. Dammann O, Leviton A (1998) Infection remote from the brain, neonatal white matter damage, and cerebral palsy in the preterm infant. *Semin Pediatr Neurol* 5: 190–201.
86. Dammann O, Leviton A (1999) Brain damage in preterm newborns: might enhancement of developmentally regulated endogenous protection open a door for prevention? *Pediatrics* 104(3 Pt 1): 541–550.
87. Yoon BH, Romero R, Yang SH, et al (1996) Interleukin-6 concentrations in umbilical cord plasma are elevated in neonates with white matter lesions associated with periventricular leukomalacia. *Am J Obstet Gynecol* 174: 1433–1440.
88. Yoon BH, Jun JK, Romero R, et al (1997) Amniotic fluid inflammatory cytokines (interleukin-6, interleukin-1beta, and tumor necrosis factor-alpha), neonatal brain white matter lesions, and cerebral palsy. *Am J Obstet Gynecol* 177: 19–26.
89. Yoon BH, Romero R, Kim CJ, et al (1997) High expression of tumor necrosis factor-alpha and interleukin-6 in periventricular leukomalacia. *Am J Obstet Gynecol* 177: 406–411.
90. Romero R, Gomez R, Ghezzi F, et al (1998) A fetal systemic inflammatory response is followed by the spontaneous onset of preterm parturition. *Am J Obstet Gynecol* 179: 186–193.
91. Chaiworapongsa T, Romero R, Kim JC, et al (2002) Evidence for fetal involvement in the pathologic process of clinical chorioamnionitis. *Am J Obstet Gynecol* 186: 1178–1182.
92. Kadhim H, Tabarki B, Verellen G, De Prez C, Rona AM, Sebire G (2001) Inflammatory cytokines in the pathogenesis of periventricular leukomalacia. *Neurology* 56: 1278–1284.
93. Kadhim H, Tabarki B, De Prez C, Sebire G (2003) Cytokine immunoreactivity in cortical and subcortical neurons in periventricular leukomalacia: are cytokines implicated in neuronal dysfunction in cerebral palsy? *Acta Neuropathol (Berl)* 105: 209–216.
94. Folkerth RD (2005) Neuropathologic substrate of cerebral palsy. *J Child Neurol* 20: 940–949.
95. Ellison VJ, Mocatta TJ, Winterbourn CC, Darlow BA, Volpe JJ, Inder TE (2005) The relationship of CSF and plasma cytokine levels to cerebral white matter injury in the premature newborn. *Pediatr Res* 57: 282–286.
96. Cai Z, Pan ZL, Pang Y, Evans OB, Rhodes PG (2000) Cytokine induction in fetal rat brains and brain injury in neonatal rats after maternal lipopolysaccharide administration. *Pediatr Res* 47: 64–72.
97. Cai Z, Pang Y, Lin S, Rhodes PG (2003) Differential roles of tumor necrosis factor-alpha and interleukin-1 beta in lipopolysaccharide-induced brain injury in the neonatal rat. *Brain Res* 975: 37–47.
98. Bell MJ, Hallenbeck JM, Gallo V (2004) Determining the fetal inflammatory response in an experimental model of intrauterine inflammation in rats. *Pediatr Res* 56: 541–546.
99. Patrick LA, Gaudet LM, Farley AE, Rossiter JP, Tomalty LL, Smith GN (2004) Development of a guinea pig model of chorioamnionitis and fetal brain injury. *Am J Obstet Gynecol* 191: 1205–1211.
100. Krishnamoorthy KS, Kuban KC, O'Shea TM, Westra SJ, Allred EN, Leviton A (2011) Early cranial ultrasound lesions predict microcephaly at age 2 years in preterm infants. *J Child Neurol [Research Support, NIH, Extramural]* 26: 188–194.
101. Kuban KC, Allred EN, O'Shea TM, et al (2009) Cranial ultrasound lesions in the NICU predict cerebral palsy at age 2 years in children born at extremely low gestational age. *J Child Neurol [Research Support, NIH, Extramural]* 24: 63–72.
102. Leviton A, Kuban K, O'Shea TM, et al (2011) The relationship between early concentrations of 25 blood proteins and cerebral white matter injury in preterm newborns: The ELGAN study. *J Pediatr* 158: 897–903 e1–5.
103. O'Shea TM, Allred EN, Dammann O, et al (2009) The ELGAN study of the brain and related disorders in extremely low gestational age newborns. *Early Hum Dev [Multicenter Study Research Support, NIH, Extramural]* 85: 719–725.
104. Leviton A, Kuban K, Allred EN, et al (2010) Antenatal antecedents of a small head circumference at age 24-months post-term equivalent in a sample of infants born before the 28th post-menstrual week. *Early Hum Dev [Multicenter Study Research Support, NIH, Extramural]* 86: 515–521.
105. Leviton A, Kuban KC, Allred EN, Fichorova RN, O'Shea TM, Paneth N (2011) Early postnatal blood concentrations of inflammation-related proteins and microcephaly two years later in infants born before the 28th post-menstrual week. *Early Hum Dev* 87: 325–330.
106. Onderdonk AB, Delaney ML, DuBois AM, Allred EN, Leviton A (2008) Detection of bacteria in placental tissues obtained from extremely low gestational age neonates. *Am J Obstet Gynecol [Research Support, NIH, Extramural]* 198: 110, e1–7.

107. Logan JW, O'Shea TM, Allred EN, et al (2010) Early postnatal hypotension and developmental delay at 24 months of age among extremely low gestational age newborns. *Arch Dis Child Fetal Neonatal Ed* 31: 524–534.
108. Tanner DC, Cherry JD, Mayer-Proschel M (2011) Oligodendrocyte progenitors reversibly exit the cell cycle and give rise to astrocytes in response to interferon-{gamma}. *J Neurosci* 31: 6235–6246.
109. Kinney HC, Back SA (1998) Human oligodendroglial development: relationship to periventricular leukomalacia. *Semin Pediatr Neurol* 5: 180–189.
110. McElrath TF, Hecht JL, Dammann O, et al (2008) Pregnancy disorders that lead to delivery before the 28th week of gestation: an epidemiologic approach to classification. *Am J Epidemiol [Multicenter Study Research Support, NI., Extramural]* 168: 980–989.
111. Back SA, Gan X, Li Y, Rosenberg PA, Volpe JJ (1998) Maturation-dependent vulnerability of oligodendrocytes to oxidative stress-induced death caused by glutathione depletion. *J Neurosci* 18: 6241–6453.
112. Back SA, Luo NL, Mallinson RA, et al (2005) Selective vulnerability of preterm white matter to oxidative damage defined by F2-isoprostanes. *Ann Neurol* 58: 108–120.
113. Boyce R (1894) A contribution to the study of descending degenerations in the brain and spinal cord, and the seat of origin and paths of conduction of the fits in absinthe epilepsy. *Proc Royal Soc London* 55: 269–275.
114. Hunt JR (1904) The retrograde atrophy of the pyramidal tracts. *J Nervous Mental Dis* 31: 504–512.
115. Jones WH, Thomas DB (1956) Trans-synaptic atrophy in the cerebral cortex. *Nature 178*: 47–48.
116. Volpe JJ (2005) Encephalopathy of prematurity includes neuronal abnormalities. *Pediatrics* 116: 221–225.
117. Pierson CR, Folkerth RD, Billiards SS, et al (2007) Gray matter injury associated with periventricular leukomalacia in the premature infant. *Acta Neuropathol* 114: 619–631.
118. Ligam P, Haynes RL, Folkerth RD, et al (2009) Thalamic damage in periventricular leukomalacia: novel pathologic observations relevant to cognitive deficits in survivors of prematurity. *Pediatr Res* 65: 524–529.
119. Iai M, Takashima S (1999) Thalamocortical development of parvalbumin neurons in normal and periventricular leukomalacia brains. *Neuropediatrics* 30: 14–18.
120. Schwartz P (1961) *Birth Injuries of the Newborn, Morphology, Pathogenesis, Clinical Pathology and Prevention*. New York: Hafner Publishing.

13
LATE FETAL AND PERINATAL BRAIN VASCULAR ABNORMALITIES AND NECROSES

Overview

In this chapter, we examine central nervous system lesions that are considered vascular or hypotensive, vascular developmental abnormalities, and late brain anomalies that follow early-life brain necrosis. We include infarcts in various supply arterial distributions, emboli to and from the brain, acute borderzone necroses, venous and sinus occlusions and their resultant hemorrhagic brain necroses, as well as neonatal vascular anomalies, pontosubicular neuronal necroses, prothrombotic conditions, and other antecedents. There are many variations of individual major cerebral arterial distributions;[1] however, we will not describe in detail occasional cases of an unusual anatomic location (such as borderzone lesions when one carotid artery is absent), which may result in diverse and unforeseen pathologic and clinical effects. Anomalous arteries or collateral circulation modify the extent of vascular lesions. Late brain anomalies that we review include lesions such as porencephaly, hydranencephaly, multicystic encephalomalacia, symmetric thalamic neuronal loss, symmetric basal ganglia lesions, and status marmoratus.

Arterial

COLLATERAL CIRCULATION

Cohnheim,[2] recognizing that tissue necrosis following cerebral artery occlusion demonstrated the intimate relationship between vascular supply and neural tissue, proposed the physiologic 'end artery' concept. Historically and clinically, the distinction between anatomical and physiologic end arteries is important. Duret[3] confirmed Cohnheim's original concept, which was accepted well into the twentieth century. During the nineteenth century, the curious location of the circle of Willis at the brain base provoked the notion that an anomalous circle could importantly modify the extent of cerebral necrosis.[4] Gradually, it became apparent that not only did potential collateral circulatory channels between internal and external cerebral arteries exist, but also that complex intracerebral capillary and arteriolar anastomoses, of most cerebral arterial systems, as well as direct arterial fetal anastomoses of anterior to middle and middle to posterior cerebral arteries, were present (see Chapter 8).[5] Therefore, except for the opossum,[6] the term 'end artery' is a physiologic term rather than an anatomic entity. Consequently, it is not surprising that major cerebral vessels sometimes gradually obstruct in early childhood without producing a neurologic deficit.[7] Moyamoya disease illustrates the developmental potential of collateral arteries at the brain base.[8,9] Collaterals also exist between external and internal carotid arteries, for instance, via ophthalmic arteries,[10] maxillary arteries,[11] or transcalvarial 'emissary' vessels.

NECROSES IN ARTERIAL BORDERZONE DISTRIBUTIONS

Arterial cortical borderzone lesions were first described in adult brains as being related to thromboangiitis obliterans[12] and later recognized as following hypotension.[13] Lesions in a similar distribution, also found in infant brains,[14] are now identified with current imaging.[15] Cruveilhier[16] (in the early nineteenth century) drew such a lesion occurring in one cerebral hemisphere (Fig. 13.1). In this case, the unilateral borderzone lesion was likely to be the result of significant neonatal hypotension in a child with a vascular anomaly at the skull base, such as carotid hypoplasia (see below). In the late gestational fetus, severe hypotension leads either to a cortical borderzone lesion or to upper brainstem, thalamic, and spinal cord damage, with cortical and cerebellar sparing.[17–19] When cerebral and cerebellar cortices are involved, the more or less symmetric lesions generally include gray and underlying white matter in borderzones between major arteries or in distal arterial supply regions, such as the dorsal thalamus (Figs. 13.2 and 13.3). The smallest lesions occur in the cortex around sulcal depths; larger lesions

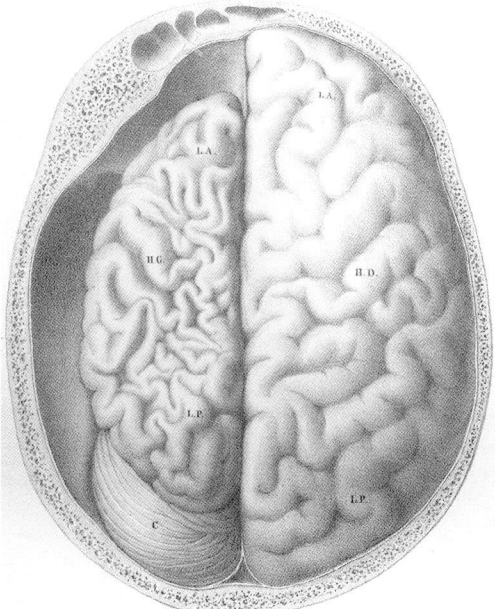

Fig. 13.1 In this image from Cruveilhier's atlas, the artist has drawn a small left hemisphere with overlying bone thickening, left frontal sinus enlargement, and a cerebellum that shows behind the small hemisphere. More important, the small shrunken gyri lie parallel to the midline between the middle and anterior cerebral arteries, a typical borderzone lesion given a small left carotid artery at the base. From Cruveilhier.[16,191]

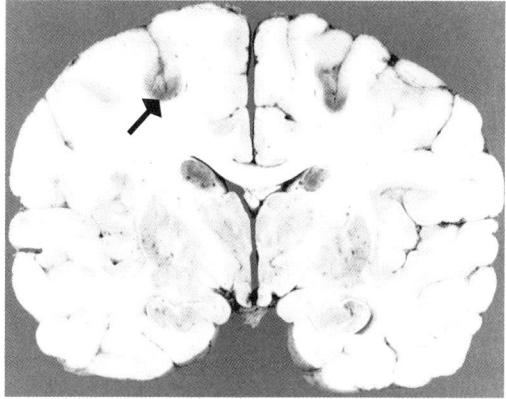

Fig. 13.2 Minimal borderzone lesions. Young child. Coronal slice through anterior thalamus. Bilaterally, there are small cortical hemorrhagic necroses at the depths of the first frontal sulcus between the first and second frontal gyri. The anterior cerebral artery supplies the first frontal gyrus; and the middle cerebral artery supplies the second frontal gyrus. Similar hemorrhagic necroses are seen in caudate bodies, the distalmost lateral striate arterial supply regions.

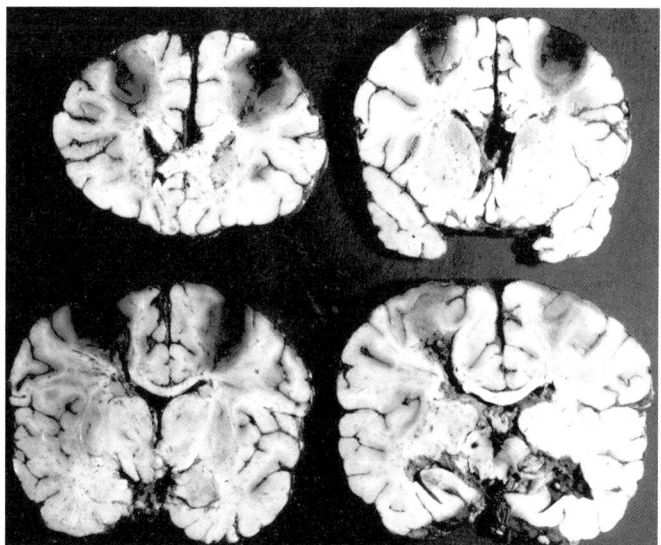

Fig. 13.3 Two-year-old child. Large borderzone lesions. Serial coronal slices from anterior (top left) through pulvinar (bottom right). Anteriorly, large hemorrhagic necroses lie symmetrically in the border-zones between anterior and middle cerebral arterial supply areas. In the pulvinar slice, the borderzone lesions are less hemorrhagic.

(a)

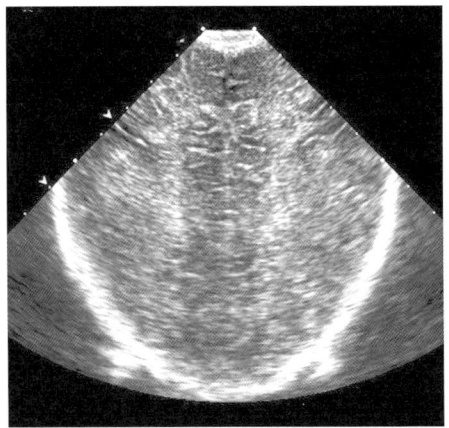

(b)

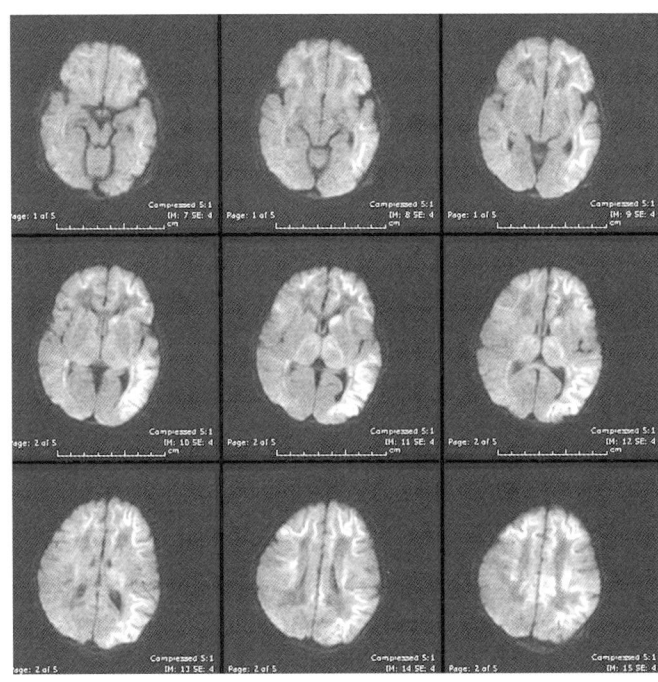

Fig. 13.4 (a) Term newborn with meconium aspiration. Coronal cranial ultrasound demonstrates patchy echogenicity in both cerebral hemispheres. (b) Diffusion-weighted MRI of same patient as in Figure 13.4a, now 7 days old, demonstrating cortical images of asymmetric deep vascular borderzone lesions, left > right. (c) Axial T1-weighted image of same child now 18 months old demonstrating sclerotic microgyria in vascular borderzones, left > right (arrows). In these regions gyri are shrunken, particularly at the gyral base. The neighboring subarachnoid space is enlarged. (d) Coronal T2-weighted images of the same patient as in Fig. 13.4a–c. Now 18 months old. Bilateral vascular borderzone lesions are present, left > right. The lower row of images demonstrate typical 'mushroom' gyri with relatively preserved cortex on gyral crests and almost total loss of cortex around sulcal bottoms (arrows). These lesions are maximal in the upper brain in the borderzones between the middle and anterior cerebral artery supply areas. There is underlying loss of white matter with prominent ventriculomegaly and a thin corpus callosum.

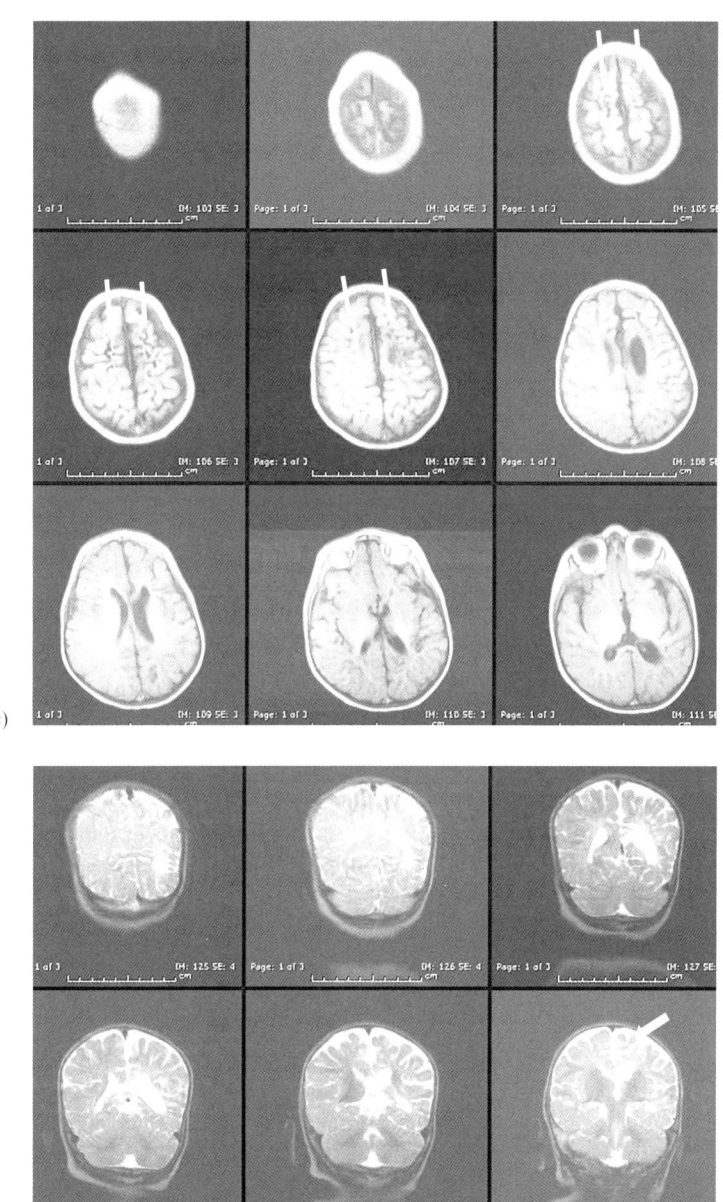

(c)

(d)

289

envelop entire gyri. Generally, cortical lesions increase in size, progressing from the frontal to the occipital lobe, depending on the duration of inadequate perfusion. Long periods of insufficient circulation result in continuous frontal to occipital lesions, gradually increasing in width (Fig. 13.4). Expected lesion symmetry is lost when the circle of Willis is asymmetric or a major cerebral artery is hypoplastic (as in Fig. 13.1), has an anomalous origin, or is otherwise constricted. Associated striatal and thalamic lesions are largest near the ventricle and in dorsal thalami. Anteriorly, borderzone necroses lie between anterior and middle cerebral arteries and posteriorly between the anterior, middle, and posterior cerebral arteries. Posteriorly, in the parietal lobe, they are usually more extensive. Sometimes, large borderzone lesions extend into the lateral temporal lobe and along the middle and posterior cerebral arterial borderzone (third temporal gyrus), forming a C-shaped necrosis on each hemispheral side with the concavity facing anteriorly. With prolonged inadequate perfusion, necrosis size increases, eventually involving the entire cerebrum. These ideas were developed from Noell and Schneider's[20] observation that, under pathologic conditions, the brain oxygen supply depends on feeding vessel length and decreases first in the most distal arterial territories, for which they coined the term 'die letzte Wiese' or 'the last meadow.' Brain oxygen supply, of course, is a function of cerebral blood flow, and thus depends on cardiac output and local arterial anomalies, which potentially constrict blood flow. The term 'die letzte Wiese,' unfortunately, was mistranslated into 'watershed.' But 'watershed,' by contrast, means the whole area or region, such as a mountainside draining into a river, and not the water supply's distal end or last field. Better terms are borderzone or endzone, referring to those brain regions in distalmost supply areas of major cerebral arteries following significant cerebral hypoperfusion.[13,21–25]

Following hypotension, bilateral brainstem lesions in the tegmentum and tectum sometimes appear in major neuronal groups, such as the inferior colliculus and motor and sensory nuclei.[17,26–30] No brainstem nucleus is spared, and, in severe cases, the entire tegmentum is necrotic with relative crural and basis pontis sparing (Fig. 13.5). The inferior colliculi deserve special attention because hypotensive episode lesions are frequent here, perhaps because of their high vascularity.[28,31] As the inferior colliculi are major auditory relay nuclei, these infantile lesions are readily detected with appropriate clinical testing.

The cerebellar borderzone peripherally lies between the superior and inferior cerebellar arteries (supplying superior and inferior hemispheral surfaces), including the horizontal fissure. Lumbosacral spinal cord gray matter shows typical necroses following cardiac arrest.[18,32] Interestingly, some childhood and adult neuronal damage, following cardiac arrest, is limited to the basal ganglia or thalamus, brainstem, or spinal cord.

MAJOR CENTRAL NERVOUS SYSTEM ARTERIAL STEM OR BRANCH
OCCLUSIONS IN NEWBORN AND EARLY CHILDHOOD
Cerebral infarcts in specific arterial beds are relatively rare neonatal or early childhood events; they occur in the left middle cerebral artery territory (57%), right middle cerebral artery (24%), vertebral–basilar (8%), multiple regions (11%),[33] and in the fetus[34–36] (Fig. 13.6). Hemiparesis is thought to be more common after childhood middle cerebral artery infarcts than after neonatal infarcts, and less likely if infarction involved only basal ganglia. For other investigators, age at infarct was less important.[37]

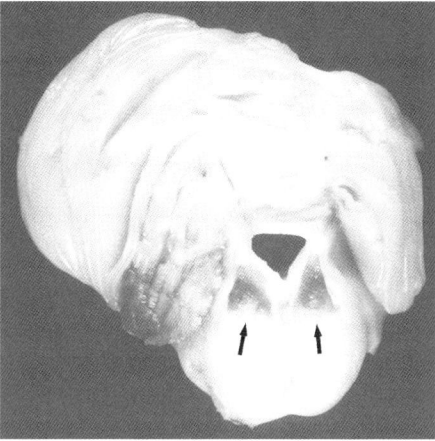

Fig. 13.5 In this pontine axial section, there is total tegmental necrosis (arrows) with cyst formation. This infant had been maintained on a respirator for several weeks following a severe neonatal hypotensive episode at birth. The lesion ceases abruptly at the basis pontis border. Similar lesions extended from the midbrain (including the inferior colliculus) to the upper medulla.

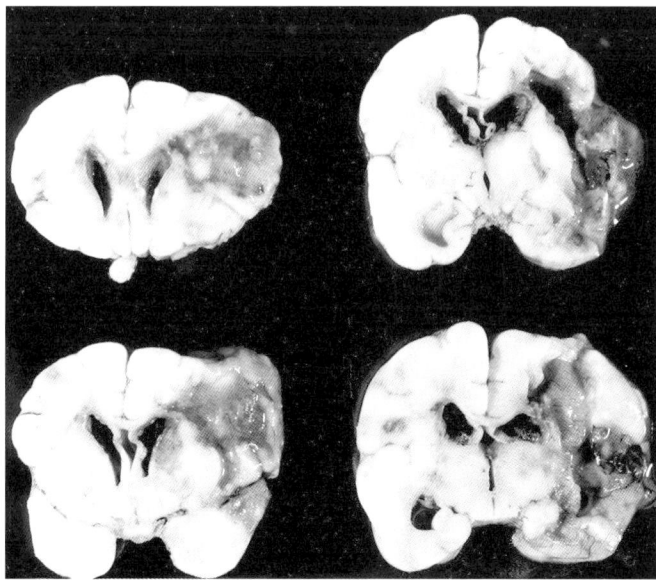

Fig. 13.6 Late third-trimester fetus with infarct in distribution of right middle cerebral artery. The large recent infarct occupies the lateral half of the second frontal gyrus, third frontal gyrus, and first, second, and third temporal gyri, as well as the putamen and caudate.

291

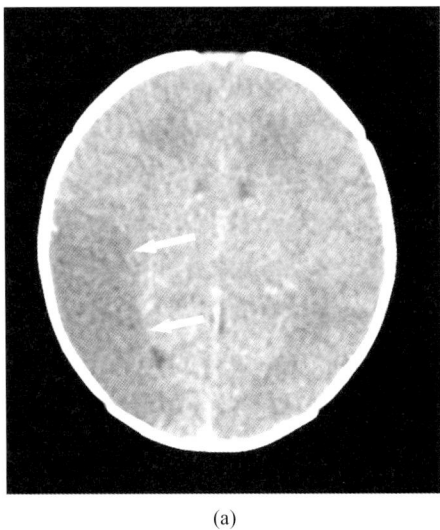

(a)

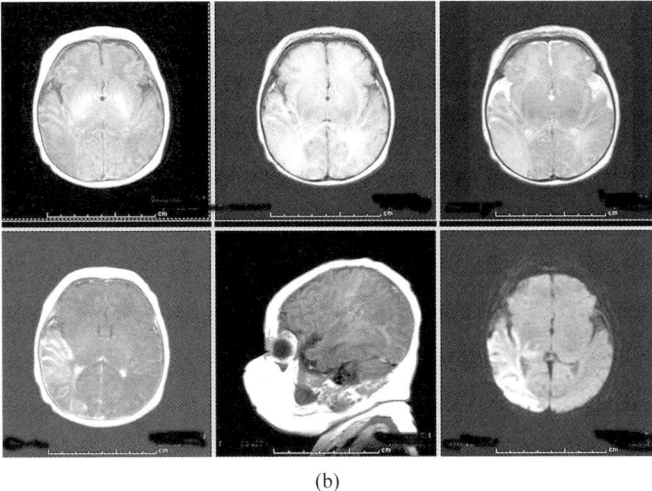

(b)

Fig. 13.7 (a) Noncontrast CT image. Acute (3 days old) right middle cerebral artery infarct. There is low attenuation (arrows) in the brain supplied by a right distal middle cerebral artery branch distribution with loss of gray/white distinction. (b) Same child, now 7 days old. MRI illustrating the acute distal right middle cerebral artery infarct in evolution. T1 weighted (top left); FLAIR (top middle); T2 weighted (top right); T1 postcontrast (bottom left); sagittal T1 (bottom middle); diffusion weighted (bottom right). (c) Same child, now 3 years old. The distal right middle cerebral artery infarct in the brain has become a cavity. The cavity is much smaller than the edematous region seen on the acute scans. T1 weighted (top left); FLAIR (top middle); T2 weighted (top right); T1 postcontrast (bottom left); sagittal T1 (botttom middle); diffusion weighted (bottom right).

292

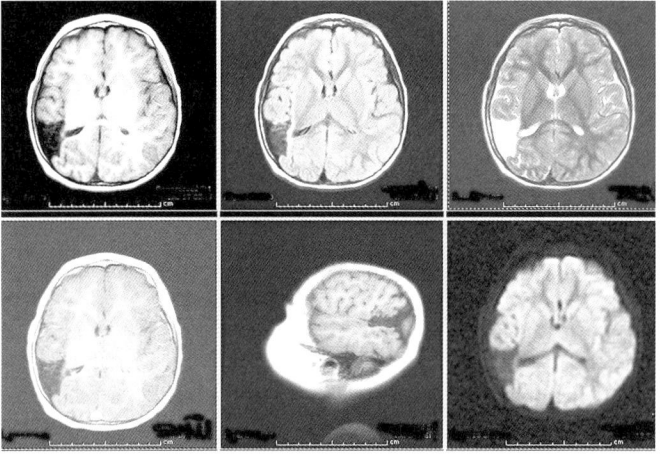

(c)

Cerebral infarcts in arterial distributions

Carotid artery occlusions, or its middle or anterior cerebral branch occlusions, causing large or small infarcts, are widely reported (Fig. 13.7).[38-43] Frequently, hemorrhage into originally ischemic infarcts occurs. Some authors concluded that cerebral arterial thromboses seemed more common than venous thromboses neonatally; others have emphasized trauma as the important inducing agent.[44,45] In preterm infants with vascular lesions elsewhere in the brain, cerebellar infarcts, particularly in the posterior inferior cerebellar artery distribution, also occur.[46] Carotid artery dissection is always suspected when infarction simultaneously occurs in both anterior and middle cerebral arterial distributions.[47,48] Infarcts appear in the context of elevated maternal anticardiolipin antibodies,[42,49] plasminogen activator inhibitor-1,[50] protein C deficiency, and their combinations;[51] birth trauma; and with underlying cardiac abnormalities accounting for about one-quarter of cases. Other conditions such as infections or collagen vascular disease; arteritis; dehydration; extracorporeal membrane oxygenation; neonatal intravascular catheters; embolism from multiple sources, including congenital or rheumatic heart disease; subacute bacterial endocarditis; intravascular catheters; sickle cell disease; maternal abnormalities such as infection, pre-eclampsia, or diabetes; and maternal drug use contribute their share of early-life infarcts. Cerebral arterial thromboses have also occurred in neonates and children secondary to atherosclerosis, granulomatous angiitis, periarteritis nodosa, lupus, subacute bacterial endocarditis, tuberculous and bacterial meningitis, sickle cell anemia, retropharyngeal abscess, and tuberous sclerosis; finally, some are cryptogenic.[52] Cerebral infarcts in late gestation or the neonate are similar to adult lesions, ending pathologically as limited defects with shaggy walls and crossing tissue bridges.

Vertebral artery birth trauma

Yates[44] found distortional trauma in the necks of 27 out of 60 infants who were stillborn or died in the neonatal period,[53] such as spinal extradural and subdural hemorrhage, hemorrhage into joint capsules, and torn ligaments and dura; occurring after all delivery methods,

293

including cesarean section. Direct spinal cord damage occurred with torn spinal roots in nine cases, usually unilaterally. Adventitial hemorrhages in one or both vertebral arteries (in 24 cases) were usually small, but others were large, either surrounding or compressing vessel lumen. These hemorrhages arose mainly from veins accompanying the vertebral arteries or from tearing of vertebral artery branches. In some cases, the compressed vertebral arteries contained thrombi. Moreover, simple neonatal head extension sometimes produced bilateral vertebral artery compression with resultant brainstem compromise.[54]

Emboli to the central nervous system
Systemic venous emboli sometimes pass through patent foramen ovale and occlude cerebral, cerebellar, or spinal cord arteries. Emboli arise from the ductus arteriosus,[55] placenta,[38,56] meconium,[57] internal carotid artery,[43] or thrombosed portal vein,[58] or are of obscure origin.[59] They often originate from umbilical vein catheterization,[60–63] central venous line thrombosis,[64,65] occasionally from portal vein thromboses,[58] and are occasionally associated with necrotic skin lesions.[66] A fibrin ring is regularly found surrounding indwelling catheter tips left in situ at death, and emboli from this source may have gone to the brain or spinal cord.[67] Rarely, they derive from thrombi at the internal carotid artery origin.[43] In some cases, the mothers have antiphospholipid antibodies.[68]

Emboli from brain
Brain tissue emboli were recognized throughout the twentieth century; they can block pulmonary arteries or enter the systemic circulation.[69–72] In one case, following a complicated breech delivery, brain tissue emboli to coronary, pulmonary, and leptomeningeal arteries originated from the left cerebellar hemisphere and entered venous blood through a left transverse sinus rupture.[73] Similar cases have been described in adults and children with head injuries.

ARTERIAL ANOMALIES

Major artery aplasia or hypoplasia
If one or more great arteries supplying the cerebrum is aplastic, alternative compensatory supply routes are established early in life and neurologic disturbance need not occur.[74–76] Less clear is when a vessel (for instance, the carotid artery) is hypoplastic and an ipsilateral cerebral tissue deficit or dysplasia exists.[77] Did the defect result from the vascular inadequacy (necessarily coupled with inadequate collateral circulation); did the vascular tree fail to develop because there was no 'demand' for blood supply from the previously deficient tissue; or did the vessel fail to continue its development after an intrauterine insult such as a thrombosis? The entire internal carotid system is sometimes hypoplastic.[78–80] As carotid intracranial portions are formed from different aortic arch regions, hypoplastic carotid portions limited to the cranium or intracranial or extracranial blood supply can occur (Fig. 13.8). Only one or several of the circle of Willis branches may be hypoplastic.[81] In any event, some carotid arterial hypoplasia cases occur without neural deficit, whereas others have widespread malformation or ipsilateral cerebral growth failure.[82,83] Occasionally, carotid aplasia is associated with intracranial aneurysms. Bilateral internal carotid hypoplasia or aplasia sometimes results

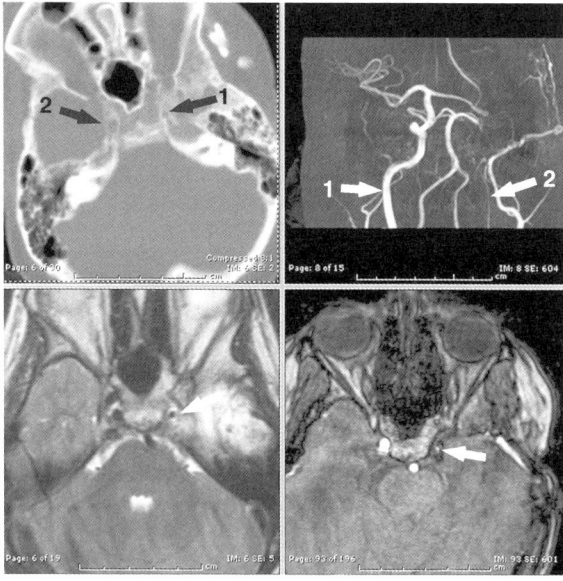

Fig. 13.8 CT image of a hypoplastic left carotid artery. Scan of skull base (top left). The left carotid canal (1) is small, ~50% the size of the right canal (2). T2-weighted MRI (bottom left). Small left carotid artery at the level of the sella (arrow). Magnetic resonance angiogram (MRA) (anterior–posterior projection) with absence of the left internal carotid artery (top right). The right internal carotid is of normal size;[1] the left should lie in the region of the fine vessel labeled 2. MRA axial three-dimensional time of flight MRA image (bottom right) showing minimal flow (white) in left internal carotid artery (arrow).

in hydranencephaly.[84,85] Additionally complicating the picture, accessory middle cerebral arteries sometimes arise from the internal carotid or proximal and/or distal anterior cerebral arteries.[86,87]

No matter the extent of capillary and sinusoidal collateral circulation between major cerebral arteries, an abrupt loss of blood supply through a major vessel usually overwhelms collaterals and the brain becomes necrotic. Furthermore, major arterial branch anomalies are sufficiently frequent that they must be kept in mind when evaluating and distinguishing fetal, neonatal, or infantile infarcts from those due to arterial occlusion or significant hypotension. Figure 13.9 shows an abnormal circle of Willis with multiple thrombi in many branches and a very small anterior cerebral artery on the left.

Persistent carotid to vertebral–basilar anastomoses
Multiple carotid to basilar (vertebral) branches sometimes persist from early embryonic life. A carotid branch coursing through the cavernous sinus medial to the trigeminal ophthalmic branch supplies the upper basilar artery in the 26-day human embryo and, while normally obliterated at about 45 days, it sometimes persists, usually asymptomatically. Although such persistent embryologic carotid–basilar anastomoses are rare, they are associated with hypoplastic or aplastic intracranial arteries or may be utilized when a major intracranial vessel is

occluded. Other carotid–vertebral anastomoses are described: proatlantal carotid to vertebral associated with vertebral aplasia or hypoplasia;[88,89] carotid to superior cerebellar artery anastomosis occurring with bilateral supraclinoid internal carotid artery hypoplasia;[90] carotid–basilar anastomosis via the primitive otic artery with vertebral and basilar arterial hypoplasia[91] (Fig. 13.10); or with moyamoya syndrome and basilar artery hypoplasia with a large anastomosis between the accessory meningeal and superior cerebellar arteries.[92,93]

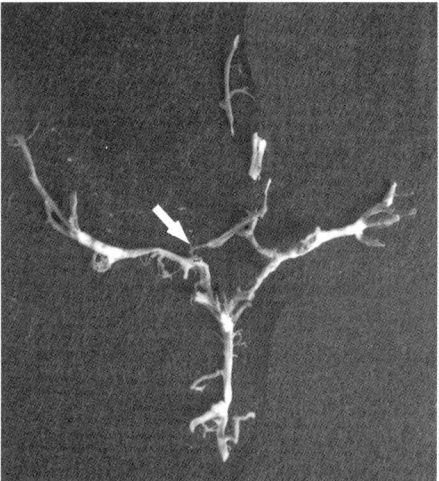

Fig. 13.9 A dissection photograph of an anomalous circle of Willis with a small anterior cerebral artery on the left (arrow). The basilar artery is at the bottom; the middle cerebral arteries lie out to either side. The white regions in both middle cerebral arteries and at the upper end of the basilar artery are organized thrombi.

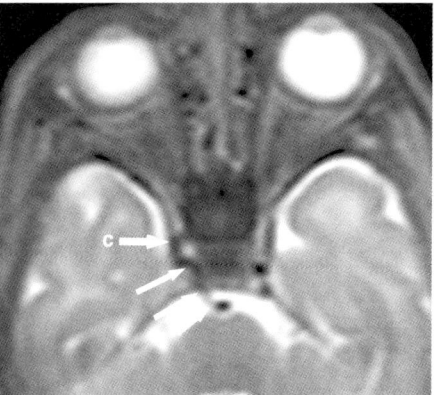

Fig. 13.10 Carotid–basilar shunt—trigeminal artery. T2-weighted axial image. There is a large vessel (small arrows) connecting the right cavernous carotid artery (c) to the basilar artery anterior to the pons.

Venous thrombotic occlusions

Cerebral venous drainage occurs largely through two systems: the external venous system, draining superficial cortical portions and much white matter; and the internal system, via the straight sinus and vein of Galen, draining basal ganglia, corpus callosum, septum pellucidum, gyrus cinguli, pineal region, quadrigeminal bodies, crura cerebri, frontal lobe base, superior cerebellar surface, and lateral and third ventricular choroid plexuses.

Venous hemorrhagic necroses vary depending on the infant's age and the extent and location of the thrombus.[94] Infantile cranial sinus and venous thrombosis reports were abundant in the nineteenth and early twentieth century; early investigators distinguished red or pale necroses from cerebral vein or sinus occlusions (Fig. 13.11).[95,96] Byers and Hass[97] found venous or sinus thromboses in 9% of neonatal, infantile, and early childhood autopsies. These venous occlusions happen in a setting of clinical dehydration, sepsis, hypernatremia, prothrombotic disorders, homocystinuria, and congenital cardiac disease.[98–100] Two distinct brain damage patterns occur following (1) superior sagittal sinus and external cerebral vein thrombosis or (2) internal cerebral vein thrombosis.[101] Occasionally, a cerebral sinus is only partially occluded and sometimes sinuses are recanalized. Currently, internal cerebral venous thromboses are uncommon in newborns and young children and, in this population, there is considerable variation in the amount of hemorrhagic necrosis in basal ganglia, thalami, and deep white matter.[102] Petrous bone infections can spread to thrombose the sigmoid, transverse, and other sinuses.

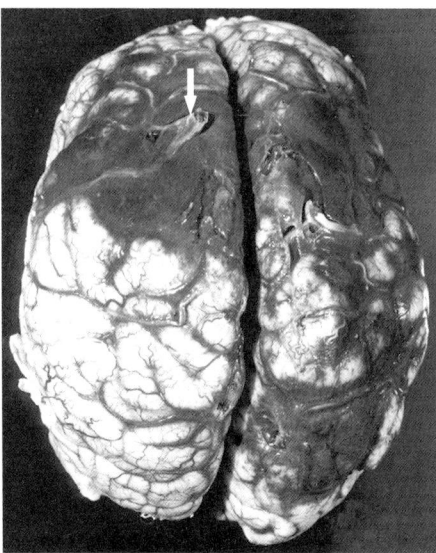

Fig. 13.11 Superior sagittal sinus thrombosis in a young child. Multiple cortical regions have undergone hemorrhagic necrosis and demonstrate superficial focal subarachnoid hemorrhage. A large superficial vein (arrow) contains organized thrombi that propagate out from the superior sagittal sinus thrombus. Other superior veins are markedly congested.

Thrombus location in superior sagittal sinus thrombosis is significant: The anterior third can usually be thrombosed or ligated without cerebral necroses;[103] the posterior third, or posterior and middle third, thrombus is likely to result in cerebral hemorrhagic necrosis. Rarely, the thrombus extends into superficial cerebral veins, leading to hemorrhagic infarction and, often, local subarachnoid hemorrhage. The hemorrhagic infarcts are usually parasagittal in location (Figs. 13.12 and 13.13), but are not necessarily symmetric. The most common risk factors include mastoiditis, persistent pulmonary hypertension, cardiac malformation, dehydration, and hypernatremia.[100,104] Occasionally, the thrombosed sinus mineralizes.[105]

Necroses of unknown origin

PONTOSUBICULAR NEURONAL NECROSIS

Friede[106] reported neuronal necrosis limited to the basis pontis and the subiculum.[107] The lesions were observed in 30-week-old preterm infants and in infants up to the age of 2 months. Others noted them even earlier at 22 weeks' gestation.[108] Newborn lesions are most severe, usually accompanying other neonatal brain damage. We have not seen it without other lesions, and the National Collaborative Perinatal Project (NCPP) material did not have this specific coupling of necroses.

Vascular organizational abnormalities

VASCULAR MALFORMATIONS

Vascular malformations are generally regarded as persistent, primitive, embryonic vascular pathways whose normal regression failed.[109] They consist of vessels that are abnormal in

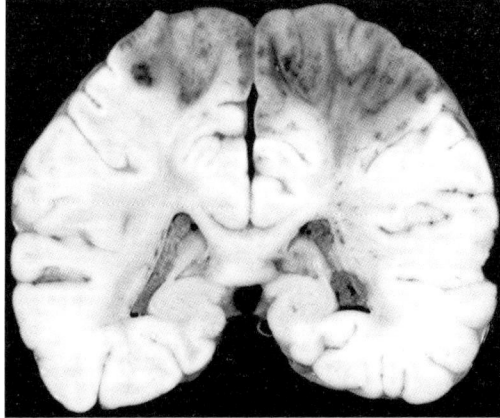

Fig. 13.12 Superior sagittal sinus thrombosis, neonate. The superior sagittal sinus thrombosis caused hemorrhagic necroses that ignored the borderzones between anterior and middle cerebral arteries and caused bilateral wedge-shaped necroses that extended from the interhemispheric fissure laterally over the convexity.

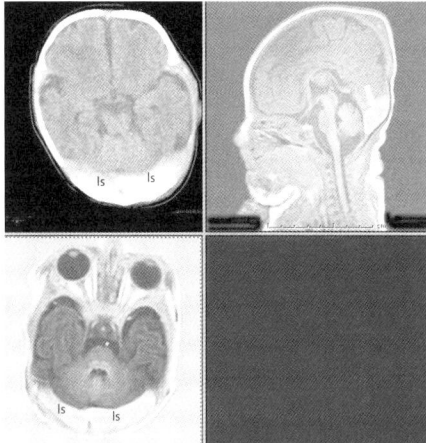

Fig. 13.13 Dural sinus thrombosis in a newborn. Noncontrast CT scan of the head (top left). There are hyperdense lateral sinuses (ls), consistent with clotted blood. Sagittal T1 MRI (top right). There is a thrombosed torcular Herophili (arrow). Axial T1 MRI (bottom left). The lateral sinuses are hyperintense, consistent with a clot within the sinus (ls).

density and/or structure and which cause alterations in neighboring tissue and vessels owing to local hemodynamic changes and are sometimes associated with local cerebral anomalies.

Malformations are classified as rapid direct shunts between arterial and venous circulations or as local slow-flow blood pools in capillary or venous ectasias. The first group includes classic arteriovenous malformations, whose rapid shunting capability is readily demonstrated angiographically, and histologically by its thick vessel walls. The second group contains malformations such as telangiectasia, cavernous angioma, and leptomeningeal venous or capillary angiomatosis (Stürge–Weber–Dimitri–Kalischer disease), all characterized by sinusoidal and thin vessel walls.[110] In capillary angiomatosis, direct blood shunting under arterial pressure is not prominent; therefore, angiographic demonstration is usually poor or impossible. Many vascular abnormalities occur together,[111] such as the Wyburn–Mason syndrome, a rare, non-hereditary neurocutaneous disorder that typically includes unilateral vascular malformations that include brain, orbits, and facial structures.[112]

Arteriovenous malformations

Arteriovenous malformations are circumscribed abnormal masses of arteries and veins, and are classified by size, location, and morphologic type.[110] Some involve the whole brain,[113] whereas others are familial.[114] Usually, the arterial shunting results in dilated draining veins and their neonatal pathology resembles that in the adult (Figs. 13.14 and 13.15). Vessel walls are duplicated, contain distorted internal elastic lamina, varying muscularis thickness, and variable fibrosis. Neural tissue is present in inconstant amounts between abnormal vessels; intervening tissue contains hemosiderin and variable chronic inflammatory infiltrates. They are located anywhere in the brain or spinal cord, but are rarely found in infants and young

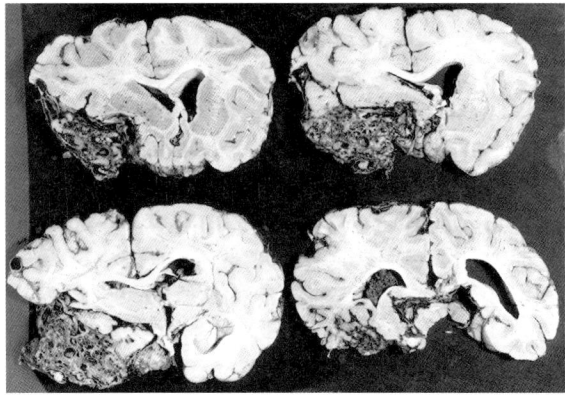

Fig. 13.14 A large arteriovenous malformation occupies the left temporal lobe, left putamen, globus pallidus, and third ventricle. In the fourth image, it extends into the left atrial choroid plexus glomus.

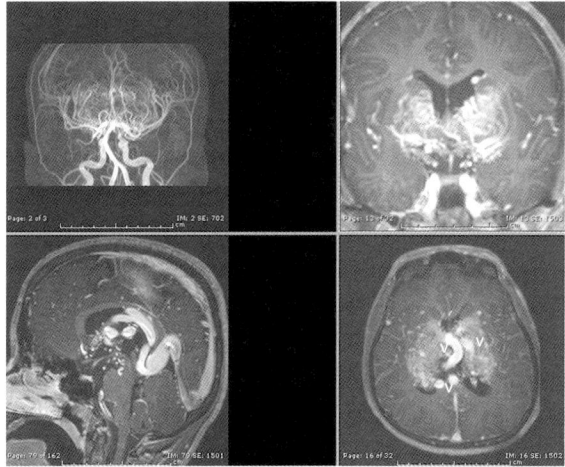

Fig. 13.15 MRI of bilateral thalamic arteriovenous malformations. Magnetic resonance angiogram demonstrating myriad abnormal vessels coursing through the basal ganglia and thalamus bilaterally (top left). Coronal postcontrast T1 magnetic resonance image showing the enhancing multiple abnormal feeding vessels coursing from the middle cerebral artery and the anterior cerebral artery through the basal ganglia (top right). Sagittal postcontrast T1 image demonstrating abnormal secondary enlargement of the internal cerebral veins, great vein of Galen, and straight sinus (bottom left). The ectasias are from the high flow shunting of blood through the arteriovenous malformation into the deep venous system. Axial postcontrast T1 MRI (bottom right) demonstrating the 'blush' of abnormal vessels of the nidus of the bithalamic arteriovenous malformation and the large draining veins (v).

300

children.[115-117] Some have abnormal expression of matrix metalloproteinases[118] and vascular endothelial growth factor.[119,120]

Vein of Galen arteriovenous aneurysm or ectasia

Neonatal great vein of Galen enlargement is usually associated with a large diencephalic arteriovenous malformation containing multiple arteriovenous connections draining into a median vein, and clinically declares itself with high-output cardiac failure (Fig. 13.16). Some have postulated that the ectatic vein is not the vein of Galen, but instead its embryonic precursor, the median prosencephalic vein of Markowski.[121] In older infants and children, the lesion may compress the aqueduct, causing ventriculomegaly. A vein of Galen saccular dilatation, communicating with a dilated straight sinus and feeding diencephalic arteries, constitute the pathologic finding. Although any major cerebral artery may shunt into this abnormality, the posterior cerebral is the common source. Occasionally, cerebral arteries shunt directly into intracranial sinuses, such as the superior sagittal or sigmoid sinus.[122]

Dural sinus arteriovenous fistula

Dural sinus malformations occur in young infants, may be multiple, and are sometimes associated with arteriovenous malformations.[123-127] A large communication between intra- and extracranial venous drainage pathways characterizes sinus pericranii, a rare, usually asymptomatic, condition in which blood circulates bidirectionally through dilated skull veins.[128,129] Later in life, traumatic fistulas can occur between the artery and sinus.

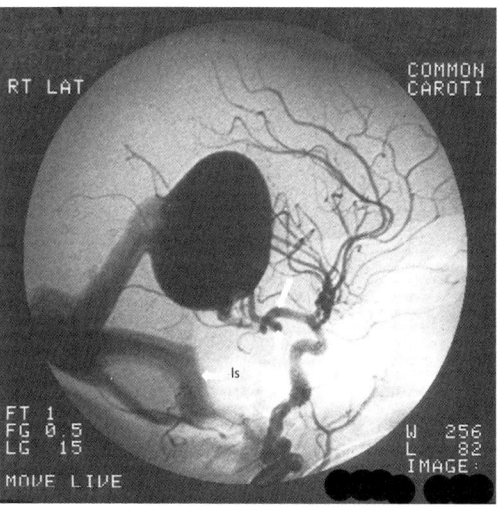

Fig. 13.16 Lateral view of distal angiogram (carotid injection) demonstrating a large vein of Galen ectasia connected with fistulous posterior cerebral artery branches. The posterior communicating and posterior cerebral arteries (arrows) are markedly dilated and feed directly into a large vein of Galen 'aneurysm.' The straight sinus and one lateral sinus (ls) are markedly enlarged.

'Congenital' arterial aneurysms

Pediatric intracranial aneurysms were described in 1939[130] (Fig. 13.17). In reviewing 1377 cerebral arterial aneurysms, 1.4% were in pediatric patients and 37% of these were giant lesions (>2cm). Male predominance was both claimed and denied, as well as location in either anterior or posterior circulations.[131,132] Saccular aneurysms are common in the first 2 years,[133] and may be neonatal[134,135] or appear in infants under 1 year of age;[132] occasionally, they are associated with other vascular malformations.[111] Cerebral arterial aneurysms may be familial,[136] but they also occur with human immunodeficiency virus,[137,138] tuberous sclerosis,[139] cerebral hemiatrophy, and internal carotid artery hypoplasia.[140] Bacterial or fungal mycotic aneurysms may occur in infants.[141]

Giant aneurysms occur on extracranial or intracranial internal carotid arteries,[142] in anterior circulation,[143] middle cerebral artery,[144,145] and in posterior circulation.[146–149] Posterior circulation giant aneurysms are more common in children under 1 year than in adults.[132]

CAVERNOUS MALFORMATIONS

Dilated sinusoidal chambers, varying in size, with thin endothelium-lined walls constitute cavernous vascular malformations which may occupy any intracranial location, including extra-axial.[150] These are spontaneous or occur as part of an autosomal dominant disorder in some families[151,152] and occur 1 to 2 years after radiation therapy.[153–155] There are differences in gene regulation of cavernous and arteriovenous malformations.[156,157] Loss of p53 sensitizes mice with a mutation in Ccm1 (KRIT1) to develop cerebral vascular malformations.[158]

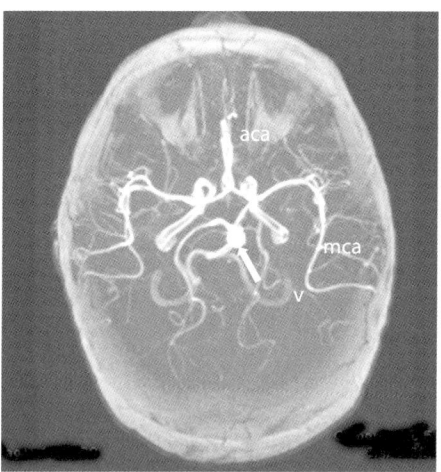

Fig. 13.17 CT angiogram. There is a large saccular aneurysm at the basilar rostral end (arrow). The middle cerebral arteries (mca) and the anterior cerebral arteries (aca) are also identified. Two large vertebral arteries (v) supply the basilar artery.

Venous malformations
Venous angiomas contain veins with abnormally thick walls and an irregular diameter converging on a large draining vein.[159] Confusion often exists between venous and cavernous angioma.[160] These are probably two distinct conditions: developmental venous anomalies and venous angiomas.[161,162] Because of their benign course, some feel they should not be excised routinely.[163]

Capillary telangiectasia
Capillary telangiectasia occur sporadically as small lesions anywhere in the brain. Usually these are incidental findings and not associated with local hemorrhage.

Meningocerebral angiodysplasia
These conditions include rare leptomeningeal vasculature abnormalities with the vascular abnormality ranging from small arterial tangles, artery and vein mixtures, and venous knots, to thin-walled sinusoidal capillary tangles. In one case, a dense small-vessel network, without distinct arteries or veins, extended over the cerebral hemispheres and replaced the circle of Willis.[164] There were widespread cortical and underlying white matter lesions associated with mineralized and dilated deep vessels. Some cases are associated with central nervous system malformations,[165] others have occurred with visceral organ agenesis or malformation,[166] and some were largely generalized leptomeningeal vessel angiectases containing dilated capillaries and terminal veins.[167] In hereditary hemorrhagic telangiectasia (telangiectases and arteriovenous malformations), an autosomal dominant disorder, vascular anomalies sometimes develop in many organs including the brain, skin, mucous membranes, lungs, and other viscera.[168,169]

Stürge–Weber–Dimitri–Kalischer disease
Facial skin, leptomeningeal, choroidal, or choroid plexus capillary hemangiomatoses in any combination constitute this well-known disease[170] (Fig. 13.18). Clinically, it presents with facial port-wine stain, glaucoma, seizures, developmental retardation, and ipsilateral

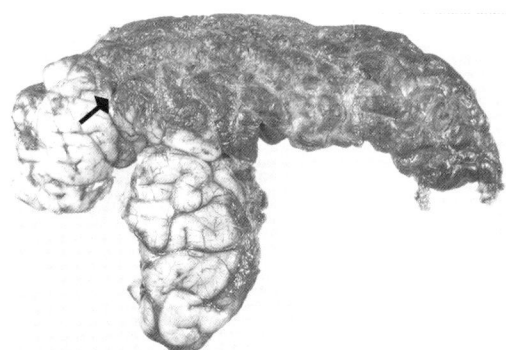

Fig. 13.18 This surgical specimen demonstrates leptomeningeal angiomatosis with its tangle of fine leptomeningeal sinusoids (the dark tissue to the right of the arrow). Note its abrupt edge.

leptomeningeal capillary hemangiomatosis. The ipsilateral affected eye is often enlarged. Involved vessels are large dilated sinuses without arterial or venous characteristics. These are low-pressure flow lesions and are usually not distinguishable on arteriography, but enhance in T1 weighted images. Eventually, the underlying brain becomes atrophic (Fig. 13.19). Early cortisectomies for seizure control demonstrate its natural history: initially, the brain underlying the hemangiomatosis is not histologically affected; during the second year, the underlying cortex begins to show proteinaceous perivascular abnormalities, which subsequently mineralize after 1 year of age (Fig. 13.20). Nearby neurons undergo necrosis with additional

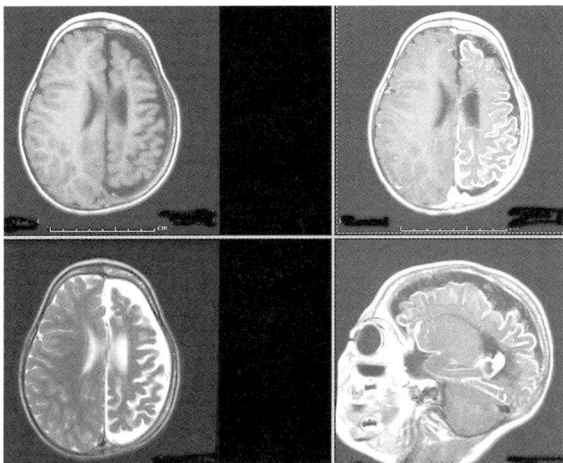

Fig. 13.19 Leptomeningeal angiomatosis in a 4-year-old. Brain MRI. T1 axial noncontrast image demonstrating atrophic left cerebral hemisphere (top left). T1 axial postcontrast image demonstrating abnormal leptomeningeal enhancement over entire hemisphere (top right). T2 axial image demonstrating atrophic left cerebral hemisphere (bottom left). T1 postcontrast sagittal image demonstrating leptomeningeal enhancement over the left cerebral cortical surface (bottom right).

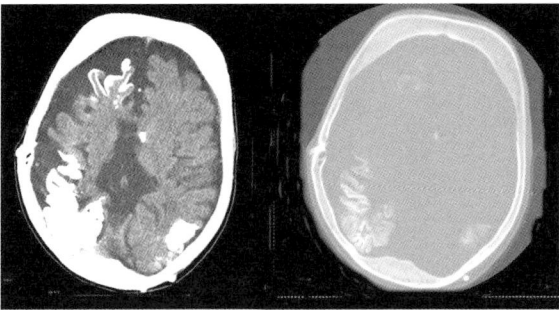

Fig. 13.20 Leptomeningeal angiomatosis. Noncontrast CT scan of the head demonstrating multiple gyral calcifications. Brain tissue windows (left); bone windows (right).

mineralization. At cortisectomy with arterial hyperoxygenation, there is no hemangiomatosis color change, whereas the remaining brain turns bright red.[170]

Harvey and Alvord[52] helped rectify our understanding of fibromuscular dysplasia: elastic and intimal hyperplasia or medial and elastic hypoplasia. Generally occurring in young adults, fibromuscular dysplasia involves renal, axillary, iliac, and hepatic arteries and rarely affects medium-to-large arteries (coronary, pulmonary, and aorta).[171,172] Histologically, fibromuscular dysplasia is a nonatheromatous, noninflammatory segmental angiopathy, involving intima, media, and, occasionally, adventitia, that narrows medium-sized arteries. Fibromuscular dysplasia has been associated with mutations in collagen, cutis laxa, and with α-1-antitrypsin deficiency, and, in children and young adults, is related to arterial dissections and aneurysms. Any major cranial vessel may be involved in the young child, leading to necrosis in the appropriate brain distribution.[172–175]

ELASTIC HYPERPLASIA
Infantile elastic hyperplasia is a rare vascular lesion, distinct from fibromuscular dysplasia.[176] All four neck arteries supplying the brain undergo marked stenosis and thickening, with dramatic internal elastic lamina duplication, but no increase in smooth muscle cells or adventitia. Brain and body vessels elsewhere are normal. Adults also develop this condition.[81]

Late cerebral consequences

SCLEROTIC MICROGYRIA 'ULEGYRIA'
Known by various names and interpretations, including ulegyria, mushroom gyri, nodular sclerosis, atrophic sclerosis, and mantle sclerosis, this condition occurs in isocortex or cerebellar cortex in bilateral symmetric or asymmetric regions. It is occasionally limited to a vascular bed distribution and, when limited to a specific arterial bed, suggests perinatal arterial occlusion, often ascribed to embolism.[38,177]

These lesions commonly occupy the borderzones between anterior and middle cerebral or between middle and posterior cerebral arteries (Figs. 13.21 and 13.22).[14,21,62] Overall gyral pattern is preserved, but individual gyri, or groups of gyri, are shrunken and sclerotic. Their magnetic resonance appearances are seen in Figure 13.4d. The parietal lobes bilaterally are the frequent location of sclerotic microgyria. Maximally, the involved territory occupies a narrow strip of cortex extending from the parieto-occipital region along the middle frontal gyrus and arching downwards at the frontal pole to include the orbital cortex. Sometimes it extends from the parietal lobe into the temporal lobe along the third temporal gyrus borderzone between the middle and posterior cerebral arterial beds. Usually, the cortex adjacent to sulcal depths is damaged most, with relatively normal gyral crest cortex. The residual gyral crest, containing large numbers of neurons, is usually only reduced in size and sits on a narrow stem lacking cortical neural elements; hence the name 'mushroom' gyrus. The sulcal cortex receives its blood supply from small intrasulcal leptomeningeal arteries. With a significant reduction in brain blood flow, brain swelling compresses these small vessels and the vulnerable sulcal

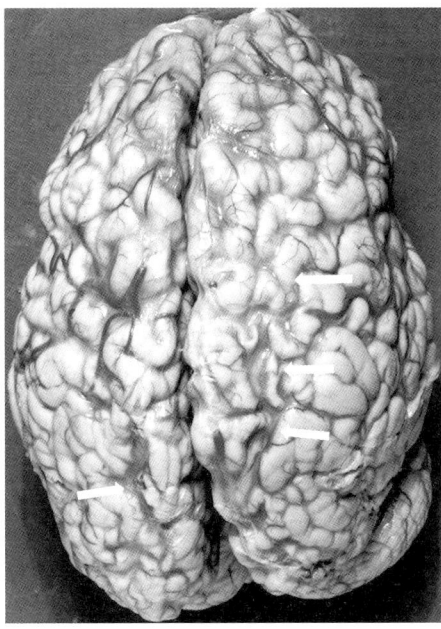

Fig. 13.21 Ulegyria. Multiple small shrunken gyri (medial to arrows) lie in the borderzone between the middle and anterior cerebral arteries bilaterally.

cortex becomes necrotic. The cortex at gyral crests is normal or contains abnormally oriented, hypermyelinated glial strands, which sometimes separate multiple preserved cortical nodules; hence the name nodular sclerosis.[178,179] Underlying white matter of the affected cortex is gliotic with depleted myelinated axons, and sometimes contains small cavities; these variations run together in some cases. Overlying leptomeninges are often thickened. Such small shrunken gyri were depicted early in the nineteenth century[62,63] and were subsequently described in many papers. Similar cerebellar lesions occur bilaterally between superior cerebellar and inferior cerebellar arteries at the periphery between convex inferior and concave superior cerebellar surfaces. Adult arterial borderzone lesions usually result from sudden severe hypotension;[180,181] similarly so in the neonate.[182] Gruenwald[183] was perhaps the first to emphasize the importance of neonatal shock as an antecedent of this condition. Usually there is an abrupt transition to more viable cortex, but if the shock is severe enough, even the gyral crowns contain glial scar islands separating cortical neurons and local cavitation.

In 1885, Sarah McNutt pointed out a condition that was seemingly an exception to the general rules promulgated above. These were cases of convexity sclerotic microgyria involving motor and sensory cortex of precentral and postcentral gyri around the central sulcus bilaterally, extending from the vertex downward and forward to the lateral sulcus (Sylvian)[184,185] (Figs. 13.23 and 13.24). These sclerotic gyri were not associated with borderzone lesions between anterior and middle cerebral arteries. The acute lesions are similar in location to the chronic lesions. They consist of typical sclerotic or nodular microgyria[102,184] and, similar to

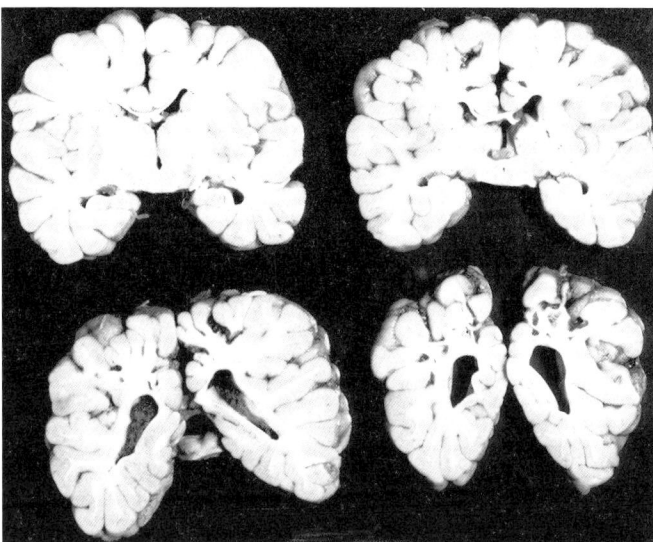

Fig. 13.22 Ulegyria. The same brain cut in coronal sections from the midthalamus to the occipital lobe. In most small gyri the cortex around the sulcal depths is missing and the crest cortex is more preserved. There is gliosis of most of these gyri. In the midthalamus photograph (top left), there is cortical thinning at sulcal depths between the superior and middle frontal gyri. In the posterior thalamus section (top right), cortical thinning at depths of sulci has become more prominent, particularly on the left. In the atrial photograph (bottom left), the cortical thinning extends well up the sides of the sulci. In the occipital photograph (bottom right), the cortical thinning of the sides of gyri is more prominent, leaving gyral caps with prominent cortex and narrow gyral stems; hence the appellation 'mushroom gyri.'

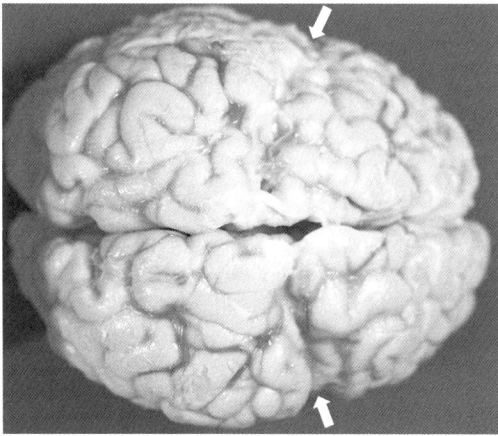

Fig. 13.23 This brain convexity photograph demonstrates a prominent atrophy of the precentral and postcentral gyri (arrows). The frontal pole is to the right. The atrophy has completely destroyed the local precentral and postcentral gyral anatomy. At the bottoms of these gutters lie typical sclerotic microgyri. The damage in this brain was limited to the precentral and postcentral gyri. There was no damage to the calcarine cortex or the thalamus.

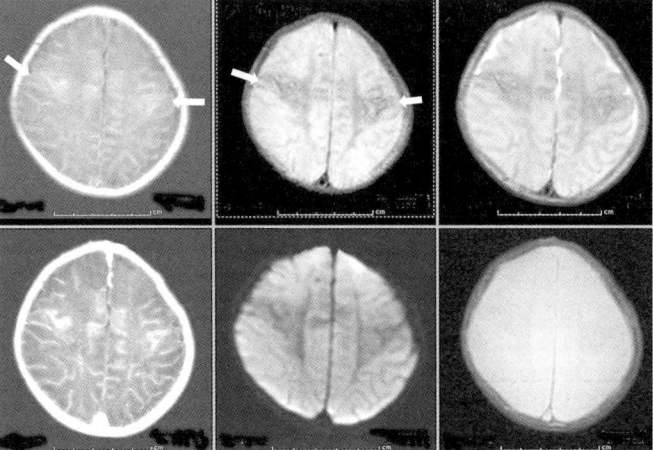

Fig. 13.24 MRI of an infant 2 days old. T1 weighted (top left); FLAIR (top middle); T2 (top right); T1 postcontrast (bottom left); diffusion weighted (botttom middle); susceptibility weighted (bottom right). There is bilateral damage to the precentral and postcentral gyral cortex (arrows) appearing bright on the T1-weighted image, dark in fluid-attenuated inversion recovery (FLAIR) and T2-weighted images, bright in T1 postcontrast image, and dark in diffusion. The susceptibility-weighted sequence is for detecting blood products such as hemosiderin and is negative.

sclerotic microgyri elsewhere, the abnormal cortical surface is shrunken around depths and walls of sulci leaving gyral crests with normal cortex, and thus forming a band of narrowed gyri along the entire central sulcus; hence the name 'girdle' atrophy.

Why should deep sulcal cortex be more vulnerable than gyral crest cortex? Cortical maturation first occurs in precentral and postcentral gyri, as well as in calcarine cortex.[186] It is unlikely that general hypoxemia or glutamate-induced excitotoxicity would affect gyral crest cortex less than sulcal cortex. Speculation as to the etiology of these cases, which often follow severe neonatal insults, suggests that more mature precentral and postcentral cortex is more susceptible to lowered blood flow at a certain time in development than the remaining less mature cortex. This idea is consistent with the simultaneous finding of sclerotic microgyria in calcarine cortex (also mature) in these individuals. Such cases continue to be reported; some of these suggest increased blood flow to this more mature cortex in the third trimester and term infants.[187–189]

HYDRANENCEPHALY

Hydranencephaly denotes thin leptomeningeal and glial membranes replacing large dorsal hemispheral regions within a relatively normal-sized cranium.[191–194] Commonly, there is relative preservation of medial occipital and temporal lobe undersurfaces as well as basal ganglia. The damaging insult, probably late in gestation, is likely to be related to significantly lowered cerebral blood flow producing supply failure in all three major arterial beds.[195] Infective agents, demonstrated in some cases, additionally complicate interpretation.

Cruveilhier[191] first described and depicted this condition, maintaining that it resulted from a destructive process because the residual tissue was yellow stained and firm (Fig. 13.25). Parè in *Les Oeuvres*[196] had briefly mentioned this lesion in 1575. He had seen four cases with only a small residual brain nugget at the skull base. In more markedly damaged regions, only a few glial remnants, left over from the widely spread hemispheral necrosis, separate lepto-meninges and ependyma.[194]

Most telencephalic structures are absent except for ventromedial hemispheral portions, basal ganglia, and thalamus (Fig. 13.26).[197] The thalamus is usually small, without pulvinar, and its atrophy pattern implicates specific corticothalamic projection pathways. Hydranencephaly is sometimes associated with optic nerve hypoplasia. Usually considered a late gestational lesion, it was described in a 30-week-old fetus.[197] A similar configuration of damage follows cardiovascular collapse in infants and young children with anterior and middle cerebral arterial distribution deficits accompanying preserved neural tissue in vertebrobasilar and posterior cerebral arterial distributions.[195]

Hydranencephaly is sometimes found in twins,[198,199] and is associated with proliferative vasculopathy,[200,201] fetofetal transfusion,[202] maternal lupus,[203] lung growth abnormalities,[204] bilateral carotid artery occlusion, and herpes simplex; it is rarely familial.[205] It appears in several domestic animals following fetal infection.[206–210] These comments do not exclude a

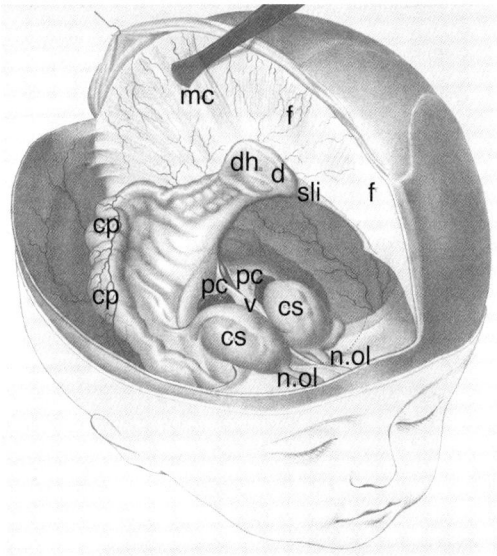

Fig. 13.25 Hydranencephaly. This hand-painted lithograph depicts an infant's head with hydranencephaly. The falx (f) lies centrally in its usual cranial position. The cranium was filled with fluid. The lateral ventricle choroid plexuses (pc) lie at the base. The only residual brain (cp) is in the posterior cerebral artery distribution, namely the inferior temporal lobe and the ventromedial and portions of the ventrolateral occipital lobe. The olfactory tracts (n.ol) are also preserved. Structurally, the cranial base is intact. From Cruveilhier.[16,191] A color version of this figure is available in the color plate section in the back of the book.

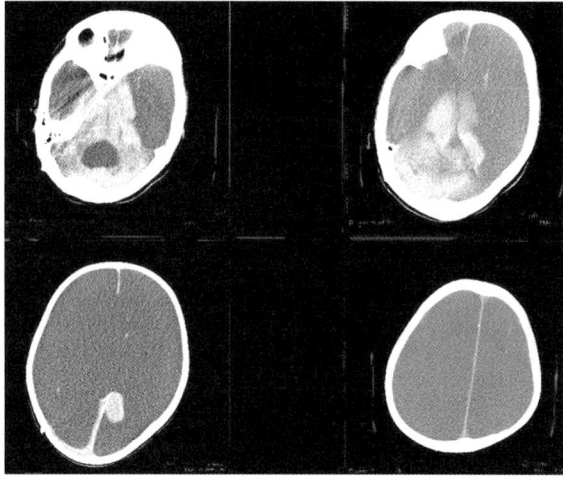

Fig. 13.26 Hydranencephaly. Axial noncontrast CT scan. The cranium is largely filled with cerebrospinal fluid (gray). The white material in the upper left image is a combination of relatively normal posterior fossa content and medial basal occipital lobes. In the section in the upper right image, residual brain lies along the medial aspect of each hemisphere posteriorly. In the lower left image there is a single fragment of residual brain.

viral infection etiology of human hydranencephaly, such as neonatal herpes simplex encephalitis;[211] but, importantly, these are cases with multiple cerebral necroses rather than a massive hemispheral necrosis. In hydranencephaly, the hemispheral wall, lying largely in the internal carotid arterial distribution, is absent or destroyed, whereas the tissue in vertebral or posterior cerebral arterial distribution is variably preserved. Bilateral carotid occlusion from paraffin injection in neonatal animals produces comparable cerebral lesions experimentally.[212,213]

PORENCEPHALY

A porus is merely a cyst. Prosencephalic cystic lesions occur in infant and childhood brains,[214,215] and frequently underlie neurologic and intellectual deficits of infancy and childhood. Rarely found after a catastrophic event during gestation or parturition, other critical antecedents leading to different cysts are not known. Large prosencephalic cysts fall into two general categories based on the presence of (1) heterotopic neuronal masses or (2) glia lining the cyst wall.

Cystic lesions with heterotopic neuronal tissue
Parenchymal cysts extending from ventricular to pial surfaces, containing neuronal nodules or layers in their walls, were recognized in the late 1800s; they are commonly ascribed to early gestational insults.[216] Usually these lesions have adjacent cortical gyral pattern or lamination abnormalities, with surrounding gyri often pointing into the deficit, as Kundrat[216] originally observed (Figs. 13.27 and 13.28). If bilateral and symmetric in site (but not necessarily in

310

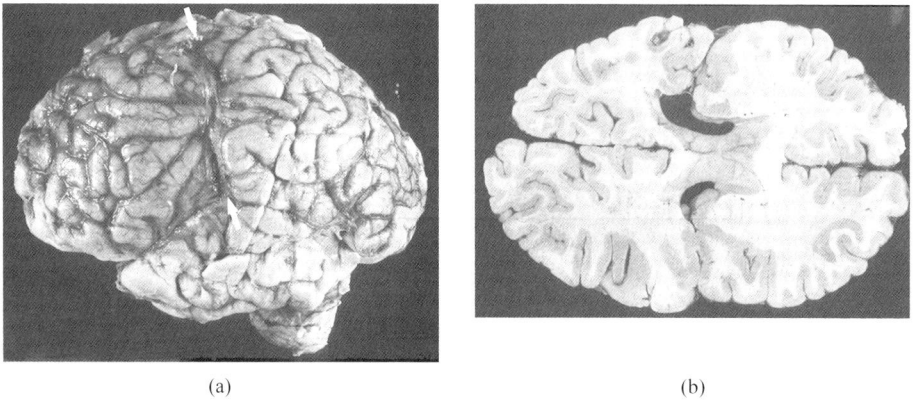

(a)   (b)

Fig. 13.27 (a) The frontal lobe lies to the left. A long mantle cleft extends down the lateral convexity between the two arrows. Nearby gyri tend to point into the defect. This is a foreshortened brain with no clear central sulcus or precentral or postcentral gyri. The opposite hemisphere contained a similar mantle defect. (b) The mantle clefts extend through the entire hemisphere to the ventricle. A pseudo-cortical layer follows the side of the cleft to the ventricle. While the layer appears to be cortex, it is a disorganized mixture of neurons, as are the heterotopic masses lining the ventricular walls as nodules in the lower hemisphere.

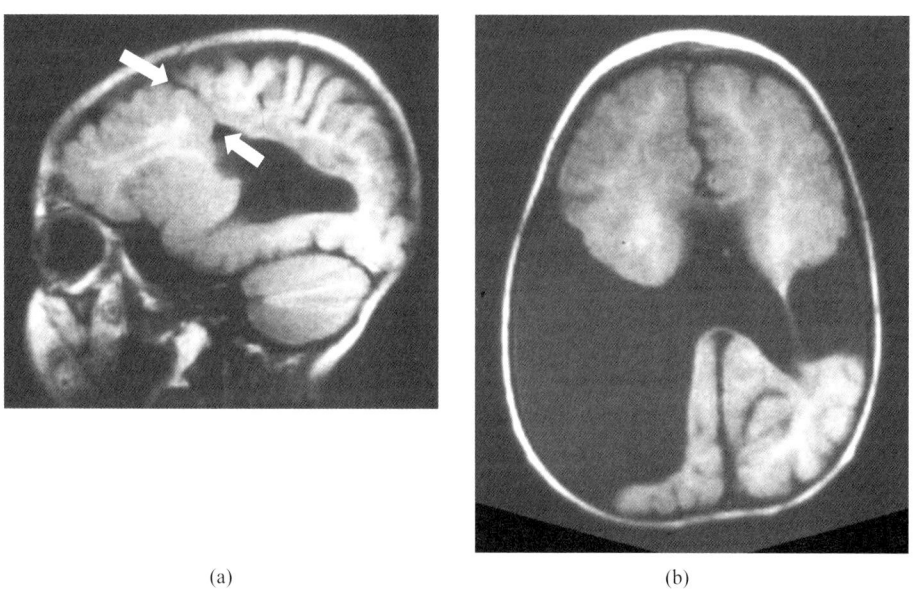

(a)   (b)

Fig. 13.28 (a) Frontal lobe to the left. Sagittal T1-weighted MRI with a gray matter-lined cleft extending from the ventricular surface completely through the cerebral tissue to the subarachnoid space (arrows). The edges of this mantle cleft are approximated and these are sometimes called closed clefts. (b) Axial T1-weighted MRI demonstrating bilateral clefts in the cerebral hemispheres that communicate with the lateral ventricles. These mantle cleft walls are not approximated and are sometimes called open clefts.

311

size), the cystic lesions constitute a 'schizencephalic' deficit.[217,218] Preferable simpler names such as 'mantle defect,' 'mantle cleft,' or 'cleft' do not imply bilaterality because these defects may be single or multiple, and unilateral or bilateral. In open-cleft deficits, the nodules or neuronal layers occupy their walls; with approximated walls, the heterotopic neuronal tissue extends from the ventricle to the surface as an 'ependymal–pial' seam, thereby simulating a closed 'cleft.' Presumably, these defects are related to developmental time of mantle formation, and heterotopic nodules along the wall reflect a local migration disorder or disorganized abortive repairs.

Cystic lesions without heterotopic neuronal tissue
Parenchymal cysts without heterotopic neuronal tissue are cerebral mantle deficits, small or large, single or multiple, involving gray and/or white matter, and are either symmetric or asymmetric in location (Figs. 13.29 and 13.30). These stand in contrast to trabeculated infarcts that sometimes communicate with ventricles (Figs. 13.31 and 13.32). Usually regarded as developing late in gestation, they lack heterotopic tissue along the cyst wall, occasionally lie in specific vascular bed distributions, and interrupt previously formed gyri within an overall normal gyral pattern.[33,214,216,219] Surrounding gyri are oriented normally. Some fetal pori follow fetal encephalitis[220] or parenchymal hemorrhage,[221,222] or are associated with an abnormal circle of Willis.[223] Familial cases are not understood.[224] Secondary lesions associated with pori include thalamic atrophy in nuclei whose axons were interrupted by the cyst and atrophy of basal forebrain complexes.[225]

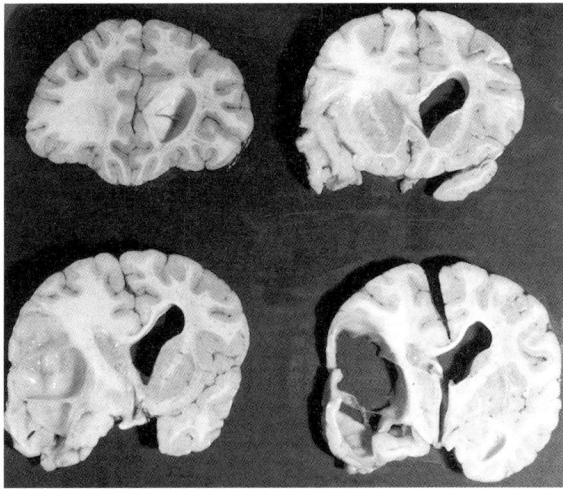

Fig. 13.29 Coronal sections with a relatively smooth walled cyst in the left hemisphere. Several trabeculae traverse the cavity. These often follow parenchymal hematomas that destroy much cerebral tissue, although few residual blood products remain.

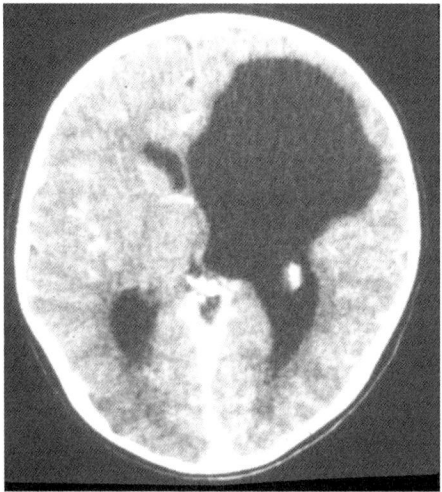

Fig. 13.30 Postcontrast CT scan with a large cerebrospinal fluid-filled smooth-walled cavity communicating with the left lateral ventricle.

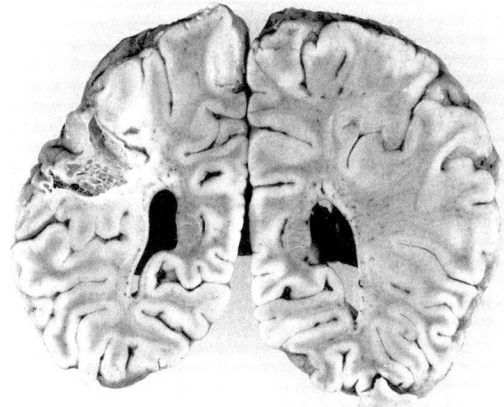

Fig. 13.31 Coronal section of posterior cerebrum with a left parietal finely trabeculated cyst in the distribution of the middle cerebral artery branch. Finely trabeculated cysts usually follow parenchymal necroses that destroy neural tissue, but spare capillaries and small vessels with their encapsulating astrocytic cells.

MULTILOCULAR CYSTIC ENCEPHALOMALACIA

Multiple varieties of asymmetric or symmetric cystic abnormalities in young brains were described throughout the late nineteenth and early twentieth century. A frequent presentation is symmetric multilocular cystic encephalopathy of infants, sometimes known as multilocular encephalomalacia (Figs. 13.33 and 13.34). This entity is distinctive because of its predominance in cerebral white matter, or, when more severe, its involvement with overlying cortex.

313

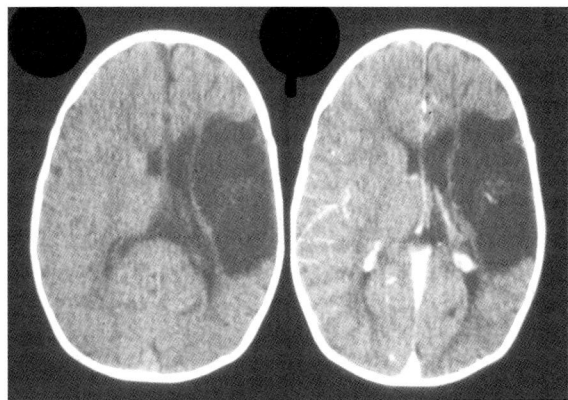

Fig. 13.32 Old left middle cerebral artery infarct. Precontrast (left) and postcontrast (right) CT scan with a large parenchymal cavity in the territory of the left middle cerebral artery. Note the intact ventricular wall and the trabeculae within the cavity.

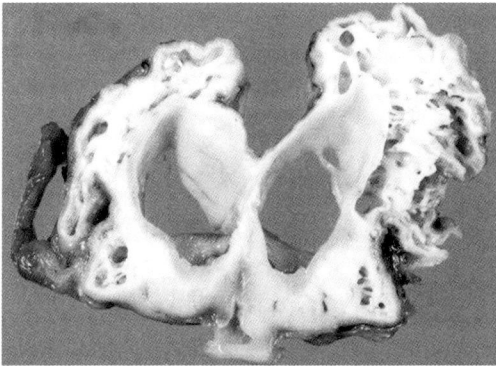

Fig. 13.33 Multilocular cystic encephalomalacia. Multiple small cysts in this shrunken cerebrum have replaced gray and white matter. Many of these cysts have collapsed. The widespread destruction has resulted in marked ventriculomegaly.

It frequently follows a late gestational or parturitional destructive process.[220,226] Some names imply a causal relationship ('parturitional' porencephaly), although cystic lesions, ipso facto, rarely identify specific antecedents. They are found in infants after severe birth trauma, venous obstruction, cerebral ischemia, or maternal carbon monoxide poisoning, or are associated with hypoplastic right ventricle or leptomeningeal vessel abnormalities.[227,228] Other reports allude to reduced blood flow, but are unable to explain lesion predominance in cerebral white matter.[195,229,230]

The brains are smaller than normal and contain multiple cavities of various sizes occupying the main bulk of both cerebral hemispheres, including the temporal lobes.[227] Trabeculated cavities generally extend from the pial surface to the ventricular wall, involve white matter

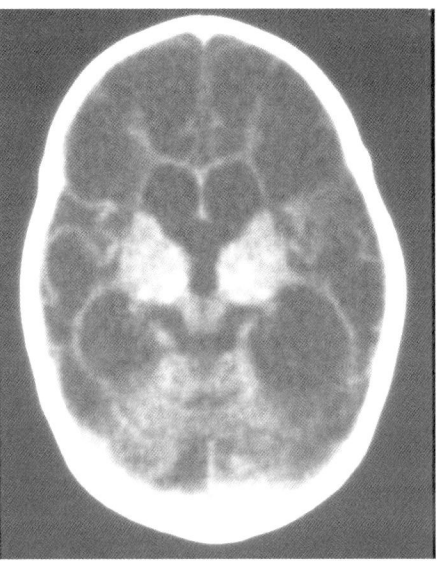

Fig. 13.34 Multilocular cystic encephalomalacia. Noncontrast CT scan of the head. There are both multiple cysts in the cerebral parenchyma and small thalami with calcifications, which are markers of old necrosis.

and overlying cortex, and commonly retain an external preserved subpial gliotic layer and a paraventricular subependymal astrocytic layer. The lesions usually lie external to the basal ganglia and thalami or may include these sites. Depending on the degree of organization post-insult, some cavities may contain phagocytes; gliotic tissue of varying thickness separates individual cysts, and fine glial and vascular trabeculae traverse many cysts. In occasional cases, posterior cerebral artery territory is relatively spared. Reticular formation and thalamic or hypothalamic neuronal loss sometimes occurs.[230] Brainstem and spinal cord are normal except for corticospinal tract absence, with a few published exceptions.[231,232] These lesions appear to develop after a maternal disaster such as cord prolapse, suicide attempt, abdominal trauma during pregnancy, or carotid artery malformation.[233] Ordinarily, there is no sign of infection, but recently it has followed human herpes simplex viral infection. Akabane virus infection in calves or sheep is associated with either multicystic encephalopathy or hydranencephaly,[234] and monkey multicystic encephalopathy follows Venezuelan equine encephalitis.[235] Some cases are associated with a vascular abnormality.[227] We agree with Friede[236] that this entity is nonspecific and results from a severe circulatory disturbance near term or during the early neonatal period.

SYMMETRIC THALAMIC AND/OR BASAL GANGLIA LESIONS—STATUS MARMORATUS
While substantial brain lesions, as described above, such as large regional cystic necroses of hemisphere, caudate, putamen, or major borderzone cortical lesions, typically follow parturitional catastrophes, lesions of less than total neuronal loss sometimes succeed these disasters.

315

The most prevalent lesion, status marmoratus, in fact, is partial loss of neurons with resultant gliosis in thalami, putamina, caudate, and globus pallidus; in isocortex, the same process has a different name—'plaque fibromyelinque.' This abnormality was recognized in the late nineteenth century[237] and consists of local neuronal loss in caudate, putamen, thalamus, or isocortex, accompanied by marked gliosis and myelination of glial fibrils and even adventitial collagen bundles[178,179,238–242] (Figs. 13.35 and 13.36). Usually the involved neuronal structure is shrunken, even when regions are solely sclerotic. For instance, the upper or lower putamen is sometimes damaged with apparent sparing of its remainder; the dorsal thalamus may be damaged without basal involvement. Usually bilateral, it is recognizable grossly as local swirls of myelinated glial fibers or whirls of myelin around small vessels, reflecting marked damage to the neuronal group. The lesions are usually in posterior cerebral artery distal thalamic branch distributions or in distal lateral striate arterial distribution, supporting the high prevalence of thalamic, putaminal, or caudate lesions following neonatal brain hypoperfusion as in placenta previa, abruptio, or torn umbilical cord. Depending on the damaged neuronal group, the common clinical deficit is a movement disorder or global intellectual retardation.

Transneuronal atrophy

Transneuronal degeneration modifies developmental brain lesions.[243] Experimentally, immature animals are more susceptible than adult animals. Retrograde inferior olivary secondary degeneration occurs after cerebellar cortical lesions.[244] Anterograde crossed cerebellar atrophy follows early-life cerebral cortical lesions or is retrograde following thalamic lesions;[245] this differs from the adult.[225] Crossed cerebellar atrophy is, nevertheless, unpredictable.

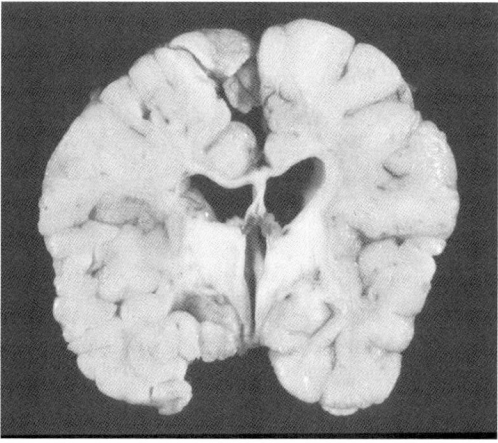

Fig. 13.35 Thalamic sclerosis (status marmoratus) in an infant. In this coronal brain section through the midthalamus, the cortical band is intact throughout. The corpus callosum is thin and the lateral (including temporal horns) and third ventricles are enlarged. The thalamus is moderately shrunken, white, and sclerotic. The white appearance comes from the dense gliosis following thalamic neuronal loss subsequent to any severe perinatal hypotensive episode.

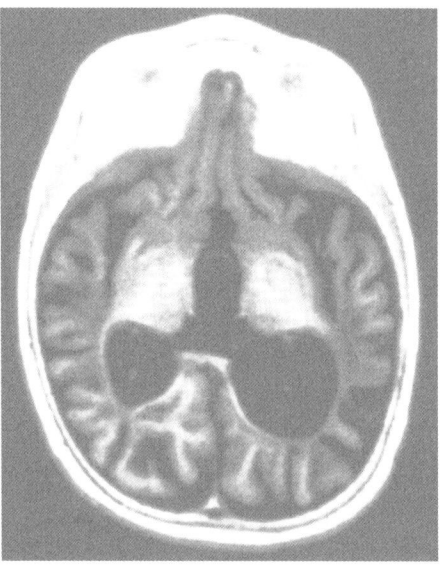

Fig. 13.36 Thalamic sclerosis. Axial inversion recovery magnetic resonance image (myelin white, gray matter gray). The increased thalamic signal intensity is evidence of the increased water content associated with thalamic gliosis and neuronal loss. Note the local widening of the third ventricle. There is widely spread cortical damage, white matter loss, and thin corpus callosum, which accounts for the lateral ventricular enlargement. As there is no cerebrospinal fluid flow obstruction, third ventricular enlargement reflects the thalamic atrophy. There are prominent sulci and shrunken gyri in both hemispheres as well as densely 'hypermyelinated' thalami bilaterally.

Neonatal extracorporeal membrane oxygenation complications

Extracorporeal membrane oxygenation (ECMO) uses prolonged cardiopulmonary bypass to reduce mortality rates in selected neonates with severe but reversible cardiorespiratory failure refractory to conventional ventilator therapy. While many cerebral deficits are later found in these children,[246] one never knows whether the deficit preceded the ECMO. For instance, veno-arterial ECMO requires unilateral carotid artery and jugular vein sacrifice, frequently resulting in altered brain blood flow, and is associated with neurologic and audiologic abnormalities in 10% to 20% of cases.[247,248] Later in infant survivors, altered cerebral blood flow, as well as infarcts, are found in about half of cases, either ipsilateral, contralateral, or bilaterally.[249,250] Even if carotid reanastomosis is accomplished, subsequent flow through the carotid system is sometimes compromised. In autopsied nonsurvivors, over half had cerebral hemorrhages or necroses and had been significantly acidotic and hypotensive.[251,252] While most infants with severe cardiorespiratory failure have significant electroencephalographic abnormalities, cerebral palsy risk is significantly increased in neonatal venoarterial ECMO survivors if the children required other cardiorespiratory support, had a systolic pressure below 39mmHg before or during ECMO, or if Pa_{CO_2} dropped below 14mmHg before ECMO (increased risk for hearing loss).[248] These authors point out that the neurologic, cognitive, and hearing defects in neonatal ECMO survivors sometimes represent defects present before ECMO.

317

Conclusions

At the autopsy table in general pediatric hospitals, and in hospitals serving the population with severe brain damage, the most prevalent brain abnormalities are hypomyelination and white matter hypoplasia. In fact, these two entities constitute a major societal cost, as the resources required to support these people are considerable. Following a neonatal disaster, the most likely lesion is upper brainstem and thalamic damage; the corpus striatum is affected far less often. Thalamic and striatal lesions commonly conclude as status marmoratus. Cortical border-zone lesions occur much less frequently and their long-term lesions are sclerotic microgyria or ulegyria. Major cerebral artery borderzones are important in understanding bilateral, usually symmetric, cortical lesions, but not in interpreting deep white matter necroses. The leptomeningeal collateral circulation is extensive; in Chapter 8 we showed that there is an extensive cerebral collateral circulation at capillary and sinusoidal level. Arterial anomalies such as major vessel aplasia, persistent carotid–basilar arteries, vascular malformations, and vessel wall abnormalities were included. Late fetal and neonatal major vascular bed infarcts and, more importantly, the high frequency of neonatal upper brainstem lesions were emphasized.

REFERENCES

1. Waddington MM (1974) *Atlas of Cerebral Angiography with Anatomic Correlation.* Boston: Little, Brown & Company.
2. Cohnheim J (1882) *Vorlesungen über allgemeine Pathologie. Pathologie: Ein Handbuch für ärtze und Studierende.* Berlin: A Hischwald.
3. Duret H (1874) Recherches anatomiques sur la circulation de l'encéphale. *Arch Physiol Norm Path S* 2: 60–91, 316–353, 664–693, 919–957.
4. Leidy J (1891) Abnormal circle of Willis. *Trans Path Soc Phil* 16: 93–94.
5. Vander Eecken HM, Adams RD (1953) The anatomy and functional significance of the meningeal arterial anastomoses of the human brain. *J Neuropathol Exp Neurol* 12: 132–157.
6. Sunderland S (1938) The production of cortical lesions by devascularization of cortical area. *J Anat* 73: 120–129.
7. Prensky AL, Davis DO (1970) Obstruction of major cerebral vessels in early childhood without neurological signs. *Neurology* 20: 945–953.
8. Suzuki J, Takaku A Cerebrovascular (1969) 'Moyomoya' disease. Disease showing abnormal net-like vessels in base of brain. *Arch Neurol* 20: 288–299.
9. Suzuki J, Kodama N (1971) Cerebrovascular 'Moyamoya' disease. 2. Collateral routes to forebrain via ethmoid sinus and superior nasal meatus. *Angiology* 22: 223–236.
10. Kerty E, Nyberg-Hansen R, Dahl A, Bakke SJ, Russell D, Rootwelt K (1996) Assessment of the ophthalmic artery as a collateral to the cerebral circulation. A comparison of transorbital Doppler ultrasonography and regional cerebral blood flow measurements. *Acta Neurol Scandinavica* 93: 374–379.
11. Damry N, Hanquinet S, Christophe C, Janssen F, Delatte P, Perlmutter N (1994) Bilateral congenital absence of the internal carotid artery with a primitive transmaxillary arterial anastomosis. *Pediatr Radiol* 24: 200–203.
12. Lindenberg R, Spatz H (1939) Über die thromboendarteriitis obliterans der Hirngefäße. (Cerebrale form der v.Winiwarter-Buergerschen Krankheit). *Virchows Arch A Pathol Anat Histopathol* 305: 531–557.
13. Lindenberg R (1959) The pathology of the arterial border zones of the brain. *J Neuropath Exp Neurol* 18: 348–349.
14. Meyer JE (1953) Über die Lokalisation frühkindlicher Hirnschäden in arteriellen Grenzgebieten. *Arch Psychiatr Nervenkr* 190: 328–341.
15. Venkataraman A, Kingsley PB, Kalina P, et al (2004) Newborn brain infarction: clinical aspects and magnetic resonance imaging. *CNS Spectr* 9: 436–444.
16. Cruveilhier J (1829–1835) *Anatomie Pathologique du Corps Humain,* part 2, XVth Liv. Paris: JB Baillière.

17. Gilles F (1969) Hypotensive brain stem necrosis. Selective symmetrical necrosis of tegmental neuronal aggregates following cardiac arrest. *Arch Pathol* 88: 32–41.
18. Sladky JT, Rorke LB (1986) Perinatal hypoxic/ischemic spinal cord injury. *Pediatr Pathol* 6: 87–101.
19. Sarnat HB (2004) Watershed infarcts in the fetal and neonatal brainstem. An aetiology of central hypoventilation, dysphagia, Moibius syndrome and micrognathia. *Eur J Paediatr Neurol* 8: 71–87.
20. Noell W, Schneider M (1942) Über die Durchblutung und Sauerstoffversorgung des Gehirns im akuten Sauerstoffmangel. *Pflügers Arch ges Physiol* 246: 181–249.
21. Norman R, Urich H, McMenemy W (1957) Vascular mechanisms of birth injury. *Brain* 80: 49–58.
22. Lindenberg R (1963) Patterns of CNS vulnerability in acute hypoxaemia, including anaesthesia accidents. In: Schadé JP, McMenemy WH, editors. *Selective Vulnerability of the Brain in Hypoxaemia*. Philadelphia: FA Davis Company, pp. 189–210.
23. Leblanc R, Yamamoto YL, Tyler JL, Diksic M, Hakim A (1987) Borderzone ischemia. *Ann Neurol* 22: 707–713.
24. Carpenter DA, Grubb RL Jr., Powers WJ (1990) Borderzone hemodynamics in cerebrovascular disease. *Neurology* 40: 1587–1592.
25. Venkataraman A, Kingsley PB, Kalina P, et al (2004) Newborn brain infarction: clinical aspects and magnetic resonance imaging. *CNS Spectr* 9: 436–444.
26. Schneider H, Ballowitz L, Schachinger H, Hanefeld F, Droszus JU (1975) Anoxic encephalopathy with predominant involvement of basal ganglia, brain stem and spinal cord in the perinatal period. Report on seven newborns. *Acta Neuropathol (Berl)* 32: 287–298.
27. Dąmbska M, Dydyk L, Szretter T, Wozniewicz J, Myers RE (1976) Topography of lesions in newborn and infant brains following cardiac arrest and resuscitation. Damage to brain and hemispheres. *Biol Neonate* 29(3–4): 194–206.
28. Leech RW, Alvord EC Jr. (1977) Anoxic–ischemic encephalopathy in the human neonatal period. The significance of brain stem involvement. *Arch Neurol* 34: 109–113.
29. Janzer RC, Friede RL (1980) Hypotensive brain stem necrosis or cardiac arrest encephalopathy? *Acta Neuropathol (Berl)* 50: 53–56.
30. Taylor SR, Roessmann U (1984) Hypotensive brain stem necrosis in a stillborn. *Acta Neuropathol (Berl)* 65: 166–167.
31. Andrew DL, Paterson JA (1989) Postnatal development of vascularity in the inferior colliculus of the young rat. *Am J Anat* 186: 389–396.
32. Gilles FH, Nag D (1971) Vulnerability of human spinal cord in transient cardiac arrest. *Neurology* 21: 833–839.
33. Barmada M, Moossy J, Shuman RM (1979) Cerebral infarcts with arterial occlusion in neonates. *Ann Neurol* 6: 495–502.
34. Govaert P, Matthys E, Zecic A, Roelens F, Oostra A, Vanzieleghem B (2000) Perinatal cortical infarction within middle cerebral artery trunks. *Arch Dis Child Fetal Neonatal Ed* 82: F59–63.
35. Ozduman K, Pober BR, Barnes P, et al (2004) Fetal stroke. *Pediatr Neurol* 30: 151–162.
36. Boardman JP, Ganesan V, Rutherford MA, Saunders DE, Mercuri E, Cowan F (2005) Magnetic resonance image correlates of hemiparesis after neonatal and childhood middle cerebral artery stroke. *Pediatrics* 115: 321–326.
37. de Vries LS, Groenendaal F, Eken P, van Haastert IC, Rademaker KJ, Meiners LC (1997) Infarcts in the vascular distribution of the middle cerebral artery in preterm and fullterm infants. *Neuropediatrics* 28: 88–96.
38. Clark RM, Linell EA (1954) Prenatal occlusion of the internal carotid artery – case report. *J Neurol Neurosurg Psychiatry* 17: 295–297.
39. Cocker J, George SW, Yates P (1965) Perinatal occlusion of the middle cerebral artery. *Dev Med Child Neurol* 7: 235–243.
40. Roodhooft AM, Parizel PM, Van Acker KJ, Deprettere AJ, Van Reempts PJ (1987) Idiopathic cerebral arterial infarction with paucity of symptoms in the full-term neonate. *Pediatrics* 80: 381–385.
41. Groenendaal F, van der Grond J, Witkamp TD, de Vries LS (1995) Proton magnetic resonance spectroscopic imaging in neonatal stroke. *Neuropediatrics* 26: 243–248.
42. Akanli LF, Trasi SS, Thuraisamy K, et al (1998) Neonatal middle cerebral artery infarction: association with elevated maternal anticardiolipin antibodies. *Am J Perinatol* 15: 399–402.
43. Alfonso I, Prieto G, Vasconcellos E, Aref K, Pacheco E, Yelin K (2001) Internal carotid artery thrombus: an underdiagnosed source of brain emboli in neonates? *J Child Neurol* 16: 446–447.

44. Yates P (1959) Birth trauma to the vertebral arteries. *Arch Dis Child* 34: 436–441.
45. Govaert P, Vanhaesebrouck P, de Praeter C (1992) Traumatic neonatal intracranial bleeding and stroke. *Arch Dis Child* 67(7 Spec No): 840–845.
46. Mercuri E, He J, Curati WL, Dubowitz LM, Cowan FM, Bydder GM (1997) Cerebellar infarction and atrophy in infants and children with a history of premature birth. *Pediatr Radiol* 27: 139–143.
47. Roessmann U, Miller RT (1980) Thrombosis of the middle cerebral artery associated with birth trauma. *Neurology* 30: 889–892.
48. Lequin MH, Peeters EA, Holscher HC, de Krijger R, Govaert P (2004) Arterial infarction caused by carotid artery dissection in the neonate. *Eur J Paediatr Neurol* 8: 155–160.
49. Silver RK, MacGregor SN, Pasternak JF, Neely SE (1992) Fetal stroke associated with elevated maternal anticardiolipin antibodies. *Obstet Gynecol* 80(3 Pt 2): 497–499.
50. Baumeister FA, Auberger K, Schneider K (2000) Thrombosis of the deep cerebral veins with excessive bilateral infarction in a premature infant with the thrombogenic 4G/4G genotype of the plasminogen activator inhibitor-1. *Eur J Pediatr* 159: 239–242.
51. Strater R, Vielhaber H, Kassenbohmer R, von Kries R, Gobel U, Nowak-Gottl U (1999) Genetic risk factors of thrombophilia in ischaemic childhood stroke of cardiac origin. A prospective ESPED survey. *Eur J Pediatr* 158 (Suppl 3): S122–125.
52. Harvey FH, Alvord EC Jr. (1972) Juvenile cerebral arteriosclerosis and other cerebral arteriopathies of childhood—six autopsied cases. *Acta Neurol Scand* 48: 479–509.
53. Jones EL, Cameron AH, Smith WT (1970) Birth trauma to the cervical spine and vertebral arteries. *J Pathol* 100: Piv.
54. Gilles FH, Bina M, Sotrel A (1979) Infantile atlantooccipital instability. *Am J Dis Child* 133: 30–37.
55. Gross RE (1945) Arterial embolism and thrombosis in infancy. *Am J Dis Child* 70: 61–73.
56. Kraus FT, Acheen VI (1999) Fetal thrombotic vasculopathy in the placenta: cerebral thrombi and infarcts, coagulopathies, and cerebral palsy. *Hum Pathol* 30: 759–769.
57. Kolker SE, Ferrell LD, Bollen AW, Ursell PC (1999) Disseminated intravascular meconium in a newborn with meconium peritonitis. *Hum Pathol* 30: 592–594.
58. Parker MJ, Joubert GI, Levin SD (2002) Portal vein thrombosis causing neonatal cerebral infarction. *Arch Dis Child Fetal Neonatal Ed* 87: F125–127.
59. Banker BQ (1961) Cerebral vascular disease in infancy and childhood. 1. Occlusive vascular diseases. *J Neuropathol Exp Neurol* 20: 127–140.
60. Larroche JC (1970) Umbilical catheterization: its complications. Anatomical study. *Biol Neonate* 16: 101–116.
61. Wigger HJ, Bransilver BR, Blanc WA (1970) Thromboses due to catheterization in infants and children. *J Pediatr* 76: 1–11.
62. Haldeman S, Fowler GW, Ashwal S, Schneider S (1983) Acute flaccid neonatal paraplegia: a case report. *Neurology* 33: 93–95.
63. Brown MS, Phibbs RH (1988) Spinal cord injury in newborns from use of umbilical artery catheters: report of two cases and a review of the literature. *J Perinatol* 8: 105–110.
64. Alkalay AL, Mazkereth R, Santulli T Jr., Pomerance JJ (1993) Central venous line thrombosis in premature infants: a case management and literature review. *Am J Perinatol* 10: 323–326.
65. Batsis JA, Craici IM, Froehling DA (2005) Central venous catheter thrombosis complicated by paradoxical embolism in a patient with diabetic ketoacidosis and respiratory failure. *Neurocrit Care* 2: 185–188.
66. Bednarek N, Morville P, Delebarre G, Akhavi A, Sommer C (2007) Necrotic skin lesions and cerebral infarction in the newborn: two case reports. *J Child Neurol* 22: 354–357.
67. Munoz ME, Roche C, Escriba R, Martinez-Bermejo A, Pascual-Castroviejo I (1993) Flaccid paraplegia as complication of umbilical artery catheterization. *Pediatr Neurol* 9: 401–403.
68. de Klerk OL, de Vries TW, Sinnige LG (1997) An unusual cause of neonatal seizures in a newborn infant. *Pediatrics* 100: E8.
69. Valdes-Dapena MA, Arey JB (1967) Pulmonary emboli of cerebral origin in the newborn. A report of two cases. *Arch Pathol* 84: 643–646.
70. Tan KL, Hwang WS (1976) Neonatal brain tissue embolism in the lung. *Aust N Z J Med* 6: 146–149.
71. Wannakrairot P, Shuangshoti S (1984) Cerebellar tissue embolism associated with birth injury. *J Med Assoc Thai* 67: 290–294.
72. Baergen RN, Castillo MM, Mario-Singh B, Stehly AJ, Benirschke K (1997) Embolism of fetal brain tissue to the lungs and the placenta. *Pediatr Pathol Lab Medn* 17: 159–167.

73. Bohm N, Keller KM, Kloke WD (1982) Pulmonary and systemic cerebellar tissue embolism due to birth injury. *Virchows Arch A Pathol Anat Histopathol* 398: 229–235.
74. Fisher A (1913) A case of complete absence of both internal carotid arteries, with a preliminary note on the developmental history of the stapedial artery. *J Anat Physiol* 48(Pt. 1): 37–46.
75. Turnbull I (1962) Agenesis of the internal carotid artery. *Neurology* 12: 588–590.
76. Hills J, Sament S (1968) Bilateral agenesis of the internal carotid artery associated with cardiac and other anomalies. Case report. *Neurology* 18: 142–146.
77. Teal JS, Rumbaugh CL, Bergeron RT, Scanlan RL, Segall HD (1972) Persistent carotid-superior cerebel-lar artery anastomosis: a variant of persistent trigeminal artery. *Radiology* 103: 335–341.
78. Lie T (1968) *Congenital Anomalies of the Carotid Arteries, Including the Carotid-Basilar and Carotid-Vertebral Anastomoses; An Angiographic Study and Review of the Literature.* Amsterdam: Excerpta Medica Foundation.
79. Smith KR Jr., Nelson JS, Dooley JM Jr. (1968) Bilateral 'hypoplasia' of the internal carotid arteries. *Neurology* 18: 1149–1156.
80. Lhermitte F, Gautier J, Poirier J (1968) Hypoplasia of the internal carotid artery. *Neurology* 18: 439–446.
81. Vuia O, Alexianu M, Gabor S (1970) Hypoplasia and obstruction of the circle of Willis in a case of atypical cerebral hemorrhage and its relationship to Nishimoto's disease. *Neurology* 20: 361–367.
82. Vogel FS, McClenahan J (1952) Anomalies of major cerebral arteries associated with congenital malfor-mations of the brain, with special reference to the pathogenesis of anencephaly. *Am J Pathol* 28: 701–723.
83. Parker J, Gaede J (1970) Occurrence of vascular anomalies in unilateral cerebral hypoplasia. 'Cerebral hemiatrophy.' *Arch Pathol* 90: 265–270.
84. Courville C (1959) Antenatal and paranatal circulatory disorders as a cause of cerebral damage in early life. *J Neuropathol Exp Neurol* 18: 115–140.
85. Muir C (1959) Hydranencephaly and allied disorders. A study of cerebral defect in Chinese children. *Arch Dis Child* 34: 231–246.
86. Abanou A, Lasjaunias P, Manelfe C, Lopez-Ibor L (1984) The accessory middle cerebral artery (AMCA). Diagnostic and therapeutic consequences. *Anat Clin* 6: 305–309.
87. Komiyama M, Nishikawa M, Yasui T (1997) The accessory middle cerebral artery as a collateral blood supply. *AJNR Am J Neuroradiol* 18: 587–590.
88. Bahsi YZ, Uysal H, Peker S, Yurdakul M (1993) Persistent primitive proatlantal intersegmental artery (proatlantal artery I) results in 'top of the basilar' syndrome. *Stroke* 24: 2114–2117.
89. Helmberger T, Spindler-Thiele S, Glatzel W, Schmitt R (1994) [A persistent carotid-basilar anastomosis: the proatlantal artery in a case of ipsilateral vertebral artery aplasia and contralateral vertebral artery hypoplasia]. *Aktuelle Radiol* 4: 153–154.
90. Okuno T, Nishiguchi T, Hayashi S, et al (1988) [A case of carotid superior cerebellar artery anastomosis associated with bilateral hypoplasia of the internal carotid artery represented as the rupture of posterior cerebral artery–posterior communicating artery aneurysm]. *No Shinkei Geka* 16: 1211–1217.
91. Huber G (1977) [The primitive otic artery, a very rare, persistent, primitive artery (author's transl.)]. *ROFO Fortschr Geb Rontgenstr Nuklearmed* 127: 350–353.
92. Komiyama M, Kitano S, Sakamoto H, Shiomi M (1998) An additional variant of the persistent primitive trigeminal artery: accessory meningeal artery–antero-superior cerebellar artery anastomosis associated with moyamoya disease. *Acta Neurochir* 140: 1037–1042.
93. Komiyama M, Nakajima H, Nishikawa M, et al (1999) High incidence of persistent primitive arteries in moyamoya and quasi-moyamoya diseases. *Neurol Med Chir (Tokyo)* 39: 416–420; discussion 20–22.
94. Ehlers H, Courville CB (1936) Thrombosis of internal cerebral veins in infancy and childhood. *J Pediatr* 8: 600–623.
95. Gerhard C (1857) Ueber Hirnsinus-Thrombosis bei Kindern. *Dtsch Klin (Berl)* 9: 45–49, 437–438.
96. Parrot MJ (1873) Etude sur le ramollissement de lencephale chez le nouveau-ne. *Arch Physiol Norm Patholol (Paris)* 5: 59–73, 176–195, 283–303.
97. Byers RK, Hass GM (1933) Thrombosis of the dural venous sinuses in infancy and in childhood. *Am J Dis Child* 45: 1161–1183.
98. Cardo E, Campistol J, Caritg J, et al (1999) Fatal haemorrhagic infarct in an infant with homocystinuria. *Dev Med Child Neurol* [Case Reports] 41: 132–135.
99. Sebire G, Tabarki B, Saunders DE, et al (2005) Cerebral venous sinus thrombosis in children: risk factors, presentation, diagnosis and outcome. *Brain* 128(Pt 3): 477–489.

100. Duran R, Aladag N, Vatansever U, Temizoz O, Genchallac H, Acunas B (2007) Cranial MR venography findings of severe hypernatremic dehydration in association with cerebral venous thrombosis in the neonatal period. *Pediatr Hematol Oncol* 24: 387–391.

101. Friede RL (1972) Residual lesions of infantile cerebral phlebothrombosis. *Acta Neuropathol (Berl)* 22: 319–332.

102. Courville C (1971) *Birth and Brain Damage*. Pasadena: Margaret Farnsworth Courville.

103. Jaeger R (1951) Observations on resection of the superior longitudinal sinus at and posterior to the Rolandic venous inflow. *J Neurosurg* 8: 103–109.

104. Carvalho KS, Bodensteiner JB, Connolly PJ, Garg BP (2001) Cerebral venous thrombosis in children. *J Child Neurol* 16: 574–580.

105. Davies RP, Slavotinek JP, James SL, Morphett AD (1989) Calcified cerebral sinus thrombosis in infancy—CT appearances with pathological correlation. *Pediatr Radiol* 20(1–2): 101–103.

106. Friede RL (1972) Ponto-subicular lesions in perinatal anoxia. *Arch Pathol* 94: 343–354.

107. Barmada M, Moossy J, Painter M (1979) Pontosubicular necrosis and hyperoxemia. *J Neuropathol Exp Neurol* 38: 304.

108. Galloway PG, Roessmann U (1986) Neuronal karyorrhexis in Sommer's sector in a 22-week stillborn. *Acta Neuropathol* 70(3–4): 343–344.

109. Aronson SM (1971) Vascular malformation. In: Minckler J, editor. *Pathology of the Nervous System*. New York: McGraw-Hill Book Co., p. 1884.

110. Jellinger K (1986) Vascular malformations of the central nervous system: a morphological overview. *Neurosurg Rev* 9: 177–216.

111. Rafalowska J, Drac H, Dziewulska D, Bojakowski J (1995) Coexistence of various vascular malformations within the brain. *Folia Neuropathol* 33: 247–250.

112. Ponce FA, Han PP, Spetzler RF, Canady A, Feiz-Erfan I (2001) Associated arteriovenous malformation of the orbit and brain: a case of Wyburn–Mason syndrome without retinal involvement. Case report. *J Neurosurg* 95: 346–349.

113. Al-Rodhan NR, Al-Mefty O, Rifai A, Fox JL (1986) Persistence of primitive cerebral vasculature in a newborn. A case report of whole brain AVM. *Clin Neurol Neurosurg* 88: 283–287.

114. van Beijnum J, van der Worp HB, Schippers HM, et al (2007) Familial occurrence of brain arteriovenous malformations: a systematic review. *J Neurol Neurosurg Psychiatry* 78: 1213–1217.

115. Takashima S, Becker LE (1980) Neuropathology of cerebral arteriovenous malformations in children. *J Neurol Neurosurg Psychiatry* 43: 380–385.

116. Hayashi N, Endo S, Oka N, Takeda S, Takaku A (1994) Intracranial hemorrhage due to rupture of an arteriovenous malformation in a full-term neonate. *Childs Nerv Syst* 10: 344–346.

117. Coulter DM, Zhou H, Rorke-Adams LB (2007) Catastrophic intrauterine spinal cord injury caused by an arteriovenous malformation. *J Perinatol* 27: 186–189.

118. Hashimoto T, Wen G, Lawton MT, et al (2003) Abnormal expression of matrix metalloproteinases and tissue inhibitors of metalloproteinases in brain arteriovenous malformations. *Stroke* 34: 925–931.

119. Sonstein WJ, Kader A, Michelsen WJ, Llena JF, Hirano A, Casper D (1996) Expression of vascular endothelial growth factor in pediatric and adult cerebral arteriovenous malformations: an immunocytochemical study. *J Neurosurg* 85: 838–845.

120. Uranishi R, Baev NI, Ng PY, Kim JH, Awad IA (2001) Expression of endothelial cell angiogenesis receptors in human cerebrovascular malformations. *Neurosurgery* 48: 359–367; discussion 67–68.

121. Gailloud P, O'Riordan D P, Burger I, Lehmann CU (2006) Confirmation of communication between deep venous drainage and the vein of galen after treatment of a vein of Galen aneurysmal malformation in an infant presenting with severe pulmonary hypertension. *AJNR American J Neuroradiol* 27: 317–320.

122. Silverman BK, Breckx T, Craig J, Nadas AS (1955) Congestive failure in the newborn caused by cerebral A-V fistula. *Am J Dis Child* 89: 539–543.

123. Gordon IJ, Shah BL, Hardman DR, Chameidcs L (1977) Giant dural supratentorial arteriovenous malformation. *AJR Am J Roentgenol* 129: 734–736.

124. Garcia-Monaco R, Rodesch G, Terbrugge K, Burrows P, Lasjaunias P (1991) Multifocal dural arteriovenous shunts in children. *Childs Nerv Syst* 7: 425–431.

125. Suh DC, Alvarez H, Bhattacharya JJ, Rodesch G, Lasjaunias PL (2001) Intracranial haemorrhage within the first two years of life. *Acta Neurochir (Wien)* 143: 997–1004.

126. van Dijk JM, TerBrugge KG, Willinsky RA, Wallace MC (2002) Multiplicity of dural arteriovenous fistulas. *J Neurosurg* 96: 76–78.

127. Zuccaro G, Arganaraz R, Villasante F, Ceciliano A (2010) Neurosurgical vascular malformations in children under 1 year of age. *Childs Nerv Syst* 26: 1381–1394.

128. David LR, Argenta LC, Venes J, Wilson J, Glazier S (1998) Sinus pericranii. *J Craniofac Surg* 9: 3–10.

129. Gandolfo C, Krings T, Alvarez H, et al (2007) Sinus pericranii: diagnostic and therapeutic considerations in 15 patients. *Neuroradiology* 49: 505–514.

130. Huang J, McGirt MJ, Gailloud P, Tamargo RJ (2005) Intracranial aneurysms in the pediatric population: case series and literature review. *Surg Neurol* 63: 424–432; discussion 32–33.

131. Krishna H, Wani AA, Behari S, Banerji D, Chhabra DK, Jain VK (2005) Intracranial aneurysms in patients 18 years of age or under, are they different from aneurysms in adult population? *Acta Neurochir (Wien)* 147: 469–476; discussion 76.

132. Buis DR, van Ouwerkerk WJ, Takahata H, Vandertop WP (2006) Intracranial aneurysms in children under 1 year of age: a systematic review of the literature. *Childs Nerv Syst* 22: 1395–1409.

133. Ferrante L, Fortuna A, Celli P, Santoro A, Fraioli B (1988) Intracranial arterial aneurysms in early childhood. *Surg Neurol* 29: 39–56.

134. Tekkok IH, Ventureyra EC (1997) Spontaneous intracranial hemorrhage of structural origin during the first year of life. *Childs Nerv Syst* 13: 154–165.

135. Tan MP, McConachie NS, Vloeberghs M (1998) Ruptured fusiform cerebral aneurysm in a neonate. *Childs Nerv Syst* 14: 467–469.

136. Kuchelmeister K, Schulz R, Bergmann M, Schwuchow R, Vollmer E (1993) A probably familial saccular aneurysm of the anterior communicating artery in a neonate. *Childs Nerv Syst* 9: 302–305.

137. Lang C, Jacobi G, Kreuz W, et al (1992) Rapid development of giant aneurysm at the base of the brain in an 8-year-old boy with perinatal HIV infection. *Acta Histochem Suppl* 42: 83–90.

138. Nunes ML, Pinho AP, Sfoggia A (2001) Cerebral aneurysmal dilatation in an infant with perinatally acquired HIV infection and HSV encephalitis. *Arq Neuropsiquiatr* 59: 116–118.

139. Beltramello A, Puppini G, Bricolo A, et al (1999) Does the tuberous sclerosis complex include intracranial aneurysms? A case report with a review of the literature. *Pediatr Radiol* 29: 206–211.

140. Afifi AK, Godersky JC, Menezes A, Smoker WR, Bell WE, Jacoby CG (1987) Cerebral hemiatrophy, hypoplasia of internal carotid artery, and intracranial aneurysm. A rare association occurring in an infant. *Arch Neurol* 44: 232–235.

141. Piastra M, Chiaretti A, Tortorolo L (2000) Ruptured intracranial mycotic aneurysm presenting as cerebral haemorrhage in an infant: case report and review of the literature. *Childs Nerv Syst* 16: 190–193.

142. Zhang J, Zhang X, Guo Q, et al (2007) Surgical treatment of giant fusiform aneurysm of extracranial internal carotid artery in a child: 1 case report and literature review. *Surg Neurol* 68: 329–333; discussion 34.

143. De Marinis P, Punzo A, Colangelo M, Ruggiero G, De Simone A, Ambrosio A (1991) Giant aneurysm of the calloso-marginal artery. *Childs Nerv Syst* 7: 353–355.

144. Cambria S, Cardia E, Macri E (1976) [Giant aneurysm of the sylvian artery in a 4-year old child (exeresis, remission)]. *Neurochirurgie* 22: 85–90.

145. Choudhury AR, al Amiri NH, al Moutaery KR, Aabed M, Strelling MK (1991) Giant middle cerebral aneurysm presenting as hemiathetosis in a child and its spontaneous thrombosis. *Childs Nerv Syst* 7: 59–61.

146. Ciceri EF, Lawhead AL, De Simone T, Valvassori L, Boccardi E (2005) Spontaneous partial thrombosis of a basilar artery giant aneurysm in a child. *AJNR Am J Neuroradiol* 26: 56–57.

147. Osenbach RK (1989) Giant aneurysm of the distal posterior inferior cerebellar artery in an 11-month-old child presenting with obstructive hydrocephalus. *Pediatr Neurosci* 15: 309–312.

148. van Donselaar CA, Stefanko SZ, van der Kwast TH, Arts WF, Koudstaal PJ (1988) Basilar artery giant fusiform aneurysms caused by congenital defect of the internal elastic lamina and media. *Clin Neuropathol* 7: 68–72.

149. Read D, Esiri MM (1979) Fusiform basilar artery aneurysm in a child. *Neurology* 29: 1045–1049.

150. Biondi A, Clemenceau S, Dormont D, et al (2002) Intracranial extra-axial cavernous (HEM) angiomas: tumors or vascular malformations? *J Neuroradiol* 29: 91–104.

151. Steichen-Gersdorf E, Felber S, Fuchs W, Russeger L, Twerdy K (1992) Familial cavernous angiomas of the brain: observations in a four generation family. *Eur J Pediatr* 151: 861–863.

152. Chen DH, Lipe HP, Qin Z, Bird TD (2002) Cerebral cavernous malformation: novel mutation in a Chinese family and evidence for heterogeneity. *J Neurol Sci* 196(1–2): 91–96.

153. Novelli PM, Reigel DH, Langham Gleason P, Yunis E (1997) Multiple cavernous angiomas after high-dose whole-brain radiation therapy. *Pediatr Neurosurg* 26: 322–325.

154. Baumgartner JE, Ater JL, Ha CS, et al (2003) Pathologically proven cavernous angiomas of the brain following radiation therapy for pediatric brain tumors. *Pediatr Neurosurg* 39: 201–207.

155. Martinez-Lage JF, de la Fuente I, Ros de San Pedro J, Fuster JL, Perez-Espejo MA, Herrero MT (2008) Cavernomas in children with brain tumors: a late complication of radiotherapy. *Neurocirugia (Astur)* 19: 50–54.

156. Shenkar R, Elliott JP, Diener K, et al (2003) Differential gene expression in human cerebrovascular malformations. *Neurosurgery* 52: 465–477; discussion 77–78.

157. Leblanc GG, Golanov E, Awad IA, Young WL (2009) Biology of vascular malformations of the brain. *Stroke* 40: e694–702.

158. Plummer NW, Gallione CJ, Srinivasan S, Zawistowski JS, Louis DN, Marchuk DA (2004) Loss of p53 sensitizes mice with a mutation in Ccm1 (KRIT1) to development of cerebral vascular malformations. *Am J Pathol* 165: 1509–1518.

159. Tannier C, Pons M, Treil J (1991) [Cerebral venous angiomas. 12 personal cases and review of the literature]. *Rev Neurol (Paris)* 147: 356–363.

160. Yamasaki T, Handa H, Yamashita J, Moritake K, Nagasawa S (1984) Intracranial cavernous angioma angiographically mimicking venous angioma in an infant. *Surg Neurol* 22: 461–466.

161. Goulao A, Alvarez H, Garcia Monaco R, Pruvost P, Lasjaunias P (1990) Venous anomalies and abnormalities of the posterior fossa. *Neuroradiology* 31: 476–482.

162. Abe M, Hagihara N, Tabuchi K, Uchino A, Miyasaka Y (2003) Histologically classified venous angiomas of the brain: a controversy. *Neurol Med Chir (Tokyo)* 43: 1–10; discussion 1.

163. Cheong WY, Tan KP (1993) Cerebral venous angioma—a misnomer? *Ann Acad Med Singapore* 22: 736–741.

164. Jellinger K, Kucsko L, Seitelberger F (1966) Diffuse meningo-cerebrale angiodysplasie mit hypoplasiogener isthmusstenose bei einem neugeborenen. [Diffuse meningo-cerebral angiodysplasia with hypoplasiogenic isthmus stenosis in a newborn infant.]. *Beitr Pathol Anat 133*: 41–72.

165. Vuia O, Pascu F (1970) [Meningo-cerebral angiomatosis in the newborn]. *Stud Cercet Neurol* 15: 69–75.

166. Valdivieso EM, Scholtz CL (1986) Diffuse meningocerebral angiodysplasia and renal agenesis: a case report. *Pediatr Pathol* 6: 119–126.

167. Potter EL (1948) Diffuse angiectasis of the cerebral meninges in the newborn infant. *Arch Pathol* 46: 87–96.

168. Memeo M, Scardapane A, Stabile Ianora AA, Sabba C, Angelelli G (2006) Hereditary haemorrhagic telangiectasia: diagnostic imaging of visceral involvement. *Curr Pharm Des* 12: 1227–1235.

169. Sabba C, Pasculli G, Cirulli A, et al (2002) Hereditary hemorrhagic telangiectasia (Rendu–Osler–Weber disease). *Minerva Cardioangiol* 50: 221–238.

170. Alexander OL, Norman TRM (1960) *Sturge–Weber Syndrome*. Bristol: Wright.

171. Leadbetter WF, Burkland CD (1938) Hypertension in unilateral renal disease. *J Urol* 39: 611–625.

172. Price RA, Vawter GF (1972) Arterial fibromuscular dysplasia in infancy and childhood. *Arch Pathol* 93: 419–426.

173. Mettinger KL (1982) Fibromuscular dysplasia and the brain. II Current concept of the disease. *Stroke* 13: 53–58.

174. Camacho A, Villarejo A, Moreno T, Simon R, Munoz A, Mateos F (2003) Vertebral artery fibromuscular dysplasia: an unusual cause of stroke in a 3-year-old child. *Dev Med Child Neurol* 45: 709–711.

175. Bowen MD, Burak CR, Barron TF (2005) Childhood ischemic stroke in a nonurban population. *J Child Neurol* 20: 194–197.

176. Thompson JA, Grunnet ML, Anderson RE (1975) Carotid arterial elastic hyperplasia in a newborn. *Stroke* 6: 391–394.

177. Hallervorden J (1937) Das Gebutrauma als Ursache der Entwicklungshemmung im Kindesalter. *Med Klinik* 33: 1224.

178. Bignami A, Ralston HJI (1968) Myelination of fibrillary astroglial processes in long term Wallerian degeneration. The possible relationship to 'status marmoratus.' *Brain Res* 11: 710.

179. Borit A, Herndon RM (1970) The fine structure of placques fibromyeliniques in ulegyria and in status marmoratus. *Acta Neuropathol* 14: 304.

180. Romanul FCA, Abramowica A (1964) Changes in brain and pial vessels in arterial border zones. *Arch Neurol* 11: 40–65.

181. Brierley JB (1979) Ischemic necrosis along brain arterial boundary zones: some aspects of its etiology. *Adv Neurol* 26: 155–162.

324

182. Perlman JM, Volpe JJ (1985) Episodes of apnea and bradycardia in the preterm newborn: impact on cerebral circulation. *Pediatrics* 76: 333–338.

183. Gruenwald P (1955) The pathology of perinatal distress. *AMA Arch Pathol* 60: 150–172.

184. McNutt S (1885) Double infantile spastic hemiplegia with the report of a case. *Am J Med Sci* 89(177): 58–79.

185. McNutt S (1885) Apoplexia neonatorum. *Am J Obstet* 18: 73–81.

186. Larroche J (1966) The development of the central nervous system during intrauterine life. In: Falkner F, editor. *Human Development*. Philadelphia: WB Saunders, pp. 257–276.

187. Korogi Y, Takahashi M, Sumi M, et al (1996) MR signal intensity of the perirolandic cortex in the neonate and infant. *Neuroradiology* 38: 578–584.

188. Maller AI, Hankins LL, Yeakley JW, Butler IJ (1998) Rolandic type cerebral palsy in children as a pattern of hypoxic–ischemic injury in the full-term neonate. *J Child Neurol* 13: 313–321.

189. Huang BY, Castillo M (2008) Hypoxic–ischemic brain injury: imaging findings from birth to adulthood. *Radiographics* 28: 417–439; quiz 617.

190. Tokumaru AM, Barkovich AJ, O'Uchi T, Matsuo T, Kusano S (1999) The evolution of cerebral blood flow in the developing brain: evaluation with iodine-123 iodoamphetamine SPECT and correlation with MR imaging. *AJNR Am J Neuroradiol* 20: 845–852.

191. Cruveilhier J (1829–1835) *Anatomie Pathologique du Corps Humain, Part 2*, XVth Liv. Paris: JB Baillière.

192. Spielmeyer W (1904–1905) Ein hydranencephales Zwillingspaar. *Arch Psychiat Nervenkr* 39: 807–819.

193. Crome L, Sylvester PE (1958) Hydranencephaly (hydrencephaly). *Arch Dis Child* 33: 235.

194. Halsey Jr. JH, Allen N, Chamberlin HR (1971) The morphogenesis of hydranencephaly. *J Neurol Sci* 12: 187–217.

195. Lindenberg R, Swanson PD (1967) 'Infantile hydranencephaly'—a report of five cases of infarction of both cerebral hemispheres in infancy. *Brain* 90: 839–850.

196. Hamby WB (1960) *Case Reports and Autopsy Records of Ambroise Paré.* Springfield: Charles C. Thomas.

197. Warner FJ (1976) The histopathology of a case of hydranencephaly in a 30 week old human fetus. *Okajimas Folia Anat Jpn* 53: 143–172.

198. Regec SP, Bernstine RL (1979) Hydranencephaly in a twin gestation. *Obstet Gynecol* 54: 369–371.

199. Hahn JS, Lewis AJ, Barnes P (2003) Hydranencephaly owing to twin–twin transfusion: serial fetal ultrasonography and magnetic resonance imaging findings. *J Child Neurol* 18: 367–370.

200. Harper C, Hockey A (1983) Proliferative vasculopathy and an hydranencephalic–hydrocephalic syndrome: a neuropathological study of two siblings. *Dev Med Child Neurol* 25: 232–239.

201. Harding BN, Ramani P, Thurley P (1995) The familial syndrome of proliferative vasculopathy and hydranencephaly–hydrocephaly: immunocytochemical and ultrastructural evidence for endothelial proliferation. *Neuropathol Appl Neurobiol* 21: 61–67.

202. Mittelbronn M, Beschorner R, Schittenhelm J, et al (2006) Multiple thromboembolic events in fetofetal transfusion syndrome in triplets contributing to the understanding of pathogenesis of hydranencephaly in combination with polymicrogyria. *Hum Pathol* 37: 1503–1507.

203. McAdams RM (2005) Maternal systemic lupus erythematosus and hydranencephaly in a neonate: a case report. *J Matern Fetal Neonatal Med* 18: 279–281.

204. Cooney TP, Thurlbeck WM (1985) Lung growth and development in anencephaly and hydranencephaly. *Am Rev Respir Dis* 132: 596–601.

205. Martin C, Allain D, Vital C, Babin JP, Demarquez JL, San Juan B (1977) [Familial hydranencephaly]. *Ann Pediatr (Paris)* 24: 673–678.

206. Richards WP, Crenshaw GL, Bushnell RB (1971) Hydranencephaly of calves associated with natural bluetongue virus infection. *Cornell Vet* 61: 336–348.

207. Osburn BI (1972) Animal model for human disease. Hydranencephaly, porencephaly, cerebral cysts, retinal dysplasia CNS malformations. Animal model: bluetongue-vaccine-virus infection in fetal lambs. *Am J Pathol* 67: 211–214.

208. Tateyama S, Yamaguchi R, Uchida K, Nosaka D, Murakami T, Otsuka H (1990) An outbreak of congenital hydranencephaly and cerebellar hypoplasia among calves in South Kyushu, Japan: a pathological study. *Res Vet Sci* 49: 127–131.

209. Binhazim AA, Buchl SJ (1994) Hydranencephaly in two rhesus monkeys (Macaca mulatta). *J Med Primatol* 23: 313–314.

210. Wintour EM, Lewitt M, McFarlane A, et al (1996) Experimental hydranencephaly in the ovine fetus. *Acta Neuropathol (Berl)* 91: 537–544.

211. Christie JD, Rakusan TA, Martinez MA, et al (1986) Hydranencephaly caused by congenital infection with herpes simplex virus. *Pediatr Infect Dis* 5: 473–478.

212. Becker H (1949) Uber Hirngefassausschatungen; intrakranielle Gefassverschlusse; uber experimentell Hydranencephalie (Blasenhirn). *Dsch Ztschr Nervenh* 161: 446–505.

213. Myers RE (1969) Brain pathology following fetal vascular occlusion: an experimental study. *Invest Ophthalmol* 8: 41–50.

214. Heschl R (1868) Neue Fälle von Porencephaly. *Prag Vierteljahrschr prakt Heilk* 100: 40.

215. Prayson RA, Hannahoe BM (2004) Clinicopathologic findings in patients with infantile hemiparesis and epilepsy. *Hum Pathol* 35: 734–738.

216. Kundrat H (1882) Die Porencephalie, eine anatomische Studie. Graz: Von Leuschner and Lubensky.

217. Yakovlev PI, Wadsworth RC (1946) Schizencephalies: a study of the congenital clefts in the cerebral mantle. I Clefts with fused lips. *J Neuropathol Exp Neurol* 5: 116–130.

218. Dekaban A (1965) Large defects in cerebral hemispheres associated with cortical dysgenesis. *J Neuropathol Exp Neurol* 24: 512–530.

219. Meyer JE (1951) Über Gefäßveränderungen beim fetalen und frühkindlichen Cerebralschaden. *Arch für Psych und Zeitschrift Neurologie* 186: 437–455.

220. Friede RL, Mikolasek J (1978) Postencephalitic porencephaly, hydranencephaly or polymicrogyria. A review. *Acta Neuropathol (Berl)* 43(1–2): 161–168.

221. Grant EG, Kerner M, Schellinger D, et al (1982) Evolution of porencephalic cysts from intraparenchymal hemorrhage in neonates: sonographic evidence. *AJR Am J Roentgenol* 138: 467–470.

222. Moinuddin A, McKinstry RC, Martin KA, Neil JJ (2003) Intracranial hemorrhage progressing to porencephaly as a result of congenitally acquired cytomegalovirus infection—an illustrative report. *Prenat Diagn* 23: 797–800.

223. Stewart RM, Williams RS, Lukl P, Schoenen J (1978) Ventral porencephaly: a cerebral defect associated with multiple congenital anomalies. *Acta Neuropathol (Berl)* 42: 231–235.

224. Mancini GM, de Coo IF, Lequin MH, Arts WF (2004) Hereditary porencephaly: clinical and MRI findings in two Dutch families. *Eur J Paediatr Neurol* 8: 45–54.

225. Strefling AM, Urich H (1986) Prenatal porencephaly: the pattern of secondary lesions. *Acta Neuropathol* 71(1–2): 171–175.

226. Wolf A, Cowen D (1955) The cerebral atrophies and encephalomalacias of infancy and childhood. *Res Publ Assoc Res Nerv Ment Dis* 34: 199–330.

227. Crome L (1958) Multilocular cystic encephalopathy of infants. *J Neurol Neurosurg Psychiatr* 21: 146–152.

228. Fowler M, Mellor G (1965) Cerebral malformation and degeneration produced in later fetal life by a primary cardiac anomaly. *J Pathol Bacteriol* 90: 523.

229. Marburg O, Casamajor L (1944) Phlebostasis and phlebothrombosis of brain in newborn and childhood. *Arch Neurol Psychiatry* 52: 170.

230. Aicardi J, Goutieres F, De Verbois AH (1972) Multicystic encephalomalacia of infants and its relation to abnormal gestation and hydranencephaly. *J Neurol Sci* 15: 357.

231. Smith JF, Rodeck C (1975) Multiple cystic and focal encephalomalacia in infancy and childhood with brain stem damage. *J Neurol Sci* 25: 377–388.

232. Adams RD, Prod'hom LS, Rabinowicz T (1977) Intrauterine brain death. Neuraxial reticular core necrosis. *Acta Neuropathol (Berl)* 40: 41–49.

233. Sendelbach KM, Gujrati M, Husain AN (1992) Web-like malformation of the carotid artery and multicystic encephalomalacia. *Pediatr Pathol* 12: 701–706.

234. Narita M, Inui S, Hashiguchi Y (1979) The pathogenesis of congenital encephalopathies in sheep experimentally induced by Akabane virus. *J Comp Pathol* 89: 229–240.

235. London WT, Levitt NH, Kent SG, Wong VG, Sever JL (1977) Congenital cerebral and ocular malformations induced in rhesus monkeys by Venezuelan equine encephalitis virus. *Teratology* 16: 285–285.

236. Friede RL (1989) *Developmental Neuropathology*, 2nd edn. New York: Springer-Verlag.

237. Anton G (1895) Ueber die bethielung der grossen basalen gehirnganlien bei bewegungsstörungen und insbesondere bei chorea. *Jahrbuch für Psychiat* 14: 141–181.

238. Malamud N (1950) Status marmoratus: a form of cerebral palsy following either birth injury of inflammation of the central nervous system. *J Pediatr* 37: 610–619.

239. Schwartz P (1958) Birth injury as a cause of status marmoratus. *Arch Pediatr* 75: 45–66.
240. Myers RE (1969) Atrophic cortical sclerosis associated with status marmoratus in a perinatally damaged monkey. *Neurology* 19: 1177–1188.
241. Friede RL, Schachenmayr W (1977) Early stages of status marmoratus. *Acta Neuropathol* 38: 123–127.
242. Parisi JE, Collins GH, Kim RC, Crosley CJ (1983) Prenatal symmetrical thalamic degeneration with flexion spasticity at birth. *Ann Neurol* 13: 94–97.
243. Norman RM, Urich H (1957) Cerebellar hypoplasia associated with systemic degeneration in early life. *J Neurol Neurosurg Psychiatry* 21: 159–166.
244. Takashima S (1982) Olivocerebellar lesions in infants born prematurely. *Brain Dev* 4: 361–366.
245. Strefling AM, Urich H (1982) Crossed cerebellar atrophy: an old problem revisited. *Acta Neuropathol* 57(2–3): 197–202.
246. Babcock DS, Han BK, Weiss RG, Ryckman FC (1989) Brain abnormalities in infants on extracorporeal membrane oxygenation: sonographic and CT findings. *AJR Am J Roentgenol* 153: 571–576.
247. Lago P, Rebsamen S, Clancy RR, et al (1995) MRI, MRA, and neurodevelopmental outcome following neonatal ECMO. *Pediatr Neurol* 12: 294–304.
248. Graziani LJ, Gringlas M, Baumgart S (1997) Cerebrovascular complications and neurodevelopmental sequelae of neonatal ECMO *Clin Perinatol* 24: 655–675.
249. Park CH, Spitzer AR, Desai HJ, Zhang JJ, Graziani LJ (1992) Brain SPECT in neonates following extracorporeal membrane oxygenation: evaluation of technique and preliminary results. *J Nucl Med* 33: 1943–1948.
250. Taylor GA, Fitz CR, Kapur S, Short BL (1989) Cerebrovascular accidents in neonates treated with extracorporeal membrane oxygenation: sonographic–pathologic correlation. *AJR Am J Roentgenol* 153: 355–361.
251. Jarjour IT, Ahdab-Barmada M (1994) Cerebrovascular lesions in infants and children dying after extracorporeal membrane oxygenation. *Pediatr Neurol* 10: 13–19.
252. Evans MJ, McKeever PA, Pearson GA, Field D, Firmin RK (1994) Pathological complications of non-survivors of newborn extracorporeal membrane oxygenation. *Arch Dis Child* 71: F88–92.

14
FETAL AND NEONATAL INTRACRANIAL HEMORRHAGE

Introduction

Newborn intracranial hemorrhage has long been a subject of importance (Willis, 1667, cited in references 1–4). Early authors separated neonatal intracranial hemorrhage into several categories depending on location or origin: (1) paradural; (2) subarachnoid; (3) cerebellum; (4) germinal matrix; (5) cerebral convexity hemorrhage; (6) terminal vein; (7) choroid plexus; (8) parenchymal; (9) tentorial laceration; (10) minor vascular ruptures; (11) isolated;[5] (12) pial hemorrhage;[6] and (13) microscopic extravasations of blood occurring anywhere in the brain.[7–9] Chessells, in 1970, recognized intracranial hemorrhages as part of secondary newborn hemorrhagic disease;[10] others downplayed disseminated intravascular coagulopathy as being significant in neonatal intracranial hemorrhage.[11]

The leptomeninges were the most prevalent site of hemorrhage in both liveborns and fetal deaths in the National Collaborative Perinatal Project (NCPP) neonatal autopsy population, occurring in about two-thirds of patients. Such hemorrhages, small or large, were rarely focal or confined to one hemisphere. Over half of stillborn neonates had leptomeningeal hemorrhages, a rate comparable to the liveborn. The second most frequent site was cerebral white matter, with hemorrhages found in 42% of fetal deaths and 47% of liveborns. The ganglionic eminence and ventricles were frequently encountered sites of hemorrhage in liveborns (44% for both sites), but these were found less frequently in fetal deaths (about 25%). One-third of liveborns had blood in the choroid plexus, and there was an approximately equal incidence among fetal deaths. Almost equal proportions of cerebellar hemorrhages were found in liveborns and fetal deaths: 14% and 12%, respectively.

Neonatal intracranial hemorrhages sometimes occur at multiple sites in one infant. One assumes that hemorrhage is more likely to occur during fetal life when cardiac output and cerebral blood flow are adequate, but less likely in the fetus dying shortly before birth. Therefore, further comparisons of rates and sites of intracranial hemorrhage in stillborn and liveborn infants potentially elucidate the relationship, if any, of hemorrhages to events other than the birth process itself.

Changes in cranial configuration during birth resulting in intracranial hemorrhage

As the infant's head is molded during labor and delivery, the fronto-occipital diameter increases and the falx and tentorium stretch, resulting in either tears of the falcine or tentorial free edge (quite rare in neonatal autopsy populations today)[3,4,12] or separation of the falcine or tentorial dural layers, causing local collection and resultant mass of blood to accumulate between the two layers (common in neonatal autopsy populations at present) (Fig. 14.1).[13–16] Hemorrhages into the potential subdural space from the falx or tentorium differ considerably from one another.[17] Falcine free edge laceration results in inferior sagittal sinus tears, located in the inferior falcine margin; tentorial free edge laceration severs the small tentorial artery in the tentorial margin.[18] In the absence of free edge laceration, one dural sheet apparently moves relative to the other dural sheet, comprising the falx and tentorium, and bleeding occurs because of the great dural vascularity.[19] These intradural falcine or tentorial hemorrhages sometimes rupture into the supratentorial or infratentorial subdural spaces,[20] resulting in symptomatic subdural hematomas.[15] The other source of subdural hemorrhage is rupture of large convexity veins, which exit the arachnoid and course in the arachnoid–dural interface for several centimeters before entering the lateral lacunes or superior sagittal sinus.

Many authors described intradural hemorrhages in great detail, including Weber,[21] Ehrenfest,[22] Von Haam,[23] Litchfield and Given,[24] Haller et al,[25] and others subsequently. Hemorrhages into the loose connective tissue between the two dural falcine or tentorial leaves are almost universal in autopsies of term or preterm neonates; they are less common in infants born after cesarean section.[26] As a rule, they consist of multiple small or large hemorrhages usually concentrated posteriorly in the falx or anteriorly in the tentorium. They are sometimes large enough to bulge or rupture into supratentorial or infratentorial subdural space, but rarely leave local traces in autopsies of older infants.[23,27]

FALX AND TENTORIUM
The dura mater constitutes the outer and most dense meningeal layer surrounding the brain. For the most part, fetal dura adheres tightly to the inner skull surface as its periosteum. Folds of pachymeningeal dura, the falx and tentorium, bridging different cranial bones,

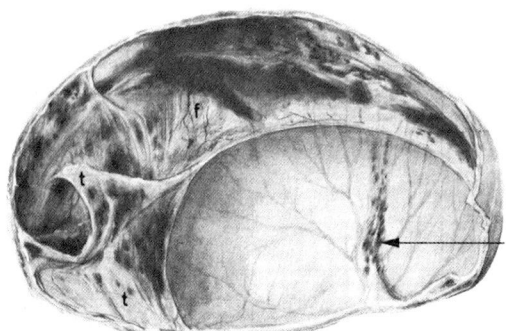

Fig. 14.1 Following normal vaginal delivery with marked occipitofrontal head elongation, there is considerable hemorrhage in the falx (f) and tentorium (t). The free tentorial or falcine edges are not torn. Note the intradural hemorrhages along the coronal suture (arrow). Reproduced with permission of S. Karger AG from Schwartz.[4] A color version of this figure is available in the color plate section at the back of the book.

traverse the vertebrate cranial cavity, compartmentalizing the brain. The supratentorial falx is formed from two dural layers, one from the dura of each cranial hemisphere; similarly, the tentorium is formed from one layer each of dura from supratentorial and infratentorial compartments. The fetal and neonatal falx and tentorium are well vascularized.[19] Superiorly, the two layers of dura enclose the superior sagittal sinus, where they are reflected from the falx onto the cranium, securing the falx and sinus superiorly. At its base, the falx is attached anteriorly to the crista galli and posteroinferiorly to the tentorial midline; the inferior sagittal sinus runs along its inferior margin and the straight sinus is secured in the midline by the falx and two tentorial leaves. The tentorium cerebelli appeared late in phylogeny as bilateral folds of dura in the cerebro–cerebellar fissure.[28] In humans, it is a broad, transverse band of dura separating the cerebrum from the cerebellum. Posteriorly and laterally, the two sheets of tentorial dura enclose lateral sinuses, where they are reflected to become the supratentorial or infratentorial dura. Anteriorly and laterally, it is anchored to the petrous ridge; anteriorly and medially, it forms the lateral cavernous sinus surface; anteriorly it is attached to the anterior clinoid process. Thus, the tentorial free edge, forming the 'tentorial notch' or incisura, sweeps occipitally and upwards from the anterior clinoid processes past the pituitary stalk and mammillary bodies, past the dorsum sellae, and past the brainstem to its anatomical apex where the tentorium and falx join. The anterior half of tentorial incisura contains the interpeduncular cistern and brainstem. There are large variations in incisural length and breadth.[29,30] In adults, the tentorium is fairly rigid; in a fetus, neonate, or young child, it is far thinner, delicate, and translucent (or even transparent), and supratentorial or infratentorial masses far more easily displace it upward or downward.[14]

Skull Fractures Associated with Intracranial Hemorrhage

Unless there is a significant disproportion between maternal pelvis and infant head or the head is pressed against the sacral promontory, the elasticity of membranous cranial bones and their movability against each other (from flexible sutures) provide unusual protection during birth against serious traumatic injury. Skull bone indentations or depressions occur, some associated with linear fractures, usually parietal, occasionally frontal, and rarely temporal. Sometimes the cranial bone is merely indented and corrects itself with time. Nevertheless, serious fractures occur in perfectly normal labors. More serious consequences follow if the fracture lacerates the dura and produces hemorrhage, such as epidural or subdural hematoma or hemorrhage within the brain. Still, serious skull fractures had become rare by 1977 and were found in only 2 of 2300 autopsies.[31]

Many authors observed neonatal diastases or fractures adjacent to the suture between the supraoccipital and exoccipital (condylar) bones.[22,32-34] The cartilaginous innominate synchondrosis between exoccipital and supraoccipital bones flexes during birth and is thought to allow cerebellar compression by the supraoccipital bone.[9,32] Nevertheless, localized hematomas were too widely distributed in the cerebellum in the NCPP population to support this hypothesis. More recently, some have claimed that supraoccipital bone fracture causes laceration of underlying cerebellum and is the result of face masks,[35] whereas others have denied the association.

Paradural hematoma

EPIDURAL

Epidural hematomas occur only if mechanical head trauma splits the dura from the bone. Neonatal epidural hemorrhage is rare. They usually assume a biconvex shape in relation to the overlying skull bone as the dura adheres firmly to the skull, particularly the coronal suture.[36] The parietal area is the most frequent location for epidural hematomas,[37] but they occasionally occur in the posterior fossa.[38,39]

SUBDURAL HEMORRHAGE

The subdural 'space' classically is considered a potential space between the arachnoid and dura. Nonetheless, the subdural potential 'space' is likely to be the weak cell layer at a continuous dural–arachnoid interface. The dural border cell layer, at this interface, is a specialized layer containing flattened fibroblasts, minimal extracellular collagen, and few cell junctions, combining to create a structurally weak inner dural layer relative to the underlying arachnoid. The arachnoid layer, in contrast, is composed of larger cells with numerous cell junctions and no extracellular collagen.[40] Thus, under normal conditions, there is no evidence of a naturally occurring space at the dura–arachnoid junction. When a space does appear, it is not subdural, but rather within a morphologically distinct layer of inner dura. While chronic subdural hematoma in infants (as a cause of large head) was a problem many years ago,[41–46] it seems to be much less of a problem at present.[47–50]

Neonatal subdural hematomas (Fig. 14.2), long recognized,[41–43,51,52] are more common than epidural hematomas and often follow breech[53] or other difficult deliveries, but sometimes follow an unremarkable delivery or caesarean section.[54] Subdural hematomas occur without a tentorial or falcine tear when superficial convexity veins, the great vein of Galen, or the straight sinus are torn.[25] Neonatal traumatic subdural hematomas have been rare for the last 30 years.[55] While uncommon in term infants, they are frequently recognized as thin collections of subdural blood. For instance, of 26 near-term neonates with subdural hematomas, seven were infratentorial, seven were supratentorial, and 12 were in both sites.[48] Vaginal delivery occurred in 25 of 26 patients and forceps were used in half of deliveries. They are occasionally found in untraumatized fetuses.[46,50,56] Small intradural hemorrhages are common in neonatal autopsy populations.

Supratentorial subdural hematoma
Death within 36 hours of birth, shock at the time of birth, irregular respirations, and absent tendon reflexes characterize the clinical picture of this entity. Infants who survive for more than 36 hours suffer from respiratory depression, early vomiting, increasing physical inactivity, nystagmus (in some), seizures (in half), and shrill or piercing crying, and constitute an alternate clinical expression. Most have irritability, seizures, coma, and collapse.[44]

Infratentorial retrocerebellar hematoma
The constrained posterior fossa space makes neonatal infratentorial subdural hematomas more serious than supratentorial, because the hematoma directly compresses and distorts the

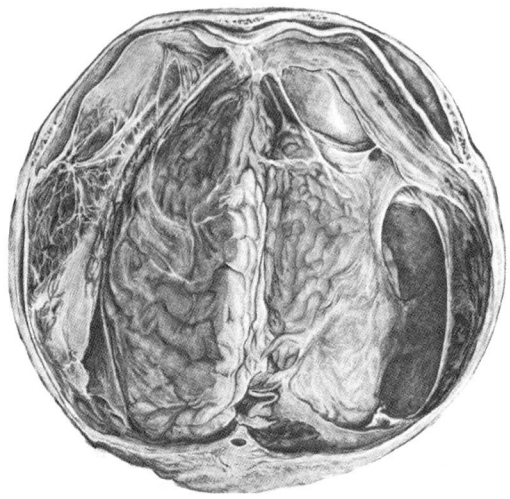

Fig. 14.2 Bilateral chronic partially organized, untreated supratentorial subdural hematomas in an infant, presumably arising from neonatal subdural hemorrhage. The underlying brain is shrunken, appears atrophic, and is surrounded by diaphanous white subdural membranes and less organized red or brown blood. Reproduced with permission of S. Karger AG from Schwartz.[4] A color version of this figure is available in the color plate section at the back of the book.

cerebellum and brainstem. While long recognized (Fig. 14.3),[15,20,51,57-67] its source has been variously attributed to free tentorial edge tears, or tears of the straight sinus or the great vein of Galen. Intratentorial hematomas sometimes rupture infratentorially. Blood from free tentorial edge tears has several routes of migration.[68] Head retraction, nuchal rigidity, and high-pitched crying characterize the clinical appearance.

Acute or chronic posterior fossa subdural hematoma potentially causes cerebellar displacement and fourth ventricular outlet occlusion.[15,63,65-67,69,70] Neonatal retrocerebellar subdural hemorrhage accumulating above the cerebellum under the tentorium or behind the cerebellum external to the cisterna magna arachnoid[8,20,71,72] potentially causes hydrocephalus.[59] The subdural blood arises from tentorial free edge tears or from blood accumulating between the two dural tentorial leaves with rupture into the retrocerebellar subdural space. Depending on location, a retrocerebellar hematoma mechanically shifts the cerebellum forward, causing the latter to envelop the medulla, and eventually occluding the midline and lateral fourth ventricular outlets. If the hematoma lies behind the cerebellum and brainstem, the latter is pressed forward and upward, occluding spinal fluid flow through the prepontine and ambient cisterns. As the aqueduct is usually dilated, along with the upper fourth ventricle, aqueductal kinking is not necessary for ventriculomegaly to occur.

In contrast to infants with large supratentorial subdural hematoma, infants with retrocerebellar subdural hematoma tend to present with marked changes in respiration and crying (high-pitched or hoarse), vomiting, poor sucking reflex, loss of Moro reflex, and usually hypotonia.[15] Ultrasonographers often have difficulty recognizing a retrocerebellar subdural hematoma when placing the transducer over the anterior fontanelle.

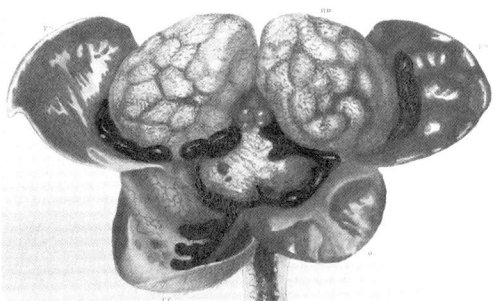

Fig. 14.3 Cruveilhier published the first image of retrocerebellar subdural hematomas in his atlas of 1828–1835. Note the black masses of blood behind the cerebellum. This hand-painted lithograph shows fine paint cracking. From Cruveilhier.[20] A color version of this figure is available in the color plate section at the back of the book.

Subarachnoid hemorrhage

GENERAL DESCRIPTION

Subarachnoid hemorrhage in autopsy populations of neonates is common,[7,8,22,23,25,73,74] and frequently not symptomatic. These hemorrhages sometimes occur as isolated, multiple large focal or local hematomas.[75] Subarachnoid hemorrhage sometimes arises from nearby intraventricular or parenchymal hemorrhage; however, subarachnoid hemorrhages, not related to intraventricular or parenchymal hemorrhage, are found anywhere in the arachnoid after preterm or term birth, but particularly over the convexity. In this chapter, we use the term subarachnoid hemorrhage only when we have excluded intraventricular or parenchymal hemorrhage as a source.

SUBARACHNOID HEMATOMA

Sometimes local subarachnoid hemorrhages accumulate sufficient blood to constitute hematomas. As far as we know, there are no clinical or pathologic studies of neonatal arachnoidal hematomas.

EPIDEMIOLOGY OF SUBARACHNOID HEMORRHAGE

Newborns who hemorrhage into the subarachnoid space in one cerebral location are at an increased risk of hemorrhage in another site. In some cases, blood moves from one area to another. The risk factors of subarachnoid hemorrhage were studied in 140 cases and 277 controls from the NCPP population.[76] Risk of subarachnoid hemorrhage was lower in infants born between 36 and 39 weeks. Infants born to primigravidas were at the same risk of subarachnoid hemorrhage as infants born to women who previously had a pregnancy that terminated in a fetal death after the twentieth gestational week. Infants born to primigravidas were twice as likely to have subarachnoid hemorrhage, as were infants whose mothers had carried at least one previous pregnancy to term and had not had any late fetal loss. Risk reduction was associated with vaginal bleeding during pregnancy and pyuria.

TABLE 14.1

Postulated scheme to explain how identified risk factors contribute to the occurrence of subarachnoid hemorrhage

Umbrella term	Risk factor
Trauma	Maternal gonococcal infection
	Late menarche
Intrapartum hypertension	Maternal gonococcal infection
	Intrapartum hypertension
	Clinic status
	Prior fetal death
Unfavorable uterine environment	Maternal gonococcal infection
	Late age at menarche
	Intrapartum hypertension
	Clinic status
	Blood type O
	Prior fetal death

Leviton et al[76] emphasized three umbrella terms under which the risk factors could be grouped (Table 14.1). First, keeping with present concepts, was 'trauma.' Schwartz[4] reviewed uncritically the history of the hypothesis that trauma contributes to the occurrences of intracranial hemorrhage in newborns. He described in detail how fragile leptomeningeal vessels were injured when the skull was pounded against the unyielding perineum. Late menarche, a correlate of increased risk of newborn subarachnoid hemorrhage, was associated with spontaneous membrane rupture. Vaginal bleeding, a correlate of reduced risk of subarachnoid hemorrhage, was associated with failure of membranes to rupture spontaneously. The mechanism by which spontaneous rupture of membranes increases the risk of subarachnoid hemorrhage remains obscure. One possibility was that women who rupture their membranes spontaneously expose their infants to a greater risk of subarachnoid hemorrhage via head trauma than do women whose membranes were cut by medical personnel to initiate or augment labor. Additional support for the 'trauma' hypothesis is that primigravidas were at greater risk of delivering a child with subarachnoid hemorrhage than were multigravidas who did not experience any late fetal wastage. This birth order effect likely conveys information about mechanisms other than trauma.

The second umbrella term emphasized in Leviton's scheme is intrapartum hypertension. Not only is intrapartum hypertension a risk factor in its own right, but also it is closely associated with three other risk factors: maternal gonococcal infection, clinic status, and previous fetal death after the twentieth week. How intrapartum hypertension is associated with an increased risk of subarachnoid hemorrhage is obscure. The possibility exists that a substance (either endogenous or exogenous) related to maternal hypertension crosses the placenta and in some way influences leptomeningeal vascular integrity.

The third umbrella term evokes the effects of an unfavorable uterine environment. Six risk factors of subarachnoid hemorrhage appeared to convey information about maternal characteristics that adversely affected the developing fetal brain. These were maternal gonococcal infection, late age at menarche, intrapartum hypertension, clinic status, blood type O (associated with low birthweight of last prior offspring), and prior fetal death.

Intracerebral parenchymal hemorrhage

CEREBRUM EXTERNAL TO GERMINAL SUBVENTRICULAR ZONE

Neonatal cerebral hemisphere hematomas are rare and, if present, suggest mechanical trauma (for instance, skull fracture), embolic infarct, venous infarct, arteriovenous malformation, or disseminated intravascular coagulopathy. Leech et al[77] found intracerebral and intracerebellar hemorrhages in 9% of 179 consecutive autopsies of preterm infants dying of respiratory distress syndrome (Fig. 14.4), and in a study by Craig, the figure was 5%.[8] Parenchymal hematomas sometimes rupture into a nearby ventricle to give intraventricular hemorrhage,[32] but are unlikely to have ruptured from a ventricle into the brain. They may be large, small, single, or multiple. Parenchymal hemorrhage did not cluster with any other brain abnormality,[78] but was associated with vaginal birth in another study.[79]

Infants who develop a parenchymal hematoma are usually unnaturally quiet and inactive. They sometimes have limb twitching, and occasionally vomit and lose weight.[8] Should the hemorrhage be limited to one hemisphere and interrupt the corticospinal system, hemiplegia with all its characteristics results.

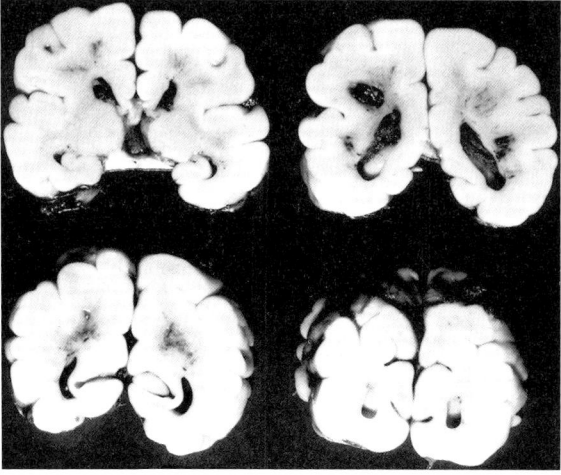

Fig. 14.4 Multiple small parenchymal petechiae and three small hematomas in posterior frontal and parietal white matter.

Subpial hemorrhage

Friede[80] brought subpial hemorrhages to our attention in 1972. They are distinct from parenchymal and subarachnoid hemorrhages, although they sometimes contribute to the latter. These small subpial glial hemorrhages or hematomas spread under the pia and are prevalent over temporal and parietal lobes and the cerebellum. Whether they are the same as small superficial hemorrhages seen in magnetic resonance images is not yet clear.[81] Rarely, small subpial arteriovenous malformations contribute to hemorrhage in this location.[82]

Cerebellar parenchymal hemorrhage

Some amount of intracerebellar hemorrhage was found in 21% of 157 newborn brains at autopsy.[83] In a review of 144 autopsied preterm neonates, cerebellar parenchymal hemorrhages were found in 16% of infants between 20 and 24 weeks' gestation, 6 of 26 (25%) infants between 26 and 28 weeks' gestation, and 2 of 24 (8%) infants between 28 and 30 weeks' gestation.[84] No preterm neonate after 32 weeks' gestation had cerebellar hemorrhage. Focal cerebellar microscopic hemorrhages sometimes coalesce and form hematomas within folia. When these resolve, small cysts sometimes remain. Clinically, large intracerebellar hemorrhages destroying at least one-third of cerebellar folia were associated with progressive loss of breathing together with a falling hematocrit.[83] Cerebellar parenchymal hemorrhages are associated with hemorrhages elsewhere in the brain.[85]

Germinal matrix hemorrhage

A frequent complication of preterm birth is bleeding into the germinal matrix with rupture into the lateral ventricle. The hemorrhages occur in the first postnatal week.[86] The main germinal mass lies anteriorly over the caudate head (see Chapters 4 and 8), rostral to the interventricular foramen. The terminal vein turns medially to become the internal cerebral vein in the posterior interventricular foramen surface. Within germinal tissue, hemorrhages are usually petechial and multiple and are located in the germinal matrix over the caudate or anywhere along the ventricular wall where there is substantial germinal matrix (Figs. 14.5 and 14.6). The hemorrhages over the caudate frequently enlarge and coalesce or rupture into the ventricle and not into the caudate, white matter, or thalamus. Multiple capillaries (or sinusoids) contain perivascular hemorrhages, yet no matter how massive the hemorrhage in one germinal matrix region, not all germinal matrix vessels bleed. Fibrinolytic activity of germinal tissue ensures continued hemorrhage once bleeding has begun.[87] The hemorrhages usually occur in the lateral ganglionic eminence.[88] Intraventricular bleeding from this location was increasingly recognized as important early in the twentieth century (Fig. 14.7),[14,89,90] even though this was not acknowledged by some concurrent pathologists,[91] and the NCPP material confirmed an association with intraventricular and basilar leptomeningeal hemorrhage, but not with convexity hemorrhage, as expected. Ylppö[89,90] noted that subependymal (i.e., germinal matrix) hemorrhage with intraventricular bleeding occurred almost exclusively in preterm infants; this was confirmed by many subsequent authors. In 78 autopsied infants who had red cells tagged with chromium during life, bleeding occurred earlier than 24 hours after birth in 16% and between 15 and 48 hours after birth in 60%.[92] Two significant hemorrhages, differing in time by more than 12 hours, were found in 16%. Although some pathologists maintain

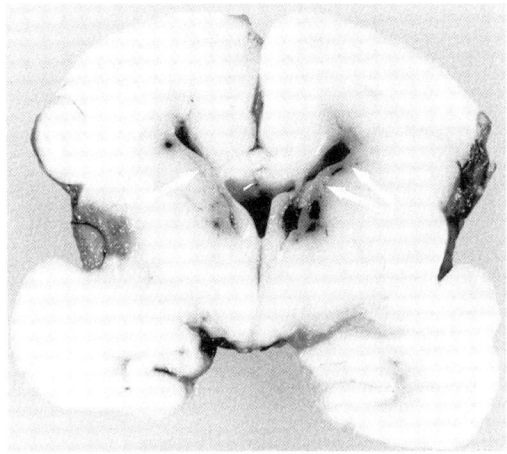

Fig. 14.5 Small germinal matrix hemorrhages (black) have been dissected between the caudate (under the arrow tips) and the germinal matrix layer (arrow tips) in this late second-trimester fetus. On the left side, two petechiae lie in the same location between the caudate and germinal matrix. There is a large cavum septi pellucidi in the midline, a normal event.

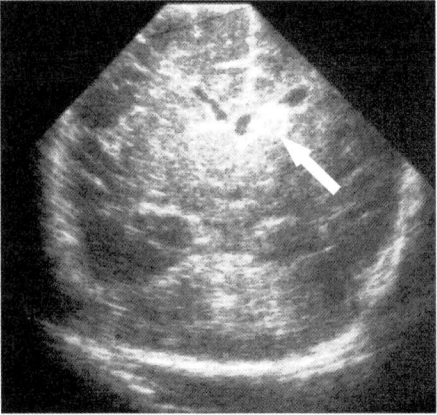

Fig. 14.6 Cranial ultrasound, coronal image, end of second trimester. There is a germinal matrix echogenic hemorrhage on the left (arrow).

that ganglionic eminence hemorrhages are rarely seen in stillborns,[93] others have found a high incidence of matrix hemorrhage in stillborns of less than 8 months' gestation.[94] This stillborn finding supports our hypothesis that prenatal factors contribute to germinal matrix hemorrhage before the onset of normal labor.

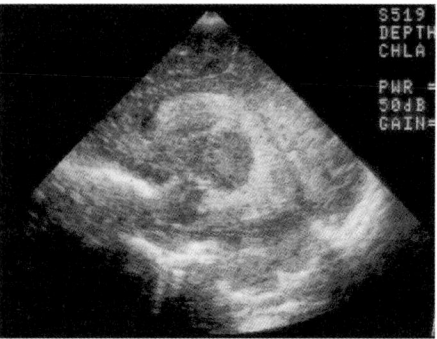

Fig. 14.7 Cranial ultrasound, sagittal view, 29 weeks. Germinal matrix hemorrhage has ruptured into the lateral ventricle and is reflected in echogenic blood filling the entire lateral ventricle.

HYPOTHESES

Currently there are eight hypotheses purporting to account for germinal matrix hemorrhage: (1) venous rupture; (2) terminal vein thrombosis with venous infarction; (3) transverse sub-ependymal caudate vein rupture; (4) immature germinal vessels or delayed vascular differentiation; (5) immature vessel–glia interaction; (6) arterial origin; (7) fibrinolytic properties of germinal tissue; and (8) polyfactorial origin.

Venous rupture

As noted, germinal matrix hemorrhages are petechial or perivascular adjacent to capillaries or sinusoids, with no particular reference to veins or arteries. There is a set of future sub-ependymal veins lying between the germinal and caudate tissue, which eventually drains into the striothalamic (or terminal) vein, but the germinal matrix vascular structures are either endothelial capillaries or sinusoids without vessel wall differentiation. Some have called these vessels veins, without identifying the veins lying between germinal matrix and caudate.[95] Rupture of terminal vein or its tributaries is rare or nonexistent.[93,96,97]

Terminal vein thrombosis with venous infarction

Thrombi in terminal veins or veins of Galen with subsequent hemorrhagic infarction of germinal matrix has been postulated,[98] yet these thrombi have been rarely found. Some have argued that the distribution of deep parenchymal hemorrhages in conjunction with germinal matrix hemorrhages supports venous infarction, but failed to demonstrate thrombosed veins.[99] Isolated cases of internal cerebral venous thrombosis occur with coagulation abnormalities.[100]

Transverse subependymal caudate vein rupture

Alkaline phosphatase staining of cerebral vessel endothelial cells is generally thought to mirror the blood–brain barrier. Alkaline phosphatase endothelial staining (also thought to indicate the afferent circulatory side) appears in some human germinal tissue vessels as early as 23 weeks and was used to separate arterioles from veins.[97,101] These investigators concluded that veins

338

were vulnerable and could rupture, giving rise to germinal matrix hemorrhage. Precapillary arteriovenous shunts (requiring alkaline phosphatase separation of arterioles from veins) were not a major influence on cerebral blood flow in infants born at 23 weeks and were present in one infant at 24 weeks, but not in 34 others.[102] Some earlier studies infrequently implicated the terminal vein or its branches in germinal matrix hemorrhage.[88]

Immature germinal vessels or delayed vascular differentiation
In 2004, Ballabh and colleagues[103] advanced the hypothesis that as three cellular elements of brain microvasculature compose the blood–brain barrier (endothelial cells, astrocyte end feet, and pericytes), germinal matrix vascular leakage of blood is related to immature tight junctions between endothelial cells or immaturity of astrocytic end feet that seem to maintain the tight junction barrier. Later, they quantitatively demonstrated that microvessel density and the percentage of blood vessel area were largest in the germinal matrix, followed by the cortex, and then white matter. Finally, they showed that the proportion of blood vessel surface covered by astrocytic end feet remained constant from 23 to 40 weeks and did not differ significantly by location.[104] There are many contributory pathogenetic factors but germinal matrix structure itself is considered significant. It contains numerous thin-walled vessels in a cellular matrix, which exhibits little fibrillary background. Early immunoreactivity was due to tanycyte fibers, and subsequently there was progressive development of a glial fiber network. The increase in glial fibers (possibly arising from tanycytes) is likely to increase capillary stabilization and contribute to the inverse relationship between gestational age and risk of intracerebral hemorrhage.[105]

Immature vessel–glia interaction (lack of astrocytic feet to support vessels)
The germinal matrix is composed of a mass of immature cells containing many thin-walled blood vessels. A major proposed factor in the occurrence of hemorrhage at this site is the absence of a fibrillary network supporting these vessels,[104–106] but some do not support this hypothesis (see above).[107] Development of such a network is not uniform and the more posterior germinal layer, lying over caudate body and tail, demonstrates more rapid maturation than that lying anteriorly, near the caudate head. Even at 35 weeks of gestation, an anterior central core of germinal layer cells remains immature with little evidence of glial differentiation.[106]

Arterial origin
The claim has been made that differently colored barium gelatin solutions injected into either carotid arteries or jugular veins allowed filling of only the arteries with one dye and the capillaries and veins with another.[93] When ganglionic matrix hemorrhages were dissected under the stereomicroscope, and serial and step sections were examined, extensive capillary bed rupture was visualized. These investigators think that germinal matrix hemorrhages are often catastrophic because increased germinal layer fibrinolytic activity in preterm infants allows hemorrhage propagation, after increased arterial blood pressure has initiated bleeding. Others opined that sudden large fluctuations in arterial blood pressure caused parenchymal hemorrhages.[14,93,108] Uterine contractions during parturition increase fetal blood pressure.[109]

Still others maintain that a low cerebral blood flow is associated with intraventricular hemorrhage.[110, 111]

Fibrinolytic properties of germinal matrix
The fibrinolytic properties of germinal tissue were reviewed in Chapter 3. Nevertheless, these studies do not answer the question of why only some capillaries or sinusoids hemorrhage, but only that they ensure continuation of bleeding once started.

Polyfactorial origin
The pathogenesis of intraventricular hemorrhages is related to intravascular, vascular, and extravascular factors. Intravascular factors primarily include control of blood flow and pressure in germinal matrix microcirculation. Particular pathogenetic importance is attached to fluctuations in cerebral blood flow; abrupt increases or decreases in flow with injury to matrix vessels; increases in cerebral venous pressure; and, in selected infants, disturbances of platelet function and coagulation. Vascular factors relate to the matrix microcirculation at the initial bleeding site; a maturation-dependent alteration in vascular integrity and a vulnerability of matrix vessels to ischemic injury also appear important. Extravascular factors include mesenchymal and glial support for matrix vessels and local germinal matrix fibrinolytic activity.[112]

Risk factors
Leviton et al[113] identified several risk factors in a multivariate analysis of germinal matrix hemorrhage in the NCPP population. The factors with the highest relative risk were 'rupture of membranes as an indication for uterine stimulation' and 'metabolic and endocrine disorders other than diabetes.' Four variables conveyed at-risk information: low gestational age; female sex; mothers with a late menarche; or mothers who gained less than one pound during the entire pregnancy. Thus, gestational age-related factors were of importance in the etiology of germinal matrix hemorrhage. It is most likely that exogenous and endogenous factors play a role in this problem. Recently, investigators developed a scoring system, based on the degree of physiologic instability in the first few postnatal hours, that predicts intraventricular hemorrhage and subsequent neurodevelopmental dysfunction.[5]

Intraventricular hemorrhage
Neonatal intraventricular hemorrhage (Fig. 14.8) arises from hemorrhage elsewhere in cerebrum with rupture into the ventricle from the parenchyma, ganglionic eminence, or choroid plexus. Hemorrhagic cerebrospinal fluid flows through the third ventricle, aqueduct, and fourth ventricle exiting through midline and lateral foramina into the perimedullary leptomeninges and covers the cerebellar undersurface, but not the dorsal subtentorial surfaces, usually stopping abruptly, approximately on the inferior cerebellar surface or along the horizontal fissure (Fig. 14.9). It fills the perimedullary and prepontine cisterns, as well as the perimesencephalic cisterns and interpeduncular fossa. At this point, it flows either through perimesencephalic cisterns (cisterna ambiens) to reach the supratentorial compartment or through the basal diencephalic cistern, around mammillary bodies, hypophyseal stalk, and the chiasm to enter the lateral sulci (Sylvian fissures), eventually arriving at the convexity. The blood from the

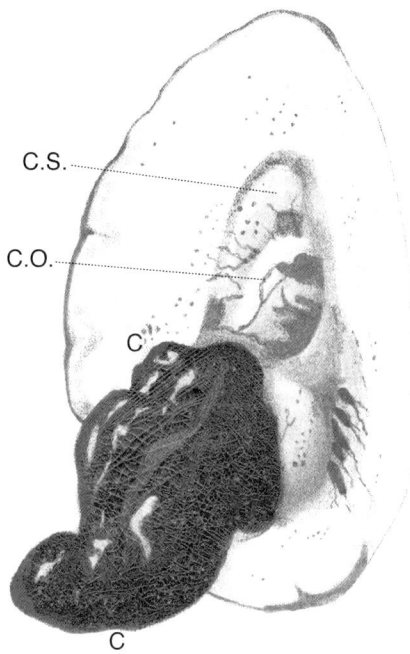

C.S.

C.O.

C'

C

C

Fig. 14.8 Cruveilhier's depiction of a left lateral intraventricular hemorrhage (C–C) in a fetus. Anterior is up. There are several small hemorrhages in the caudate (C.S.), as well as intraventricular hemorrhage overlying the thalamus (C.O.). In this lithograph from the atlas of 1828–35, colors were applied by hand and small paint cracks have appeared in this large intraventricular hemorrhage. The lateral ventricle is markedly dilated. From Cruveilhier.[20]

perimesencephalic cisterns flows up into subarachnoid space within the interhemispheric fissure and then over either hemisphere. Even in fetal brains with intraventricular hemorrhage, leptomeningeal blood in other distinct anatomic locations is usually from separate subpial or parenchymal origins. Absorption of extensive leptomeningeal hemorrhage is a poorly understood subject and will not be dealt with here.

When postintraventricular hemorrhage ventriculomegaly follows, it results from either cerebrospinal fluid flow obstruction or still unknown factors causing white matter loss.

HISTOLOGIC CHANGES IN LATERAL VENTRICLE WALL FOLLOWING
INTRAVENTRICULAR HEMORRHAGE

Preterm fetuses need a different set of histologic criteria for intermediate and late stages of organization following hemorrhage than those used in the adult.[114] Four days after intraventricular hemorrhage, mononuclear phagocytes around the hemorrhage evolve to become iron-containing macrophages. Astrocytic proliferation is delayed to about 11 days along with ependymal disruption and only scanty glial fibril production.[86] At sites of ependymal disruption, glial cells proliferate and extend into the ventricle as small nodules. Ventricular

341

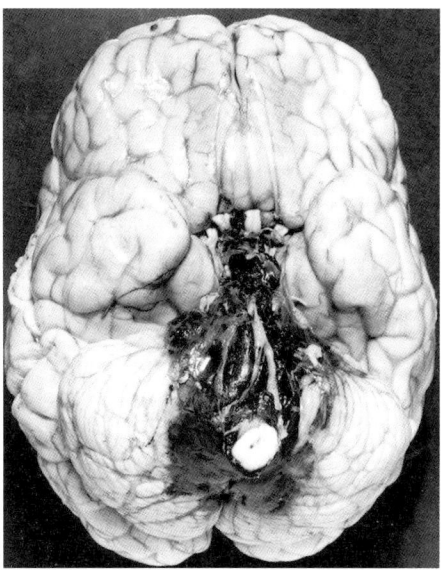

Fig. 14.9 In this term fetus, a large intraventricular hemorrhage has emerged from the fourth ventricle through the midline and lateral apertures and flows in the subarachnoid space into the prepontine, perimesencephalic, and perichiasmatic cisterns. Note that the blood flows only a short distance on the inferior cerebellar undersurface, a cerebrospinal flow distribution identified by Key and Retzius in 1875.

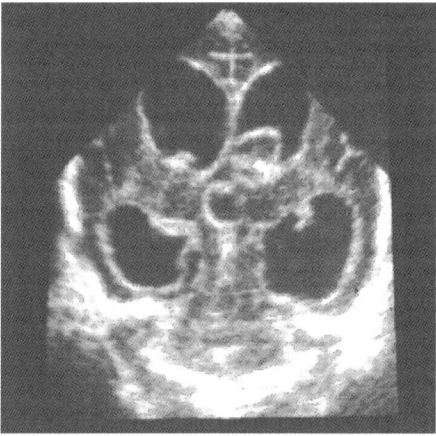

Fig. 14.10 Cranial ultrasound 2 weeks after intraventricular hemorrhage. Red cell debris lines the dilated ventricles, resulting in the prominent echogenic band throughout all ventricular walls.

wall echogenicity develops about 7 days after the intraventricular hemorrhage and usually disappears in about 6 weeks (Fig. 14.10).[115] Some attribute the echogenicity to the proliferated astrocytic layer, but we are more inclined to consider the macrophage and glial hemosiderin as responsible.

Conclusion

Intracranial hemorrhages occur in the late gestational fetus, during delivery or shortly after birth. While the proclivity of infants with hemorrhage in one nervous system region is to have a hemorrhage in another region, the risk factors of hemorrhage in one region are likely to differ from those of another region. We have reviewed the underlying anatomy of the regions that are susceptible to hemorrhage in the hope of understanding why hemorrhage occurs in each location; however, as there are essentially no epidemiologic studies (except for subarachnoid hemorrhage) of hemorrhages and location, we continue to work without a clear understanding of risk factors for many of these hemorrhages.

Fetal intracranial hemorrhages occur in several locations. They are not associated with hemiplegia or paraplegia unless in an anatomically appropriate location. For instance, ganglionic eminence hemorrhage occurs at a time when this mass of germinal cells is being depleted, long after the great neuronal and glial migrations from the ventricular wall; thus, hemorrhage in this location cannot be expected to be associated with any neurologic deficits. Deep parenchymal hemorrhages, on the other hand, can interrupt the posterior limb of the internal capsule and cause hemiplegia. Posthemorrhagic paraplegia is a different story. Unless ventricles dilate excessively and interrupt both posterior limb radiations, they usually do not cause paraplegia (see Chapter 15). Paraplegia following intracranial hemorrhage is more likely to be the result of a cervical cord or lower brainstem lesion during delivery.

One concept, 'periventricular hemorrhage,' we find confusing and misleading as it groups deep parenchymal hemorrhages together with germinal matrix hemorrhage. Each of these entities should be kept separate until we have more knowledge of their risk factors.

REFERENCES

1. Caulfield E (1928) A full view of all the diseases, incident to children. *Ann Med History* 10: 409.
2. Courant F (1804) *Dissertation sur l'apoplexie de l'enfant nouveau-né*. Paris.
3. Denis P (1826) *Recherches d'anatomie et de physiologie pathologiques sur plusier maladies des enfants nouveau-nés*. Commercy: CF Denis.
4. Schwartz P (1961) *Birth Injuries of the Newborn, Morphology, Pathogenesis, Clinical Pathology and Prevention*. New York: Hafner Publishing.
5. Dammann O, Naples M, Bednarek F, et al (2010) SNAP-II and SNAPPE-II and the risk of structural and functional brain disorders in extremely low gestational age newborns: the ELGAN study. *Neonatology* 97: 71–82.
6. Gröntoft O (1953) Intracerebral and meningeal haemorrhages in perinatally deceased infants. II Meningeal hemorrhages. A pathologico-anatomical and obstetric study. *Acta Obstet Gynecol Scand* 32: 458–498.
7. Hemsath FA, Canavan MM (1932) Microscopic cerebral hemorrhage in stillbirths and newborn deaths. A study of fifty-three infants with relation to minute hemorrhages of the medulla oblongata. *Am J Obstet Gynecol* 23: 471–478.
8. Craig WS (1938) Intracranial hemorrhage in the newborn. A study of diagnosis and differential diagnosis based on pathological and clinical findings in 126 cases. *Arch Dis Child* 13: 89–124.
9. Pape KE, Wigglesworth JS (1979) *Haemorrhage, Ischemia and the Perinatal Brain*. London: Heinemann.
10. Chessells JM, Wigglesworth JS (1970) Secondary haemorrhagic disease of the newborn. *Arch Dis Child* 45: 539–543.
11. Margolis CZ, Orzalesi MM, Schwartz AD (1973) Disseminated intravascular coagulation in the respiratory distress syndrome. *Am J Dis Child* 125: 324–326.
12. Sims J (1846) Trismus nascentium. Its pathology and treatment. *Am J Med Sci* 11: 363.
13. Holland EL (1922) Cranial stress in the foetus during labour. *J Obstet Gynaecol Br Empire* 29: 551–571.

14. Rydberg E (1932) Cerebral injury in new-born children consequent on birth trauma. With an inquiry into the normal and pathological anatomy of the neuroglia. *Copenhagen: Acta Path et Microbiol Scand* Suppl. X.

15. Gilles FH, Shillito JS (1970) Infantile hydrocephalus: retrocerebellar subdural hematoma. *J Pediatr* 76: 529–532.

16. Gilles FH (1991) Perinatal neuropathology. In: Davis R, Robertson D, editors. *Textbook of Neuropathology*. Baltimore: Williams & Wilkins, pp. 281–330.

17. Pott R (1911) Über Tentoriumzerreißungen bei der Geburt. *Z Geburtsülfe Gynäkol (Stuttgart)* 69: 674–718.

18. Tubbs RS, Loukas M, Louis RG Jr., et al (2007) Surgical anatomy and landmarks for the basal vein of Rosenthal. *J Neurosurg* 106: 900–902.

19. Mack J, Squier W, Eastman JT (2009) Anatomy and development of the meninges: implications for subdural collections and CSF circulation. *Pediatr Radiol* 39: 200–210.

20. Cruveilhier J (1829–1835) *Anatomie Pathologique du Corps Humain*, Part 2, XVth Liv. Paris: JB Baillière.

21. Weber F (1851–1854) *Beiträge zur pathologischen Anatomie des Neugeborenen*. Kiel: Karl Schroder & Co.

22. Ehrenfest H (1922) *Birth Injuries of the Child*. New York: D. Appleton & Co.

23. Von Haam E (1934) Pathology of intracranial hemorrhage in the newborn child. *Am J Obstet Gynecol* 27: 184–194.

24. Litchfield HR, Given TB (1934) Pathology of intracranial hemorrhage of the new-born. *Arch Pediatr* 51: 186–191.

25. Haller ES, Nesbitt REL, Anderson G (1956) Clinical and pathologic concepts of gross intracranial hemorrhage in perinatal mortality. *Obstet Gynecol Surv* 11: 179–204.

26. Leviton A, Gilles F, Strassfeld R (1977) The influence of route of delivery and hyaline membranes on the risk of neonatal intracranial hemorrhages. *Ann Neurol* 2: 451–454.

27. Friede RL (1989) *Developmental Neuropathology*, 2nd edn. New York: Springer-Verlag.

28. Klintworth GK (1968) The comparative anatomy and phylogeny of the tentorium cerebelli. *Anat Rec* 160: 635–642.

29. Corsellis JAN (1958) Individual variation in the size of the tentorial opening. *J Neurol Neurosurg Psychiatry* 21: 279–283.

30. Osborn AG (1977) The medical tentorium and incisura: normal and pathological anatomy. *Neuroradiology* 13: 109–113.

31. Larroche JC (1977) *Developmental Pathology of the Neonate*. Amsterdam: Excerpta Medica.

32. Hemsath FA (1934) Ventricular cerebral hemorrhage in the newborn infant. *Am J Obstet Gynecol* 28: 343–353.

33. Potter EL, Craig JM (1975) *Pathology of the Fetus and the Infant*, 3rd edn. Chicago: Year Book Medical Publishers.

34. Rothballer AB (1962) Traumatic cerebellar hematoma in the newborn. Case report of operative removal with survival. *J Neurosurg* 19: 913–915.

35. Pape KE, Armstrong DL, Fitzhardinge PM (1976) Central nervous system pathology associated with mask ventilation in the very low birthweight infant: a new etiology for intracerebellar hemorrhages. *Pediatrics* 58: 473–483.

36. Choux M, Grisoli F, Peragut J-C (1975) Extradural hematomas in children. *Childs Brain* 1: 337–347.

37. Heyman R, Heckly A, Magagi J, Pladys P, Hamlat A (2005) Intracranial epidural hematoma in newborn infants: clinical study of 15 cases. *Neurosurgery* 57: 924–929; discussion 9.

38. Choux M, Grisoli F, Peragut JC (1975) Extradural hematomas in children. 104 cases. *Childs Brain* 1: 337–347.

39. Esparza J, Portillo JM, Mateos F, Lamas E (1982) Extradural hemorrhage in the posterior fossa in neonates. *Surg Neurol* 17: 341–343.

40. Haines DE, Harkey HL, al-Mefty O (1993) The 'subdural' space: a new look at an outdated concept. *Neurosurgery* 32: 111–120.

41. Sherwood D (1930) Chronic subdural hematoma in infants. *Am J Dis Child* 39: 980.

42. Peet MM, Kahn EA (1932) Subdural hematoma in infants. *JAMA* 98: 1851.

43. Ingraham FD, Heyl HL (1939) Subdural hematoma in infancy and childhood. *JAMA* 112: 198–204.

44. Ingraham FD, Matson DD (1944) Subdural hematoma in infancy. *J Pediatr* 24: 1–37.

45. McDonald R (1967) Large heads in small children. Notes on the causes of increased head circumference. *Clin Pediatr (Phila)* 6: 47–50.

46. MacDonald JT, Weitz R, Sher PK (1977) Intrauterine chronic subdural hematoma. *Arch Neurol* 34: 777–778.

47. Hayashi T, Hashimoto T, Fukuda S, Ohshima Y, Moritaka K (1987) Neonatal subdural hematoma secondary to birth injury. Clinical analysis of 48 survivors. *Childs Nerv Syst* 3: 23–29.

48. Chamnanvanakij S, Rollins N, Perlman JM (2002) Subdural hematoma in term infants. *Pediatr Neurol* 26: 301–304.

49. Whitby EH, Griffiths PD, Rutter S, et al (2004) Frequency and natural history of subdural haemorrhages in babies and relation to obstetric factors. *Lancet* 363(9412): 846–851.

50. Powers CJ, Fuchs HE, George TM (2007) Chronic subdural hematoma of the neonate: report of two cases and literature review. *Pediatr Neurosurg* 43: 25–28.

51. McNutt S (1885) Apoplexia neonatorum. *Am J Obstet* 18: 73–81.

52. Rosenberg O (1921) Die pachymeningitis hemorrhagica interna im kindesalter. *Ergebn d inn Med u Kinderh* 20: 549–638.

53. Abroms IF, McLennan JE, Mandell F (1977) Acute neonatal subdural hematoma following breech delivery. *Obstet Gynecol Surv* 32: 594–595.

54. Haase R, Kursawe I, Nagel F, Sitka U, Burdach S (2003) Acute subdural hematoma after caesarean section: a case report. *Pediatr Crit Care Med* 4: 246–248.

55. Leech RW, Kohnen P (1974) Subependymal and intraventricular hemorrhages in the newborn. *Am J Pathol* 77: 465–475.

56. Mateos F, Esteban J, Ramos JT, et al (1987) Fetal subdural hematoma: diagnosis in utero. Case report. *Pediatr Neurosci* 13: 125–128.

57. Willis T (1667) *Pathologiae Cerebri et Nervosi Generis Specimen. In quo Agitur de Morbis Convulsivis, et de Scorbuto.* Oxford: Gui Hall.

58. Patridge J (1886) Intracranial hemorrhage in the newborn. *Arch Pediatr* 3: 501.

59. Coblentz RG (1940) Cerebellar subdural hematoma in an infant two weeks old with secondary hydrocephalus. *Surgery* 8: 771.

60. Nelson TY (1960) Acute subdural haematoma in the posterior fossa. *Med J Aust* 2: 792.

61. Schreiber MS (1963) Intraspinal tumours in infancy and childhood. *Med J Aust* 50: 186–190.

62. Norlén G, Granholm L (1964) Infantile hydrocephalus and hematoma in the posterior fossa. *J Neurosurg* 21: 309–310.

63. Pitlyk PJ, Miller RH, Stayura LA (1967) Subdural hematoma of the posterior fossa: report of a case. *Pediatrics* 40: 436–439.

64. Carter LP, Pittman HW (1971) Posterior fossa subdural hematoma of the newborn. Case report. *J Neurosurg* 34: 423–426.

65. Scotti G, Flodmark O, Harwood-Nash DC, Humphries RP (1981) Posterior fossa hemorrhages in the newborn. *J Comput Assist Tomogr* 5: 68–72.

66. French BN, Dublin AB (1977) Infantile chronic subdural hematoma of the posterior fossa diagnosed by computerized tomography. Case report. *J Neurosurg* 47: 949–952.

67. Huang CC, Shen EY (1991) Tentorial subdural hemorrhage in term newborns: ultrasonographic diagnosis and clinical correlates. *Pediatr Neurol* 7: 171–177.

68. Welch K, Strand R (1986) Traumatic parturitional intracranial hemorrhage. *Dev Med Child Neurol* 28: 156–164.

69. Blank NK, Strand R, Gilles FH, Palakshappa A (1978) Posterior fossa subdural hematomas in neonates. *Arch Neurol* 35: 108–111.

70. Serfontein GL, Rom S, Stein S (1980) Posterior fossa subdural hemorrhage in the newborn. *Pediatrics* 65: 40–43.

71. Virchow R (1846) Über das granulirte Ansehen der Wanderungen der Gehirnventrikel. *Allg Z Psychiat Berlin* 3: 242–250.

72. Beneke R (1910) Über tentoriumzerreitzungen bei der geburt, sowie die bedeutung der duraspannung für chronische gehirnerkrankungen. *Münch Med Wschr* 57: 2125.

73. Gruenwald P (1951) Subependymal cerebral hemorrhages in premature infants and its relation to various injurious influences at birth. *Am J Obstet Gynecol* 61: 1285–1292.

74. Dooling EC, Gilles FH (1983) Intracranial hemorrhage: Topography. In: Gilles FH, Leviton A, Dooling EC, editors. *The Developing Human Brain: Growth and Epidemiologic Neuropathology*. Boston: Wright-PSG, pp. 193–203.

75. Vlasiuk VV, Keshelava SD (1986) [Pathomorphology and pathogenesis of leptomeningeal hemorrhages in fetuses and newborn infants]. *Arkh Patol* 48: 36–42.

76. Leviton A, Gilles FH, Dooling EC (1983) The epidemiology of subarachnoid hemorrhage. In: Gilles FH, Leviton A, Dooling EC, editors. *The Developing Human Brain: Growth and Epidemiologic Neuropathology*. Boston: Wright-PSG, pp. 217–226.

77. Leech RW, Olson MI, Alvord EC Jr. (1979) Neuropathologic features of idiopathic respiratory distress syndrome. *Arch Pathol Lab Med* 103: 341–343.

78. Gilles FH, Leviton A, Golden JA, Paneth N, Rudelli RD (1998) Groups of histopathologic abnormalities in brains of very low birthweight infants. *J Neuropathol Exp Neurol* 57: 1026–1034.

79. Looney CB, Smith JK, Merck LH, et al (2007) Intracranial hemorrhage in asymptomatic neonates: prevalence on MR images and relationship to obstetric and neonatal risk factors. *Radiology* 242: 535–541.

80. Friede RL (1972) Subpial hemorrhage in infants. *J Neuropathol Exp Neurol* 31: 548–556.

81. Huang AH, Robertson RL (2004) Spontaneous superficial parenchymal and leptomeningeal hemorrhage in term neonates. *AJNR Am J Neuroradiol* 25: 469–475.

82. Lasjaunias P, Hui F, Zerah M, et al (1995) Cerebral arteriovenous malformations in children. Management of 179 consecutive cases and review of the literature. *Childs Nerv Syst* 11: 66–79; discussion.

83. Martin R, Roessmann U, Fanaroff A (1976) Massive intracerebellar hemorrhage in low-birth-weight infants. *J Pediatr* 89: 290–293.

84. Grunnet ML, Shields WD (1976) Cerebellar hemorrhage in the premature infant. *J Pediatr* 88(4 Pt. 1): 605–608.

85. Gilles FH, Leviton A, Dooling EC (1983) *Developing Human Brain: Growth and Epidemiologic Neuropathology*. Boston: John Wright-PSG Publishing Co.

86. Sherwood A, Hopp A, Smith JF (1978) Cellular reactions to subependymal plate haemorrhage in the human neonate. *Neuropathol Appl Neurobiol* 4: 245–261.

87. Gilles FH, Price RA, Kevy SV, Berenberg W (1971) Fibrinolytic activity in the ganglionic eminence of the premature human brain. *Biol Neonate* 18: 426–432.

88. Ross JJ, Dimmette RM (1965) Subependymal cerebral hemorrhage in infancy. *Am J Dis Child* 110: 531–542.

89. Ylppö A (1919) Pathologisch-anatomische studien bei frühgeborenen. *Zeitschrift für Kinderheilkunde* 19: 212–431.

90. Ylppö A (1924) Origin of hemorrhages in prematures and the newborn. *Zeit Kinderheilk* 38: 32–45.

91. Ballantyne JW (1920) Cerebral ventricular haemorrhages at and soon after birth. *Edinb, Med J* 25: 63–71.

92. Tsiantos A, Victorin L, Relier JP, et al (1974) Intracranial hemorrhage in the prematurely born infant. Timing of clots and evaluation of clinical signs and symptoms. *J Pediatr* 85: 854–859.

93. Hambleton G, Wigglesworth JS (1976) Origin of intraventricular haemorrhage in the preterm infant. *Arch Dis Child* 51: 651–659.

94. Larroche JC (1964) [Intraventricular cerebral hemorrhages in the premature infant. I. Anatomy and physiopathology.]. *Biol Neonat* 7: 26–56.

95. Moody DM, Brown WR, Challa VR, Block SM (1994) Alkaline phosphatase histochemical staining in the study of germinal matrix hemorrhage and brain vascular morphology in a very-low-birth-weight neonate. *Pediatr Res* 35(4 Pt 1): 424–430.

96. Nakamura Y, Okudera T, Fukuda S, Hashimoto T (1990) Germinal matrix hemorrhage of venous origin in preterm neonates. *Hum Pathol* 21: 1059–1062.

97. Ghazi-Birry HS, Brown WR, Moody DM, Challa VR, Block SM, Reboussin DM (1997) Human germinal matrix: venous origin of hemorrhage and vascular characteristics. *AJNR Am J Neuroradiol* 18: 219–229.

98. Towbin A (1968) Cerebral intraventricular hemorrhage and subependymal matrix infarction in the fetus and premature newborn. *Am J Pathol* 52: 121–140.

99. Gould SJ, Howard S, Hope PL, Reynolds EO (1987) Periventricular intraparenchymal cerebral haemorrhage in preterm infants: the role of venous infarction. *J Pathol* 151: 197–202.

100. Friese S, Muller-Hansen I, Schoning M, Nowak-Gottl U, Kuker W (2003) Isolated internal cerebral venous thrombosis in a neonate with increased lipoprotein (a) level: diagnostic and therapeutic considerations. *Neuropediatrics* 34: 36–39.

346

101. Anstrom JA, Brown WR, Moody DM, Thore CR, Challa VR, Block SM (2004) Subependymal veins in premature neonates: implications for hemorrhage. *Pediatr Neurol* 30: 46–53.
102. Anstrom JA, Brown WR, Moody DM, Thore CR, Challa VR, Block SM (2002) Anatomical analysis of the developing cerebral vasculature in premature neonates: absence of precapillary arteriole-to-venous shunts. *Pediatr Res* 52: 554–560.
103. Ballabh P, Braun A, Nedergaard M (2004) Anatomic analysis of blood vessels in germinal matrix, cerebral cortex, and white matter in developing infants. *Pediatr Res* 56: 117–124.
104. El-Khoury N, Braun A, Hu F, et al (2006) Astrocyte end-feet in germinal matrix, cerebral cortex, and white matter in developing infants. *Pediatr Res* 59: 673–679.
105. Gould SJ, Howard S (1987) An immunohistochemical study of the germinal layer in the late gestation human fetal brain. *Neuropathol Appl Neurobiol* 13: 421–437.
106. Gould SJ, Howard S (1988) Glial differentiation in the germinal layer of fetal and preterm infant brain: an immunocytochemical study. *Pediatr Pathol* 8: 25–36.
107. Bass T, Singer G, Slusser J, Liuzzi FJ (1992) Radial glial interaction with cerebral germinal matrix capillaries in the fetal baboon. *Exp Neurol* 118: 126–132.
108. Lou HC, Lassen NA, Friis-Hansen B (1979) Is arterial hypertension crucial for the development of cerebral haemorrhage in premature infants? *Lancet* 1(8128): 1215–1217.
109. Oh W, Lind J, Gessner IH (1966) The circulatory and respiratory adaptation to early and late cord clamping in newborn infants. *Acta Paediatr Scand* 55: 17–25.
110. Ment LR, Duncan CC, Ehrenkranz RA, et al (1984) Intraventricular hemorrhage in the preterm neonate: timing and cerebral blood flow changes. *J Pediatr* 104: 419–425.
111. Meek JH, Tyszczuk L, Elwell CE, Wyatt JS (1999) Low cerebral blood flow is a risk factor for severe intraventricular haemorrhage. *Arch Dis Child Fetal Neonatal Ed* 81: F15–F18.
112. Volpe JJ (1989) Intraventricular hemorrhage in the premature infant—current concepts. Part I. *Ann Neurol* 25: 3–11.
113. Leviton A, Gilles FH, Dooling EC (1983) The epidemiology of ganglionic eminence hemorrhage. In: Gilles FH, Leviton A, Dooling EC, editors. *The Developing Human Brain: Growth and Epidemiologic Neuropathology*. Boston: Wright-PSG, pp. 204–216.
114. Darrow VC, Alvord EC Jr., Mack LA, Hodson WA (1988) Histologic evolution of the reactions to hemorrhage in the premature human infant's brain. A combined ultrasound and autopsy study and a comparison with the reaction in adults. *Am J Pathol* 130: 44–58.
115. Gaisie G, Roberts MS, Bouldin TW, Scatliff JH (1990) The echogenic ependymal wall in intraventricular hemorrhage: sonographic–pathologic correlation. *Pediatr Radiol* 20: 297–300.

15
VENTRICULOMEGALY, LARGE HEAD, MEGALENCEPHALY, AND HYDROCEPHALUS

Introduction

In this chapter, we consider ventriculomegaly without head enlargement, large head, mega-lencephaly, and hydrocephalus. Ventriculomegaly is ventricular enlargement beyond that expected for the child's age, whether or not the head is also enlarged. The head is necessarily enlarged in hydrocephalus. The prevalences of ventriculomegaly without head enlargement and large heads with or without megencephalic brains are unknown. Hydrocephalus occurs in 0.4 to 0.8 per 1000 liveborns and stillbirths, with X-linked hydrocephalus constituting approximately 5% of cases.[1] Normal embryonic and early fetal ventricular development is discussed along with fetal ventriculomegaly in Chapter 3.

Ventriculomegaly secondary to white matter or neuronal loss with normal or small head size

WHITE MATTER HYPOPLASIA

Ventriculomegaly accompanying white matter paucity with relatively normal gray matter was recognized a century later than patients with normal or small head circumferences and ventriculomegaly accompanying gray and white matter damage and loss.[2] McClelland[3] demonstrated this in the case of a child who died at the age of 11 months with ventriculomegaly and a 'normal' cortex, basal ganglia, and thalami with 'hydromicrocephaly.' This is probably the first case of white matter hypoplasia.

VENTRICULOMEGALY SECONDARY TO LOSS OF NEURONAL TISSUE

Ventricular regions will dilate locally if adjacent neural tissue is lost (see Fig. 13.36). For instance, fetal and neonatal thalami are frequently damaged (see Chapter 13), leaving residual thalamic atrophy with a widened adjacent third ventricle. With regional cortical or cortical and white matter damage (as in middle cerebral artery infarct), there is an attendant loss of axons, and appropriate ventricular regions dilate. Symmetric striatal atrophy (for instance, Huntington disease) is associated with bilateral local rostral frontal horn enlargement, or, if it is asymmetric (for instance, a lateral striate artery infarct), the resulting ventricular dilatation is asymmetric. The same simple rules apply to the third ventricular enlargement without

348

lateral ventricular enlargement accompanying thalamic atrophy (the specific third ventricular enlargement following thalamic mass loss in Morquio disease).

FETAL AND NEONATAL VENTRICULOMEGALY ASSOCIATED WITH WHITE
MATTER FOCAL NECROSES

Newborns frequently have focal necroses in white matter (see Chapter 12). Included in these necrotic zones are axons and oligodendrocytes or glial cells destined to become oligodendrocytes. Widespread destruction of these components in a fetal or term brain results in a diminished bulk of cerebral white matter and ventriculomegaly,[4-10] but the subsequent paucity of white matter in living children who had focal necroses is sometimes considerably greater than would be expected, leading to the speculation that there is, in addition, more widely spread white matter damage.

The very-low-birthweight infant with ventriculomegaly unassociated with hemorrhage often has histologic evidence of white matter damage.[4,11-14] Some children (especially those born preterm) with motor impairment have scans with or without evidence of earlier focal necroses (including paucity of white matter and corpus callosum thinning).[15-20] Infants who died a few weeks after the first ultrasonographic expression of focal necroses have evidence of 'markedly depressed rates of white-matter growth'.[21]

Ventriculomegaly also occurs in neonates who sustained intraventricular hemorrhage (IVH). Many preterm infants who develop ventriculomegaly do so with or after IVH.[22] The assumption is that the hemorrhage and its consequences diminish the ability of arachnoid granulations to absorb cerebrospinal fluid. The resulting increased cerebrospinal fluid pressure causes ventricular enlargement. However, newborn ventriculomegaly is not necessarily associated with increased intraventricular pressure.[23] A period of 'clinically asymptomatic ventricular dilation',[24] which sometimes lasts several weeks, occurs in 35% of very-low-birthweight infants who sustain IVH.[25] In 65% of these infants, the progression arrests spontaneously, but sometimes the lateral ventricles do not return to a normal size. Fetal and early life ventriculomegaly need not be due to posthemorrhagic hydrocephalus, even in infants who sustained IVH.

OUTCOME OF FETAL VENTRICULOMEGALY

Hypoplastic white matter, of necessity, leads to ventriculomegaly. Sonographically enlarged fetal ventricles (>95th centile) are associated with chromosomal and other ultrasonic defects.[26-28] In the fetus, ventriculomegaly beyond normal fetal ventriculomegaly (see Chapter 3) is important and conveys prognostic information. Very-low-birthweight infants who develop ventriculomegaly (whether or not associated with intracranial hemorrhage) during the first postnatal week of age are at an increased risk of motor and other disabilities.

Large head

A neonatal term infant's head is 33 to 35.5cm in circumference. During the first year it grows about 10cm, and from 1 to 5 years it grows at a rate of about 1.25cm per year.[29] A larger or smaller growth rate implies a bony cranial or intracranial cerebral abnormality. Healthy preterm infants' head growth is more rapid than that of term infants, and sick preterm infants' heads grow much more slowly.[30,31]

Megalencephaly, hydrocephalus, microencephaly with large chronic subdural hematomas (subdural hygromas or empyema), and hydrencephaly sometimes occur with large heads. In a young child, a large head and a large brain sometimes follows intoxication from lead, vitamin A, or tetracycline, an endocrinologic abnormality such as hypoparathyroidism or hypoadreno-corticism, or galactosemia. The cranioskeletal dysplasias are associated with skull thickening.

Chronic Subdural Hematoma in Infants
While chronic supratentorial subdural hematoma in infants (as a cause of large head) was a problem many years ago, it seems much less of a problem at present (see Chapter 14).

Neonatal posterior fossa subdural hematomas
Acute or chronic posterior fossa subdural hematoma potentially causes cerebellar displacement, fourth ventricular outlet occlusion, and hydrocephalus (see Chapter 14).

Megalencephaly
Megalencephaly is an overweight brain that exceeds the mean by more than two standard errors or is above the ninety-fifth centile (for instance, a brain weight over 1600g),[32] or macrocephaly with normal-sized ventricles and subarachnoid space.[33,34] DeMeyer[35] grouped megalencephaly into two types: anatomic and metabolic. Anatomic megalencephaly includes those brains enlarged because of an increased number of cells, an increased size of cells, or both, but without known metabolic abnormality. A metabolic megalencephaly includes those brains enlarged because of an accumulation of a metabolic product.

Anatomic megalencephaly
The most common category consists of normal brains at the upper limits of the normal distribution of brain weight. Some families have abnormally large and heavy brains, as is sometimes found in outstanding individuals, for instance Byron (1807g), Turgenev (2012g), and Bismarck (1790g).[36] However, megalencephaly is usually associated with mental retardation[a] and sometimes other brain abnormalities, and is bilateral or unilateral. Bilateral megalencephalies include those with gigantism (Sotos syndrome, arachnodactyly, Weaver–Smith syndrome), with dwarfism (multiple endocrinopathies, muscular dystrophy, achondroplasia, and thanatophoric dwarfism),[37] neurocutaneous syndromes, or a chromosomal anomaly (Klinefelter syndrome). Other syndromes with megalencephaly include those with broad corpus callosum, excessive white matter, and pachygyria,[38] Cowden disease,[39,40] dwarfism,[41] Apert syndrome,[42,43] familial megalencephaly,[44] ipsilateral linear nevus sebaceous syndrome,[45–47] organoid nevus syndrome,[48] some megalocornea syndromes,[49] FG syndrome,[50] ataxia telangiectasia,[51] Collins–Hashino syndrome,[52,53] megalencephaly with L1 adhesion molecule disorder,[54] and megalencephaly with Donohue syndrome.[41] The pathologic abnormalities in anatomic megalencephaly include gyral abnormalities, neuronal heterotopias, corpus

---

[a]UK usage: learning disability.

350

callosum dysgenesis, neuronal surplus, glial overgrowth, and general enlargement of all cortical layers. Unilateral megalencephalies are associated with somatic hemihypertrophy, such as simple hemimegalencephaly,[55] and Klippel–Trénaunay–Weber and Proteus syndromes.

Metabolic megalencephalies

The metabolic megalencephalies include maple syrup urine disease, leukodystrophies [Canavan disease (spongy brain degeneration, sometimes associated with increased *N*-acetylaspartate),[56] Alexander disease[57] and metachromatic leukodystrophy], lysosomal diseases (Tay–Sachs disease, generalized gangliosidosis, mucopolysaccharidosis), hypoparathyroidism and hypo-adrenocorticoidism,[58–61] some spongiform leukoencephalies, some organic acid disorders, and glutaric aciduria type 1.[62,63]

Hydrocephalus

HISTORY

Occasional cases of hydrocephalic crania date to about 10 000 BC.[64] The Hippocratic writers (Hippocrates ~460–370 BC) were the first to apply the name hydrocephalus to children with large heads.[65,66] There is confusion about whether they referred to fluid collections outside the brain or within the ventricles. Galen (129–200 BC) thought they were subdural, extradural or extracranial in location, and both Albucasis (tenth century), and Sabuncuoglu (fifteenth century) described draining of superficial intracranial fluid.[66–68] Sometimes Sabuncuoglu is given credit for draining the ventricles, but his descriptions sound more like he drained superficial intracranial fluid[69,70] (Fig. 15.1). However, in markedly hydrocephalic heads, the brain

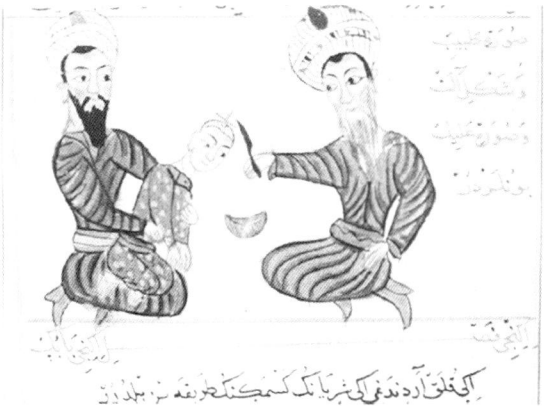

Fig. 15.1 Sabuncuoglu draining the head of a hydrocephalic child into a bowl. Albucasis (tenth century) and Sabuncuoglu (fifteenth century) described draining of superficial intracranial fluid, but whether they drained superficial subdural collections or dilated ventricles is unclear. A color version of this figure is available in the color plate section at the back of the book.

351

convexity is noticeably thinned and surgeons in the middle ages probably did not recognize that the fluid source was within the lateral ventricles.

Galen (~130–200 AD)[71] quoted Erasistratus (c. 310–250 BC) as having described two cerebral lateral ventricles, each with an interventricular foramen into a third ventricle connected with the fourth ventricle. Galen also provided descriptions of ventricular anatomy, cerebrospinal fluid, and the midline fourth ventricular foramen (later redescribed by Magendie in 1825) in animals.[72] The human ventricular system was not depicted until da Vinci drew a dissected human brain in 1510 (Fig. 15.2);[73] however, he did not recognize Magendie's foramen.

Vesalius (1543) observed that in children with large heads the fluid collected within the ventricles rather than external to the brain:

> I observed (a disease) at Augsburg in a two year old girl whose head had grown in seven months, more or less, to such a size that I never saw any man's head which was not surpassed by it in bulk. This disease was what the ancients [sic] called hydrocephalus, from the water which is stored in the head and gradually collects. In this girl's case, however, the water had not collected between the skull and its outer surrounding membrane... but in the cavity of the brain itself, and actually in the right and left ventricles of the brain.[74]

This observation disposed of two millennia of confusion about fluid location in children with hydrocephalus and was confirmed two centuries later in 1769.[75] At the same time, internal and external hydrocephalus were separated.[76]

In 1664, Willis[77] proposed that the choroid plexus produces cerebrospinal fluid. Pacchioni,[78] in contrast, thought that arachnoid granulations were the source of spinal fluid,

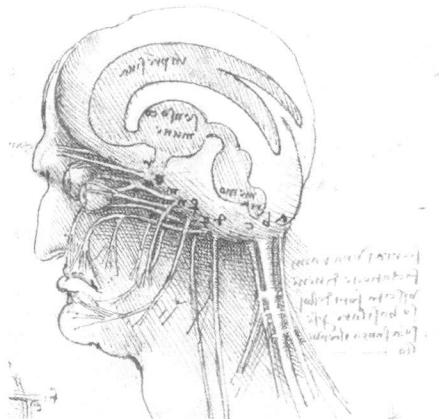

Fig. 15.2 In this drawing from 1510 of the human ventricular system, Leonardo DaVinci he demonstrates the fourth and third ventricles connected with a tube, and from the third ventricle a curious structure, probably depicting two lateral ventricles.

a misconception that Fantoni[66] corrected in 1738. Morgagni (eighteenth century) described cranial enlargement, suture separation, and skull thinning in children with large heads, but he also recognized that ventriculomegaly could occur without head enlargement.[75] He also described one case of hydrocephalus with low-lying cerebellar tonsils and hydromyelia, 120 years before Arnold and Chiari (1894–95).[66] Von Haller first presented the modern idea of cerebrospinal fluid flow and demonstrated the foramina of Luschka (1747).[72,79] Magendie, in 1842, demonstrated the midline foramen at the caudal fourth ventricular end (which Galen had previously described, but Vesalius and Willis overlooked), described the cerebrospinal fluid circulation within the brain as flowing from the brain surface into the ventricular system, and postulated that cerebrospinal flow obstruction causes hydrocephalus.[66] von Luschka, in 1855,[80] redescribed the lateral foramina of exit from the fourth ventricle [see Virchow's depiction of obstructed lateral foramina (see Chapter 10)]. Key and Retzius[81] characterized the meninges, subarachnoid space, and cisterns, ventricles, and arachnoid villi, and documented that the choroid plexus produced spinal fluid that circulated throughout the ventricular system, exited from the fourth ventricle via the midline and lateral foramina, and flowed throughout the subarachnoid space to the cerebral convexity where arachnoidal villi or Pacchionian granulations absorbed it. Dandy and Blackfan[82] blocked the aqueduct in dogs and provided the first animal model of hydrocephalus.

Pacchionian granulation development

In 1705, Pacchioni published his observations on Pacchionian granulation development and later acknowledged Mery, who had published a thesis on these granulations in 1701.[78] Other anatomists, including Vesalius in 1543,[83] had mentioned them. von Luschka[80] pointed out that the granulations were hypertrophied arachnoidal villi normally present in all brains. Key and Retzius[81] considered them passive filters of cerebrospinal fluid into venous channels (Fig. 15.3). Arachnoidal granulations are not visible grossly at birth, but are present as microscopic arachnoidal villi. They first become apparent with a hand lens at 6 months, and at 18 months are grossly visible, appearing first in regions where the parieto-occipital and central veins open into the superior sagittal sinus near the vertex.[84,85] They then spread anteriorly and posteriorly and by the third or fourth year are widely distributed as conspicuous nodules in dural venous channels. More recent investigators have shown that a second pathway exists through the regional lymphatics.[86]

The location of granulations in adults is, in order of number, superior sagittal sinus (including lateral lacunae), transverse, cavernous, and superior petrosal sinuses; middle cerebral vein; sphenoparietal and straight sinuses; and occasionally the torcular Herophili.[81,84] The superior sagittal sinus contains the largest number of granulations per given volume of any sinus. In 3- to 4-year-old children with nonneurologic disease, more than 50 large arachnoidal granulations are present along the superior sagittal sinus.[85] In younger children, arachnoidal granulations are more cellular and less numerous.[87] Under light microscopy, arachnoidal granulations are sagittal sinus or lateral lacuna dural wall invaginations with a core of cellular leptomeningeal tissue and have been demonstrated in an 80mm fetus.[88] Their ultrastructural appearance in adult *Macaca* consists of a core of arachnoidal cells and attenuated collagen bundles, a subendothelial space continuous with the subarachnoid

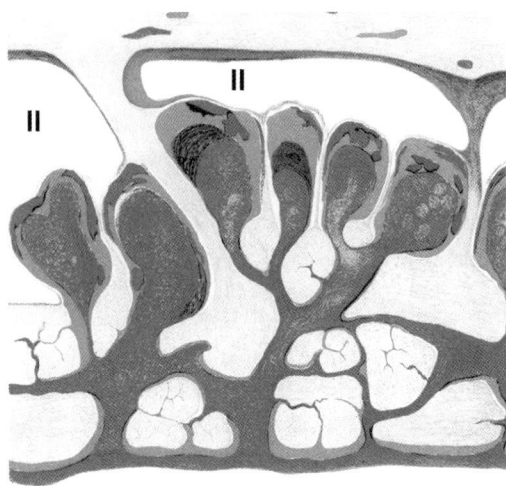

Fig. 15.3 Key and Retzius figure of the arachnoid villi or Pacchonian granulations containing Prussian blue-stained cerebrospinal fluid bulging into the superior sagittal sinus lateral lacuna (ll). Subdural space is red. The iron-containing substance had been injected into the lateral ventricles and freely communicated with the subarachnoid space via the midline and lateral fourth ventricle apertures. They also demonstrated that blue cerebrospinal fluid could be transferred to the intracranial veins. From Key and Retzius.[81] A color version of this figure is available in the color plate section at the back of the book.

space via lacunae between arachnoidal cells, and an endothelial covering continuous with the sinus lining.[89]

Cerebrospinal fluid flow
Cerebrospinal fluid emerges from the fourth ventricle via the midline and lateral apertures into the perimedullary leptomeninges and flows anteriorly to the brainstem to follow a pathway in front of the upper medulla, pons, and midbrain to the interpeduncular fossa. It does not flow over the cerebellar hemisphere under the tentorium. The flow of hemorrhagic cerebrospinal fluid from the fourth ventricle in a preterm neonate or an older child with IVH demonstrates this limitation to the flow of cerebrospinal fluid (see Chapter 14), which had originally been described by Key and Retzius.[81] In 1914, Weed[90] introduced isotonic solutions of iron ammonium citrate and potassium ferrocyanide into the spinal subarachnoid space in dogs and cats and at various intervals sacrificed his specimens, perfusing the carotid vessels with a formalin and acid mixture. The arachnoidal granulations contained precipitated Prussian blue and this work established the basis for the spinal fluid flow concept, which most authors accept; that is, the Pacchionian granulation is a structure necessary for cerebrospinal fluid absorption. There are two pathways from the interpeduncular fossa to the Pacchionian granulations. The first is from the interpeduncular fossa through the perichiasmatic cisterns and laterally past limen insulae, gaining cerebral convexity through the Sylvian fissure (lateral sulcus). The second is through the cisterna ambiens around the midbrain to parasagittal and subtemporal leptomeninges. The Pacchionian granulations remove spinal fluid, depositing it in the sagittal

sinus using either bulk flow or an active secretory process. Alternative pathways of absorption via the orbit or the cranial nerve perineural lymphatics and arachnoid vessels to regional lymphatics exist in some experimental animals.[81,90,91]

Change from a plastic head to a rigid skull during growth

Late fetal and neonatal ventriculomegaly occurs in a very different setting from that in the older child and adult. The neonatal brain is undergoing a large number of growth processes, each of which is differently influenced by ventricular dilatation and which, in turn, differently influence the course of dilatation. As we saw in Chapter 2, the brain attains its greatest growth rate at term and acquires most of its adult weight by the second year. Some embryologic anatomic components are undergoing depletion (such as germinal tissue lining the ventricular wall), some are just beginning to appear (such as the normal layer of subependymal glial fibrils lining the ventricles), and some are undergoing major rearrangements (such as microvascular bed), to name only a few. Most white matter is immature and is a mixture of differentiated and undifferentiated glia, early and mature oligodendroglia, and a few myelinated tracts. Much lateral ventricular ependymal cell layer is mature, but in several regions it is discontinuous (see Chapter 3). The choroid plexus is completing its maturational change from a glycogen-rich organ to a glycogen-poor organ. Finally, the chondrocranium and membranous cranium are far from mature and the sutures are mere connective tissue strips, providing entirely different support and resistance to an expanding brain. Cranial elements respond differently to increasing ventricular and brain size, depending on the state of craniofacial development. In older children and adults whose crania cannot expand in the same way as an infant's, ventricular expansion eventually results in prominent sulcal and gyral impressions on the skull inner table and dorsum sellae erosion including its posterior clinoids.[92] However, in contrast, the fetal and neonatal cranium consists of a firm skull base including the orbital frontal bone. Thus, when the fetal or neonatal lateral ventricles expand as the brain enlarges, the enlargement takes place disproportionately parietally and posteriorly (as fetal and neonatal parietal bone merely floats in connective tissue sutures and is not attached to the skull base) as well as frontally along upper frontal bone (Fig. 15.4). The face partakes very little in skull enlargement, although distorted. The common 'setting sun' sign (Fig. 15.5) is caused by cranial convexity upward displacement away from frontal bone, and, because it is so thin, orbital plate downward displacement, depressing the globes. The eyes are also displaced by a change in orbital direction. Between the two movements, frontal skin is stretched upward pulling upper and lower eyelids over the globe. At any neonatal or early childhood age, rapidly expanding lateral ventricles can separate sutures (Fig. 15.6).

Hydrocephalus: antecedents

Aqueductal Narrowing

Aqueductal size and shape in children
The normal aqueduct changes its embryonic round shape to a slit during late embryonic and fetal growth and decreases its relative size.[93] Some have attributed the slit shape to lateral

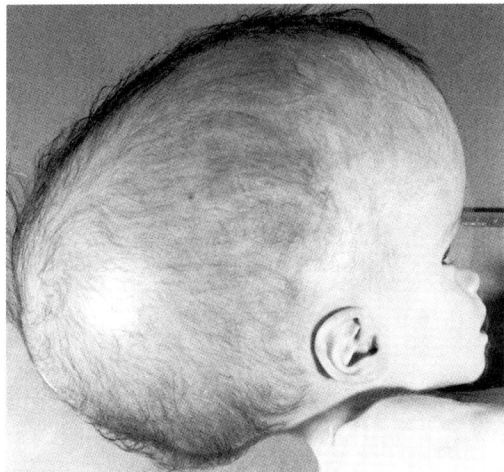

Fig. 15.4 Lateral view of a large hydrocephalic head showing the marked expansion of parietal portions but the relative lack of basal frontal expansion.

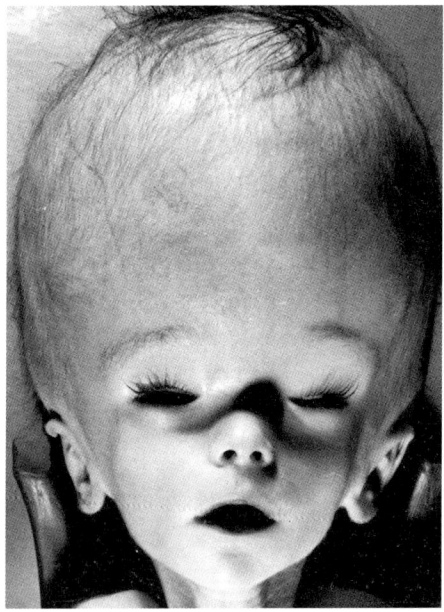

Fig. 15.5 Frontal view of the large head of the same untreated child with hydrocephalus (see Fig. 15.4). The upper eyelids are stretched. The convexity frontal bone has moved up, relative to the cranial base, which is relatively preserved. The ears are relatively low.

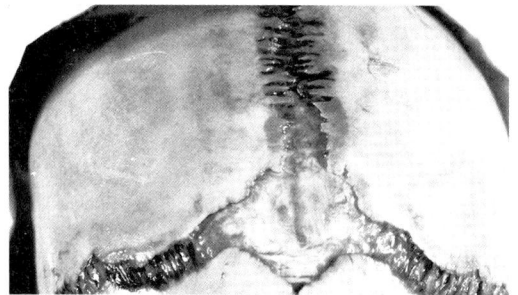

Fig. 15.6 The coronal and sagittal sutures are 'split,' that is they are separated and exhibit recent hemorrhage along the lines of separation.

compression.[94] The normal aqueductal shape varies at different midbrain levels, ranging from a slit or rhomboid to trapezoid. It is normally narrowest subjacent to the superior colliculi and under the intercollicular sulcus. A round-to-oval aqueduct is part of a generalized ventricular enlargement, or reflects local periaqueductal gray matter atrophy.[74,95] The normal aqueduct varies from 0.2mm² to 1.8mm²; in stenotic aqueducts the lumen is reduced below the lower figure somewhere along its length.[96] In midbrain midline, small ependymal rosettes occasionally occur immediately dorsal or ventral to the aqueduct. Although they amount to small tubules, these normal variants are not considered as 'forking' (multiple blind outpouchings without a patent aqueduct).

Other potentially confusing ependyma-lined spaces exist at aqueductal rostral ends. At the midbrain and pons juncture, there is occasionally a ventral slit from the caudal aqueduct, which divides the rostral pontine tegmentum, specifically the nucleus supratrochlearis (normally an unpaired midline reticular nucleus) and the nucleus centralis superior. It often extends deeply enough into the tegmentum to lie between the medial longitudinal fasciculi. Although not rare, it is not associated with other anomalies. Dorsal to the rostral aqueductal end, there is normally a blind pouch in the fetal brain (see Chapter 3), the mesocoelic recess, which is obliterated by birth, and leaves behind several small ependymal rosettes or glial islands in tectal midline, which are not aqueductal 'forks'.[97,98]

Stenosis
Hydrocephalus is associated with a stenotic aqueduct or with an intra-aqueductal glial mass with or without entrapped ependymal islands (Figs. 15.7 and 15.8). At times, the aqueduct seems merely compressed from side to side into a slit oriented in a sagittal direction from the bilateral medial temporal horn ventricular diverticuli (see below).[94,99,100] In other circumstances, a suprapineal recess diverticulum causes tectal distortion and a secondary aqueductal stenosis.[101]

Stenosis: postinfectious
Aqueductal stenosis often follows bacterial or fungal ventriculitis, as expected. Moreover, aqueductal stenosis follows mumps,[102,103] rheovirus, arborvirus, and influenza virus.[102–105]

357

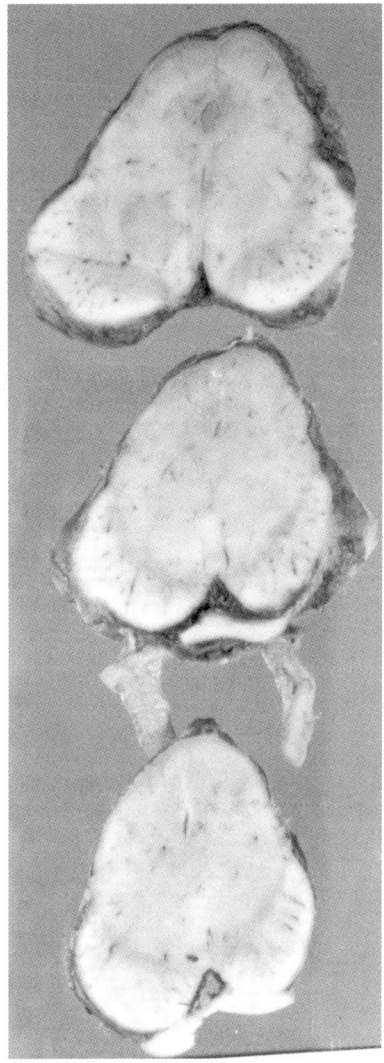

Fig. 15.7 In these three midbrain levels, the aqueduct is closed in the upper two and is slit-like in the lower.

Stenosis: the result of marked ventriculomegaly?

As the lateral ventricles enlarge, for example, from arachnoid or Pacchionian granulation obstruction or an Arnold–Chiari malformation, the thin, medial, enlarging cerebral hemispheres compress the entire midbrain externally, forcing midbrain elongation and aqueduct compression from side to side.[101] Penfield[106] first described pulsion diverticuli of medial trigonal surfaces below the splenium where white matter fiber tracts do not protect the ventricular wall.[107] The diverticuli bulge through the incisura and also symmetrically or asymmetrically

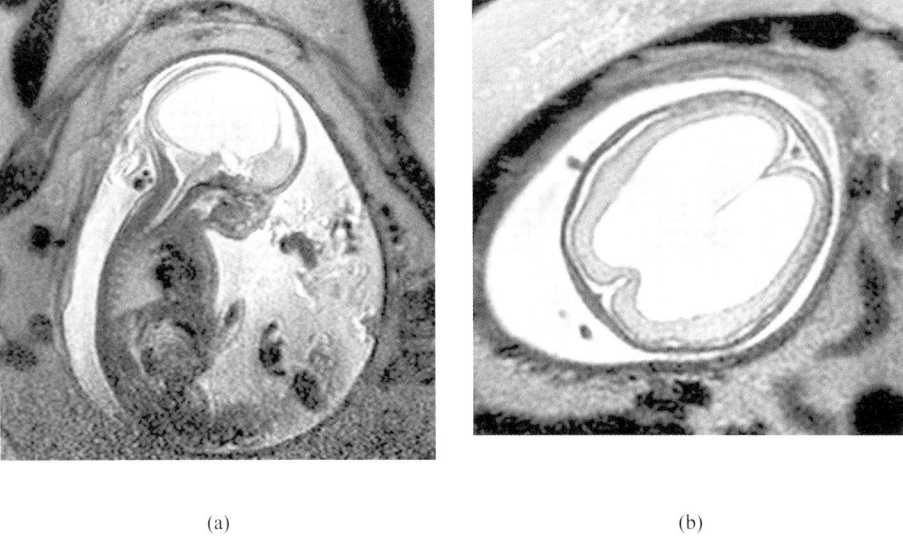

Fig. 15.8 Aqueductal stenosis, fetal MRI at 19 weeks. (a) Sagittal. (b) Axial through cerebral hemisphere. The lateral and third ventricles are markedly enlarged. No aqueduct was identified on any image.

compress the cerebellar anterior lobe and superior surface. The tectal compression seems to occur from the medial temporal lobes herniating and expanding below the great vein of Galen while bulging through the tentorial incisura. Axial tectal compression causes further distortion between the third and fourth ventricles and secondary closure and gliosis.[99] These effects act particularly on the midbrain, and occur even when primary events act at some distance from the aqueduct. They are more important to the infant in whom the skull and dural membranes are easily movable.[94,108]

Forking

Some degree of forking is within the normal range.[108] When forking occurs, the channels usually lie sagittally rather than side by side. Aqueductal forking implies two or more channels of small size inadequate for handling cerebrospinal fluid flow.[109] Aqueductal forks become significant only when all forks end as blind pouches, or when the cerebrospinal fluid channel is so markedly reduced in cross-sectional area as to impair bulk flow.[74]

Septum formation

Posterior third ventricular glial cysts or membranes sometimes occlude cerebrospinal fluid access to the aqueduct (Fig. 15.9). In other cases, a thin glial membrane partially or completely occludes the aqueduct, commonly the caudal end. The source of this membrane is not clear. It is thought to be developmental, the result of granular ependymitis from remote inflammation, or associated with tectal or tegmental vascular malformations.[74,104] Occasionally, glial cysts lying in paraventricular regions enlarge and obstruct spinal flow. In one example, a large pineal

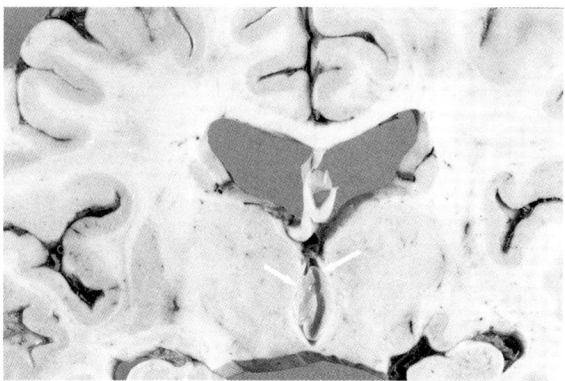

Fig. 15.9 There is a glial cyst wall obstructing the posterior third ventricle between the two thalami (arrows) and the entrance into the aqueduct. The lateral ventricles are moderately enlarged.

glial cyst filled the caudal third ventricle, without obstructing flow into the aqueduct until the child developed generalized cerebral edema secondary to a cardiac arrest. She subsequently developed lateral and rostral third ventricular dilatation.

Gliosis
Aqueductal gliosis follows infection, blood, or other debris within the ventricular system. Islands of ependymal cells always accompany gliosis and there is no lumen with an ependymal lining. The gliosis often extends the length of the aqueduct, unlike the simple glial membrane.

X-linked hydrocephalus
This condition is associated with many cerebral abnormalities in addition to aqueductal stenosis, such as anterior vermian atrophy, flat corpora quadrigemina, small brainstem, corpus callosum aplasia or hypoplasia, and hemispheral white matter hypoplasia.[110,111] The aqueduct is patent in some cases. Ventricular shunting does not improve the neurologic outcome. Gene mutations at Xq28 encoding for L1, a neural cell adhesion molecule, cause this condition.[1,112,113]

Other common antecedents of hydrocephalus
Large lateral ventricles are an integral component of many varieties of malformation: those thought to occur early or late in gestation, both as part of general cerebral malformations and as local rhombencephalic malformations. For instance, the malformations called lissencephaly, holoprosencephaly, Cleland–Arnold–Chiari, Dandy–Walker, many kinds of so-called porencephaly, schizencephaly, agenesis of corpus callosum (complete or partial), and encephaloceles, as well as encephaloclastic processes occurring later in gestation, such as other kinds of pori and hydranencephaly, are sometimes associated with ventriculomegaly or frank hydrocephalus. Many of the former malformations have gyral abnormalities, such as broad, wide gyri (pachygyria); excessive numbers of small gyri containing normally laminated isocortex

(polygyria); or the distinct migration abnormality of micropolygyria, with its abnormality of lamination. The encephaloceles, particularly in the occipital region, seemingly originating in the mesencephalon and the rhombencephalon, are often associated with dilated ventricles, as are those in the frontal ethmoid region.[114,115]

ARNOLD–CHIARI MALFORMATION

While Arnold[116] recognized caudal tongue-like cerebellar protrusions in cases of spina bifida (they had been previously described by Morgagni),[75] Chiari[117,118] presented many cases in great detail and classified them. The classic description includes elongation of the pons, medulla, and fourth ventricle and a caudal cerebellar tongue protruding dorsally far down the cervical spinal cord as well as a caudal choroid plexus tuft (Fig. 15.10). The posterior fossa volume is markedly decreased. The cervical spinal cord is caudally displaced with its rootlets running rostrally toward their foramina. Usually overlooked are small posterior fossa size, abnormality of cerebellar folial arrangement (Fig. 15.11), aqueductal and midbrain malformations or distortions, and multiple malformations elsewhere in the brain, including gyral pattern. The association of these abnormalities with severe spina bifida has been the subject of many manuscripts.

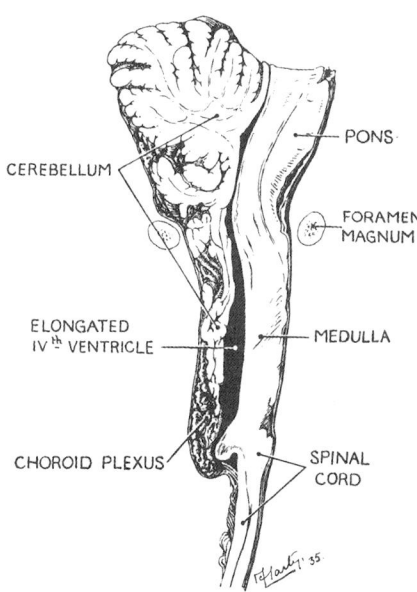

Fig. 15.10 Diagram of Arnold–Chiari malformation in Russell's monograph. The small pons and cerebellum and the elongated medulla and cerebellum are associated with a small posterior fossa. The foramen magnum bony edges are indicated. The elongated fourth ventricle with its caudal choroid plexus tuft sometimes extends down to the midcervical vertebral bodies. From Russell.[74]

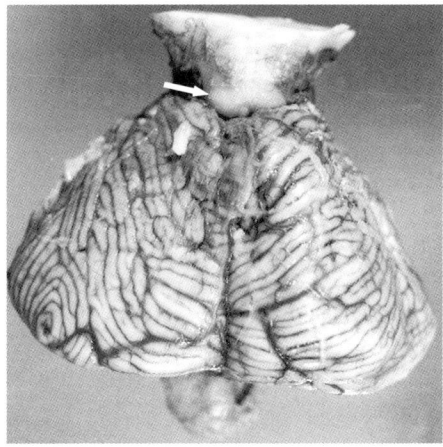

Fig. 15.11 Arnold–Chiari malformation with abnormal cerebellar folial pattern. The cerebellum is elongated in a caudal direction and has an abnormal folial pattern, particularly on the left. The inferior colliculi (arrow) are fused across the midline and the superior colliculi are flat and indistinct.

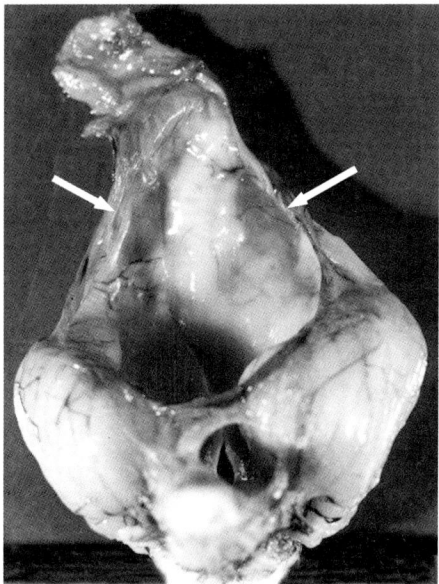

Fig. 15.12 Dorsal and caudal view of Dandy–Walker malformation. The cerebellar hemispheres are markedly laterally displaced, replaced by a large diaphanous cyst (arrows) containing in its most rostral portion a thin remnant of cerebellar vermis. The foramen of Magendie opening is an artifact. The caudal medulla is out of focus at the bottom of the photograph.

Dandy–Walker Malformation

A large fourth ventricle, partial or complete cerebellar vermis absence, and closed lateral and midline fourth ventricular foramina characterize the Dandy–Walker malformation (Fig. 15.12).[119] Other nervous system malformations are likely with this malformation, ranging from the cortex to the caudal spinal cord.[120,121] The ZIC family of genes is implicated in some Dandy–Walker familial cases.[122]

Deficient Dysplastic Parasagittal Arachnoid Granulations

In some instances of 'communicating' hydrocephalus, parasagittal granulations are apparently congenitally absent or dysplastic.[85,123] In 1914, without citing specific cases, Cushing[124] mentioned that hydrocephalus in some of his patients could be attributed to an 'absence of arachnoidal projections or villi.' Winkelman and Fay, in 1930,[125] in discussing the 'Pacchionian system' and its possible relation to epilepsy, listed three patients with hydrocephalus and Pacchionian granulation 'aplasia,' although they did not mention concurrent problems potentially causing the hydrocephalus.

Posthemorrhagic ventriculomegaly

Bleeding into the subarachnoid space sometimes impairs absorption of spinal fluid in both infants and adults. No satisfactory explanation of this phenomenon has been advanced. The usual explanation is that there is posthemorrhage basal arachnoidal fibrosis and thickening,[126] but autopsy studies do not always support this interpretation. One suggestion is that blood, or attendant arachnoidal villus inflammation-induced arachnoid cap cell proliferation, reduces the ability of arachnoidal villi to transport spinal fluid into the superior sagittal sinus lateral lacunae.[127] Forty-four percent of liveborns from the National Collaborative Perinatal Project (NCPP) who lived fewer than 7 days and 25% of stillborns had IVH,[128] sometimes leading to in utero ventriculomegaly. While most preterm IVH is related to germinal matrix hemorrhage, late gestational IVH is related to choroid plexus hemorrhage.[126,129–131]

Intraventricular hemorrhage results in a granular ependymitis that increases with time. The granular ependymitis contains the debris of red cell breakdown pathologically, and sonographically the hyperechoic ependyma persists for at least 2 months.[132] Increased intraventricular pressure sometimes accompanies the ventriculomegaly following IVH.[23] The outcome in these children includes seizures and developmental delays.[133]

Intraventricular hemorrhage occurs in 31% to 43% of infants who weigh less than 1500g. IVH is rarely an isolated lesion at autopsy. To document associated cerebral abnormality, 24 brains of infants with IVH and who survived for at least 1 week were examined.[134] Choroid plexus hemorrhage and brain calcification had been misdiagnosed as IVH in two infants, while in two other infants IVH was not evident. Eleven infants (46%) had choroid plexus hemorrhage. Twenty-two infants (92%) had additional cerebral abnormalities: periventricular leukomalacia, brainstem necrosis, hydrocephalus, or cerebellar necrosis. This study demonstrates that preterm IVH is rarely an isolated abnormality. The associated brain lesions should be considered in attempts to prevent or treat IVH and their presence should be suspected during the clinical assessment of survivors.

BASAL MENINGITIS: CHRONIC GRANULOMATOUS INFLAMMATION

Neonatal purulent meningitis differs in its pathology from purulent meningitis in older children and adults. First, the choroid plexus is likely to be a route of invasion of organisms, with immediate production of a plexitis and ventriculitis, and eventually meningitis.[135] The plexitis leads to the production of much intraventricular exudate and debris that eventually plugs spinal fluid flow pathways, resulting in ventricular enlargement.

Subsequent to the neonatal period, basal and hemispheral meningitis leads to a leptomeningeal fibrosis with hydrocephalus. A wide variety of invasive agents cause the meningitis, and these change with the child's age.

TUMORS OR MALFORMATIONS OBSTRUCTING SPINAL FLUID FLOW

Neoplasms and vascular malformations distort the brain and obstruct spinal fluid flow in a variety of ways, in both the neonate and the older child. Within the cerebrum, lateral ventricular constriction or obliteration leads to ventricular dilation when cut off from the interventricular foramen. Midline shifts from a unilateral glioma potentially cause opposite lateral ventricle dilation from compression of its interventricular foramen. During herniation, cerebral tumors sometimes compress the midbrain, causing aqueductal obstruction. Tumors bulging into the third ventricle sometimes obstruct spinal fluid flow. When in an appropriate location, midbrain tumors, vascular malformations, or great vein of Galen aneurysms occlude the aqueduct. When growing into or compressing the fourth ventricle, intrinsic or extrinsic brainstem or cerebellar tumors constrain the flow of spinal fluid. Finally, diffuse leptomeningeal tumors potentially have the same effect.

OTHER CONGENITAL MALFORMATIONS

Many congenital malformations of the brain are associated with ventriculomegaly or hydrocephalus, such as 'occlusion of foramina of Luschka and Magendie' and the Chiari malformation. Recent texts have dealt with the neuropathology of brain malformations, and retrocerebellar cysts are dealt with in Chapter 10 of this volume and recent publications.[115,136]

SKULL BASE DEFORMITIES

Hydrocephalus occurs with a number of skull base abnormalities such as achondroplasia,[137] osteopetrosis,[138] Crouzon disease,[139,140] osteogenesis imperfecta,[141] Chiari malformation,[142] Pfeiffer syndrome,[143] cloverleaf skull,[10,143] and other craniosynostoses.[144]

ARACHNOIDAL CYSTS

In this condition, the arachnoid is split into the inner and outer arachnoidal layer (see Chapter 10).[145–148] Arachnoidal trabeculae extend from the inner cyst arachnoidal layer to the underlying pia, but there are no trabeculae between the inner and outer cyst layers.[149–151] The outer layer is composed of fibroconnective tissue and arachnoid, the inner layer mainly of arachnoid. Many of these cysts occur in association with normal arachnoidal cisterns.[152]

Arachnoidal or glioependymal cysts are associated with ventriculomegaly in utero.[153,154] Later in life they occur in the middle cranial fossa,[155,156] the lateral sulcus (Sylvian fissure),[157] quadrigeminal cistern,[158–160] suprasellar,[161–163] retroclival,[164] or at the craniospinal junction.[165–167] Some suprasellar cysts are related to an imperforate arachnoidal membrane of Liliequist.[168] Occasionally an arachnoidal cyst is found within the fourth ventricle. They have also been found in association with glutaric aciduria type I,[169] polycystic kidney disease,[170] mucopolysaccharidoses,[171] and cri du chat syndrome. Clinically, arachnoid cysts are associated with hydrocephalus, seizures, headache, weakness, sexual precocity, cranial neuropathy, scoliosis, cognitive decline, and visual loss.[172,173]

The anatomic results of hydrocephalus
Symmetric or asymmetric ventricular dilatation occurs at the expense of the immediately adjacent tissue, whether it is white or gray matter. When lateral ventricles dilate during obstructive hydrocephalus, they do not do so initially at cortical expense but at the expense of white matter until the late stages (Fig. 15.13), regardless of cause, whether it be tumor, hemorrhage, or postinflammatory leptomeningeal fibrosis.[74,174–176] Generalized neonatal lateral ventricular enlargement occurs unequally throughout lateral ventricular regions, in contrast to the more proportional ventricular enlargement when it occurs at an older age. Fetal or infantile lateral ventricular horn enlargement occurs in the occipital horns and atria first and to the greatest extent. The dorsolateral ventricle angle above the caudate and thalamus at the

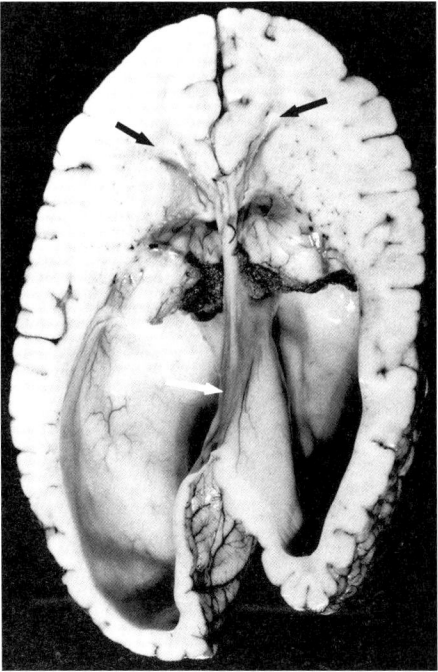

Fig. 15.13 Axial view of neonatal brain with hydrocephalus. The occipital, parietal, and atrial portions of lateral ventricles are markedly enlarged. In contrast, frontal horns (black arrows) are not. The medial hemispheres are thinned to a diaphanous membrane (white arrow).

365

coronal interventricular foramen becomes blunted either in parallel with or shortly after atrial and occipital horn enlargement. In contrast, ventricular dilatation acquired later in life generally involves all lateral ventricular regions equally. The medial ventricular walls are thinned disproportionately.

Several developmental conditions contribute to disproportionate parieto-occipital horn enlargement. Throughout the last half of gestation, the occipital horn ependyma is discontinuous, particularly on its lateral surface, potentially reducing lateral ventricular wall structural support.[98] Second, during the last half of gestation, the temporal, parietal, and occipital lobes grow rapidly in all directions except toward the skull base; that is, toward the relatively stable body, and the greater and lesser sphenoidal wings and the basiocciput.[177] In conjunction with this growth, there is a major discrepancy between the relative frontal bone 'rigidity' and the parietal and supraoccipital bone 'fluidity' throughout the last half of gestation. The orbital frontal bone base is fixed to the cranial portion across the supraorbital ridge; the frontal bone grows only along its coronal and sagittal sutures, a far different situation to that found in parietal and supraoccipital bony plates. Sutures surround the parietal bone on all sides, suspending it within membranous tissue. Thus, while in the advanced hydrocephalic head the cranial vault convexity enlarges markedly, the skull base remains small and stable except for the enlargement of the basal foramina and the erosion of the posterior clinoids.[74] The supraoccipital bone is quite similar in that it rides in connective tissue on all sides except at the innominate suture, where it lies free within the suture membrane. Third, a specific anatomic event is the change in brain growth pattern that occurs at the end of the second trimester (see Chapter 2). The parietal lobes undergo a growth spurt, resulting in progressive biparietal enlargement starting at about the end of the second trimester. Fourth, the choroid plexus's main mass is the atrial glomus. It seems possible that the pulsatile pressure wave originating from the glomus arterial bed is maximal within the atrium and occipital horn; the glomus cardiac pulsation is apparent in real-time ultrasonography.

The paraventricular effects in acute hydrocephalus consist of an increase in water content and, both histologically and experimentally, destruction of axons and myelin sheaths, and an increase in cerebrospinal fluid myelin basic protein,[175,178–180] although changes in glial cell density with myelination take place as expected.[181] The long-term effect in some cases of treated hydrocephalus is a diffuse, fine paraventricular white matter fibrillary gliosis. Despite these findings, the fresh hydrocephalic brain weight (without cerebrospinal fluid) is maintained until a considerable degree of hydrocephalus is attained. Yakovlev[182] pointed out that stretching and disintegration of the corona radiata lateral to the lateral ventricular body in advanced hydrocephalus accounts for the accompanying paraparesis. Myelination progresses normally in the remaining brain portions, except for the midcorpus callosum, where the hydrocephalus is increasing.[178,181] When shunting relieves hydrocephalus, corpus callosum cell and myelination activity return to a normal range. Loss of ependymal lining and deep white matter astrocytosis is prominent in human hydrocephalus.[74]

The morphologic abnormalities, both nature and location, depend on the age at onset of ventricular enlargement, the velocity and magnitude of enlargement, and its duration. The paraventricular white matter in experimental and human obstructive hydrocephalus is similar. Acutely, edema and nerve fiber damage are present, and chronically there is gliosis both experimentally and in needle biopsies along shunt tracts in infants. There is little cortical abnormality in these biopsies. The edema apparently subsides if the ventricular dilatation is present for a long enough period. Myelin debris fills deeply located macrophages. Occasionally, there is astrocytic process myelination.[175,176] With advanced hydrocephalus there are many hypothalamic effects as the third ventricle dilates and the hypothalamus atrophies. The basal ganglia and thalamus are preserved size-wise, but displaced basally. Interventricular foramina are markedly enlarged and there is marked septum pellucidum fenestration. In advanced hydrocephalus, the choroid plexuses become more or less atrophic and the ependyma is destroyed over variable amounts of lateral ventricular surface with variable degrees of supependymal gliosis. Finally, there are lateral ventricular wall bulges or ruptures forming false diverticuli. Some of these are spontaneous and dissect through the lateral ventricular wall adjacent to the lateral ventricles and some bulge into the posterior fossa, compressing the midbrain and upper cerebellar surfaces.

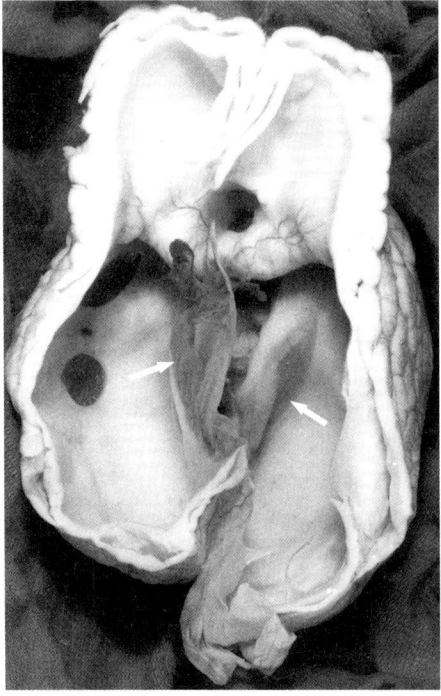

Fig. 15.14 The entire ventricular system is markedly enlarged. The medial walls are thinned to mere membranes and can bulge past the tentorial edge to form diverticuli extending into the posterior fossa (arrows).

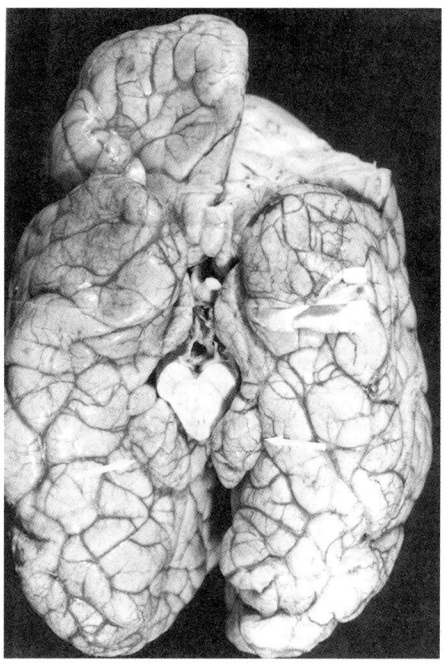

Fig. 15.15 The parahippocampal gyri bulge past the indentation left by the tentorial edges (arrows) into the posterior fossa.

LATERAL VENTRICULAR DIVERTICULI

The most frequent anatomic complications are diverticuli into paraventricular white matter (Figs. 15.14 and 15.15), medial posterior temporal horn wall thinning and herniation, and septum pellucidum fenestration. Paraventricular clefts that communicate with a lateral (or rarely, the fourth) ventricle develop in paraventricular white matter (or, rarely, tegmentum) in advanced degrees of hydrocephalus.[183] The cysts are astroglia lined and partially loculated, bilateral and symmetric or asymmetric, and occur adjacent to any lateral ventricular region except the striatum, thalamus, or corpus callosum, and, depending on location, are symptomatic.

Medial lateral ventricular thinning and herniation usually occur adjacent to the atrium where the temporal and occipital horns join, and rarely adjacent to the lateral ventricle body.[184] When these ventricular diverticuli attain great size, they often herniate through the tentorial incisura or under the falx to compress the cerebellum or opposite cerebrum, or even to separate the mesencephalic tectum from the vermis posteriorly. They occur in at least one-quarter of cases with advanced hydrocephalus,[185] are either symmetric or asymmetric, and are occasionally associated with clinical cerebellar deficits. In a similar fashion, when the suprapineal recess enlarges, it secondarily distorts and displaces the mesencephalic tectum.[101] The medial herniations sometimes rupture and provide a spontaneous ventriculostomy.[74]

368

Puncture pori

In hydrocephalic brains, enlargement of a penetrating tract, whether from a surgical needle or a penetrating wound, often occurs.[88,186]

RELATIONSHIP BETWEEN VENTRICULAR AND HEAD SIZE

The little information available about the correlation of ventricular width and the rate of fronto-occipital circumference growth in preterm infants indicates that head size increase lags behind ventricular enlargement.[187–189] The widely used criterion of a head growth rate of more than 2cm/week[129] is a poor criterion for the definition of posthemorrhagic hydrocephalus.[24]

EXPERIMENTAL HYDROCEPHALUS

Although data from experimental studies are not directly applicable to humans, spinal fluid flow obstruction (interventricular foramina, aqueduct, or interpeduncular cistern) through the ventricular system produces ventriculomegaly.[82,190] In experimental acute obstructive hydrocephalus, the lateral ventricles enlarge very rapidly,[191] and fragmentation of deep white matter axons and structural abnormalities of cortical neurons occurs.[192] A relationship exists between ventricle pressure and ventricular size.[193] A reduction in the number and caliber of capillaries in deep white matter and basal ganglia occurs in rats.[194] Shunting reduces secondary astrocytosis and microgliosis, particularly in deep white matter and periaqueductal gray matter.[195]

Experimentally, acute ventricular dilatation is associated with white matter edema adjacent to the lateral ventricles and nerve fiber degeneration. Asymmetric lateral ventricular enlargement follows necrosis or local atrophy in deep white matter, choroid plexus papilloma, or is sometimes cryptogenic.[196] Whereas many hydrocephalic brains have less tissue when cerebrospinal fluid is drained, some have more.[197]

In both human and experimental animals there is ependymal stretching and breaking, microvasculature reduction and distortion, deep white matter axonal and myelin damage, with edema, and, sometimes, neuronal distortion or damage. Occasionally, macrophages are found in deep white matter near the ventricle.[198] Some early studies failed to detect most of these changes.[199] The damage appears to result from mechanical brain distortion combined with impaired cerebral blood flow.[200] Puppies with induced hydrocephalus have histologic changes that correlate roughly with the intraventricular pressures, and they consist of ependymal disruptions, deep white matter edema, and tissue destruction around the ventricle.[201]

PATHOLOGIC FINDINGS IN SHUNTED HYDROCEPHALUS

In successfully shunted hydrocephalus, there is a reduction in ventricle size and cortical and underlying white matter widening.[202] Ventricular dilatation sometimes regresses completely after shunting.[203] The gyral pattern is often more complicated than usual, although it is likely to be related to the original cause of the dilatation. The corpus callosum seems not to recover and remains thin. The arachnoid thickens somewhat. The subdural–arachnoid interface widens, fills with loose connective tissue, and bridging veins stretch, sometimes leading to subdural hemorrhage. The thin tentorium is pushed downward around the anterior cerebellum, and the upper brainstem and cerebellum stand high as the skull base is pushed in a basal direction. Restitution of squamous bone erosion, cranial base, and sellar shrinkage occurs.[204]

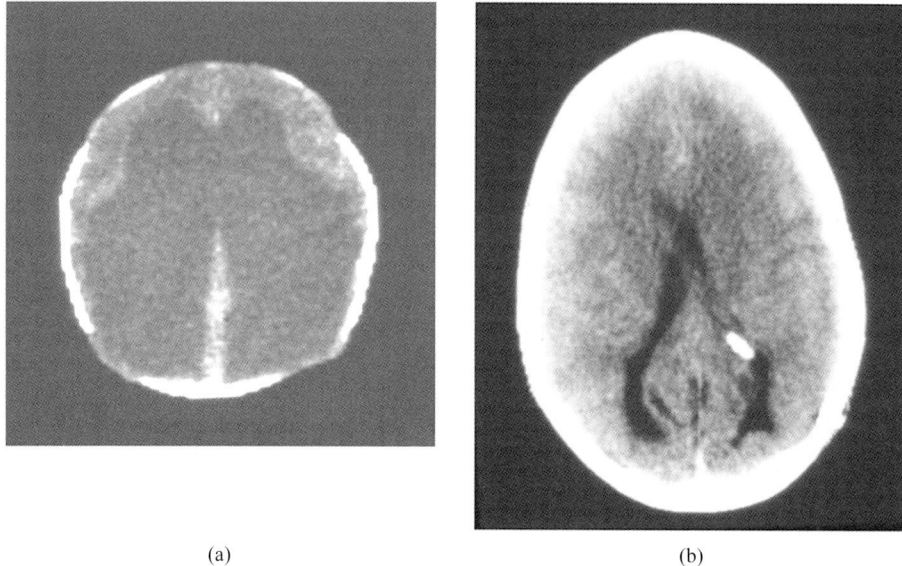

(a)   (b)

Fig. 15.16 Noncontrast CT of the head. (a) Newborn with acute hydrocephalus with markedly thinned cerebral mantle. (b) Same patient as in (a) 6 months after placing ventriculoperitoneal shunt. Note the cerebral parenchymal expansion.

CEREBRAL REBULKING FOLLOWING SHUNTING

Frequently, a very impressive paraventricular effect follows shunting in early life. The paraventricular white matter rebulks, or recovers, at a very rapid rate and to a considerable degree (Fig. 15.16).[202] This phenomenon is without explanation except for the hypotheses that postulate that brain water shifts in opposite directions, that is, a decrease in extracellular water during advancing hydrocephalus and an increase in extracellular water as the ventricle comes down to normal size following shunting.[205,206] Unfortunately, the latter study ignored the white matter hypodense regions near the frontal horn angle, and therefore the question remains unsettled. The rebulking, or recovery, of cerebral white matter following shunting parallels clinical observations of an apparent progressive decrease in size of paraventricular white matter cysts in infants,[207] and the reconstitution of cerebral bulk following extensive white matter lesions in neonatal kittens.[208] In adult hydrocephalic cats, there is prompt reduction of ventricular size when shunted. The regions most severely affected, such as the corpus callosum, contained a paucity of myelinated fibers and numerous reactive astrocytes, without evidence of replacement of lost myelinated fibers. Ultrastructurally, the white matter edema persisted for weeks, even when the ventricles were of a normal size.[209] This is a topic demanding extensive investigation.

STRUCTURAL COMPLICATIONS OF THERAPY

Infection within the ventricles is the most common complication of shunting. Plexitis, ventriculitis, ventricular septae, and/or loculi within the ventricles are all well documented. The second most common complication of the shunt procedure is the inadvertent shunt placement into the septum pellucidum, thalamus, hypothalamus, or through the cerebral wall into the subarachnoid space, particularly at the brain base. Uncommonly, the shunt cranial end is lost within the ventricular system, or the distal end perforates bowel or organ,[210] forms an abdominal cyst or ascites,[211] or migrates into the umbilical and scrotal canals.[212,213]

COLPOCEPHALY

Colpocephaly (enlarged occipital horns, microcephaly, and absence of corpus callosum) is sometimes considered a separate developmental brain disorder.[214] Unfortunately, it is too often confused with the normal occipital horn enlargement in early hydrocephalus. It has been found in a wide variety of malformations including optic nerve hypoplasia, chorioretinal coloboma, micrognathia, cleft palate, hypoplastic nails, simian creases, cerebellar atrophy, cisterna magna enlargement, microgyria, macrogyria, pachygyria, lissencephaly, Pierre Robin syndrome, neurofibromatosis, meningomyelocele, and schizencephaly, but colpocephaly is variably present in these abnormalities.

Conclusions

In this chapter we have reviewed fetal ventriculomegaly, ventriculomegaly occurring without head enlargement, particularly if there is loss or hypoplasia of white matter, the anatomic and metabolic megalencephalies, and pathologic brain changes in hydrocephalus. Perhaps the most important observation is the rebulking following early-life shunting of hydrocephalic children, a subject which is in need of further study.

A most important distinction was made in this chapter between ventriculomegaly and hydrocephalus. There is little point in shunting simple ventriculomegaly from neuronal or white matter loss from a previous insult or from white matter hypoplasia. The ventriculomegaly etiology must be fully understood. Hydrocephalus, on the other hand, is historically ventriculomegaly and head enlargement.

REFERENCES

1. Schrander-Stumpel C, Fryns JP (1998) Congenital hydrocephalus: nosology and guidelines for clinical approach and genetic counselling. *Eur J Pediatr* 157: 355–362.
2. Cruveilhier J (1829–1835) *Anatomie Pathologique du Corps Humain*, Part 2, XVth Liv. Paris: JB Baillière.
3. McClelland JE (1940) The syndrome of hydromicrocephaly. *J Pediatr* 16: 36–51.
4. Gilles F, Murphy SF (1969) Perinatal telencephalic leukoencephalopathy. *J Neurol Neurosurg Psych* 32: 404–413.
5. Chattha AS, Richardson EP Jr. (1977) Cerebral white-matter hypoplasia. *Arch Neurol* 34: 137–141.
6. Palmer P, Dubowitz LMS, Levene MI, Dubowitz V (1982) Developmental and neurological progress of preterm infants with intraventricular hemorrhage and ventricular dilatation. *Arch Dis Child* 57: 748–753.
7. Stewart AL, Thorburn RJ, Hope PL, Goldsmith M, Lipscomb AP, Reynolds EO (1983) Ultrasound appearance of the brain in very preterm infants and neurodevelopmental outcome at 18 months of age. *Arch Dis Child* 58: 598–604.
8. DeVries LS, Dubowitz LM, Dubowitz W, et al (1985) Predictive value of cranial ultrasound in the newborn baby: a reappraisal. *Lancet* 2: 137–140.

9. DeVries LS, Dubowitz LMS, Pennock JM, Bydder GM (1989) Extensive cystic leukomalacia: correlation of cranial ultrasound, magnetic resonance imaging and clinical findings in sequential studies. *Clin Radiol* 40: 158–166.

10. Squires LA, Krishnamoorthy KS, Natowicz MR (1995) Delayed myelination in infants and young children: radiographic and clinical correlates. *J Child Neurol* 10: 100–104.

11. Hope PL, Gould SJ, Howard S, Hamilton PA, Costello AM, Reynolds EO (1988) Precision of ultrasound diagnosis of pathologically verified lesions in the brains of very preterm infants. *Dev Med Child Neurol* 30: 457–471.

12. Paneth N, Rudelli R, Monte W, et al (1990) White matter necrosis in very low birth weight infants: neuropathologic and ultrasonographic findings in infants surviving six days or longer. *J Pediatr* 116: 975–984.

13. Hansen A, Leviton A (1999) Labor and delivery characteristics and risks of cranial ultrasonographic abnormalities among very-low-birth-weight infants. The Developmental Epidemiology Network Investigators. *Am J Obstet Gynecol* 181: 997–1006.

14. Kuban K, Sanocka U, Leviton A, et al (1999) White matter disorders of prematurity: association with intraventricular hemorrhage and ventriculomegaly. The Developmental Epidemiology Network. *J Pediatr* 134: 539–546.

15. Schellinger D, Grant EG, Manz HJ, Lavenstein BL, Patronas NJ (1986) Ventricular shapes, distortions, and deformities: mirrors of past cerebral insults. A study based on early sonographic follow-up studies. *Pediatr Neurol* 4: 193–201.

16. Schouman-Claeys E, Picard A, Lalande G, et al (1989) Contribution of computed tomography in the aetiology and prognosis of cerebral palsy in children. *Br J Radiol* 62: 248–252.

17. Krageloh-Mann I, Hagberg B, Petersen D, Riethmuller J, Gut E, Michaelis R (1992) Bilateral spastic cerebral palsy. Pathogenetic aspects from MRI. *Neuropediatrics* 23: 46–48.

18. Truwit CL, Barkovich AJ, Koch TK, Ferriero DM (1992) Cerebral palsy: MR findings in 40 patients. *AJNR Am J Neuroradiol* 13: 67–78.

19. DeVries LS, Eken P, Groenendaal F, van-Haastert IC, Meiners LC (1993) Correlation between the degree of periventricular leukomalacia diagnosed using cranial ultrasound and MRI later in infancy in children with cerebral palsy. *Neuropediatrics* 24: 263–268.

20. Skranes JS, Vik T, Nilsen G, et al (1993) Cerebral magnetic resonance imaging (MRI) and mental and motor function of very low birth weight infants at one year of corrected age. *Neuropediatrics* 24: 256–262.

21. de la Monte SM, Hsu FI, Hedley-Whyte ET, Kupsky W (1990) Morphometric analysis of the human infant brain: effects of intraventricular hemorrhage and periventricular leukomalacia. *J Child Neurol* 5: 101–110.

22. Levene MI, Starte DR (1981) A longitudinal study of post-haemorrhagic ventricular dilatation in the newborn. *Arch Dis Child* 56: 905–910.

23. Hill A, Volpe JJ (1981) Normal pressure hydrocephalus in the newborn. *Pediatrics* 68: 623–629.

24. Muller WD, Urlesberger B (1992) Correlation of ventricular size and head circumference after severe intra-periventricular haemorrhage in preterm infants. *Childs Nerv Syst* 8: 33–35.

25. Volpe JJ (1994) *Neurology of the Newborn*. Philadelphia: WB Saunders.

26. Bromley B, Frigoletto FD Jr., Benacerraf BR (1991) Mild fetal lateral cerebral ventriculomegaly: clinical course and outcome. *Am J Obstet Gynecol* 164: 863–867.

27. Goldstein RB, La Pidus AS, Filly RA, Cardoza J (1990) Mild lateral cerebral ventricular dilatation in utero: clinical significance and prognosis. *Radiology* 176: 237–242.

28. Nicolaides KH, Berry S, Snijders RJ, Thorpe-Beeston JG, Gosden C (1990) Fetal lateral cerebral ventriculomegaly: associated malformations and chromosomal defects. *Fetal Diagn Ther* 5: 5–14.

29. McDonald R (1967) Large heads in small children. Notes on the causes of increased head circumference. *Clin Pediatr (Phila)* 6: 47–50.

30. Sher PK, Brown SB (1975) A longitudinal study of head growth in pre-term infants. II: differentiation between 'catch-up' head growth and early infantile hydrocephalus. *Dev Med Child Neurol* 17: 711–718.

31. Sher PK, Brown SB (1975) A longitudinal study of head growth in pre-term infants, I: normal rates of head growth. *Dev Med Child Neurol* 17: 705–710.

32. Laurence KM (1964) Megalencephaly. *Dev Med Child Neurol* 6: 638–640.

33. Gooskens RH, Willemse J, Bijlsma JB, Hanlo PW (1988) Megalencephaly: definition and classification. *Brain Dev* 10: 1–7.

34. Gooskens RH, Willemse J, Faber JA, Verdonck AF (1989) Macrocephalies—a differentiated approach. *Neuropediatrics* 20: 164–169.

35. DeMeyer W (1972) Megalencephaly in children. Clinical syndromes, genetic patterns, and differential diagnosis from other causes of megalocephaly. *Neurology* 22: 634–643.
36. Wilson SA (1934) Megalencephaly. *J Neurol Psychopathol* 14: 193–216.
37. Ho KL, Chang CH, Yang SS, Chason JL (1984) Neuropathologic findings in thanatophoric dysplasia. *Acta Neuropathol* 63: 218–228.
38. Gohlich-Ratmann G, Baethmann M, Lorenz P, et al (1998) Megalencephaly, mega corpus callosum, and complete lack of motor development: a previously undescribed syndrome. *Am J Med Genet* 79: 161–167.
39. Nelen MR, Kremer H, Konings IB, et al (1999) Novel *PTEN* mutations in patients with Cowden disease: absence of clear genotype–phenotype correlations. *Eur J Hum Genet* 7: 267–273.
40. Nelen MR, Padberg GW, Peeters EA, et al (1996) Localization of the gene for Cowden disease to chromosome 10q22–23. *Nat Genet* 13: 114–116.
41. Hayashi M, Kurata K, Suzuki K, Hirasawa K, Nagata J, Morimatsu Y (1998) Megalencephaly, hydrocephalus and cortical dysplasia in severe dwarfism mimicking leprechaunism. *Acta Neuropathol (Berl)* 95: 431–436.
42. Cohen MM Jr., Kreiborg S (1990) The central nervous system in the Apert syndrome. *Am J Med Genet* 35: 36–45.
43. Cohen MM Jr., Kreiborg S (1994) Cranial size and configuration in the Apert syndrome. *J Craniofac Genet Dev Biol* 14: 153–162.
44. Orstavik KH, Stromme P, Ek J, Torvik A, Skjeldal OH (1997) Macrocephaly, epilepsy, autism, dysmorphic features, and mental retardation in two sisters: a new autosomal recessive syndrome? *J Med Genet* 34: 849–851.
45. Sarwar M, Schafer ME (1988) Brain malformations in linear nevus sebaceous syndrome: an MR study. *J Comput Assist Tomogr* 12: 338–340.
46. Hager BC, Dyme IZ, Guertin SR, Tyler RJ, Tryciecky EW, Fratkin JD (1991) Linear nevus sebaceous syndrome: megalencephaly and heterotopic gray matter. *Pediatr Neurol* 7: 45–49.
47. Gurecki PJ, Holden KR, Sahn EE, Dyer DS, Cure JK (1996) Developmental neural abnormalities and seizures in epidermal nevus syndrome. *Dev Med Child Neurol* 38: 716–723.
48. Clancy RR, Kurtz MB, Baker D, Sladky JT, Honig PJ, Younkin DP (1985) Neurologic manifestations of the organoid nevus syndrome. *Arch Neurol* 42: 236–240.
49. Verloes A, Journel H, Elmer C, et al (1993) Heterogeneity versus variability in megalocornea–mental retardation (MMR) syndromes: report of new cases and delineation of 4 probable types. *Am J Med Genet* 46: 132–137.
50. Opitz JM, Kaveggia EG, Adkins WN Jr., et al (1982) Studies of malformation syndromes of humans XXXIIIC: the FG syndrome—further studies on three affected individuals from the FG family. *Am J Med Genet* 12: 147–154.
51. Scott RE (1969) Ataxia–telangiectasia. Its association with megalencephaly and mesenteric lymphangiectasia. *Arch Pathol* 88: 78–84.
52. Collins JO, Falk M, Guibone R (1966) Benign lymphoid polyposis of the colon. A case report. *Pediatrics* 38: 897–899.
53. Hoshino A (1981) [Megalencephaly: a report of 4 children including a previously undescribed congenital syndrome and review of the literature (author's transl)]. *No To Shinkei* 33: 377–384.
54. Tsuru A, Mizuguchi M, Uyemura K, Becker LE, Takashima S (1997) Immunohistochemical expression of cell adhesion molecule L1 in hemimegalencephaly. *Pediatr Neurol* 16: 45–49.
55. DeLone DR, Brown WD, Gentry LR (1999) Proteus syndrome: craniofacial and cerebral MRI. *Neuroradiology* 41: 840–843.
56. Aydinli N, Caliskan M, Calay M, Ozmen M (1998) Use of localized proton nuclear magnetic resonance spectroscopy in Canavan's disease. *Turk J Pediatr* 40: 549–557.
57. Deprez M, D'Hooghe M, Misson JP, et al (1999) Infantile and juvenile presentations of Alexander's disease: a report of two cases. *Acta Neurol Scand* (1999) 99: 158–165. *Erratum in Acta Neurol Scand* 100: 354.
58. Goutieres F, Boulloche J, Bourgeois M, Aicardi J (1996) Leukoencephalopathy, megalencephaly, and mild clinical course. A recently individualized familial leukodystrophy. Report on five new cases. *J Child Neurol* 11: 439–444.
59. van der Knaap MS, Barth PG, Vrensen GF, Valk J (1996) Histopathology of an infantile-onset spongiform leukoencephalopathy with a discrepantly mild clinical course. *Acta Neuropathol (Berl)* 92: 206–212.

60. Topcu M, Saatci I, Topcuoglu MA, Kose G, Kunak B (1998) Megalencephaly and leukodystrophy with mild clinical course: a report on 12 new cases. *Brain Dev* 20: 142–153.
61. Topcu M, Gartioux C, Ribierre F, et al (2000) Vacuoliting megalencephalic leukoencephalopathy with subcortical cysts, mapped to chromosome 22qtel. *Am J Hum Genet* 66: 733–739.
62. Iafolla AK, Kahler SG (1989) Megalencephaly in the neonatal period as the initial manifestation of glutaric aciduria type I [see comments]. *J Pediatr* 114: 1004–1006.
63. Hoffmann GF, Gibson KM, Trefz FK, Nyhan WL, Bremer HJ, Rating D (1994) Neurological manifestations of organic acid disorders. *Eur J Pediatr* 153: S94–100.
64. Vallois H-V (1971) Le Crâne trépané magdalénien de Rochereil. *Bull Soc Préhist Française* 68: 485–495.
65. Aronyk KE (1993) The history and classification of hydrocephalus. *Neurosurg Clin N Am* 4: 599–609.
66. Aschoff A, Kremer P, Hashemi B, Kunze S (1999) The scientific history of hydrocephalus and its treatment. *Neurosurg Rev* 22(2–3): 67–93; discussion 4–5.
67. al-Qasim Khalaf A (1973) *Albucasis on Surgery and Instruments* (Spink MS, Lewis GL, transl.). London: The Wellcome Institute of the History of Medicine.
68. Elmaci I (2000) Color illustrations and neurosurgical techniques of Serefeddin Sabuncuoglu in the 15th century. *Neurosurgery* 47: 951–955.
69. Erbengi A (1993) History and development of neurosurgery in Anatolia (part one). *Turk Neurosurg* 3: 1–5.
70. Aciduman A, Belen D (2007) Hydrocephalus and its management in Avicenna's Canon of Medicine. *J Neurosurg* 106 (6 Suppl): 513–516.
71. Clarke E, O'Malley C (1996) *The Human Brain and Spinal Cord; A historical study illustrated by writings from antiquity to the twentieth century*. San Francisco: Norman Publishing.
72. Torack RM (1982) Historical aspects of normal and abnormal brain fluids. II Hydrocephalus. *Arch Neurol* 39: 276–279.
73. Gjerris F, Snorrason E (1992) The history of hydrocephalus. *J Hist Neurosci* 1: 285–312.
74. Russell DS (1949) *Observations on the Pathology of Hydrocephalus*. London: Her Majesty's Stationery Office.
75. Morgagni G (1769) *The Seats and Causes of Diseases*. London: A. Millar, T. Cadell, and Johnson and Payne.
76. Whytt R (1768) *Observations on the Dropsy in the Brain*. Edinburgh: J Balfour.
77. Willis T [1664] *Cerebri anatome: cui accessit nervorum descriptio et usus.* Feindel W, editor, tercentenary edition, 1964. London: J Martyn and J Allestry, pp. 1–104. Willis T [1664] *The Anatomy of the Brain and Nerves*. Feindel W, editor, tercentenary edition, 1965. Montreal: McGill University Press, pp. 1–192.
78. Pacchioni A (1705) *Dissertatio epistolaris ad Lucam Schroeckium de glandulis conglobatis durae meningis humanae*. Rome: Francesco Buagni.
79. Torack RM (1982) Historical aspects of normal and abnormal brain fluids. III Cerebral edema. *Arch Neurol* 39: 355–357.
80. von Luschka H (1855) *Die Adergeflechte der menschlichen Gehirnes. Eine Mongraphie*. Berlin: Reimer.
81. Key A, Retzius G (1875) *Studien in der Anatomie des Nerversystems und des Bindegewebes*. Stockholm: Samson and Wallin.
82. Dandy WE, Blackfan KD (1914) Internal hydrocephalus: an experimental, clinical, and pathological study. *Am J Dis Child* 8: 406–482.
83. Vesalius A (1543) *De Humani Corporis Fabrica Libri Septem*. ex off. Ioannis Oportini, Basel.
84. LeGros Clark W (1920) On the Pacchionian bodies. *J Anat* 55: 40–48.
85. Gilles FH, Davidson RI (1971) Communicating hydrocephalus associated with deficient dysplastic parasagittal arachnoidal granulations. *J Neurosurg* 35: 421–426.
86. McComb JG, Davson H, Hyman S, Weiss MH (1982) Cerebrospinal fluid drainage as influenced by ventricular pressure in the rabbit. *J Neurosurg* 56: 790–797.
87. Turner L (1961) The structure of arachnoidal granulations with observations under physiologic and pathologic significance. *Ann R Coll Surg Engl* 29: 237–264.
88. Salmon JH (1967) Puncture porencephaly. *Am J Dis Child* 114: 72–79.
89. Shabo AL, Maxwell DS (1968) The morphology of the arachnoid villi: a light and electron microscopic study in the monkey. *J Neurosurg* 29: 451–463.
90. Weed LH (1917) An anatomical consideration of the cerebrospinal fluid. *Anat Rec* 12: 461–496.
91. McComb JG, Hyman S, Weiss MH (1983) Cerebrospinal fluid drainage following acute obstruction of the fourth ventricle in the rabbit. In: Humphries RR, editor. *Concepts in Pediatric Neurosurgery*. Basel: S. Karger, pp. 90–101.

92. New PF, Weiner MA (1971) The radiological investigation of hydrocephalus. *Radiol Clin N Am* 9: 117–140.
93. Turkewitsch N (1935) Die Entwicklung des Aquaeductus cerebri des Menschen. *Morphol Jahrb (Leipzig)* 76: 421–447.
94. Williams B (1973) Is aqueduct stenosis a result of hydrocephalus? *Brain* 96: 399–412.
95. Emery JL, Staschak MC (1972) The size and form of the cerebral aqueduct in children. *Brain* 95: 591–598.
96. Woollam DHM, Millen JW (1953) Anatomical considerations in the pathology of stenosis of the cerebral aqueduct. *Brain* 76: 104–112.
97. Fredericks EJ, van Nuis C (1967) Diverticulum of the rostral cerebral aqueduct with ocular dysfunctions. *Arch Neurol* 16: 621–629.
98. Dooling EC, Chi JG, Gilles FH (1983) Developmental change in ventricular epithelia. In: Gilles FH, Leviton A, Dooling EC, editors. *The Developing Human Brain: Growth and Epidemiologic Neuropathology*. Boston: Wright-PSG, pp. 113–117.
99. Shellshear I, Emery JL (1975) The tectum and the aqueduct of Sylvius in hydrocephalus unassociated with myelomeningocele. *Dev Med Child Neurol* 35 (Suppl): 26–34.
100. Shellshear I, Emery JL (1976) Gliosis and aqueductule formation in the aqueduct of Sylvius. *Dev Med Child Neurol* 37 (Suppl): 22–28.
101. Masters CL (1978) Pathogenesis of the Arnold–Chiari malformation: the significance of hydrocephalus and aqueduct stenosis. *J Neuropathol Exp Neurol* 37: 56–74.
102. Johnson RT, Johnson KP (1968) Hydrocephalus following viral infection: The pathology of aqueductal stenosis developing after experimental mumps virus infection. *J Neuropathol Exp Neurol* 27: 591–606.
103. Cinalli G, Spennato P, Ruggiero C, Aliberti F, Maggi G (2004) Aqueductal stenosis 9 years after mumps meningoencephalitis: treatment by endoscopic third ventriculostomy. *Childs Nerv Syst* 20: 61–64.
104. Jellinger G (1986) Anatomopathology of non-tumoral aqueductal stenosis. *J Neurosurg Sci* 30(1–2): 1–16.
105. Conover PT, Roessmann U (1990) Malformational complex in an infant with intrauterine influenza viral infection. *Arch Pathol Lab Med* 114: 535–538.
106. Penfield W (1929) Diencephalic autonomic epilepsy. *Arch Neurol Psychiatry* 22: 358–374.
107. Pennybacker J, Russell DS (1943) Spontaneous ventricular rupture in hydrocephalus, with subtentorial cyst formation. *J Neurol Psychiatry* 6: 38–45.
108. Beckett RS, Netsky MG, Zimmerman HM (1950) Developmental stenosis of the Aqueduct of Sylvius. *Am J Path* 26: 755–771.
109. Russell DS, Donald C (1935) The mechanism of internal hydrocephalus in spina bifida. *Brain* 58: 203–215.
110. Ko TM, Hwa HL, Tseng LH, Hsieh FJ, Huang SF, Lee TY (1994) Prenatal diagnosis of X-linked hydrocephalus in a Chinese family with four successive affected pregnancies. *Prenat Diagn* 14: 57–60.
111. Yamasaki M, Arita N, Hiraga S, et al (1995) A clinical and neuroradiological study of X-linked hydrocephalus in Japan. *J Neurosurg* 83: 50–55.
112. Takahashi S, Makita Y, Okamoto N, Miyamoto A, Oki J (1997) L1CAM mutation in a Japanese family with X-linked hydrocephalus: a study for genetic counseling. *Brain Dev* 19: 559–562.
113. Senat MV, Bernard JP, Delezoide A, et al (2001) Prenatal diagnosis of hydrocephalus-stenosis of the aqueduct of Sylvius by ultrasound in the first trimester of pregnancy. Report of two cases. *Prenat Diagn* 21: 1129–1132.
114. David DJ, Sheffield L, Simpson D, White J (1984) Fronto-ethmoidal meningoencephaloceles: morphology and treatment. *Br J Plast Surg* 37: 271–284.
115. Golden JA, Harding BN, editors (2004) *Developmental Neuropathology*. Basal: International Society of Neuropathology.
116. Arnold J (1894) Myelocyste transposition von gewebs, gewebskenmen und Sympodic. *Beitr Pathol Anat* 16: 1–16.
117. Chiari H (1891) Uber die Veranderungen des Kleinhirns, des Pons und der Medulla Oblongata infolge von kongenitaler hydrocephalic des Grosshirns. *Deutsch Med Wochenschr* 56: 825–836.
118. Chiari H (1896) Uber die Veranderungen des Kleinhirns, des Pons und der Medulla Oblongata infolge von kongenitaler hydroephlic des Grosshirns. *Drukschriften der Akademie der Wissenschaften* 63: 71–116.
119. Taggert JK Jr., Walker AE (1942) Congenital atresia of the foramens of Luschka and Magendie. *Arch Neurol Psychiatry* 48: 583–612.
120. Hirsch JF, Pierre-Kahn A, Renier D, Sainte-Rose C, Hoppe-Hirsch E (1984) The Dandy–Walker malformation. A review of 40 cases. *J Neurosurg* 61: 515–522.

121. Golden JA, Rorke LB, Bruce DA (1987) Dandy–Walker syndrome and associated anomalies. *Pediatr Neurosci* 13: 38–44.
122. Grinberg I, Millen KJ (2005) The *ZIC* gene family in development and disease. *Clin Genet* 67: 290–296.
123. Gutierrez Y, Friede RL, Kaliney WJ (1975) Agenesis of arachnoid granulations and its relationship to communicating hydrocephalus. *J Neurosurg* 43: 553–558.
124. Cushing H (1914) Studies on cerebrospinal fluid. 1. Introduction. *J Med Res* 31: 1–19.
125. Winkelman N, Fay T (1930) The Pacchionian system: histologic and pathologic changes with particular reference to the idiopathic and symptomatic convulsive states. *Arch Neurol Psychiat* 23: 44–64.
126. Larroche JC (1972) Post-haemorrhagic hydrocephalus in infancy. Anatomical study. *Biol Neonate* 20: 287–299.
127. Massicotte EM, Del Bigio MR (1999) Human arachnoid villi response to subarachnoid hemorrhage: possible relationship to chronic hydrocephalus. *J Neurosurg* 91: 80–84.
128. Dooling EC, Gilles FH (1983) Intracranial hemorrhage: topography. In: Gilles FH, Leviton A, Dooling EC, editors. *The Developing Human Brain: Growth and Epidemiologic Neuropathology*. Boston: Wright-PSG, pp. 193–203.
129. Leviton A, Gilles F, Strassfeld R (1977) The influence of route of delivery and hyaline membranes on the risk of neonatal intracranial hemorrhages. *Ann Neurol* 2: 451–454.
130. Donat JF, Okazaki H, Kleinberg F, Reagan TJ (1978) Intraventricular hemorrhages in full-term and premature infants. *Mayo Clin Proc* 53: 437–441.
131. Allan WC, Holt PJ, Sawyer LR, Tito AM, Meade SK (1982) Ventricular dilation after neonatal periventricular–intraventricular hemorrhage. Natural history and therapeutic implications. *Am J Dis Child* 136: 589–593.
132. Rypens E, Avni EF, Dussaussois L, et al (1994) Hyperechoic thickened ependyma: sonographic demonstration and significance in neonates. *Pediatr Radiol* 24: 550–553.
133. Ment LR, Duncan CC, Scott DT, Ehrenkranz RA (1984) Posthemorrhagic hydrocephalus. Low incidence in very low birth weight neonates with intraventricular hemorrhage. *J Neurosurg* 60: 343–347.
134. Armstrong DL, Sauls CD, Goddard-Finegold J (1987) Neuropathologic findings in short-term survivors of intraventricular hemorrhage. *Am J Dis Child* 141: 617–621.
135. Gilles FH, Jammes JL, Berenberg W (1977) Neonatal meningitis. The ventricle as a bacterial reservoir. *Arch Neurol* 34: 560–562.
136. Shoja MM, Tubbs RS (2007) The history of anatomy in Persia. *J Anat* 210: 359–378.
137. Pierre-Kahn A, Hirsch JF, Renier D, Metzger J, Maroteaux P (1980) Hydrocephalus and achondroplasia. A study of 25 observations. *Childs Brain* 7: 205–219.
138. Amacher AL (1977) Neurological complications of osteopetrosis. *Childs Brain* 3: 257–264.
139. Kawai K, Shigemori M, In K, Kuga S, Kuramoto S (1980) [A case of cranio-facial dysostosis (Crouzon's disease) associated with hydrocephalus (author's transl)]. *No Shinkei Geka* 8: 1093–1099.
140. Rohatgi M (1991) Cloverleaf skull—a severe form of Crouzon's syndrome: a new concept in aetiology. *Acta Neurochir (Wien)* 108(1–2): 45–52.
141. Frank E, Berger T, Tew JM Jr. (1982) Basilar impression and platybasia in osteogenesis imperfecta tarda. *Surg Neurol* 17: 116–119.
142. Raynor RB (1986) The Arnold–Chiari malformation. *Spine* 11: 343–344.
143. Kroczek RA, Muhlbauer W, Zimmermann I (1986) Cloverleaf skull associated with Pfeiffer syndrome: pathology and management. *Eur J Pediatr* 145: 442–445.
144. Collmann H, Sorensen N, Krauss J (2005) Hydrocephalus in craniosynostosis: a review. *Childs Nerv Syst* 21: 902–912.
145. Bright R (1831) *Serous Cysts in the Arachnoid. Reports of Medical Cases Selected with a View of Illustrating the Symptoms and Cure of Diseases by a Reference to Morbid Anatomy*, Vol. 2. London: Longman, Rees, Orme, Brown and Green.
146. Scherer E (1935) Über Cystenbildung der weichen Hirnhäute im Liquorraum der Sylvischen Furche mit hochgradiger Deformierung des Gehirns. *Zeitschrift für die gesamte Neurologie und Psychiatrie* 152: 787–799.
147. Starkman SP, Brown TC, Linell EA (1958) Cerebral arachnoid cysts. *J Neuropath Exp Neurol* 17: 484–500.
148. Anderson FM, Landing BH (1966) Cerebral arachnoid cysts in infants. *J Pediatr* 69: 88–96.
149. Rengachary SS, Watanabe I, Brackett CE (1978) Pathogenesis of intracranial arachnoid cysts. *Surg Neurol* 9: 139–144.

150. Schachenmayr W, Friede RL (1979) Fine structure of arachnoid cysts. *J Neuropathol Exp Neurol* 38: 434–446.
151. Rengachary SS, Watanabe I (1981) Ultrastructure and pathogenesis of intracranial arachnoid cysts. *J Neuropathol Exp Neurol* 40: 61–83.
152. Friede RL (1975) *Developmental Neuropathology*. Vienna: Springer.
153. Hassan J, Sepulveda W, Teixeira J, Cox PM (1996) Glioependymal and arachnoid cysts: unusual causes of early ventriculomegaly in utero. *Prenat Diagn* 16: 729–733.
154. Acar O, Kocaogullar Y, Guney O (2003) Arachnoid cyst within the fourth ventricle: a case report. *Clin Neurol Neurosurg* 105: 93–94.
155. von Wild K, Gullotta F (1987) Arachnoid cyst of the middle cranial fossa—aplasia of temporal lobe? *Childs Nerv Syst* 3: 232–234.
156. Levy ML, Meltzer HS, Hughes S, Aryan HE, Yoo K, Amar AP (2004) Hydrocephalus in children with middle fossa arachnoid cysts. *J Neurosurg* 101 (1 Suppl): 25–31.
157. Lange M, Oeckler R, Beck OJ (1990) Surgical treatment of patients with midline arachnoid cysts. *Neurosurg Rev* 13: 35–39.
158. Grollmus JM, Wilson CB, Newton TH (1976) Paramesencephalic arachnoid cysts. *Neurology* 26: 128–134.
159. Hayashi T, Kuratomi A, Kuramoto S Arachnoid cyst of the quadrigeminal cistern. *Surg Neurol* (1980) 14: 267–273.
160. Topsakal C, Kaplan M, Erol F, Cetin H, Ozercan I (2002) Unusual arachnoid cyst of the quadrigeminal cistern in an adult presenting with apneic spells and normal pressure hydrocephalus—case report. *Neurol Med Chir (Tokyo)* 42: 44–50.
161. Kasdon DL, Douglas EA, Brougham MF (1977) Suprasellar arachnoid cyst diagnosed preoperatively by computerized tomographic scanning. *Surg Neurol* 7: 299–303.
162. Krawchenko J, Collins GH (1979) Pathology of an arachnoid cyst. Case report. *J Neurosurg* 50: 224–228.
163. Starshak RJ, Meyer GA, Choi SK, Sty JR, Kovnar EA, Dunn DK (1986) Arachnoid cyst of the collicular cistern. *Childs Nerv Syst* 2: 144–148.
164. Rousseaux M, Lesoin F, Dhellemmes P, Jomin M (1986) Retroclival cysts. Report of two cases. *Neurochirurgia (Stuttg)* 29: 244–247.
165. Fukushima Y, Sato M, Taguchi J, Sasaki M, Kanai N, Hayakawa T (1996) Craniospinal arachnoid cyst: case report [in Japanese]. *No Shinkei Geka* 24: 75–79.
166. Balci S, Oguz KK (2001) Cri-du-chat syndrome associated with arachnoid cyst causing triventricular hydrocephalus. *Clin Dysmorphol* 10: 289–290.
167. Price SJ, David KM, O'Donovan DG, Aspoas AR (2001) Arachnoid cyst of the craniocervical junction: case report. *Neurosurgery* 49: 212–215.
168. Fox JL, Al-Mefty O (1980) Suprasellar arachnoid cysts: an extension of the membrane of Liliequist. *Neurosurgery* 7: 615–618.
169. Martinez-Lage JF, Casas C, Fernandez MA, Puche A, Rodriguez Costa T, Poza M (1994) Macrocephaly, dystonia, and bilateral temporal arachnoid cysts: glutaric aciduria type 1. *Childs Nerv Syst* 10: 198–203.
170. Schievink WI, Huston J 3rd, Torres VE, Marsh WR (1995) Intracranial cysts in autosomal dominant polycystic kidney disease. *J Neurosurg* 83: 1004–1007.
171. Neuhauser EBD, Griscom T, Gilles FH, Crocker AC (1968) Arachnoid cyst in the Hurler—Hunter syndrome. *Ann Radiol (Paris)* 11: 453–470.
172. Wang PJ, Lin HC, Liu HM, Tseng CL, Shen YZ (1998) Intracranial arachnoid cysts in children: related signs and associated anomalies. *Pediatr Neurol* 19: 100–104.
173. Pradilla G, Jallo G (2007) Arachnoid cysts: case series and review of the literature. *Neurosurg Focus* 22: E7.
174. Fraser J, Dott NM (1922) Hydrocephalus. *Br J Surg* 10: 165–191.
175. Weller RO, Shulman K (1972) Infantile hydrocephalus: clinical, histological, and ultrastructural study of brain damage. *J Neurosurg* 36: 255–265.
176. Weller RO, Williams BN (1975) Cerebral biopsy and assessment of brain damage in hydrocephalus. *Arch Dis Child* 50: 763–768.
177. Gilles FH (1983) Telencephalon medium and the olfacto-cerebral outpouching. In: Gilles FH, Leviton A, Dooling EC, editors. *The Developing Human Brain*. Littleton, MA: Wright-PSG, pp. 59–86.
178. Gadsdon DR, Variend S, Emery JL (1978) The effect of hydrocephalus upon the myelination of the corpus callosum. *Z Kinderchir* 25: 311–319.

179. Gadsdon DR, Variend S, Emery JL (1979) Myelination of the corpus callosum. II The effect of relief of hydrocephalus upon the processes of myelination. *Z Kinderchir Grenzgeb* 28: 314–321.

180. Sutton LN, Wood JH, Brooks BR, Barrer SJ, Kline M, Cohen SR (1983) Cerebrospinal fluid myelin basic protein in hydrocephalus. *J Neurosurg* 59: 467–470.

181. Friede RL (1962) A quantitative study of myelination in hydrocephalus. *J Neuropath Exp Neurol* 21: 645–648.

182. Yakovlev PI (1947) Paraplegias of hydrocephalics. *Am J Ment Defic* 51: 561–576.

183. Northfield D, Russell DS (1939) False diverticulum of a lateral ventricle causing hemiplegia in chronic internal hydrocephalus. *Brain* 62: 311–320.

184. Childe AE, McNaughton FL (1942) Diverticula of the lateral ventricles extending into the cerebellar fossa. *Arch Neurol Psychiatry* 47: 768–778.

185. Naidich TP, McLone DG, Hahn YS, Hanaway J (1982) Atrial diverticula in severe hydrocephalus. *AJNR Am J Neuroradiol* 3: 257–266.

186. Cairns H, Daniel P, Johnson RT, Northcroft GB (1947) Localized hydrocephalus following penetrating wounds of the ventricle. *Br J Surg War Surgery Suppl* 1: 187–197.

187. Korobkin R (1975) The relationship between head circumference and the development of communicating hydrocephalus in infants following intraventricular hemorrhage. *Pediatrics* 56: 74–77.

188. Rumack CM, McDonald MM, O'Meara OP, Sanders BB, Rudikoff JC (1978) CT detection and course of intracranial hemorrhage in premature infants. *AJR Am J Roentgenol* 131: 493–497.

189. D'Souza SW, Gowland M, Richards B, et al (1986) Head size, brain growth, and lateral ventricles in very low birthweight infants. *Arch Dis Child* 61: 1090–1095.

190. Thomas WT (1914) Experimental hydrocephalus. *J Exp Med* 19: 106–120.

191. Milhorat TH, Clark RG, Hammock MK (1970) Experimental hydrocephalus. Part 2. Gross pathological findings in acute and subacute obstructive hydrocephalus in the dog and monkey. *J Neurosurg* 32: 390–399.

192. Aoyama Y, Kinoshita Y, Yokota A, Hamada T (2006) Neuronal damage in hydrocephalus and its restoration by shunt insertion in experimental hydrocephalus: a study involving the neurofilament-immunostaining method. *J Neurosurg (5 Suppl Pediatrics)* 104: 332–339.

193. Edvinsson L, West KA (1971) Relation between intracranial pressure and ventricular size at various stages of experimental hydrocephalus. *Acta Neurol Scand* 47: 451–457.

194. Oka N, Nakada J, Endo S, Takaku A, Shinohara H, Morisawa S (1985) Angioarchitecture in experimental hydrocephalus. *Neurologia Medico-Chirurgica (Tokyo)* 25: 701–706.

195. Miller JM, McAllister JPI (2007) Reduction of astrogliosis and microgliosis by cerebrospinal fluid shunting in experimental hydrocephalus. *Cerebrospinal Fluid Res* 4: 5.

196. Cohen MD, Slabaugh RD, Smith JA, et al (1984) Neurosonographic identification of ventricular asymmetry in premature infants. *Clin Radiol* 35: 29–31.

197. Potter EL, Craig JM (1975) *Pathology of the Fetus and the Infant*, 3rd ed. Chicago: Year Book Medical Publishers.

198. Ulfig N, Bohl J, Neudorfer F, Rezaie P (2004) Brain macrophages and microglia in human fetal hydrocephalus. *Brain Dev* 26: 307–315.

199. Nyberg-Hansen R, Torvik A, Bhatia R (1975) On the pathology of experimental hydrocephalus. *Brain Res* 95(2–3): 343–350.

200. Del Bigio MR (1993) Neuropathological changes caused by hydrocephalus. *Acta Neuropathol (Berl)* 85: 573–585.

201. Weller RO, Wisniewski H, Shulman K, Terry RD (1971) Experimental hydrocephalus in young dogs: histological and ultrastructural study of the brain tissue damage. *J Neuropathol Exp Neurol* 30: 613–626.

202. Emery JL (1965) Intracranial effects of long-standing decompression of the brain in children with hydrocephalus and meningomyelocele. *Dev Med Child Neurol* 7: 302–309.

203. Shenkin H, Perryman C (1946) Reversibility of cerebral ventricular dilatation. *J Neurosurg* 3: 234–238.

204. Kaufman B, Weiss M, Young H, Nulsen F (1973) Effects of prolonged cerebrospinal fluid shunting on the skull and brain. *J Neurosurg* 38: 288–297.

205. Hakim S, Venegas JG, Burton JD (1976) The physics of the cranial cavity, hydrocephalus and normal pressure hydrocephalus: mechanical interpretation and mathematical model. *Surg Neurol* 5: 187–210.

206. Penn RD, Bacus JW (1984) The brain as a sponge: a computed tomographic look at Hakim's hypothesis. *Neurosurgery* 14: 670–675.

207. Ordia IJ, Strand R, Gilles F, Welch K (1981) Computerized tomography of contusional clefts in the white matter in infants. Report of two cases. *J Neurosurg* 54: 696–698.
208. Gilles FH, Averill Jr. DR, Kerr CS (1977) Changes in neonatally induced cerebral lesions with advancing age. *J Neuropathol Exp Neurol* 36: 666–679.
209. Rubin RC, Hochwald GM, Tiell M, Epstein F, Ghatak N, Wisniewski H (1976) Hydrocephalus: III Reconstitution of the cerebral cortical mantle following ventricular shunting. *Surg Neurol* 5: 179–183.
210. Patel CD, Matloub H (1973) Vaginal perforation as a complication of ventriculoperitoneal shunt. Case report. *J Neurosurg* 38: 761–762.
211. Pierce KR, Loesser JD (1973) Perforation of the intestine by a Raimondi peritoneal catheter: case report. *J Neurosurg* 43: 112–113.
212. Bristow DL, Buntain WL, James HL (1978) Ventriculoperitoneal (VP) shunt migration causing an acute scrotum: a case report of Doppler evaluation. *J Pediatr Surg* 13: 538–539.
213. Chaplin ER, Goldstein GW, Myerberg DZ, Hunt JV, Tooley WH (1980) Posthemorrhagic hydrocephalus in the preterm infant. *Pediatrics* 65: 901–909.
214. Yakovlev PI, Wadsworth RC (1946) Schizencephalies: a study of the congenital clefts in the cerebral mantle. I Clefts with fused lips. *J Neuropathol Exp Neurol* 5: 116–130.

16
DEVELOPING BRAIN REACTIONS DURING CHRONIC CHILDHOOD DISEASE

Introduction

The child's brain is not spared during chronic childhood disease. There are three brain changes that seem unrelated to any specific illness as they appear to occur only after years of a number of chronic illnesses. The first change is neuroaxonal spheroids or dystrophic changes of terminal axonal synaptic structures in the medullary gracile and cuneate nuclei. These structures terminate the gracile and cuneate spinal cord fasciculi, which contain the longest and largest axons in the body. The second change is delayed neuromelanin deposition in midbrain substantia nigra, and the third is lipofuscin deposition in globus pallidus glial cells.

All three changes are seen in a child's brain in the context of longstanding congenital biliary atresia, cystic fibrosis, severe prenatal or perinatal brain damage, central nervous system malformations, congenital heart disease, Williams syndrome, Hunter disease, Fanconi aplastic anemia, craniopharyngioma, Duchenne dystrophy, lymphosarcoma, chronic leukemia of several varieties, lupus erythematosus, diabetes, dysgammaglobulinemia, Hodgkin disease, neurofibromatosis, chronic renal failure, dermatomyositis, or Morquio disease.

Gracile and cuneate nuclear neuroaxonal spheroids

The medullary gracile and, to a lesser extent, cuneate nuclei are normally the sites of large, elongated, bulbous structures constituting the large polymorphic terminal synaptic portion of gracile or cuneate fasciculi axons.[1] Axons entering the gracile nuclei originate in the lower thoracic, lumbar, and sacral dorsal root ganglia; cuneate axons originate from dorsal root ganglia supplying the brachial plexus. Dorsal root ganglion peripheral processes receive proprioceptive and cutaneous information from the body, including lower legs and feet as well as arms. Thus, some single gracile axonal processes extend, without synaptic interruption, from the toes to the medullary gracile nucleus, making these the longest, if not the largest, human body cells. This implies that a large number of supporting Schwann cells are necessary to support the myelin sheaths of these axons peripherally and a large number of oligodendroglia centrally in addition to amphicytes or dorsal root ganglia satellite cells. The distal ends of these dorsal root neuronal axons terminate in the medullary gracile nuclei in large polymorphic synaptic structures that are long and wide, contacting several neurons in the gracile medullary nuclei before terminating.[2,3] Normally, central nervous system terminal synapses have a wide range of shapes and sizes; those in the gracile nucleus, arising from lumbosacral dorsal root ganglia, for instance, are many microns wide and long. These synaptic structures are not seen in usual histologic preparations of normal medulla, but require ultrastructural or Golgi preparations. While dorsal root ganglion long neuronal peripheral and proximal processes are vulnerable to a number of environmental agents resulting in 'dying-back' neuropathies, the latter are not the concern of this chapter as there is usually no axonal damage in these chronically ill children.

In chronically ill children, gracile nuclei become filled with large eosinophilic masses known as neuroaxonal spheroids or dystrophic axons (Fig. 16.1); to a lesser extent, the cuneate nuclei also contain these same abnormal structures. Sung[4,5] first reported gracile and cuneate spheroids in congenital biliary atresia and cystic fibrosis; the same changes that occur in older patients with advancing age, but not in those aged under 20 years. They have also been called axonal bodies[6] and are similar to the spheroids seen in these same locations in adult rats maintained on vitamin E-deficient diets.[6,7] The posterior funiculi remain intact in axonal and myelin preparations. These changes are similar to those in neuroaxonal dystrophy (Seitelberger disease) or in Hallervorden–Spatz disease,[8] in which large numbers of dystrophic axons or spheroids are found throughout the brain, including in the cortex; nonetheless, the deposits discussed here are limited almost exclusively to the gracile nuclei and, to a lesser degree, the cuneate nuclei. These nuclei also contain dystrophic axons in many species during aging.[9]

POSTERIOR COLUMN SIGNS IN CHRONICALLY ILL CHILDREN

While one might expect posterior column neurologic deficits, most chronically ill children do not have a posterior column clinical neurologic evaluation. A small proportion of children with cystic fibrosis do have anatomic posterior column changes, as well as gracile and cuneate neuroaxonal spheroids.[10] In addition, a progressive clinical neurologic syndrome has been described in children with chronic liver disease.[11]

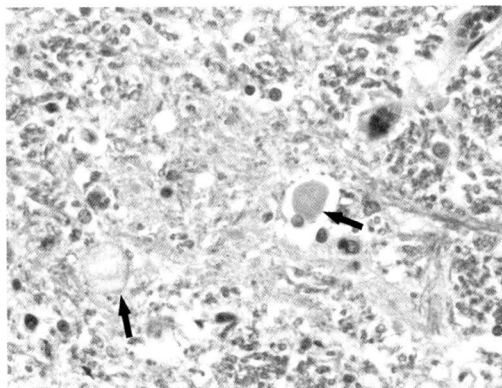

Fig. 16.1 This photomicrograph of the caudal nucleus gracilis contains two large neuroaxonal spheroids (arrows). Spheroids have various appearances ranging from granular (left) to more homogeneous (right).

Failure of neuromelanin deposition in substantia nigra neurons during early-onset chronic childhood illness

Substantia nigra brown–black melanin granules mark the adult midbrain. While a large number of other brainstem nuclei contain microscopic melanin, the presence of this gross streak of black melanin in the midbrain, extending from the pontine base to the diencephalic subthalamic nucleus, is a distinguishing landmark; this pigment is not grossly present at birth.[12,13] Intracellular melanogenesis is a fundamental genetically controlled physiologic process.[14] Neuromelanin is present in albino midbrains, but not in leptomeningeal melano-cytes.[15] Neuromelanin forms in human substantia nigra dopamine neurons and first becomes manifest at various times from midterm to 3 years microscopically then increases gradually over the next 17 years, depending on the investigative technique used.[15–18] While the normal nigra pigment is noted histologically much earlier when special stains are used, grossly visible pigment is not seen until the fifth to seventh year.

Children whose chronic illness started early in life fail to deposit neuromelanin in nigral neurons by the expected time of 5 to 7 years or even the tenth year (Fig. 16.2).[19] A similar failure is seen in Rett syndrome.[20] Their nigral neuronal cellular population is normal histologi-cally, unlike Parkinson disease in which nigral neurons are lost along with their pigment, and thus accelerated breakdown seems unlikely. No common therapy, drug exposure, hereditary or geographic factor, or prior disease exposure stands out as being shared among the affected group. There are no known behavioral or neurologic events paralleling these substantia nigra changes.

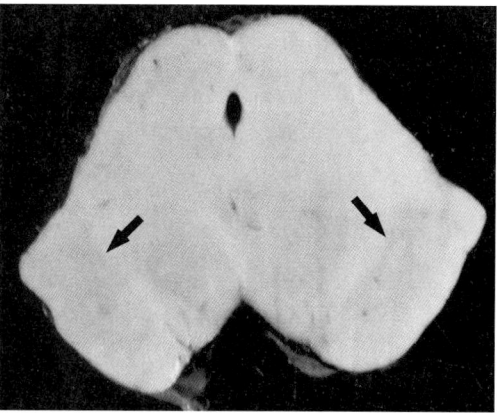

Fig. 16.2 Midbrain axial slice with the aqueduct located at the top centrally below the quadrigeminal plate, and the red nuclei located anteriorly on either side of the interpeduncular fossa. The crus pedunculi lies in front of the substantia nigra (arrows). There is no nigral pigment whatsoever in this chronically ill adolescent.

Accumulation of lipofuscin in pallidal glial cells during early-onset chronic childhood illness

Neuronal lipofuscin deposition has been known for a century and a half;[21,22] whereas glial lipofuscin deposition has been known for a somewhat shorter period.[23] The mature brain globus pallidus stands in distinct contrast to most neuronal aggregates in that considerable quantities of yellow–brown pigment are located in extraneuronal sites.[24-26] Generally, lipofuscin pigment in the glia is thought to follow its appearance in neurons.[27] Nonetheless, in the chronic childhood diseases previously listed, there is considerable accumulation of glial pigment in the absence of pigment in nearby neurons.

In one chronic illness, glial lipofuscin developed before neuronal lipofuscin and occurred in two morphologic forms (large globules and clustered small yellow–brown granules) (Fig. 16.3). It appeared to a greater extent than in children dying of an acute illness, and there was a marked acceleration in deposition at the end of the first decade.[28] The pigment did not contain iron over the ages investigated. The granular form developed earlier and had a steeper slope with age than the globular form. No glial cell contained both forms. The abrupt increase in the rate of deposition at the end of childhood suggests some additional glial cell environmental change, beyond the effects of age and chronic illness. No glial cell morphologic changes suggested a reactive process. While the increases in globus pallidus pigment occurred in proximity to major spurts of bone growth, intelligence, and social or school stress in these children, other clinical signs of puberty were usually delayed, often to the end of the second decade.

Conclusion

We have shown in this chapter that the developing child's brain is not spared the stresses imposed by chronic illness. Changes include the appearance of medullary gracile and cuneate neuroaxonal spheroids, the failure of mesencephalic substantia nigra neuromelanin pigmentation, and lipofuscin deposition in globus pallidus glia without neuronal lipofuscin deposition.

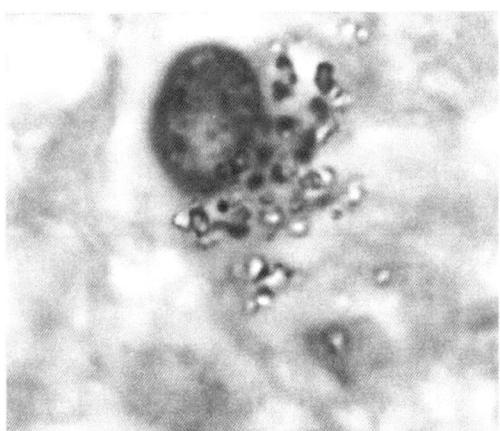

Fig 16.3 Globus pallidus glial cell with cluster of golden-brown granules. Nissl stain. Reproduced with permission of Wolters Kluwer Health from Gilles and Tavaré.[28] A color version of this figure is available in the color plate section at the back of the book.

REFERENCES

1. Rustioni A, Sotelo C (1974) Synaptic organization of the nucleus gracilis of the cat. Experimental identification of dorsal root fibers and cortical afferents. *J Comp Neurol* 155: 441–468.
2. Hashimoto P, Palay S (1965) Peculiar axons with enlarged endings in nucleus gracilis (Abst). *Anat Rec* 151: 454.
3. Walberg F (1966) The fine structure of the cuneate nucleus in normal cats and following interruption of afferent fibers. An electron microscopical study with particular reference to findings made in Glees and Nauta sections. *Exp Brain Res* 2: 107–128.
4. Sung JH (1964) Neuroaxonal dystrophy in mucoviscidosis. *J Neuropath Exp Neurol* 23: 567–583.
5. Sung JH, Stadlan EM (1966) Neuroaxonal dystrophy in congenital biliary atresia. *J Neuropathol Exp Neurol* 25: 341–361.
6. Lampert P, Blumberg JM, Pentschew A (1964) An electron microscopic study of dystrophic axons in the gracile and cuneate nuclei of vitamin E-deficient rats. *J Neuropathol Exp Neurol* 23: 60–77.
7. Pentschew A, Schwarz K (1962) Systemic axonal dystrophy in vitamin E deficient adult rats with implication in human neuropathology. *Acta Neuropathol* 1: 313–334.
8. Cowen D, Olmstead EV (1963) Infantile neuroaxonal dystrophy. *J Neuropathol Exp Neurol* 22: 175–236.
9. Bronson RT, Sweet HO, Spencer CA, Davisson MT (1992) Genetic and age related models of neuro-degeneration in mice: dystrophic axons. *J Neurogenet* 8: 71–83.
10. Geller A, Gilles F, Shwachman H (1977) Degeneration of fasciculus gracilis in cystic fibrosis. *Neurology* 27: 185–187.
11. Rosenblum JL, Keating JP, Prensky AL, Nelson JS (1981) A progressive neurologic syndrome in children with chronic liver disease. *N Engl J Med* 304: 503–508.
12. Scherer H (1939) Melanin pigmentation of the substantia nigra in primates. *J Comp Neurol* 71: 91–98.
13. Adler A (1939) Melanin pigment in the central nervous system vertebrates. *J Comp Neurol* 70: 315–329.
14. Nicolaus BJ (2005) A critical review of the function of neuromelanin and an attempt to provide a unified theory. *Med Hypotheses* 65: 791–796.
15. Foley J, Baxter D (1958) On the nature of pigment granules in the cells of the locus coeruleus and substantia nigra. *J Neuropath Exp Neurol* 17: 586–598.
16. Cooper ERA (1946) The development of the substantia nigra. *Brain* 69: 22–33.
17. Halliday GM, Fedorow H, Rickert CH, Gerlach M, Riederer P, Double KL (2006) Evidence for specific phases in the development of human neuromelanin. *J Neural Transm* 113: 721–728.
18. Fenichel G, Bazelon M (1968) Studies on neuromelanin. II Melanin in the brainstems of infants and children. *Neurology* 18: 817–820.
19. Spence AM, Gilles FH (1971) Underpigmentation of the substantia nigra in chronic disease in children. *Neurol* 21: 386–390.
20. Jellinger K, Seitelberger F (1986) Neuropathology of Rett syndrome. *Am J Med Genet Suppl* 1: 259–288.
21. Hannover A (1842) Mikroskopische undersoegelser af nerversystemet. *Kgl Danske Videns Kabernes Selskobs Naturv og Math Afh* 10: 1–112.
22. Virchow R (1847) Die pathologischen pigmente. *Virch Arch Path Anat* 1: 379–486.
23. Robertson WF (1897) The normal histology and pathology of the neuroglia (in relation specially to mental diseases). *J Ment Sci* 43: 733–752.
24. Wolf A, Pappenheimer A (1945) Occurrence and distribution of acid-fast pigment in the central nervous system. *J Neuropathol Exp Neurol* 4: 402–406.
25. Friede RI (1962) The relation of the formation of lipofuscin to the distribution of oxidative enzymes in the human brain. *Acta Neuropathol* 2: 113–125.
26. Friede RI, Knoller M (1965) A quantitative mapping of acid phosphatase in the brain of the rhesus monkey. *J Neurochem* 12: 441–450.
27. Cavanagh JB, Nolan CC, Brown AW (1990) Glial cell intrusions actively remove detritus due to toxic chemicals from within nerve cells. *Neurotoxicol* 11: 1–12.
28. Gilles FH, Tavare CJ (2002) Globus pallidus glial pigment and its changes with age and chronic illness in childhood. *J Neuropathol Exp Neurol* 61: 351–357.

17
CONCLUDING REMARKS

Despite the last two 'decades of the brain,' our understanding of how the human brain develops and functions is still a work in progress. We hope we have provided a foundation for continued study of normal human brain development. The brains of most individuals have survived complicated developmental events and avoided a large number of adverse events. While we think this points to brain plasticity, we have outlined in this book many adverse events, some of which can potentially be clinically modified during fetal or infantile life, for instance the distant effects of maternal infections on the developing fetus, or the effects of malnutrition on developing white matter.

The careful work of Davenport Hooker and Tryphena Humphreys early in the twentieth century (see Chapter 9) beautifully demonstrated the simultaneous appearance of human reflexes and responsiveness in momentarily viable human embryos and early fetuses. They showed that physiologic responses occur shortly after the first axonal connections are made between the fifth cranial nerve and cervical spinal cord motoneurons at the second gestational month end, long before any myelination. These axonal connections become functional without myelin. They contribute to the embryonic cephalic movement repertoire: avoid, squint, sneer, and pucker. The development of spinal, upper, and lower extremity local reflexes, and stretch, trunk, and feeding reflexes follows these events in Hooker's narrative. Subsequent fetal real-time ultrasound reveals bursts of fetal limb movements; thumb sucking and handedness; breathing movements; swallowing; hiccups; sleep–wakefulness cycles; gastric and bladder emptying; auditory responses; responses to light on maternal abdomen; fetal sexual dimorphism; behavior states; and maternal stress effects on the embryo.

The importance of peripheral and autonomic nervous systems during embryonic and fetal growth is often overlooked in central nervous system considerations. These systems, estimated at substantial portions of brain weight, constitute essential features of neural function: sensory input for the spinal cord and the brain from the peripheral sensory nervous system; and sensory input and organization and motor output throughout the entire body for the autonomic nervous system.

At the completion of the second trimester, brain weight accretion is accelerating maximally. Primary gyri begin their individual maturation, forming distinctive secondary patterns in each hemisphere, which are not mirror images forming left–right asymmetries, while the total surface area remains comparable in both hemispheres throughout gestation. Gyri grow outward from the brain surface in patterns unique to each hemisphere and, probably, to each individual, leading to considerable difficulties for functional imaging studies, information known for more than a century. At the same time, the myelination accelerates, to be maximized almost a year later in the last half of the first postnatal year. Early myelination occurs in groups related to vestibular connections to the upper cervical cord via the medial longitudinal fasciculus and cerebellum; auditory connections with the brainstem, inferior colliculus, and medial geniculate; and peripheral sensory systems ascending from the body to the brainstem, cerebellum, diencephalon, and eventually to the isocortex. Surprisingly, the tractus and nucleus solitarius, vital brainstem sites of central pattern generators for respiratory, cardiac, and visceral function, myelinate very late. Also late to myelinate are the fornix, hippocampus, and cingulum, given that they lie at the medial hemispheral edge, which first forms during embryonic life. Again, there is considerable variance in timing for any individual tract.

Many other developmental events are reaching full expression at the end of the second trimester. The microvasculature, which first penetrated pia at embryonic period termination, is, as brain size increases, continuously remodeling itself and extending the blood–brain barrier to new cerebral territories. The vasculature supporting the rapidly forming nervous system develops pari passu with the nervous system: never too fast or too slow. Based on three data sets, the Carniege, Boston, and Los Angeles material, we feel that current concepts of fetal vasculature development are outdated and that the Bär model best fits the data.

Pineal pigmentation recedes and various paraventricular organs and the mesocoelic recess are established at the end of the second trimester. The embryologically massive ventricular zone germinal tissue has reached its maximal size and rapidly regresses thereafter. In Chapter 7, we showed the normal developmental curves for a large number of chemicals that are vital to brain function.

During nervous system remodeling, many excess neurons are lost and, if not lost, their dendritic trees and axonal beds are extensively pruned. Nevertheless, continuing brain growth past midgestation, and particularly after the end of the second trimester, is subject to numerous additional deleterious maternal and environmental events. Before midgestational end, it seems unlikely that there is much brain cellular reaction, except for a few features of an immature inflammatory response; necrosis and hemorrhage early in the second trimester do not elicit the same kinds of response as they do months or years later when they occur in the older child or adult. Late fetal and neonatal brain does not become edematous except when necrotic or hemorrhagic; nor does herniation occur except with frank necrosis or hemorrhage.

Microglia swarm through the brain, beginning in the third trimester and continuing throughout the first postnatal year. Macrophages, while present around the twelfth gestational week during cavum septi formation, are infrequent before the end of the second trimester and frank infarcts in specific arterial beds of the brain are not prominent until this same time. Myelinating white matter is exquisitely vulnerable to a large number of factors. The most likely factor is endotoxin or the proinflammatory cytokines induced by its presence in the mother or fetus. Widespread cerebral diffuse white matter astrocytosis with glial fibril production is common (and distinct from 'myelination gliosis' or the dense gliosis around focal necroses) and, although less prevalent than diffuse white matter astrocytosis, white matter focal necroses occur with appreciable frequency. Both of these pathologic findings reflect adverse white matter events that interrupt long-distance axonal connections established earlier in gestation and result in white matter paucity, hypomyelination, and ventriculomegaly. As expected with telencephalic white matter axonal interruption, anterograde, retrograde, and trans-synaptic neuronal loss result in volumetric cortical and thalamic depletion.

Within this setting of normal and abnormal developmental events, we detail potential lesions that occur throughout gestation, and spell out the evidence that damage to neurons and glial cells varies dramatically throughout this period. Delays in neuroanatomic component acquisition must be differentiated from loss of such a component. Brain responses to insult change throughout gestation—for example, fetal, neonatal, and infantile necrosis—evolve differently. The concept of late fetal and neonatal edema, without other damage, should be rethought, as nonnecrotic late fetal or neonatal brain is not likely to swell without necrotizing or hemorrhagic insult.

The perinatal telencephalic leukoencephalopathies, their histologic varieties, and their relationships to inflammation are detailed. The importance of hypertrophic astrocytes, amphophilic globules, acutely damaged glial cells, and focal necroses are emphasized. Histologic feature clustering in groups of autopsy brains helps synthesize the risk factors of these four histologic features and to create testable hypotheses.

Borderzone lesions between the supply regions of the larger cerebral arteries become more prevalent in the third trimester, exaggerated by hypoplastic or abnormally formed vessels at the skull base. Large infarcts in specific arterial beds, venous occlusions, or emboli from an abnormal process elsewhere in the fetus and neonate also become more prevalent.

Birth complications include paradural hematomas, hemorrhage into subarachnoid space, parenchyma, germinal matrix, and ventricles. Some are minor, leaving no long-term footprint; others are quite serious and permanently damage hemispheric long-distance connections established earlier in gestation. Other hemorrhages occur during a structural involution, such as ganglionic eminence, and some lead to ventriculomegaly.

Another marginalizing event in late gestation occurs with simple failure of spinal fluid to reach the subarachnoid space, because of either an aqueductal stenosis or a failure to open the midline or lateral fourth ventricle foramina with subsequent development of a persistent retrocerebellar cyst (Blake's pouch). Bland posterior fossa cysts are also important, such as arachnoidal duplications or fibrous arachnoidal cysts. Such cysts are quite distinct from Dandy–Walker abnormalities and usually are not associated with other nervous system abnormalities. Other antecedents of ventriculomegaly include Arnold–Chiari malformation, deficient dysplastic parasagittal arachnoidal granulations, intraventricular hemorrhage, basal meningitis, arachnoidal cysts, or skull base malformations. Probably the most important and least studied effect of shunted hydrocephalus is the remarkable cerebral rebulking that can occur.

The late neuropathologic events marginalizing the developing human brain are all well known: delayed myelination; hypoplastic white matter with ventriculomegaly; pori; hydranencephaly; multicystic encephalomalacia; sclerotic microgyri; borderzone cortical necroses between major vascular beds or along the central sulcus bilaterally; upper brainstem lesions, particularly the inferior colliculi, thalami, and basal ganglia; and lower spinal cord lesions.

Even the infant or child who, escaping the above, succumbs to a chronic illness in childhood develops a number of brain markers over the years in his or her brain: gracile nuclei dystrophic axons; failure of nigral pigmentation; and pallidal glial lipofuscin deposition.

Beyond the conceptual limitations of many of our assumptions and hypotheses about the maturing human brain, the current decline in autopsy rates forces us into greater reliance on neuroimaging. The autopsy rate decline forces dependence on older databases with clinical data collected prospectively, such as the National Collaborative Perinatal Project database. In the future we will need to have better conceptual understanding of normal and abnormal developmental events in the human embryo and fetus. Without better autopsy rates and better conceptual understanding of the fetus and its acquired abnormalities, we will be unable to assist neuroimaging conceptually. For the present, we need to rely on older data sets and historic descriptions to assist our understanding of these developmental processes. Fortunately, magnetic resonance imaging (MRI) has improved sufficiently in both resolution and sequence development to replace ultrasound as the imaging method of choice for neonates. MRI is the only imaging modality that can assess subtle migration abnormalities and myelination, and depict the small focal white matter coagulation necroses. Ultrasound remains adequate for the cribside assessment of intraventricular hemorrhage. However, despite the great strengths of imaging, more pathologic and imaging correlative work, as discussed in this book, is required to understand what the images mean for the future of the individual neonate.

INDEX

Notes
Page number in *italics* refer to material in tables or figures. vs indicates a comparison or differential diagnosis.
The following abbreviations have been used:
    CNS, central nervous system
    MRI, magnetic resonance imaging
    MRS, magnetic resonance spectroscopy

394

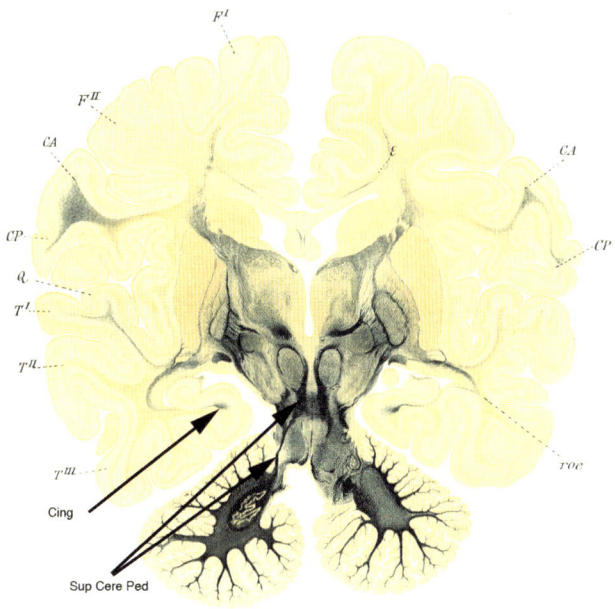

Plate 6.6 Coronal section through basal ganglia, red nucleus, and cerebellum, 7 postnatal weeks. Down is inferior or toward feet. Early auditory radiation myelination occupies the superior temporal gyrus (T^I) subjacent to the transverse gyrus (Q). Sup Cere Ped, superior cerebellar peduncle. As the superior cerebellar peduncle enters the midbrain, it encompasses the red nucleus. Early optic radiation myelination (roe) shows the optic radiation as it curves around the temporal lateral ventricular horn. T^I, T^{II}, and T^{III} indicate the first, second, and third temporal gyri. The T^I marker points to the myelinated auditory radiation. Cing, cingulum; e, cingulum myelin in gyrus cinguli; F^I and F^{II} indicate the first and second frontal gyri; CA and CP, pre- and postcentral gyri. This coronal section angle is tipped forward at the top sufficiently to include the face area of the central sulcus. The sulcus appears minute because of a large annectant gyrus crossing the central sulcus. Myelin stain. The myelin in the pre- (CA) and postcentral (CP) gyri constitutes the distal corona radiata. Weigert–Pal myelin stain. The cingulum, optic radiation (roe), and auditory radiation [myelin in transverse temporal gyrus (Q)] are partially myelinated. The superior cerebellar peduncle is well myelinated and forms a capsule around the red nucleus (the large oval structure above the arrowhead). Modified from Flechsig.[6]

A

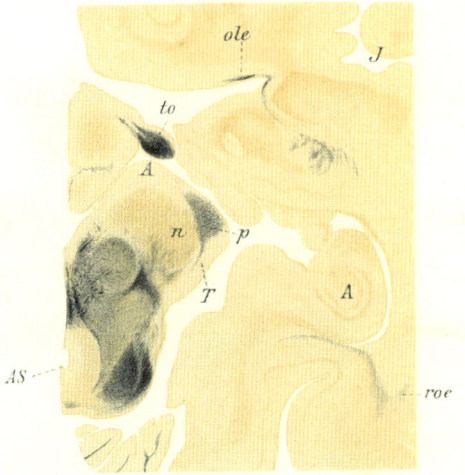

Plate 6.7 Horizontal section through midbrain, 8-month fetus. The direction toward the face is to the top in the image. The only myelinated fibers in the cerebral peduncle are the corticospinal fibers (p). The frontopontine (left A) and the parieto-occipital-temporal (T) fibers are unmyelinated. The mammillary body lies to the left of A. AS, aqueduct; n, substantia nigra; to, optic tract; ole, lateral olfactory tract; right A, Ammon's horn or hippocampus; J, insula; roe, a portion of optic radiation. Modified from Flechsig.[6]

Plate 6.8 (a) Sagittal section through lateral geniculate body, term brain. Anterior or nose to the left. Myelinated thalamocortical and corticospinal fibers are present in the internal capsule between the thalamus and globus pallidus. These same fibers are seen myelinated in the distal corona radiata inferior to the central sulcus and pre- and postcentral gyri. (b) Sagittal section through lateral putamen, term brain. The black myelinated fibers of the corona radiata sweep past the putamen in the internal capsule. (c) Sagittal section, term brain + 9 weeks postnatal age. In the interval since the above photographs, the amount of myelin in the corona radiata has increased considerably. The corpus callosum (cc) subjacent to the central sulcus is partially myelinated. The anterior limb of the internal capsule is partially myelinated. (d) Sagittal section, term + 9 weeks postnatal age. More laterally, the continuity between the internal capsule (between putamen and pulvinar) and the corona radiata below the pre and postcentral gyri is seen. (e) Sagittal section. Term + 4.5 months. In the few months between the above images and this one, the amount of hemispheral myelin has increased markedly. Note that occipital, parietal, posterior frontal, and posterior temporal myelination exceeds that in the anterior temporal and frontal lobes considerably. The most intense myelin staining is in the internal capsule (between Pu and pu), the corona radiata [particularly well seen in the pre- and postcentral gyral white matter cores (CA and CP)] and the optic radiation (particularly well seen below the calcarine sulcus fca). A, Ammon's horn; β, cingulum; CA and

B

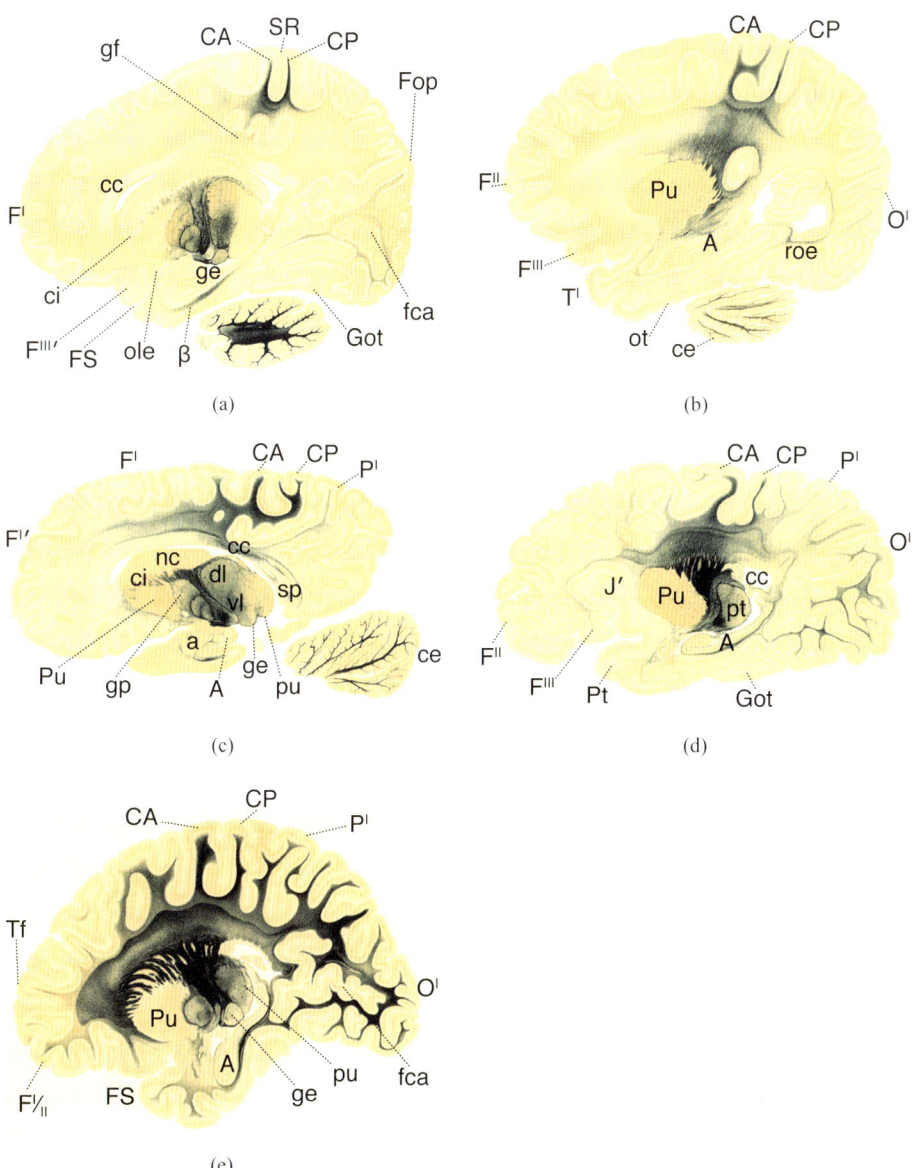

CP, pre- and postcentral gyri; cc, corpus callosum; ce, cerebellum; ci, internal capsule, anterior limb; dl, thalamus, dorsolateral nucleus; F^I and F$^{I'}$, first or superior frontal gyrus; F$^{I/II}$, superior and middle (first and second) frontal gyri; F^{II}, middle frontal gyrus; F^{III}, inferior or third frontal gyrus; F$^{III'}$, inferior frontal gyrus; fca, calcarine sulcus; Fop, occipito-parietal sulcus; FS, lateral sulcus; ge, lateral geniculate body; gf, gyrus cinguli; Got, occipitotemporal gyrus; gp, globus pallidus; J', insula; nc, caudate nucleus; O^I, first occipital gyrus; ole, lateral olfactory stria; ot, occipitotemporal gyrus; PI, superior parietal gyrus; Pt, temporal pole; Pu, putamen; pu, pulvinar; roe, external optic radiation; sp, splenium; SR, central sulcus; T^I, superior temporal gyrus; Tf, frontal pole; vl, thalamus, ventrolateral nucleus. Modified from Flechsig.[6]

C

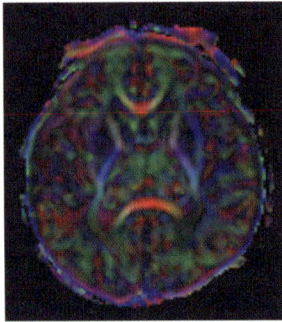

Plate 7.4(e)(iii) DTI color map. In this format, the tensor information is color-coded and all three planes are presented on one image. Red is the *x*-axis (left/right), green is the *y*-axis (superior/inferior), and blue is the *z*-axis (anterior/posterior.

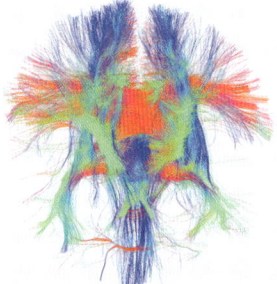

Plate 7.4(e)(iv) Magnetic resonance tractography. By connecting voxels with their neighbors with a similar tensor, large groups of axons may be configured into 'tracts' and color coded by direction.

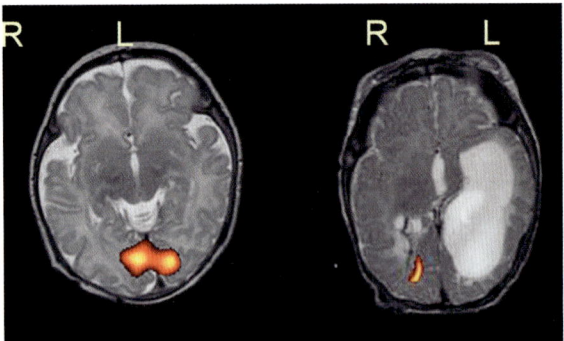

Plate 7.5 Functional magnetic resonance imaging (MRI) study of two neonates exposed to a flashing strobe light. On the left is a normal response with activation around the primary visual cortex in the occipital lobes. On the right is a former preterm neonate with extensive parenchymal damage in which the strobe light evokes only weak activation in the right medial occipital lobe, indicating compromise of the visual pathways.

D